PSYCHIATRIC SECRETS

PSYCHIATRIC SECRETS

JAMES L. JACOBSON, M.D.
Clinical Assistant Professor
Department of Psychiatry
University of Colorado School of Medicine
Associate Medical Director, The Alternatives Program
Colorado Psychiatric Hospital
Denver, Colorado

ALAN M. JACOBSON, M.D.
Associate Professor
Department of Psychiatry
Harvard Medical School
Chief, Psychiatry Service
Joslin Diabetes Center
Boston, Massachusetts

HANLEY & BELFUS, INC./ Philadelphia
MOSBY/ St. Louis • Baltimore • Boston • Carlsbad • Chicago • London
Madrid • Naples • New York • Philadelphia • Sydney • Tokyo • Toronto

Publisher: HANLEY & BELFUS
                    210 S. 13th Street
                    Philadelphia, PA 19107
                    (215) 546-7293
                    FAX (215) 790-9330

North American and worldwide sales and distribution:

                    MOSBY
                    11830 Westline Industrial Drive
                    St. Louis, MO 63146

In Canada: Times Mirror Professional Publishing, Ltd.
                    130 Flaska Drive
                    Markham, Ontario L6G 1B8
                    Canada

Library of Congress Cataloging-in-Publication Data

Psychiatric secrets / [edited by] Alan Jacobson, James Jacobson.
        p.   cm.
    Includes bibliographical references and index.
    ISBN 1-56053-107-X (soft cover : alk. paper)
        1. Psychiatry—Examinations, questions, etc.   I. Jacobson, Alan,
    1944–   .   II. Jacobson, James, 1951–   .
        [DNLM: 1. Mental Disorders—diagnosis.   2. Mental Disorders—
    therapy.   WM 141 P97375 1995]
    RC457.P76   1995
    616.89'0076—dc20
    DNLM/DLC   95-35461
    for Library of Congress   CIP

PSYCHIATRIC SECRETS   ISBN 1-56053-107-X

Last digit is the print number: 9   8   7   6   5   4   3   2   1

DEDICATION

To our parents
whose support and encouragement
helped us to pursue our fascination
with the brain and behavior

CONTENTS

CONTRIBUTORS

C. Alan Anderson, M.D.
Chief Resident, Department of Neurology, University of Colorado School of Medicine, Denver, Colorado

Elissa M. Ball, M.D.
Senior Instructor, Department of Psychiatry, University of Colorado School of Medicine, Denver; Staff Psychiatrist, Colorado Mental Health Institute at Pueblo, Pueblo, Colorado

Jon A. Bell, M.D.
Associate Professor and Director, Anxiety and Mood Disorders Clinic, Department of Psychiatry, University of Colorado School of Medicine, Denver, Colorado

Loisa Bennetto, M.A.
Doctoral Candidate, Department of Psychology, University of Denver, Denver, Colorado

Carol S. Birnbaum, M.D.
Instructor in Psychiatry, Harvard Medical School; Assistant in Psychiatry, Massachusetts General Hospital, Boston, Massachusetts

Mark Alan Blais, Psy.D.
Instructor in Psychology, Department of Psychiatry, Harvard Medical School, Boston; Staff Psychologist, Massachusetts General Hospital, Boston, Massachusetts

Kerry L. Bloomingdale, M.D.
Department of Psychiatry, Harvard Medical School, Boston; New England Deaconess Hospital, Boston, Massachusetts

Archie Brodsky, B.A.
Senior Research Associate, Program in Psychiatry and the Law, Department of Psychiatry, Harvard Medical School at Massachusetts Mental Health Center, Boston, Massachusetts

Andrew W. Brotman, M.D.
Associate Professor of Psychiatry, Harvard Medical School, Boston; Chief, Department of Psychiatry, Deaconess Hospital, Boston, Massachusetts

Randall D. Buzan, M.D.
Instructor, and Director of Electroconvulsive Therapy Service, Department of Psychiatry, University of Colorado School of Medicine, Denver, Colorado

Harold J. Bursztajn, M.D.
Co-director of the Program in Psychiatry and the Law, and Associate Clinical Professor, Department of Psychiatry, Harvard Medical School at Massachusetts Mental Health Center, Boston, Massachusetts

Carl Clark, M.D.
Assistant Clinical Professor, Department of Psychiatry, University of Colorado School of Medicine, Denver; Medical/Clinical Director, Mental Health Corporation of Denver, Denver, Colorado

Sherry Tziporah Cohen, M.D.
Psychiatry Resident, The Cambridge Hospital, Cambridge; Harvard Medical School, Boston, Massachusetts

C. Munro Cullum, Ph.D.
Associate Professor, Department of Psychiatry, University of Texas Southwestern Medical Center, Dallas, Texas

Sharon L. Elliott, M.S.
Pain Management Center, Department of Anesthesia, Harvard Medical School, Boston, Massachusetts

Jane L. Erb, M.D.
Instructor in Psychiatry, Harvard Medical School; Beth Israel Hospital of Boston, Boston, Massachusetts

Gordon K. Farley, M.D.
Professor, Department of Psychiatry, Associate Head and Clinical Director, Division of Child Psychiatry, University of Colorado School of Medicine, Denver; Medical Director, Children's Day Psychiatric Hospital, Denver, Colorado

Christopher M. Filley, M.D.
Associate Professor of Neurology and Psychiatry, Department of Neurology, University of Colorado School of Medicine, Denver, Colorado

Judith Ellen Fox, Ph.D.
Assistant Clinical Professor, Department of Psychiatry, University of Colorado School of Medicine, Denver, Colorado

Michael H. Gendel, M.D.
Clinical Associate Professor, Department of Psychiatry, University of Colorado School of Medicine, Denver; Medical Director of Chemical Dependency Treatment Services, West Pines at Lutheran Medical Center, Denver, Colorado

Alexis A. Giese, M.D.
Assistant Professor, Department of Psychiatry, University of Colorado School of Medicine, Denver, Colorado

Benjamin P. Green, M.D.
Assistant Clinical Professor, Department of Psychiatry, University of Colorado School of Medicine, Denver, Colorado

Doris Christine Gundersen, M.D.
Instructor, Department of Psychiatry, University of Colorado School of Medicine, Denver, Colorado

Frederick B. Hebert, M.D.
Clinical Associate Professor, Department of Psychiatry, University of Colorado School of Medicine, Denver; Associate Director, Psychiatric Services, Denver General Hospital, Denver, Colorado

Robert M. House, M.D.
Associate Professor, Director of Residency Training, and Director of Consultation/Liaison Psychiatry, Department of Psychiatry, University of Colorado School of Medicine, Denver, Colorado

Alan M. Jacobson, M.D.
Associate Professor, Department of Psychiatry, Harvard Medical School, Boston; Chief, Psychiatry Service, Joslin Diabetes Center, Boston, Massachusetts

James L. Jacobson, M.D.
Clinical Assistant Professor, Department of Psychiatry, University of Colorado School of Medicine, Denver; Associate Medical Director, The Alternatives Program of Colorado Psychiatric Hospital, Denver, Colorado

Robert N. Jamison, Ph.D.
Assistant Professor, Departments of Anesthesia and Psychiatry, Harvard Medical School, Boston, Massachusetts

Michael A. Jenike, M.D.
Associate Professor, Department of Psychiatry, Harvard Medical School, Boston; Associate Chief of Psychiatry, Massachusetts General Hospital, Boston, Massachusetts

Michael Kahn, M.D.
Instructor, Department of Psychiatry, Harvard Medical School, Boston; New England Deaconess Hospital, Boston, Massachusetts

Marita J. Keeling, M.D.
Clinical Associate Professor, Department of Psychiatry, University of Colorado School of Medicine, Denver, Colorado

Jane A. Kennedy, D.O.
Assistant Professor, Department of Psychiatry, University of Colorado School of Medicine, Denver, Colorado

Steven Kick, M.D., M.S.P.H.
Assistant Professor, Departments of Psychiatry and Medicine, University of Colorado School of Medicine, Denver, Colorado

Mary Lou Klem, Ph.D.
Postdoctoral Fellow, Department of Epidemiology, University of Pittsburgh School of Medicine, Pittsburgh, Pennsylvania

Joyce Seiko Kobayashi, M.D.
Associate Professor, Department of Psychiatry, University of Colorado School of Medicine, Denver; Director, Neuropsychiatric Consultation Service, Denver General Hospital, Denver, Colorado

Andrew B. Littman, M.D.
Instructor in Psychiatry, Harvard Medical School; Director, Behavioral Medicine Division, Preventive Cardiology, Massachusetts General Hospital, Boston, Massachusetts

Theo C. Manschreck, M.D., M.P.H.
Professor, Department of Psychiatry and Human Behavior, Brown University School of Medicine, Providence, Rhode Island

Harold P. Martin, M.D.
Associate Professor, Department of Psychiatry, University of Colorado School of Medicine, Denver

Mary Jane Massie, M.D.
Professor of Clinical Psychiatry, Cornell University Medical College, New York, New York

Robin April McCann, Ph.D.
Staff Psychologist, Institute of Forensic Psychiatry, Colorado Mental Health Institute, Pueblo, Colorado

John A. Menninger, M.D.
Assistant Professor, Department of Psychiatry, University of Colorado School of Medicine, Denver, Colorado

Jeffrey L. Metzner, M.D.
Clinical Associate Professor of Psychiatry, University of Colorado School of Medicine, Denver, Colorado

Herbert T. Nagamoto, M.D.
Assistant Professor, Department of Psychiatry, University of Colorado School of Medicine, Denver, Coloradopy

Kim Elliot Nagel, M.D.
Assistant Clinical Professor, Department of Psychiatry, University of Colorado School of Medicine, Denver, Colorado

Richard L. O'Sullivan, M.D.
Instructor in Psychiatry, Harvard Medical School, Boston; Clinical Assistant in Psychiatry, Massachusetts General Hospital, Boston, Massachusetts

William H. Polonsky, Ph.D.
Clinical Psychologist, Diabetes Management and Research Center, Sharp Healthcare, San Diego, California

Michael K. Popkin, M.D.
Professor of Psychiatry and Medicine, University of Minnesota Medical School; Chief of Psychiatry, Hennepin County Medical Center, Minneapolis, Minnesota

William H. Redd, Ph.D.
Professor, Department of Psychiatry, Cornell University Medical College, and Memorial Sloan-Kettering, New York, New York

Martin Reite, M.D.
Professor, Department of Psychiatry, University of Colorado School of Medicine, Denver, Colorado

Roberta M. Richardson, M.D.
Assistant Clinical Professor, Department of Psychiatry, University of Colorado School of Medicine, Denver, Colorado

Paula DeGraffenreid Riggs, M.D.
Assistant Professor, and Director of Psychiatric Services for Adolescents, Department of Psychiatry, University of Colorado School of Medicine, Denver, Colorado

Margaret Roath, M.S.W., L.C.S.W.
Assistant Professor, Department of Psychiatry, University of Colorado School of Medicine, Denver, Colorado

Sally J. Rogers, Ph.D.
Associate Professor, Department of Psychiatry, University of Colorado School of Medicine, Denver, Colorado

Andrew J. Roth, M.D.
Assistant Professor of Clinical Psychiatry, Cornell University Medical College, New York; Assistant Attending Psychiatrist, Memorial Sloan-Kettering Cancer Center, New York, New York

Jacqueline A. Samson, Ph.D.
Assistant Professor of Psychology, Department of Psychiatry, Harvard Medical School, Boston; McLean Hospital, Belmont, Massachusetts

Ronald Schouten, J.D., M.D.
Instructor, Department of Psychiatry, Harvard Medical School, Boston; Director, Law and Psychiatry Service, and Assistant Director, Somatic Therapies Consultation Service, Massachusetts General Hospital, Boston, Massachusetts

Stephen R. Shuchter, M.D.
Professor of Clinical Psychiatry, and Director of Outpatient Psychiatric Services, University of California at San Diego, San Diego, California

Thomas D. Stewart, M.D.
Associate Clinical Professor, Department of Psychiatry, Yale University School of Medicine, New Haven; Chairman, Department of Psychiatry, Hospital of St. Raphael, New Haven, Connecticut

Marshall R. Thomas, M.D.
Assistant Professor, Department of Psychiatry, University of Colorado School of Medicine, Denver, Colorado

Hubert Hiram Thomason, Jr., M.D.
Assistant Clinical Professor, Department of Psychiatry, University of Colorado School of Medicine, Denver, Colorado

Laetitia L. Thompson, Ph.D.
Associate Professor, Departments of Psychiatry and Neurology, University of Colorado School of Medicine, Denver, Colorado

Russell George Vasile, M.D.
Assistant Professor, Department of Psychiatry, Harvard Medical School, Boston; Director of Outpatient Psychiatry, Deaconess Hospital, Boston, Massachusetts

Robert J. Waldinger, M.D.
Assistant Professor of Psychiatry, Harvard Medical School, Boston; Director of Residency Training, Massachusetts Mental Health Center, Boston, Massachusetts

Garry William Welch, B.Sc., M.A., Ph.D.
Research Associate, Mental Health Unit, Joslin Diabetes Center, Boston; Department of Psychiatry, Harvard Medical School, Boston, Massachusetts

Rena R. Wing, Ph.D.
Professor of Psychiatry, Psychology and Epidemiology, Department of Psychiatry, University of Pittsburgh School of Medicine, Western Psychiatric Institute and Clinic, Pittsburgh, Pennsylvania

Lawson Reed Wulsin, M.D.
Associate Professor, Department of Psychiatry, University of Cincinnati College of Medicine, Cincinnati, Ohio

Claire Zilber, M.D.
Assistant Professor, Departments of Psychiatry and Internal Medicine, University of Colorado School of Medicine, Denver, Colorado

Sidney Zisook, M.D.
Professor and Director of Residency Training Program, Department of Psychiatry, University of California at San Diego, San Diego, California

John F. Zrebiec, M.S.W.
Senior Clinical Social Worker, Joslin Diabetes Center, Boston; Lecturer on Group Psychotherapy, Harvard Medical School, Boston, Massachusetts

PREFACE

Psychiatric Secrets presents an up-to-date approach to the assessment and treatment of psychiatric disorders in children, adults, and the elderly. It uses a question and answer format to address key principles in clinical practice in keeping with the concept of *The Secrets Series®*. The questions raise central issues and provide the organizational structure for each chapter. This process of question and answer yields a dialogue through which the expert clinicians who authored each chapter can provide their best "pearls of wisdom" often gained from years of experience as researchers, educators, and practicing clinicians.

Psychiatric Secrets is divided into twelve sections that address in systematic fashion the steps in the treatment process. The book has a heavy emphasis on diagnosis, for it is the belief of the editors that careful, thoughtful diagnosis is the "springboard" to treatment. The first two sections outline a general approach to gathering and presenting clinical information. The next three sections on major psychiatric syndromes and clinical problems focus primarily on issues related to diagnosis, including careful descriptions of common clinical characteristics, etiology, course of illness, and, when appropriate, basic features of treatment. The section devoted to therapeutic approaches presents introductions to both psychotherapeutic and biologic treatments, and includes indications, contraindications, and side effects of interventions. The final section provides integrating information related to common problems and settings, such as child psychiatry, assessment and treatment of suicidal and violent patients, and consultation-liaison psychiatry, as well as ethical and legal aspects of psychiatry.

This text is intended to reinforce concepts for the mental health professional, yet is geared primarily for the medical student, house officer, and general practitioner. The chapters are designed to be read independently, and thus there is occasional overlap of information. Each author was given complete freedom to utilize his or her expertise in expressing views about assessment or treatment. Thus, *Psychiatric Secrets* presents both basic information as well as the approach of experienced practitioners to specific topics.

We are grateful to the authors for contributing their knowledge, time, and talent. In addition, we would like to thank Linda Belfus and Polly E. Parsons, who encouraged us to undertake this project, and the many unsung heroes who typed, re-typed, re-re-typed, critiqued, proofread, and helped us move the book to completion. Without all of their efforts, this book would not have happened.

James L. Jacobson, M.D.
Alan M. Jacobson, M.D.

I. Approach to Clinical Interviewing and Diagnosis in Psychiatry

1. THE INITIAL PSYCHIATRIC INTERVIEW

Robert Waldinger, M.D., and Alan M. Jacobson, M.D.

1. What are the goals of the first psychiatric interview?

The primary aims of the first psychiatric interview are to make an initial differential diagnosis and to formulate a treatment plan. These goals are achieved by:

1. Gathering information about the patient's current difficulties and past experiences. This includes information about:

- Chief complaint
- History of presenting problem(s)
- Precipitating factors
- Symptoms
  - (1) Affective
  - (2) Cognitive
  - (3) Physical
- Substance use and abuse
- Changes in role and social functioning
- Current and past history of suicidality and aggression
- Past psychiatric history, including treatment and response
- Past social and developmental history
- Family psychiatric and social history
- Mental status
- Medical history

2. Arriving at an empathic understanding of how the patient feels. This understanding supplements descriptive data by imparting a strong sense of the patient's own experience. It is a critical base for building a relationship with the patient and establishing rapport. When the clinician experiences and then communicates an appreciation of the patient's worries and concerns, the patient gains a sense of being understood. This sense of being understood is the bedrock of all subsequent treatment. The task for the clinician is to initiate a human relationship in which an alliance for treatment can be established. The ability to place oneself in the patient's shoes assists in this process.

The initial diagnosis and treatment plan may be rudimentary. Indeed, when patients present in a crisis, the history may be confused, incomplete, or narrowly focused. As a result, some interventions are started even while basic information about current and past history, family relationships, and ongoing stressors is being gathered. It is critical to remember that emotional difficulties are often isolating. The experience of sharing one's problem with a concerned listener can be enormously relieving in and of itself. Thus, the initial interview is the start of treatment even before a formal treatment plan has been established.

2. How should the initial interview be organized?

There is no single ideal, but it is useful to think of the initial interview as having three components:

1. The first part involves establishing initial rapport with the patient and asking about the presenting complaint or problems, i.e., what has brought the patient to the first meeting. Some patients tell their stories without much guidance from the interviewer, whereas others require explicit instructions in the form of specific questions to help them to organize their thoughts. During this phase of the first interview the patient should be allowed to follow as much as possible his or her own thought patterns.

1

2. Some specific information should be elicited during the initial interview, including a review of past history, pertinent medical information, family background, social history, and specific symptom and behavioral patterns. Formal mental status testing also should be included (see chapter 2).

3. Finally, the interview is ended by asking the patient if he or she has any questions or unmentioned concerns. Initial recommendations are then made to the patient for further evaluation and/or beginning treatment.

Although the three parts of the interview can be considered separately, they often weave together, e.g., mental status observations can be made from the moment the clinician meets the patient. Furthermore, pertinent medical and family history may be brought up in the course of presenting other concerns, and patients may pose important questions about treatment recommendations as they present their initial history.

The initial psychiatric assessment may require more than one session for complex situations such as evaluation of children or families and of suitability for particular therapeutic approaches such as brief psychotherapy. The initial assessment also may require information gathering from other sources: parents, children, spouse, best friend, teacher, police officers, and/or other health care providers. Depending on the situation, this step may be incorporated in the first visit. Alternatively, such contacts may occur after the first meeting. The first step in making such arrangements is to explain the reason for them to the patient and to obtain explicit permission for the contact. Before contact is made with outside sources (e.g., other physicians, teachers), written permission should be obtained.

It is almost always appropriate to call the referral source to gather information and to explain the initial diagnostic impressions and treatment plan. Exceptions may occur when the referral comes from other patients, friends, or other nonprofessionals, whom the patient wishes to exclude from treatment.

Specific theoretical orientations may dictate important variations in the initial assessment. For example, a behavioral therapist guides discussion to specific analyses of current problems and spends little time on early childhood experiences. The psychopharmacologic evaluation places heavy emphasis on specific symptom patterns, responses to prior medication treatment, and family history of psychiatric illness. The approach presented in this chapter is designed as a broadly applicable set of principles that can be used in evaluating most patients.

3. How is information gathered from an interview?

To be effective in evaluating a patient's problems, the interviewer must discover as much as possible about how the patient thinks and feels. During the clinical interview, information is gathered from what the patient tells the interviewer; critically important clues also come from how the history unfolds. Thus both the content of the interview (i.e., what the patient says) and the process of the interview (i.e., how the patient says it) offer important routes to understanding the patient's problems. A patient may describe information about job loss, difficulties with a spouse, or problems with a small child. The order of information, the degree of comfort in talking about it, the emotions associated with the discussion, the patient's reactions to questions and initial comments, the coherence of the presentation, and the timing of the information may be the route to a deeper level of understanding about why the patient is seeking help and how he or she functions. The full elaboration of such information may take one or several sessions over the course of days, weeks, or months, but in the first interview hints of deeper concerns may be suggested by both the content and process of the conversation.

For example, a 35-year-old woman presented with worries about her son's recurrent asthma and associated difficulties in school. She talked freely about her worries and sought advice on how to help her son. When asked about her husband's thoughts, she became momentarily quiet. She then said that he shared her concern and switched the discussion back to the decisions that she felt must be made to help her son. The hesitancy hinted at problems that were left unaddressed in the initial session. Indeed, she began the next session by asking, "Can I talk about something else besides my son?" After being reassured, she returned to the topic of her husband

and his chronic anger at their son for his "weakness." His anger and her own feelings in response became an important focus of subsequent treatment.

4. How should the interview be started?

The here and now is the place to begin all interviews. Any one of a number of simple questions can be used: "What brings you to see me today? Can you tell me what has been troubling you? How is it that you decided to make this appointment?" For anxious patients, structure is useful; early inquiry about age, marital status, and living situation may give them time to become comfortable before embarking on a description of their problems. If the anxiety is evident, a simple comment about the anxiety may help patients to talk about their worries.

5. What types of questions are best to ask?

Patients must be given some opportunity to organize their information in the way that they feel most comfortable. The interviewer who prematurely subjects the patient to a stream of specific questions limits guidance from and information about the patient's own process of thinking. The interviewer does not learn how the patient handles silences or sadness and closes off the patient's opportunities to hint spontaneously at or bring up new topics for discussion. Furthermore, the task of formulating one specific question after another may intrude on the clinician's ability to listen and to understand the patient. This does not mean that specific questions should be avoided. Many times patients provide elaborate answers to specific questions such as "When were you married?" Their responses may open new avenues to the inquiry. The key is to avoid a rapid-fire approach and to provide patients time to elaborate their thoughts.

Questions should be phrased in a way that invites patients to talk. Open-ended questions that do not indicate an answer tend to allow people to elaborate more than specific or leading questions. In general, leading questions (e.g., "Did you feel sad when your girlfriend moved out?") can be conversation stoppers, because they may give the impression that the interviewer expects the patient to have certain feelings. Nonleading questions ("How did you feel when your girlfriend moved out?") are as direct and more effective.

When patients need help in elaborating, a simple statement and/or request may elicit more information: "Tell me more about that: Oh, I see." Repeating or reflecting what patients say also encourages them to open up and elaborate when they become hesitant (e.g., "You were talking about your girlfriend."). Sometimes comments that specifically reflect the clinician's understanding of the patient's feelings about events may help the patient to elaborate. This approach provides confirmation for both the interviewer and the patient that they are on the same wavelength. When the interviewer correctly responds to their feelings, patients frequently confirm the response by further discussion. The patient discussing the discouragement and pessimism that developed after his girlfriend left may feel understood and freer to discuss the loss after a comment such as "You seem discouraged about your girlfriend moving out."

An elderly man was referred for increasing despondency. In the initial interview, he first described financial difficulties and then brought up the recent development of medical problems, culminating with the diagnosis of prostatic carcinoma. As he began talking about the cancer and his wish to give up, he fell silent. At this point in the interview, the clinician expressed his recognition that the patient seemed to feel overwhelmed by the build-up of financial and, most of all, medical reversals. The patient nodded quietly and then elaborated his particular concerns about how his wife would get on after he died. He did not feel that his children would be helpful to her. It was not yet clear whether his pessimism reflected a depressive overreaction to the diagnosis of cancer or accurate appraisal of the prognosis. Further assessment of his symptoms and mental state and brief discussion with his wife later in the meeting revealed that the prognosis was quite good. The treatment then focused on his depressive reactions to the diagnosis.

The interviewer should use language that is not technical and not overly intellectual. Furthermore, the patient's own words should be used in commenting on or asking questions about the patient's history. This is particularly important in dealing with intimate matters such as sexual concerns. People may describe their sexual experiences in a language that is quite varied.

If a patient says that he or she is gay, one should use that exact term rather than an apparently equivalent term such as homosexual. People may use some words and not others because of the specific connotations that different words carry for them; at first, such distinctions may not be apparent to the interviewer.

The interviewer must remain aware at all times of what is going on during the interview. If the patient is currently hallucinating or intensely upset, failure to acknowledge the upset or the disconcerting experience may elevate the patient's anxiety. Discussing the patient's current upset helps to alleviate tension and tells the patient that the clinician is listening. If the patient's story rambles or is confusing, it is important to acknowledge the difficulty of understanding the patient and also to evaluate the possible reasons for the difficulty (e.g., psychosis with loosened associations vs. anxiety about coming to the visit).

When patients have difficulties in answering general questions such as, "Tell me something about your background," it may be necessary to follow up with specific questions about parents, schooling, and dates of events. It is important to realize, however, that it can be tempting to ask endless questions to alleviate one's own anxiety rather than the patient's.

In sum, allowing the patient freedom to tell his or her story must be balanced by attending to the patient's ability to focus on relevant topics. Some people require guidance from the interviewer to avoid getting lost in tangential themes. Others may need consistent structure because they have trouble ordering their thoughts or have such a high degree of anxiety that they find it difficult to collect their thoughts. In the second situation, an empathic comment about the patient's anxiety may lead to the feeling of being listened to; this feeling may reduce the anxiety and thus lead to clearer communication.

Do's and Don'ts of Interviewing

- Let the first part of the initial interview follow the patient's train of thought.
- Provide structure to help patients who have trouble with ordering their thoughts or to finish obtaining specific data.
- Phrase questions to invite the patient to talk (e.g., open-ended, nonleading questions).
- Use the patient's words.
- Be alert to early signs of loss of behavioral control (e.g., standing up to pace).
- Identify the patient's strengths as well as problem areas.
- Avoid jargon and technical language.
- Avoid questions that begin with "why?"
- Avoid premature reassurance.
- Do not allow patients to act inappropriately (e.g., break or throw an object).

6. What specific pitfalls should be avoided during the initial interview?

Avoid jargon or technical terms, unless clearly explained and necessary. Patients may use jargon, for example, "I was feeling paranoid." If patients use a technical word, ask about their own meaning for the term. The clinician may be quite surprised by the patient's understanding. For example, patients may use "paranoid" in a way that suggests fear of social disapproval or pessimism about the future. One must also be careful about assigning too quickly a diagnostic label to the patient's problems during the interview. The patient may be frightened and confused by the label.

In general, avoid asking questions that begin with "why." Patients may or may not know why they have certain experiences or feelings. However, they may feel put on the spot and stupid if they do not believe that they have good answers. Asking why may also imply that the clinician expects the patient to provide quick explanations. Patients discover more about the roots of their problems as they reflect on their lives during the interview and in subsequent sessions. When tempted to ask why, it is often helpful to rephrase the question so that it elicits a more detailed response. Alternatives include "What happened?" "How did that come about?" or "What thoughts do you have about that?"

Avoid premature reassurance. When patients are upset, as they often are during first interviews, the interviewer may be tempted to allay the patient's fears with such assurances as

"Everything will be fine" or "There is nothing really seriously wrong here." However, reassurance is genuine only when the clinician (1) has explored the precise nature and extent of the patient's problems and (2) is certain of what he or she is telling the patient. Premature reassurance may heighten the patient's anxiety by giving the impression that the clinician has jumped to a conclusion without a thorough evaluation or is just saying what he or she thinks the patient wants to hear. It also leaves patients alone with their fears about what is really wrong. Furthermore, premature reassurance tends to close off discussion rather than encourage further exploration of the problem. It may be more reassuring to ask what the patient is concerned about than to try to provide direct reassurance. For example, patients who are worried about having an incurable disease are likely to be more reassured when the clinician asks questions about their concerns rather than provides a quick reassurance that "things will be okay." The process (i.e., the nature of the interaction) helps the patient to feel comforted more than any single thing the interviewer may say to take away the patient's pain or emotional upset.

Do not let the patient act in inappropriate ways during the session. Because of their psychiatric problems, some patients may lose control of their behavior in the session. Although the approach described here emphasizes letting the patient direct much of the verbal discussion, at times patients need to have limits set on their inappropriate behavior. Patients who are aroused and want to take off their clothes or threaten to throw an object need to be controlled. This goal is most often accomplished by commenting on the increasing arousal, discussing it, inquiring about sources of upset, and letting patients know the limits of acceptable behavior. On rare occasions outside help may be necessary (e.g., security guards in an emergency department). This should be done if the behavior is escalating, especially if the interviewer feels that he or she may be harmed. The interview should be stopped until the patient's behavior can be managed so that it is safe to proceed.

7. What is commonly forgotten in evaluating patients?
The new patient initiates context with the clinician because of problems and worries; these are the legitimate first topics of the interview. Whether in the first interview or shortly after, it also may be helpful to gain an understanding of the patient's strengths, which are the foundation on which treatment will build. These strengths include ways in which the patient has coped successfully with past and current distress, accomplishments, sources of inner value, friendships, work accomplishments, and family support. Strengths also include important hobbies or other interests that patients use to battle the worries that bring them for treatment. Questions such as "What are you proud of?" or "What do you like about yourself?" may help to bring out such information. Often the information comes out as an afterthought in the course of conversation. For example, one patient took great pride in his volunteer work through his church. He mentioned it only in passing as he discussed his activities of the week before the meeting. Yet this volunteer work was his only current source of personal value. He turned to it when he became upset about his lack of success in his career.

8. What is the role of humor in the interview?
Patients may use humor to deflect the conversation from anxiety-provoking or troubling topics. It may be useful to allow such deviations to help patients to maintain emotional equilibrium. It also may be helpful to ask about concerns related to the topic if the humor seems to lead to a radical change in focus from something that seemed important and/or emotionally relevant. Humor also may help to direct the interviewer toward new topics of importance. A light joke by the patient may be the first step in introducing a topic that takes on later importance.

On the part of the interviewer, humor may be protective and defensive. Just as the patient may feel anxious or uncomfortable, so may the interviewer. As a consequence, one must be careful, because humor can backfire. It may be misunderstood as ridicule and also allow both patient and interviewer to avoid important topics. Sometimes humor is a wonderful way to show the human qualities of the interviewer and thus helps to build a therapeutic alliance. Nonetheless, it is important to keep in mind the problematic aspects of humor, especially before the patient and interviewer have come to know each other well.

9. How does one assess suicidal intent?

Because of the frequency of depressive disorders and their association with suicidality, it is almost always necessary to address the possibility of suicidal intent in a first interview. Asking about suicide will not provoke a person to try to hurt him- or herself. If the subject does not come up spontaneously, several types of questions can be used to draw out the patient's thoughts on suicide. Such questions are listed in the order that they may be used in beginning a discussion about suicide:

- How badly have you been feeling?
- Have you thought of hurting yourself?
- Have you wanted to die?
- Have you thought of killing yourself?
- Have you tried?
- How, when, and what led up to your attempt?
- If you have not tried, what led you to hold back?
- Do you feel safe to go home?
- What arrangements can be made to increase your safety and to decrease your risk of acting on suicidal feelings?

Such discussion may need to be extended and elaborated until it is clear whether the patient may safely leave or needs hospital admission (see chapters 74 and 75).

10. What is the best way to bring a first evaluation interview to a close?

It is always important to leave time for the patient's own questions, concerns, or comments. One way to begin the ending phase of an interview is to ask the patient if he or she has any specific questions or concerns that have not been addressed. After addressing such issues, the clinician should briefly summarize important impressions and diagnostic conclusions and then suggest the course of action. The clinician should be as clear as possible about formulation of the problem, its diagnosis, and the next steps. At this time the clinician may begin to lay out the need for any tests, including laboratory examinations, further psychological assessments, and getting permission for meeting or talking with important others who may provide needed information or should be included in the treatment plan. Both clinician and patient should recognize that the plan is tentative and may include alternatives that need further discussion. If medication is recommended, the clinician should describe the specific benefits and expected time course as well as inform the patient about potential side effects, adverse effects, and alternative treatments. Often patients want to think over suggestions, get more information about medications, or ask family members about their thoughts. In most instances, the clinical situation is not so emergent that clear action must be taken in the first interview. However, the clinician should be clear in presenting recommendations, even if they are tentative and primarily oriented to further diagnostic assessment.

At this point it is tempting to provide false reassurance, such as, "I know everything is going to be okay." It is perfectly legitimate—and indeed better—to allow for uncertainty where uncertainty exists. Patients can tolerate uncertainty, if they see that the clinician has a plan to elucidate the problem further and to arrive at a sound plan for treatment.

BIBLIOGRAPHY

1. MacKinnon R, Yudofsky S: The Psychiatric Evaluation in Clinical Practice. Philadelphia, J.B. Lippincott, 1986.
2. Morrison J: The First Interview. New York, Guilford Press, 1993.
3. Orthmer E, Orthmer SC: The Clinical Interview Using DSM IV. Washington, DC, American Psychiatric Association Press, 1994.
4. Stone E: American Psychiatric Glossary. Washington, DC, American Psychiatric Press, 1988.
5. Sullivan HS: The Psychiatric Interview. New York, Norton, 1954.
6. Waldinger R: Psychiatry for Medical Students, 3rd ed. Washington, DC, American Psychiatric Press, 1996.

2. THE MENTAL STATUS EXAMINATION

Robert M. House, M.D.

1. What is the mental status examination?

The mental status examination (MSE) is a component of all medical exams. It is especially important in neurologic and psychiatric evaluations. It may be viewed as the psychological equivalent of the physical exam. The purpose is to evaluate, quantitatively and qualitatively, a range of mental functions and behaviors at a specific point in time. The MSE provides important information for diagnosis as well as assessing the course of the disorder and response to treatment. Information and observations noted throughout the interview become part of the MSE, which begins when the clinician first meets the patient. Information is gathered about the patient's behaviors, thinking, and mood. At an appropriate point in the evaluation the formal MSE is undertaken to compile specific data. Earlier informal observations about mental state are woven together with the results of specific testing. For example, the interviewer will have considerable information about attention span and memory from the process of the interview. Specific questions during the formal exam are used to clarify more precisely the degree of attention or memory dysfunction.

Case. A 55-year-old man presented with recent complaints of sadness and fear of being alone. He also expressed thoughts about death. As he presented his concerns, he rambled to unrelated topics and seemed to lose track of the interviewer's questions. During the formal inquiry he was able to recall only 1 of 3 objects he was asked to memorize and made several mistakes in serial subtractions of 7 from 100. Specific questioning about suicidal wishes and actions revealed that he had overdosed with aspirin 1 month earlier and still experienced suicidal thoughts and wishes to die. The cognitive tests were compatible with mild dementia and differential diagnosis including major depression. Further work-up and treatment supported this diagnosis. Cognitive functioning improved with antidepressants.

2. Is the MSE a separate part of the patient evaluation?

The MSE must be interpreted along with the presenting history, physical exam, and laboratory and radiologic studies. Not to do so leaves one vulnerable to erroneous conclusions. Collateral information from families and friends is also invaluable to confirm or supply missing data.

Case. A 27-year-old man presented to the psychiatric emergency department with somewhat grandiose behavior, pressured speech, irritability, and psychomotor agitation. The initial diagnostic impression was bipolar disorder, manic or drug-induced mania. The patient denied drug abuse. However, questioning of his wife uncovered a history of substance abuse, and laboratory evaluation revealed the presence of amphetamine metabolites. The correct diagnosis was amphetamine-induced mood disorder.

3. What key factors should be considered along with the MSE?

To assess properly the patient's mental status, it is important to have some understanding of the patient's social, cultural, and educational background. What may be abnormal for someone with higher intellectual abilities may be normal for someone with less intellectual abilities. Patients for whom English is a second language may have difficulty understanding various components of the MSE, such as the proverbs. Age may be a factor. In general, patients over the age of 60 years tend to do less well on the cognitive elements of the MSE. Often this is related to less education rather than to aging alone.

4. What are the major components of the MSE?

Components vary somewhat from author to author. However, most detailed MSEs include information about appearance, motor activity, speech, affect, thought content, thought process, perception, intellect, and insight.

Major Components of the Mental Status Examination

Appearance	Age, sex, race, body build, posture, eye contact, dress, grooming, manner, attentiveness to examiner, distinguishing features, prominent physical abnormalities, emotional facial expression, alertness.
Motor	Retardation, agitation, abnormal movements, gait, catatonia
Speech	Rate, rhythm, volume, amount, articulation, spontaneity
Affect	Stability, range, appropriateness, intensity, affect, mood
Thought content	Suicidal ideation, death wishes, homicidal ideation, depressive cognitions, obsessions, ruminations, phobias, ideas of reference, paranoid ideation, magical ideation, delusions, overvalued ideas
Thought process	Associations, coherence, logic, stream, clang associations, perseveration, neologism, blocking, attention
Perception	Hallucinations, illusions, depersonalization, derealization, déjà vu, jamais vu
Intellect	Global impression: average, above average, below average
Insight	Awareness of illness

Adapted from Zimmerman M: Interviewing Guide for Evaluating DSM–IV Psychiatric Disorders and the Mental Status Examination. Philadelphia, Psychiatric Press Products, 1994, pp 121–122.

5. What is the first step in the MSE?

A determination of consciousness must be the first step in the MSE. Basic brain function determines the patient's ability to relate and cooperate with the surroundings and the interviewer. Disturbance of this basic function affects higher level mental processes that make up the major portions of the exam. The Glasgow Coma Scale was developed by Teasdale and Jennett in 1974 to assess impaired consciousness. It is based on eye opening and motor and verbal responses to stimuli. The scale ranges from 3 (deep coma) to 14 (full alert wakefulness).

Glasgow Coma Scale

CATEGORY	SCORE
Eyes open (E)	
Spontaneously	4
To speech	3
To pain	2
None	1
Best motor response (M)	
Obeys commands	5
Localizes pain	4
Flexion to pain	3
Extension to pain	2
None	1
Best verbal response (V)	
Oriented	5
Confused	4
Inappropriate words	3
Incomprehensible sounds	2
None	1
Summed coma scale = E + M + V	

6. Are there short forms of the MSE?

Several shortened forms of the MSE have been developed as screening instruments. All are composed of a combination of measures to detect cognitive impairments more accurately. Although helpful, such exams must be combined with clinical history. The diagnosis of dementia and delirium also requires the demonstration of a decline in cognitive functioning from a higher baseline. All screening exams have difficulty in identifying patients with mild cognitive impairment and patients with focal neurologic lesions, such as subdural hematomas or meningiomas. The key point is that MSEs should not be used as the sole criteria for diagnosing delirium or dementia.

7. What are some of the more common screening exams?

The Mini-Mental State Examination (MMSE) is probably he best known. The MMSE tests orientation, immediate and short-term memory, concentration, arithmetic ability, language, and praxis. It takes about 10 minutes to administer. The Cognitive Capacity Screening Examination (CCSE) tests orientation, serial subtraction, memory, and similarities. It is less sensitive to delirium or dementia in the elderly. The Mental Status Questionnaire (MSQ) stresses orientation and long-term memory. The Neurobehavioral Cognitive Status Examination (NCSE) is especially good for medically ill patients; it focuses on consciousness, orientation, attention, language, construction, memory, calculations, and reasoning. Because it is more detailed, it tends to be more sensitive in detecting cognitive impairment.

Mini-Mental State Exam

MAXIMAL SCORE	SCORE	
		Orientation
5	( )	What is the (year) (season) (date) (day) (month)?
5	( )	Where are we: (state) (county) (town) (hospital) (floor)?
		Registration
3	( )	Name 3 objects: take 1 second to say each. Then ask patient to repeat them. Give 1 point for each correct answer.
		Attention and Calculation
5	( )	Serial 7s from 100. 1 point for each correct answer. Stop after 5 answers. Alternatively, spell "world" backward.
		Recall
3	( )	Ask for the 3 objects named above. 1 point for each correct answer.
		Language
9	( )	Ask patient to name a pencil and watch. (2 points)
		Repeat the following "No ifs, ands, or buts." (2 points)
		Follow a 3-stage command: "Take a paper in your right hand, fold it in half, and put it on the table." (3 points)
		Read and obey the following:
		Close your eyes (1 point)
		Write a sentence (1 point)
		Copy a drawing of intersecting pentagons (1 point)

Adapted from Folstein MF, Folstein SE, McHugh PR: Mini-mental State: A practical method for grading the cognitive states of patients for the clinician. J Psychiatr Res 12:189–198, 1975.

Additional questions can be used to extend and expand the components of a screening exam. For example:

Attention can be tested with counting by 2s to 20. This task is easier and can be used for patients with poor arithmetic skills.

Calculation abilities can be tested by asking the patient to add simple combinations of two digit numbers. The task can be graded in difficulty.

Immediate recall can be assessed by asking patients to repeat number sequences up to seven forward and four in reverse order. Start with shorter sequences.

Memory can be assessed by asking about news events, sports, television shows, or recent meals.

Long-term memory can be assessed by using past events confirmed by family members and also be repeating names of important historical figures, such as presidents of the U.S.

Language ability can be assessed by asking patients to explain similarities and differences between common objects and concepts (e.g., tree-bush, car-plane, air-water).

Thinking processes can be assessed by asking patients to explain common proverbs with which they are familiar.

8. Can the MSE help to detect organic brain disease?
Emotional and behavioral change is frequently the first presentation of organic brain disease, especially in patients with frontal and temporal tumors, hydrocephalus, or cortical atrophy. Brain tumors, subdural hematomas, small infarcts, and cerebral atrophy may be undetected on routine neurologic exam, whereas the cognitive effects of such lesions may be apparent on mental status examination. For patients with known brain lesions, a thorough MSE documents cognitive or emotional changes.

9. Does a normal MSE or MMSE score mean competence?
No. Competency relates to patients' ability to make reasonable decisions for themselves and others. Such decisions include ability to provide food and shelter, to manage money, and to participate in activities such as deciding a course of medical care. Patients who score well on an MSE may have deficits in understanding or completing common tasks of daily living. Among a population with a probable diagnosis of Alzheimer's disease, 50% of patients scoring between 26 and 30 on the MMSE had difficulty with basic tasks such as coping with small sums of money or finding their way around familiar streets. The MSE is only one component needed to assess competency. Medical condition, current ability for self-care, and corroborating information from family or friends must be taken in consideration. A more detailed discussion of competency and its evaluation is provided in chapter 82.

Probability of Alzheimer's Disease among Patients with Specific Problems of Daily Living

SPECIFIC ABILITY	MMSE RANGE (%)*			
	0–10	11–20	21–25	26–30
Cope with small sums of money	98	78	53	50
Perform household tasks	97	87	63	56
Recall recent events	97	92	89	91
Remember short lists of items	95	89	83	84
Find way around familiar streets	92	72	59	53
Recognize surroundings	82	44	30	19
Dress self	82	38	15	16
Find way about indoors	68	40	20	16
Tendency to dwell in the past	50	57	48	34
Feed self	44	05	02	06
Bowel and bladder continence	41	14	17	12

* Values are percentages of probable Alzheimer's disease among patients with MMSE scores falling in each range and difficulty performing the indicated activities.
Adapted from Mungas D: In-office mental status testing: A practical guide. Geriatrics 46:54–66, 1991, with permission.

10. Does an abnormal MSE or MMSE score mean incompetence?
Not necessarily. Many patients with cognitive limitations develop alternative means of coping with their deficits that allows them to live fairly independent and satisfying lives. As with patients with a normal MSE or MMSE score, collateral history helps to determine whether the patient is able to provide for basic needs.

11. What are the major limitations of MSE screening questionnaires?
Although structured, screening questionnaires are still subject to interpretive bias and depend on the skill and experience of the interviewer. All screening questionnaires have a fairly significant false-negative rate, especially in patients with focal lesions of the right hemisphere. Age (especially > 60 years), education (< 9th grade), cultural experience, and low socioeconomic standing limit the usefulness of MSE screening questionnaires. Unlike a detailed mental status exam, screening questionnaires are less sensitive to subtle cognitive impairment.

12. What are executive functions?
Complex cognitive abilities mediated primarily by the frontal lobes, dorsolateral prefrontal cortex, head of the caudate nucleus, and medial thalamus are referred to as executive functions. To assess such disorders, one may evaluate the patient's ability to self-regulate and plan. For example, can the patient inhibit impulsive responses to a stimuli and deliberate before acting. Failure to do so suggests a frontal lobe disorder. Similarly, perseveration of motor activity is another example of frontal lobe dysfunction; for example, asking the patient to perform an alternating task such as palm up–palm down and later inserting a third task: palm up–palm down–fist. The impaired patient may be able to repeat only two components of the assigned task. Focal lesions or degenerative disorders, such as Huntington's chorea, that affect these structures may lead to disorders of executive function.

13. Is the MSE important to perform in patients who appear cognitively intact?
Yes. The exam may be abbreviated, but testing of cognitive functions provides a useful baseline. Patients may deteriorate during follow-up. The initial exam provides a point for comparison. Furthermore, mental status observations are a key tool for psychiatrists. Honing observational skills through informal assessment and formal exams helps to key the clinician to subtle aspects of affect, speech, and behavior, especially as the change during the course of meetings. Subtle fluctuations are important sources of information throughout treatment. Learning to detect subtleties is a critical component of learning to become a skilled psychiatric clinician.

GLOSSARY

Aphasia: inability to communicate by speech, writing, or symbols.
Apraxia: inability to complete purposeful movements.
Catatonia: form of schizophrenia marked by periods of rigidity, excitement, and stupor.
Clang association: speech in which words are repeated based on similarity of sound without regard to meaning.
Déjà vu: sense that one is seeing or experiencing something that has been seen before.
Delusion: a false belief that is not shared by others.
Dysarthria: difficulty in speech production.
Echolalia: imitative repetition of speech of another person.
Flight of ideas: rapid shifting from one topic to another, often with a common theme.
Loosening of association: disturbance of associations that render speech vague and unfocused.
Neologism: creation of new words; often a mixture of other words.
Perseveration: Excessive continuation of a response or action, usually verbal.
Thought insertion: a delusion that thoughts are placed in one's mind by an outside source.

BIBLIOGRAPHY

1. Beresford T, Holt R, Hall R, et al: Cognitive screening at the bedside: Usefulness of a structured examination. Psychosomatics 26:319–326, 1985.
2. Cummings JL: The mental status examination. Hosp Pract 28:56–68, 1993.
3. Folstein MF, Folstein SE, McHugh PR: "Mini-Mental State": A practical method for grading the cognitive state of patients for the clinician. J Psychiatr Res 12:189–198, 1975.
4. Kiernan RJ, Mueller J, Langston JW, et al: The neurobehavioral cognitive status examination: A brief but differentiated approach to cognitive assessment. Ann Intern Med 107:481–485, 1987.
5. Mungas D: In-office mental status testing: A practical guide. Geriatrics 46:54–66, 1991.
6. Nelson A, Fogel B, Faust D: Bedside cognitive screening instruments: A critical assessment. J Nerv Ment Disease 174:73–83, 1986.
7. O'Neill DO: Brain stethoscopes: The use and abuse of brief mental status schedules. Postgrad Med J 69:599–601, 1993.
8. Strub RL, Black FW: The Mental Status Examination in Neurology, 2nd ed. Philadelphia, F.A. Davis, 1985.
9. Teasdale G, Jennett B: Assessment of coma and impaired consciousness: A practical scale. Lancet 2:81–84, 1974.
10. Zimmerman M: Interview Guide for Evaluating DSM–IV Psychiatric Disorders and the Mental Status Examination. Philadelphia, Psychiatric Press Products, 1994.

3. ORGANIZATION AND PRESENTATION OF PSYCHIATRIC INFORMATION

Michael Kahn, M.D.

1. Which principles guide the organization and presentation of clinical data?

After you have done the initial interview(s), performed the mental status, and gathered the results of various tests, you are left with the task of organizing and presenting the data coherently. This task often appears more daunting than it is. Keep in mind that your primary goal is to be able to tell a concise yet sufficiently detailed story about the patient's current state so that (1) you yourself have at least a few working hypotheses about the patient's problems, and (2) a person hearing (or reading) about the patient has enough information to arrive at his or her own hypotheses. The success of any effort toward organization and presentation of information is founded on *the clearest presentation of the most relevant facts* about a given case.

2. Sounds daunting. Where does one start?

You already know much of what you need to know. The psychiatric presentation differs little from the standard way of presenting a medical patient, and is often organized in the following order:

- Chief complaint
- History of present illness
- Past psychiatric history
- Past medical history
- Psychosocial history
- Family psychiatric history
- Physical exam
- Mental status exam
- Assessment and plan

3. How is it different to write up someone with schizophrenia than someone with diabetes?

In theory, nothing is different; in practice, however, psychiatrists tend to work more effectively when they have even a rudimentary grasp of who the patient is *as a person,* and not just as the vehicle for an array of signs and symptoms. Of course, this could be said to be true for *all* physicians, not just psychiatrists; yet because psychiatrists deal so much with disturbances in patients' behavior, thoughts, moods, and feelings generally, a vivid and lifelike description of the patient's history can be especially helpful in diagnosing and treating psychiatric problems.

4. What does that mean in practice?

Compare these two hypothetical histories of present illness:

A. Mr. Jones is a 54-year-old married white man who was in his usual state of health until three weeks prior to admission, when he lost his job. He then noted the subacute onset of early morning awakening, weight loss, fatigue, decreased concentration, and depressed mood. His wife, noticing that he had suicidal ideation, brought him to the hospital.

B. Mr. Jones is a 54-year-old married white man who derived much of his sense of self-esteem and accomplishment from the job as an accountant which he had held for over thirty years. Three weeks ago, when he was laid off (due to cutbacks at the firm where he worked), he felt that "The rug was pulled out from under me." He had always made his job the center of his life, and was left with nothing to do at home. His wife was overwhelmed as well. He says that he began to feel that "Nothing made sense any more . . . I felt all washed-up," and gradually lost his appetite as well as his interest in and energy for the few hobbies he had. He developed insomnia with early-morning awakening, and after a while began to tell his wife that "I'm no use to anyone any more." When he asked his wife if she'd miss him if he "were gone," she brought him to the hospital.

Although both histories give a clear picture of someone developing an episode of major depression, the second one conveys a more detailed and useful assessment of the patient *as a person*, as well as of the circumstances leading up to hospital admission. History "B" presents at least the beginning of an understanding of the patient's personality and home life. The use of direct quotations greatly contributes to the sense of vividness and immediacy, and begins to help the listener empathize with the patient's suffering. When thinking about or hearing such a presentation, important questions may more readily come to mind: Had Mr. Jones seen the cutbacks coming but failed to plan for them? Why was the job the center of his life? Why couldn't his wife have been more of a support? Why does he frame his anguish in terms of his not being any "use" to anyone?—and so forth.

The essential point is to make the "history of present illness" as *vivid and richly detailed* as possible, making use of direct patient quotations when applicable and useful, and minimizing use of standard "boiler-plate" jargon about symptoms and behavior.

5. What sort of boiler-plate jargon?

The kind that represents the tendency to describe symptoms in concise but impoverished ways that lack important complexity. For example, rather than saying that

> *"The patient demonstrated intense affect when faced with his illness."*

Consider saying instead that

> *"The patient became tearful and sad when discussing the isolation caused by his psychotic thinking."*

Rather than saying that

> *"The patient exhibited agitated and threatening behavior in her relationship."*

Consider saying that

> *"The patient shouted angrily and shook her fist at her boyfriend."*

Once again, the more successful one is in depicting a clear, detailed, and evocative history, the greater the chances will be of reaching a more accurate assessment that leads directly to a rational treatment plan. Avoid clinical clichés!

6. What about the past psychiatric history?

This part of the presentation should document not only what prior treatment the patient has received, but also the *circumstances* and *outcome* of such treatment. Outlining *untreated* episodes of illness can also be very helpful, as can describing the initial onset of symptoms.

Hospitalizations: Note precipitating factors, length of stay, success/failure of different treatments used, working diagnoses.

Somatic treatments: Note dosage of medication, duration, usefulness, and side effects. If appropriate, mention whether electroconvulsive therapy (ECT) has been used.

Therapy: Note session length, frequency, duration, focus (e.g., supportive, exploratory, behavioral, cognitive, etc.), and its usefulness.

Suicidality/Homicidality: Note stressors, prior attempts (in detail), and treatment measures that proved effective. Classifying prior attempts in terms of relative risk and rescue potential can be particularly helpful. For example: the patient who lightly lacerated a wrist in full view of a family member would be considered a low-risk/high-rescue attempt; taking an overdose of acetaminophen behind a locked bathroom door would be high-risk/low-rescue; and so forth.

Remember: eliminate vagueness! Saying "The patient failed a lithium trial" is less helpful than saying "A two-month trial of lithium at therapeutic plasma levels resulted in intolerable tremor and polyuria." Direct patient quotations can be quite useful here as well.

7. Is taking a past medical history in a psychiatric setting different than in nonpsychiatric settings?

Not substantially. Clearly, any illness with possible psychiatric complications (e.g., Parkinson's disease, multiple sclerosis, stroke, hypothyroidism) should be explored in some detail. Given the protean psychiatric manifestations of several different types of seizures, the presence or absence of a seizure disorder is especially important to determine. Mood disorders, hallucinations, delusions, and unusual character traits may be sequelae of a seizure focus, often, if not always, in the temporolimbic area. Because these symptoms may represent ictal manifestations of a *nonconvulsive* seizure, a patient's seizures may have gone undiagnosed. It is therefore important to inquire about any history of head trauma, particularly if it led to loss of consciousness.

8. What about differences in the psychosocial history?

Given the importance of early relationships to personality development and the ways in which one will be able to cope with an illness in later life, a few essential facts about the patient's upbringing can shed much useful light on his or her current functioning. A brief outline of the structure of the patient's family is essential, and should include the place of the patient in the birth order, whether or not the parents were ever married or remained married, and whether either parent is deceased. Patients will often fail to mention spontaneously losses of other family members and it can be useful to ask about whether any siblings or grandparents were lost to the patient either recently or in childhood.

Physical and sexual abuse—two obviously sensitive subjects—should be mentioned tactfully but candidly if they are clinically relevant. Clearly, taking a history of abuse must be done with care, with special attention paid to the patient's clinical condition and whether or not discussion of such events could be traumatizing or intrusive.

The psychosocial history can convey information about the patient's **work history** and **relationships** invaluable for an accurate assessment of personality functioning. How does the patient respond to the responsibility of a job? How does he or she deal with interpersonal conflict and intimacy? Similarly, even a brief history of how the patient performed in **school** can convey a sense of early social relationships as well as any possible learning difficulties that may have gone undetected.

Substance abuse is often presented in this section. The same overall suggestions for detail and richness apply, e.g.: "The patient typically drinks alone, on weekends only, consuming 'anything I can get my hands on' until he passes out. He has never had seizures or DTs, and does not like AA because 'it's hard to be around so many strangers.'" How much more evocative this is than is "Patient is alcohol-dependent."

The patient's **religion** and whether it is important should also be mentioned. This assumes special importance if the patient is struggling with suicidal impulses.

Finally, taking **military** and **legal** elements of a history is important and should not be neglected.

9. What about the family psychiatric history?

A careful exploration of the family's history of mental illness frequently offers much helpful data. Not uncommonly, patients will remember that a family member was psychiatrically ill, without knowing what diagnosis was given. Learning certain facts can therefore be revealing:

"Patient's mother was 'nervous a lot' and was in fact hospitalized 5 times for 'shock treatments.'"

"Patient's uncle was 'always hyper,' 'drank too much,' and was arrested three times for passing bad checks."

Not surprisingly, such data are often more revealing than the "diagnosis" remembered by the patient.

10. What are the pitfalls in presenting the mental status exam?
This is where "boiler-plate jargon" can easily get out of hand. "Patient has auditory hallucinations" can be true, if the examiner was careful, or quite false, if the exam was cursory. Be specific! If a patient mentions hearing voices, you need to ask: How many voices? Are they there all the time? Do they comment on the patient? Are they perceived as coming from inside or outside the head? Do they tell the patient to do anything? Are they threatening or comforting? . . . and so forth. *"Don't just mention the symptom—describe it"* would be good advice here. *Describe* the patient's appearance, interpersonal style, and mannerisms or idiosyncrasies. This principle applies to all portions of the mental status exam, including cognitive testing.

11. So how do you "pull everything together" in the formulation (or assessment) section?
Remarkably little consensus exists about what it means to formulate a case. A common belief is that formulation involves coming up with an esoteric and sophisticated explanation of the patient's difficulties which somehow will display the examiner's ability to extrapolate more from details of the case than meets the eye. Perhaps the essence of the formulation is rather that it arranges facts in such a way as to suggest a differential diagnosis and a treatment plan. A focus on *basic* psychiatric knowledge, common sense, and a willingness to think in terms of *hypotheses* rather than *conclusions* will usually allow one to come up with a formulation which is both clarifying and useful. Where does one begin?
  Remember first of all that one main function of the formulation is to summarize known pertinent clinical facts, emphasizing the *stressors* and *sequence of events* that led to the patient seeking help. Thus, a simple but nonetheless useful formulation might be something like this:

> In summary, Ms. Smith is a 19-year-old woman with the new onset of a psychotic disorder that has developed over the past 3 weeks. The symptoms appeared to begin fairly abruptly after she was fired from her job and began using cocaine daily to avoid her feelings of shame and disappointment. Her grandiosity, irritability, sleeplessness, and pressured speech all suggest the diagnosis of bipolar disorder, manic phase; however, given the amount of cocaine she was using, it is worth considering the possibility of a substance-induced mood disorder with manic features, secondary to cocaine.

Nothing elaborate is involved here, yet this simple example includes features essential to any formulation:
  • An indication of baseline functioning (no prior psychosis)
  • A description of a likely stressor (the loss of the job)
  • A response to that stressor (humiliation, followed by cocaine use)
  • A summary of the salient symptomatic phenomenology (grandiosity, irritability, etc.)
  • A differential diagnosis

  The hypothesis that the patient used cocaine "to avoid the pain of her loss" is clearly based more on common sense and empathy rather than on any formula concerning human behavior.
  A somewhat more complex formulation (referring to the patient in Question 4) might look like this:

> In summary, Mr. Jones is a man without prior psychiatric history whose self-esteem was closely tied to his ability to be an effective worker and to provide for his family. The loss of his job was a tremendous blow to his self-image and quickly led to his feeling worthless, guilty, and hopeless. He developed all the signs of a major depressive episode. His suicidality may have been the outcome both of his hopelessness as well as his turning his rage about the layoff onto himself.

12. Explain "turning his rage onto himself."
That is a hypothesis based on psychodynamic theory, which holds that human behavior is, to a large extent, governed by hidden (or, more specifically, *unconscious*) meanings and forces within the mind. Psychodynamic principles can be useful tools for probing and unraveling patients' difficulties; these principles are most helpful when used to generate *hypotheses,* which then require further data to be confirmed or refuted. In this case, for example, further discussions with this

patient while he was recovering clinically might reveal the rage (perhaps directed against a harsh and over-demanding father) masked by the acute symptoms, the exploration and venting of which might lead to further improvement and reduced vulnerability to future depression.

13. Are there other hypotheses that can be used as tools in case formulation?

Three other sets of hypotheses, which are well-summarized by Lazare,[1] are the *sociocultural,* the *behavioral,* and the *biologic/syndromal.* Although a complete description of each of these hypotheses would be beyond the scope of this chapter, some familiarity with each can greatly enhance a clinician's skill in reaching an accurate and thorough formulation. The biologic/syndromal approach underlies the classification system contained in the Diagnostic and Statistical Manual (DSM-IV) of the American Psychiatric Association, which is the prevailing diagnostic system within American psychiatry.

14. What if the formulation is wrong?

You revise it. The value of a formulation is that it provides a starting point for an informed understanding and discussion of the case at hand. It is less important to be "right" than to be flexible. One should think of the initial formulation as leading to a *working diagnosis* that will guide the initial work-up and treatment and may be modified as you become more familiar with the patient. In summary:

- Emphasize clinical detail and richness.
- Avoid clinical clichés and "boiler-plate jargon."
- Quote the patient where applicable.
- Describe symptoms.
- Use the formulation to summarize the facts, to generate hypotheses, and to arrive at a working diagnosis.

APPENDIX: A SAMPLE WRITEUP

Chief complaint: "I think I can go home; I'm feeling fine."

History of present illness: Mr. Williams is a 36-year-old single white man well-known to our system who carries the diagnosis of bipolar affective disorder. He was doing well living in his own apartment and working as a salesman, and was coming to see his therapist weekly for psychotherapy and lithium. About 2 weeks ago, his girlfriend of 3 years broke up with him; he began to drink daily (6 to 10 beers) and failed to show up for his appointments. The therapist estimates he should have run out of lithium 1 week before. On the night of admission Mr. Williams arrived at his girlfriend's house intoxicated; he was verbally threatening, and tried to break down her door. The police were called and he was taken to the emergency room at a city hospital. There his blood alcohol level was initially .256 and he was placed in restraints overnight. When sober, he continued to be pressured, hyperalert, and grandiose, and showed markedly impaired insight and judgment, with plans to "charge two tickets on the Concorde to take my girlfriend to Paris" despite the fact that he has no money left in the bank. He was sent to this hospital on a temporary commitment paper because of severely impaired judgment and the inability to care for himself.

Past psychiatric history: First hospitalization was at age 22 for 4 weeks for typical manic symptoms. Responded well to lithium 1200 mg q.d. and complied with follow-up treatment.

Second hospitalization was at age 26 for severe depression that seemed to begin after stopping lithium "to see if I needed it any more." He overdosed on aspirin but immediately called his doctor and then an ambulance; there were no medical sequelae. Depression responded well to fluoxetine, although he had some hypomania; dose of fluoxetine stabilized at 10 mg q.d. Lithium level was 1.0 mEq/L on 1200 mg q.d.

Third hospitalization was for mania at age 34, again after stopping medication because "It was making me sleepy." Quickly improved when lithium was restarted.

He has never had electroconvulsive therapy (ECT) or received valproic acid or carbamazepine. Had a significant acute dystonic reaction to haloperidol during first admission.

Weekly psychotherapy sessions have focused on helping the patient accept his illness and improve self-esteem. Only suicide attempt was the aspirin overdose mentioned above.

Past medical history: No known allergies or significant medical problems. Lost consciousness for "about 10 seconds" after a childhood accident. No resulting headaches, behavior changes, or seizures. Twice-yearly creatinine levels have been stable. No evidence exists of impaired renal function due to lithium. Thyroid function has been normal.

Psychosocial history: He is the oldest of two sons born to a still-married retired couple. Younger brother is healthy and works as an engineer. Mother and father are in good health.

Patient did well in school and "always had friends." Received a degree in history from a state college and has worked as an appliance salesman. He has never married but has had several long-term relationships. He was arrested for driving recklessly during a manic episode but otherwise has had no legal problems. He was never in the military. He is Protestant and does not attend church.

When manic he tends to drink to excess, but otherwise drinks socially. As a teenager, he experimented with marijuana.

Family psychiatric history: Father has had problems with depression and is on desipramine, but has never been hospitalized. Maternal grandmother had clear-cut bipolar illness, and was hospitalized over 20 times for both depression and mania until she began taking lithium in 1972; since then she has had two hospitalizations and is doing well.

Mental status exam: On admission he was a gaunt, dishevelled young man who was pacing around the room throughout the interview and was very difficult to interrupt. He showed clear pressured speech and flight of ideas: "I wanted to take the Concorde but they wouldn't let me . . . you seem to be a brilliant doctor . . . Maybe I'll just move to Hollywood . . ." etc. He was irritable when asked questions. Claims he hears "God's voice every morning when I wake up" but otherwise denies auditory or visual hallucinations. Mood is described as "terrific," but affect is irritable and elated. He has no homicidal or suicidal thoughts: "Why should I hurt anyone?"

He is hyper-alert and oriented in all three spheres. He refused cognitive testing: "I hate remembering those three things and doing those sevens." When asked about proverbs he said "A rolling stone is a rolling stone is Mick Jagger." Analogies were deferred. Judgment and insight were both obviously severely compromised.

Formulation: This is the fourth hospitalization in fourteen years for this 36-year-old man with what appears to be clear-cut bipolar disorder, with a history of both mania and depression following discontinuation of lithium. This present episode seems to have been precipitated by his sense of helplessness after a girlfriend left him. He ran out of medicine and began drinking heavily; his anger at the girlfriend came out while he was manic and intoxicated. Because he has never had mania or depression while actually taking lithium, it would make sense to start this medication again. Because of a history of dystonia with high-potency neuroleptics, thorazine is prescribed to control the acute manic symptoms.

Diagnoses: Axis I: Bipolar I disorder, most recent episode manic, 296.44
Axis II: No diagnosis
Axis III: No diagnosis
Axis IV: Loss of important relationship
Axis V: GAF: 20

Plan: Lithium 600 mg b.i.d.
Thorazine 100 mg t.i.d.
Daily meetings as tolerated by patient to monitor side effects and develop alliance.

BIBLIOGRAPHY

1. Clinical hypothesis testing. In Lazare A (ed): Outpatient Psychiatry. Baltimore, Williams & Wilkins, 1989.

4. INTRODUCTION TO DSM-IV

Michael Kahn, M.D.

1. What is the conceptual orientation of DSM-IV?

The Diagnostic and Statistical Manuals (DSM) are handbooks developed by the American Psychiatric Association. They contain listings and descriptions of psychiatric diagnoses, analogous to the International Classification of Diseases (ICD) manuals. The DSMs have changed as the prevailing concepts of mental disorder have changed. DSM-I (1952) reflected Adolf Meyer's influence on American psychiatry, and classified mental disorders as various "reactions" to stressors. DSM-II (1968) dropped the concept of "reactions," but maintained a perspective strongly influenced by psychodynamic theory. DSM-III (1980) marked a watershed in the development of the classification system, in that it outlined a research-based, empirical, and phenomenologic approach to diagnosis, which attempted to be atheoretical with regard to etiology. DSM-IV continues this tradition, which some writers would characterize as the "biologic" or "syndromal" approach to diagnosis.

2. What is the purpose of the multiaxial system?

The five-axis classification system was developed in order to provide a systematic framework for the thorough descriptive assessment of a given patient's psychiatric condition and overall functioning. The axes are specified as follows:

- Axis I: Clinical disorders
- Axis II: Personality disorders
  Mental retardation
- Axis III: General medical conditions
- Axis IV: Psychosocial and environmental problems
- Axis V: Global assessment of functioning

3. What are the characteristics of axis I disorders?

Axis I diagnoses comprise those *clinical syndromes* that generally develop in late adolescence or adulthood. Schizophrenia, bipolar disorder, panic disorder, posttraumatic stress disorder, and alcohol abuse are all diagnoses coded on axis I. One can think of axis I diagnoses as "illnesses," as opposed to the persistently maladaptive *behavior patterns* that characterize personality disorders.

4. How do these differ from axis II disorders?

Axis II comprises *personality disorders,* and *mental retardation.* One may also note maladaptive personality traits on axis II (see below).

5. Can one make multiple diagnoses on axes I and II?

Definitely. A patient with well-controlled schizophrenia may develop a problem with alcohol abuse, and would therefore warrant *both* diagnoses on axis I. A patient with mental retardation may also meet criteria for obsessive-compulsive personality disorder, and would therefore receive both diagnoses on axis II. One may include several diagnoses on each axis, if needed.

6. What if a patient's signs and symptoms don't fit neatly into one or more categories?

Several ways exist to deal with this very common situation. On axis I, most clinical syndromes described have one variant called [syndrome name] *not otherwise specified* (or NOS). Psychosis NOS, adjustment disorder NOS, and bipolar disorder NOS are all diagnoses which may be used when although not all criteria characterizing a given syndrome are met, that syndrome seems closest to describing the patient's difficulties.

If the clinical picture is even less clear, one has the option of *deferring* diagnoses on either axis I or II until one is able to gather the information needed to make a more definitive diagnosis. The code for a deferred diagnosis on either axis I or II is 799.90.

Finally, one may make a *provisional* diagnosis if enough information is available to make a reasonable formulation, but some doubt or uncertainty remains. In these cases, one merely writes "provisional" following the suspected diagnosis.

7. Do these issues apply to personality disorders as well?
Yes. If a patient seems to have several of the characteristics of, for example, antisocial personality disorder, but does not meet *all* criteria for that diagnosis, one may record that the patient has antisocial *traits*. Likewise, a patient may have traits of more than one personality disorder; in this situation one would make a diagnosis of, for example, *mixed personality disorder with borderline and histrionic traits.*

8. How does axis III function?
Axis III primarily records *medical* problems *relevant* to the ongoing treatment of the patient. Examples are glaucoma in a patient requiring antidepressants, asthma in a patient with anxiety who is taking theophylline, AIDS in a patient with new-onset psychosis, and cirrhosis of the liver in a patient with alcohol dependence.

9. What about axes IV and V?
Axis IV records psychosocial stressors encountered by the patient within the previous 12 months that have contributed to (1) the development of a new mental disorder; (2) the recurrence of a previous mental disorder; or (3) the exacerbation of an ongoing mental disorder. The stressor should be described in as much detail as needed to indicate how it affects the patient's functioning. Even mild stressors should be noted if they figure into the clinical presentation.

Axis V records the patient's global level of functioning both at the time of evaluation and during the past year. The clinician consults the Global Assessment of Functioning (GAF) scale in the manual and determines the patient's current GAF score as well as the highest one obtained during a relatively prolonged period within the past year.

10. Does the DSM system provide a good way to diagnose psychiatric disorders?
Compared to what? would probably be the first reply to this thorny question. So long as psychiatry lacks definitive tests to diagnose illness, arguments about which criteria should form the basis of the diagnostic system will continue to flourish. The publication of DSM-III in 1980 was widely hailed both inside and outside the field for at last providing diagnoses which relied on what people *observed* rather than what they *believed* on the basis of theory. A wide variety of mental health (and general medical) practitioners found that DSM-III provided a straightforward, comprehensible, and "user-friendly" tool for making sense of (or at least classifying) psychopathology.

The DSM system has some clear shortcomings, however, and some well-regarded clinicians have called it parochial, reductionistic, adynamic (i.e., not sensitive to the dynamic hypothesis mentioned above), and clumsy in its difficulty distinguishing between "state" and "trait" behaviors.[2] The DSM system was designed to have high reliability among different raters; that is, it was fashioned so that two different clinicians would have a high likelihood of arriving at the same diagnosis for a given patient. Yet it is clear that *reliability* and *validity* of diagnosis remain distinct. Some would say that the DSM system favors the former at the expense of the latter, whereas others would reply that so long as validity remains elusive, we should do our best to at least improve reliability, which can be empirically tested in field trials. DSM-IV creates some problems and helps to solve others; a nondogmatic, open-minded, and pragmatic approach to this complicated issue probably serves *patients* best.

BIBLIOGRAPHY

1. American Psychiatric Association: Diagnostic and Statistical Manual–IV. Washington, DC, American Psychiatric Association, 1994.
2. Klerman GL, Vaillant GE, Spitzer RL, Michels R: A debate on DSM-III. Am J Psychiatry 141:4, 1984.

II. Diagnostic Procedures

5. PROJECTIVE TESTING

Judith E. Fox, Ph.D.

1. What are projective tests?

Projective tests are individually administered tests generally used to obtain information about emotional functioning. Projective tests are founded on the idea that in ambiguous, unstructured, and open-ended situations aspects of the individual's internal, emotional world are projected onto the environment to influence his or her perception and experience of it. Test responses are understood as samples of the individual's emotional life.

Murray was one of the first psychologists to offer a description of how the process of projection works. Murray's ideas about projection were derived largely from Freud: To cope with what is felt to be personally threatening, individuals defensively turn what they experience internally to be dangerous into external dangers. Once the experienced dangers are perceived to be external, they are easier to cope with. Rather than viewing this process of projection necessarily as a defensive maneuver, Murray viewed it more as people's tendency to be influenced in the cognitive mediation of perceptual inputs by their needs, interests, and overall psychological organization.[4] The label *projective methods* is applied to various techniques that present the examinee with such psychological activity.

2. What are the most commonly used projective techniques?

Among the many projective tests, the Rorschach, Thematic Apperception Test (TAT), and Draw-A-Person Test are perhaps the most commonly used. Sentence completion tests, in which the patient is asked to complete sentences such as "my mother . . ." or "the best time I ever had was . . ." are also common. Although many tests have been developed to uncover inner thoughts and feelings, Lindzey[14] long go suggested a way to classify projective tests based on the nature of the projective activity:

1. **Associations**: The patient is asked to verbalize a response to some stimuli. The Rorschach, in which the subject views several ink blots and responds verbally to each, is one such example. Word association test, in which the patient is asked to indicate the word that comes to mind in response to another word, is another example.

2. **Completions**: The patient completes an unfinished stimulus. Sentence completion tasks are an example.

3. **Constructions**: The patient is required to form or develop a production out of a stimulus. The story-telling task of the TAT, for example, requires the patient to construct a story from a picture.

4. **Choice or ordering**: Patients are asked to place objects in categories or rank order choices or preferences for items.

5. **Self-expression**: The patient creates something without a stimulus to initiate the response. Drawing tasks or dramatic play are examples.

All of these projective methods are based on the assumption that the patient's responses and creations reflect some aspect of his or her inner world; thus they are viewed as vehicles that lend articulation to a person's inner experiences.

3. What are the differences between objective and projective personality tests?

"When the subject is asked to guess what the examiner is thinking, we call it an objective test; when the examiner tries to guess what the subject is thinking, we call it a projective device."[11]

The utility of dichotomizing "objective" and "projective" tests is controversial. This dichotomy sometimes refers to the way in which a test has been developed, the degree to which the results involve clinician subjectivity, and/or whether or not test questions are open-ended. It often is used to classify tests based on the degree to which they were developed in accordance with fundamental principles of measurement. This affects the degree to which a test is a reliable and valid indicator of the personality variables that it purports to measure. Objective measures are developed through lengthy empirical testing and group comparison. An individual's score can be represented on a graph and compared with scores obtained from a normative sample. Projective measures may lack these advantages.

Personality tests, such as the Minnesota Multiphasic Personality Inventory (MMPI), also may be termed objective when they do not require the clinician to exercise a great deal of individual judgment in ascertaining a subject's test score and personality profile. Projective tests tend to require greater subjectivity on the part of the clinician. Even with objective tests, however, subjectivity of the examiner affects interpretation of the test profile. Exner, the developer of a major scoring and interpretation system for the Rorschach, notes the the objective-projective dichotomy is grossly over-simplified: "Any stimulus situation that evokes or facilitates the process of projection can be considered a projective method. This is quite independent of whether or not basic rules of measurement have been employed in developing or establishing the test.[4] Exner developed a comprehensive system of scoring and interpreting the Rorschach. This, then, is an example of a projective test that has been developed in a fashion similar to the objective test.

In yet another common usage, objective tests are structured to elicit a specific class of responses (for example, true-false inventories), whereas projective tests elicit more open-ended responses. Questions on objective tests tend to be fairly direct and self-evident, whereas answers to projective items tend to be obscure and unstructured. Regardless of whether a test utilizes a projective task or is categorized as nonobjective and less open-ended, contemporary psychologists generally interpret the findings in the context of history, behavior, and interpersonal relationships.

4. Describe the Rorschach test.

The Rorschach (one of the most widely used projective tests) is a projective test originally developed in 1921 by Hermann Rorschach. It consists of a set of ten ink blots. Each block is sequentially presented to the patient, who is asked to describe what the ink blot suggests. The examiner then asks about the various details of the perceptions to understand the key factors associated with their creation.

Of the numerous scoring systems developed for Rorschach data, many involve looking at at least three general categories: (1) the location or area of the ink blot on which the response is based; (2) the specific aspects or determinants of the blot used to form the percept (e.g., shape, color, shading), and (3) the content of the percept (e.g., whether it is human or animal). Some systems also attempt to capture the fashion by which the individual organized the response. The degree to which a percept represents an integrated and/or well-formed response is often one indicator of the intactness of the person's thinking.

The major premise of the Rorschach is that a person organizes stimuli from the environment based on needs, motives, conflicts, and perceptual processes. Ambiguous stimuli, like ink blots, promote cognitive disorganization and represent the fashion and ease by which the individual draws from internal resources to organize and confront ambiguous situations.

5. What are the assets and limitations of the Rorschach?

Since its initial development, the Rorschach has been a controversial psychological testing instrument. Criticisms of the Rorschach, as is true of most projective tests, focus on the validity and reliability of the test instrument and the conclusions based on test results. Although both reliability and validity have reached acceptable levels on the Rorschach, more objective psychological tests reach superior levels of validity.

The most contemporary, data-based system of scoring and interpreting the Rorschach is the Exner Comprehensive System,[5] which provides many scores and formulas of varying reliability and validity. The examiner must be aware of the differences among scores in terms of psychometric properties to interpret test productions adequately.

The Rorschach is a complex test. Extensive training is required to evaluate its findings, and some graduate school programs lack such training. Furthermore, the Rorschach may have limited value as an assessment tool for children, in whom its reliability may be adequate for short-term evaluation but limited for longer-term predictions. Lastly, because its administration and interpretation are relatively complex compared with some other psychological tests, it allows an increased possibility for error.

On the positive side, highly trained Rorschach clinicians can describe a person's characteristics accurately based on responses to the test.[10] The Rorschach is also thought to assist in the evaluation of underlying personality structure because its ambiguity bypasses conscious awareness and defensiveness. It is often used to evaluate an individual who outwardly presents as well-adjusted but inwardly may experience psychopathology. Edell[3] has shown, for example, that individuals with borderline personality disorder may perform normally on structured tests but demonstrate psychopathology on the less structured Rorschach. Lastly, the Rorschach is relatively easy to administer.

6. Describe the Thematic Apperception Test (TAT) and discuss its assets and limitations.
The TAT is a projective test developed by Henry Murray in the mid 1930s. It consists of 20 cards that depict a variety of ambiguous scenes. The subject is instructed to make up a story about each card and to include a beginning, middle, and end to the story as well as to describe the thoughts and feelings of the characters.

Unlike the Rorschach, the TAT presents more structured test stimuli. It requires a different kind of organization and verbal response. Its interpretation is largely based on Murray's theory of personality, which emphasizes both biologic and socioenvironmental determinants of behavior. Murray believed that the way in which individuals deal with their environment involves both how their environment affects them and how their unique set of needs, attitudes and values affect their reaction to the environment. The TAT grew from Murray's motivation to assess individuals' psychological needs.

Generally, the interpretation of TAT responses is based on content analysis of the story. Quantitative analysis of the TAT is generally not attempted, even though some scoring systems have been successfully applied.[15] Because scoring systems are generally not applied, the reliability and validity of the measure are difficult to ascertain. The effectiveness of the technique often depends more on the clinician's skill than on the quality of the test.

On the positive side, the TAT provides material related to various aspects of psychological functioning, including mood, interpersonal themes, problem-solving style, and motivational variables. Patients generally find the test interesting and nonthreatening, and it is easy to administer. Like all projective techniques, the TAT may bypass conscious defenses and facilitate self-revelation.

7. What are projective drawings? How are they used?
One common assumption of projective drawing tests of personality is that individuals create symbolically in their productions important themes, dynamics, and attitudes and they project images, feelings, and thoughts important to understanding them.

Projective drawings were most popular during the 1950s and 1960s when psychoanalytic theory was dominant. Goodenough's Draw-A-Man Test, developed in 1926,[7] was the first projective drawing test; it was used to estimate a child's level of intellectual maturity. Machover[16] extended projective drawings into the area of personality assessment. Such characteristics as size of drawing and placement on the page were interpreted as indicators of self-esteem and/or mood.

Koppitz[12] expanded the developmental and personality aspects of human figure drawings by creating scoring systems reflecting various cognitive and emotional attributes. The House-Tree-Person Test was concurrently developed by Buck. In 1987 Burns developed the Kinetic House-Tree-Person Test, in which the patient is asked to make the person in the drawing "do something." This is probably the most popular form of projective drawings used today. Similarly, the Burn's Kinetic Family Drawing, in which the patient draws his family "doing something," has been used to assess interpersonal relationships and family dynamics.

In interpreting drawings, clinicians tend to depend on clinical intuition, judgment, and experience. In a review of projective drawings, Grath-Marnat[8] concludes that projective drawings have been used most successfully as a rough measure of intellectual maturation. They are moderately successful in measuring global estimates of adjustment, impulsivity, and anxiety. They are least successful in assessing specific aspects of personality or in making clear diagnoses.

8. What important factors should be considered in evaluating the efficacy of results produced by projective test techniques?

1. **Test reliability**. Many projective tests have been criticized for the degree to which they provide stable, consistent, and predictable results. Reliability refers to the extent to which an individual will achieve the same score if the test is administered again. Although one expects some variability between scores obtained on the same test at different times, a test is thought to be most reliable when variability is at a minimum. In evaluating the reliability of a test, one expects higher reliabilities when stable variables are measured (e.g., stable personality traits) and lower reliabilities when unstable aspects (e.g., current emotional states) are measured.

Some projective tests (e.g., the TAT) lack normative data; the clinician must rely on his or her own experience to interpret the responses. The effectiveness of the technique often depends more on the clinician's skills than on the quality of the test. Patient responses to projective tests also have been found to be affected by such variables as mood, stress, sleep deprivation, and differences in instruction. Such variables may limit the degree to which one obtains a reliable measure of personality traits. Furthermore, when a personality test does not use standardized administration and scoring, its reliability is severely reduced.

2. **Test validity**. Projective tests also have been criticized for the degree to which they actually measure what they intend to measure. Validity involves the relationship between the test and some external, independently observed event. Thus, a score on impulse control on a particular projective test should correlate highly with some observed criterion of impulse control, i.e., how the patient behaves when experiencing strong emotions. Validity data on projective tests are limited.

3. **Test-taking factors**. Projective techniques are viewed generally as less susceptible to "faking," because they present the subject with an ambiguous situation in which the underlying concepts are covert or unknown. Individuals, therefore, are less able to manipulate their responses to be viewed in a particular light. Projective tests also are nonthreatening to most subjects because they are intrinsically interesting and have no "wrong" answers.

9. When should patients be referred for projective testing?

In general, projective testing is used to address referral questions about emotional functioning. Examples include (1) the nature and level of depression, anxiety, and/or anger; (2) level and style of impulse control; (3) quality and clarity of thinking (e.g., does the patient experience disordered thinking and/or psychosis); (4) coping styles and capacities; (5) style and capacity for relatedness to others; (6) experience of others; (7) style of solving problems; (8) originality and integrative capacities; (9) emotional responses to stress; (10) emotional reactivity; (11) defensiveness and style of defense; (12) level of personal adjustment or ego functioning; (13) ability to tolerate stress; (14) adequacy of daily functioning; (15) reality testing; (16) level of self-esteem; and (17) experience of family dynamics.

Although some psychologists may use projective testing alone to answer some of the above questions, it is more often used as part of a battery of tests and interpreted in the context of responses to several tests, history, and present described functioning. Projective tests are viewed as often versatile and rich in their findings but not as self-sufficient. Several authors, such as Anastasi,[1] have emphasized that projective tests give optimal results when used in a battery of tests and/or as a type of structured clinical interview. Others have noted, however, that test results have not been shown to increase in validity with the addition of other tests.[6]

Personality tests are often used to identify the patient's verbal responses to structured vs. unstructured situations. Such information may be invaluable to understand how someone who generally appears to function well in a structured interview would handle an ambiguous situation that may be more stressful and disorganizing. Individuals with borderline personality disorder, for example, may perform well on structured tests but evidence disorganized thinking on ambiguous, projective tests. Projective tests may address certain diagnostic questions pertaining to the intactness of thinking and reality testing.

Projective testing also may be useful in gaining information about emotional functioning in situations in which the individual is highly defensive and/or motivated to appear in particular ways during interview or on more direct, objective tests. Such an approach to test-taking may be part of patients' overt personality style or related more to their situation, e.g., feeling a need to present well because of a pending legal situation. In such instances, the ambiguity of projective testing may bypass the patient's reluctance to provide personal material.

BIBLIOGRAPHY

1. Anastasi A: Psychological Testing, 6th ed. New York, Macmillan, 1988.
2. Bellak L: The TAT, CAT and SAT in Clinical Use, 4th ed. New York, Grune & Stratton, 1986.
3. Edell WS: Role of structure in disordered thinking in borderline and schizophrenic disorders. J Pers Assess 51:23–41, 1987.
4. Exner JE: Rorschach assessment. In Weiner LB (ed): Clinical Method in Psychology. New York, John Wiley & Sons, 1983.
5. Exner JE: The Rorschach: A Comprehensive System, vol 1, 2nd ed. New York, John Wiley & Sons, 1986.
6. Garb HN: The incremental validity of information used in personality assessment. Clin Psychol Rev 4:641–655, 1985.
7. Goodenough F: Measurement of Intelligence by Drawings. New York, World Book, 1926.
8. Grath-Marnat G: Handbook of Psychological Assessment, 2nd ed. New York, John Wiley & Sons, 1990.
9. Handler L: The clinical use of the Draw-A-Person Test (DAP). In Newmark CS (ed): Major Psychological Assessment Instruments. Newton, MA, Selyn & Bacon, 1985.
10. Karon BP: Projective tests are valid. Am Psychol 33:764–765, 1978.
11. Kelly GA: The theory and technique of assessment. Annu Rev Psychol 9:325–352, 1958.
12. Koppitz EM: Psychological Evaluation of Human Figure Drawings by Middle School Pupils. New York, Grune & Stratton, 1984.
13. Leiter E: The role of projective testing. In Wetzler S, Katz M (eds): Contemporary Approaches to Psychological Assessment. New York, Brunner/Mazel, 1989.
14. Lindzey G: Projective Techniques and Cross-Cultural Research. New York, Appleton-Century-Crofts, 1961.
15. McClelland DC: The Achieving Society. NJ, Van Nostrand, 1961.
16. Machover K: Personality Projection in the Drawings of the Human Figure. Springfield, IL, Charles C Thomas, 1949.
17. Oster GD, Gould P: Using Drawings in Assessment and Therapy. New York, Brunner/Mazel, 1987.
18. Rabin I (ed): Assessment with Projective Techniques. New York, Springer, 1981.
19. Weiner IB: Conceptual and empirical perspectives on the Rorschach assessment of psychopathology. J Pers Assess 50:472–479.

6. NEUROPSYCHOLOGICAL TESTING

Laetitia L. Thompson, Ph.D.

1. What is neuropsychological testing?

Neuropsychological testing uses behavioral measures to assess skills and abilities that relate to brain functioning. Most neuropsychological tests have been developed to measure "higher cerebral functioning," so the tests usually focus on cognitive skills and abilities. These tests have been developed to help diagnose brain damage or brain dysfunction in some patients and to help ascertain the behavioral effects of known brain damage in others. Such evaluation can provide information about cognitive strengths and weaknesses within an individual and the areas in which an individual's functioning may differ from that of the normal population. This type of evaluation is most commonly conducted on patients with neurologic disorders.

2. How does it differ from clinical psychological evaluation?

Clinical psychological evaluation uses tests designed to provide information about the personality and emotional functioning of patients. Measures may include objective personality tests or so-called projective techniques such as the Rorschach or the Thematic Apperception Test. Procedures used in clinical psychological evaluations generally differ from those used in neuropsychological evaluations, although there may occasionally be a little overlap. For example, clinical evaluations frequently include an intelligence test, which is essentially a measure of cognitive function, and many neuropsychological evaluations have a personality measure to screen for emotional difficulties. The focus of the two types of evaluations differs, however, so the referring person must think about the goal of the evaluation in deciding where to refer.

3. What is neuropsychological testing like for the patient? (or, How to prepare your patient for a neuropsychological evaluation.)

Neuropsychological tests are behavioral. They are not invasive and present no physical risk to the patient. Typically, the patient will work with one or two testing examiners (sometimes, all or part of the testing will be done by the neuropsychologist).

The tests may require reading or listening to verbal information, viewing nonverbal visual information, or palpating stimuli. Some tasks require pencil and paper, whereas others need only verbal responses from the patient. Some tasks require manipulation of objects, puzzle assembly, drawing of objects, or writing. If a patient has impaired vision or hearing, testing usually can be modified to enable the patient to complete it. If a patient has any such peripheral impairment, however, it is helpful to discuss this with the neuropsychologist at the time of the referral.

The testing *can* be fatiguing, and precautions should be taken to administer the tests in an order that: (1) intersperses easier and harder tests; (2) begins the testing with tasks that reduce rather than increase anxiety; and (3) places tests with demanding attentional/speed requirements when the patient is fresh and well rested, yet past the initial anxiety.

In referring a patient for neuropsychological evaluation, it can be reassuring to talk briefly with the patient about the type of situation to be encountered. Patients sometimes telephone or arrive for their appointments wondering if they are going to be "stuck with needles or probed with electrodes." After they realize the testing is behavioral, they frequently are quite relieved.

4. What are appropriate questions to consider in referring a psychiatric patient for neuropsychological testing?

Several issues may be addressed by neuropsychological testing. First, neuropsychological testing can help with diagnostic issues in certain cases, as when there are considerations of depression or dementia. In addition to overall level of performance, the neuropsychologist can look at patterns of test performance. For example, some patterns are more frequently associated with depression, whereas others are more likely to be seen in dementia. Of course, in some individuals, elements of *both* depression and dementia may co-exist, and neuropsychological evaluation may confirm this. Another type of diagnostic situation might involve a psychiatric patient for whom there is also a suspicion of a neurologic problem, such as early dementia or traumatic brain injury.

Second, as views about psychopathology change, and more psychiatric conditions are found to have biologic components, more interest exists in understanding the neuropsychological characteristics of psychiatric disorders themselves. The psychiatric disorder that has received the most attention to date has been schizophrenia, but now there are also studies of neuropsychological functioning in patients with bipolar, obsessive-compulsive, panic, post-traumatic stress, attention-deficit-hyperactivity, and conduct disorders, among others. It may be helpful to obtain information about the neurocognitive strengths and weaknesses of individual patients with these disorders and to learn whether their pattern of performance is similar to those of other patients with the same disorder.

Third, a practical area of concern is the everyday implications of neurocognitive function (or dysfunction) for psychiatrically ill patients. Neuropsychological evaluation helps clarify these issues and provides important information about long-term planning.

When referring a patient for evaluation, the referring person ought to communicate the major question(s) to the neuropsychologist rather than simply indicating "neuropsychological testing" on a referral form. This facilitates a more useful battery of tests, as well as a more focused report. Some specific referral questions are listed in the table.

Examples of Common Referral Questions

1. Is the patient depressed, demented, or both?
2. Does this patient with schizophrenia have cognitive impairment? Is the impairment typical of that seen in schizophrenia?
3. A 59-year-old patient has a history of schizophrenia. Is there also evidence for early dementia?
4. The patient complains of memory problems. Is there evidence of memory problems or other cognitive deficits?
5. Does the patient have the cognitive capabilities to: live independently? comply with a medication regimen? work in a competitive or sheltered capacity?
6. The patient does not follow through with treatment planning? Is this related to memory or other cognitive deficits?

5. What should a neuropsychological evaluation include?

Many tests are now available from which the neuropsychologist may select. This may result in some confusion to the referring person who sees little apparent rhyme or reason to the specific tests used. It may be helpful to keep in mind *areas of cognition* that usually are covered to evaluate the comprehensiveness of a particular evaluation. The table below lists the major areas of cognition likely to be included.

Major Cognitive Areas Assessed in a Comprehensive Evaluation

General intelligence	Perceptual functioning
Attention and concentration	Spatial analysis
Learning and memory	Sensory motor functioning
Language	Psychological/emotional status
Reasoning, planning and problem solving	

The last area listed (psychological/emotional status) may be assessed during an interview and/or through formal testing.

Most neuropsychologists stress the use of standardized measures with high reliability and validity as well as normative guidelines to assist interpretation. Most emphasize that level of performance is only part of the process of interpretation, and that the pattern of performance across several tests is important. Some psychologists emphasize the quality of the patient's performance or the types of errors made.

In addition to the formal testing, the evaluation ought to include history taking, either from the patient, family, physician, and/or records, paying particular attention to background information and any medical history relating to possible neuropsychological risk factors.

The report should include discussion of the history, a report and discussion of the patient's behavior during testing, and an assessment of whether the test results are considered valid measures of the patient's neurocognitive functioning. Most reports will also include a test-by-test description of the results, followed by conclusion(s), recommendations, and/or a discussion of the overall meaning and implications of the results for the patient.

6. When is it appropriate to refer a patient for a neuropsychological screening rather than a comprehensive evaluation?

Many times, psychiatrists and other referrers hope that a screening evaluation will suffice for their patients. In some cases, relatively brief screening (i.e., 1–2 hour battery) can adequately answer the question and, in some cases, a brief evaluation will be all a patient can tolerate because of acute psychiatric symptoms.

When there are questions regarding an in-patient with acute psychiatric symptoms, limited testing may be the only feasible alternative. Such testing provides information about the general level of intellectual functioning or presence of clear dementia, but it is unlikely to answer more specific questions, especially in younger adults where questions about relatively subtle neurocognitive deficits may exist. If complex questions are being asked which would indicate the need for more comprehensive testing, it may be better to defer testing until the patient is as stable as possible in terms of medication and psychiatric symptoms.

Screening may be appropriate to answer questions about presence or absence of neurocognitive dysfunction. More intensive evaluation is necessary if there are specific questions about nature, localization, or the functional implications of deficits.

Describing the patient to the neuropsychologist and discussing the issues and questions will often be the best way to determine the most appropriate battery of tests to be given.

7. What are the effects of depression on neuropsychological testing?

The former answer to this question was that patients presenting with depression but without any "organic" dysfunction would show few, if any, deficits on classic neuropsychological batteries of tests such as the Halstead-Reitan. More recent studies, however, using newly developed measures of attention, information processing speed, and learning have shown that depression can cause slowing of information processing, decreased attention and concentration abilities, and learning inefficiency. Research findings are inconsistent about the existence of a high correlation between severity of depression and test performance. Groups of severely depressed patients are likely to perform more poorly than mildly depressed patients, but these findings are not sufficiently consistent to enable the clinician to predict the degree of cognitive inefficiency by knowing severity of depression.

In many cases, deficits in depressed individuals are subtle, but they may still affect interpretation of results. For example, in a patient with a clinical depression who has had a mild traumatic brain injury (TBI), it can be very difficult to know whether mild deficits in areas of concentration and/or learning are caused by the TBI, the depression, or a combination. Frequently, the practical approach to such a case is to treat the depression and then reevaluate the patient for any residual neurocognitive deficits. Other areas of cognition are generally not impaired in depressed patients (language, problem solving, visual spatial analysis, executive functioning, visual or auditory perception, for example), but, of course, individual patients may present as exceptions to the rule.

In a few instances, severe depression may render the patient untestable. If the patient has severe agitation or psychomotor retardation, he or she may not be able to comply with test requirements and fail to put forth sufficient effort to yield valid results. In my experience, this is not a common occurrence but it does happen. In such instances, neuropsychological evaluation will have to be postponed until the acute depression improves.

8. What are the effects of anxiety on neuropsychological testing?

Most people who undergo neuropsychological testing experience some anxiety about the process. Part of a good testing procedure involves establishing rapport with the patient and providing a reassuring atmosphere to minimize anxiety about testing. In most situations, this will suffice to enable the patient to be validly tested. Very little systematic investigation has been done, however, to explore the effects of especially high levels of anxiety on test performance. To date, the few studies that have been done have found little in the way of specific effects. Clinically, neuropsychologists rely on behavioral observation of the patient to help determine whether unusual levels of anxiety interfere with the patient's effort on the testing. Occasionally, undue anxiety may produce an invalid result (which should, of course, be noted), but in my experience, most patients can control their anxiety sufficiently to produce valid results. Frequently, putting the tests in an order to minimize stress to the patient is enough to permit the patient to complete the evaluation. Whether or not a particular evaluation is valid must be determined by the neuropsychologist.

In some cases, patients with formal anxiety disorders may be referred for neuropsychological evaluation. Research into the effects of formal anxiety disorders is currently at an early stage, and few definite conclusions can be drawn, but the following provides a brief summary of select diagnoses.

9. How do different disorders show an impact on testing?

Patients with panic disorder typically have been found to fall below normative guidelines for impairment on a few tests, but across studies, cognitive deficits have been inconsistent. Currently more evidence exists for memory problems than for other cognitive deficits, thus suggesting possible involvement of the temporal regions of the brain in panic disorder, but additional research is needed to replicate previous findings.

A few studies have assessed neurocognitive functioning in patients with obsessive-compulsive disorder (OCD). Results showing impaired memory and executive functioning suggest possible bilateral frontal and temporal involvement, with considerable disagreement from study to study as to whether the left or right hemisphere is more implicated.

Post-traumatic stress disorder (PTSD) is another anxiety disorder that has recently received attention, mostly in individuals with combat-related PTSD. Most studies have not included well-matched control groups but rather have compared patient performance to available normative guidelines. Such studies have not found large deficits in groups of patients, but have shown that individuals may perform in the below average to borderline range on some tests of memory and attentional function.

Good neuropsychological testing involves administration of the tests in a supportive way to minimize state anxiety and behavioral observation of the patient to determine whether efforts to minimize anxiety have been successful. In patients with panic disorder, OCD, or PTSD, careful analysis of the pattern of test results can help determine: (1) whether deficits appear related to the anxiety disorder alone; and (2) the extent to which any cognitive deficits will have an impact on the patient's everyday life.

10. Is neuropsychological testing indicated in schizophrenia? How do patients with schizophrenia perform?

Schizophrenia is now thought to be a brain disorder, and in a subset of patients, there are neurocognitive effects. Research on the neuropsychological profiles of patients with schizophrenia has revealed considerable heterogeneity. Some patients will, in fact, perform normally on testing, whereas others will be quite diffusely impaired. Commonly, the individual earns mildly impaired scores on a number of measures but looks somewhat more impaired on verbal learning measures. This more pronounced verbal learning deficit superimposed upon diffuse mild impairment has now been found in several studies evaluating groups of schizophrenic patients, but specific individuals do not always, or even routinely, produce this profile. Little evidence exists for a decline in general intellectual functioning following the onset of symptoms, and it is rare for schizophrenic patients to have severe impairment without the presence of some coexisting dementia.

Because of the lack of a unique neuropsychological profile in patients with schizophrenia, interest has evolved in understanding patterns of deficits in subgroups of schizophrenic patients. Groups of paranoid patients generally perform better on neuropsychological testing than groups of non-paranoid patients. Studies of groups of patients with either predominantly positive or negative symptoms have produced similar results, with those patients showing more positive symptoms generally performing better. Additionally, a few studies have found that positive symptoms tend to be associated with deficits on verbal measures, whereas negative symptoms are associated with visual-perceptual deficits.

Neuropsychological test results may be useful in predicting functional outcome in patients with schizophrenia. One study[9] found that test scores were more powerful predictors of outcome measures than were ratings of psychiatric symptoms when Walker et al. looked at patients 1.5 years after the assessment. Therefore, extent of cognitive impairment may be important in predicting everyday functioning parameters such as treatment compliance, independent living, and employability.

11. What effects do medications have on testing?

This is obviously a very complex question, the answer to which depends on what medication or medications at what dosages. Medications that have central nervous system effects may, in some cases, affect neuropsychological test results.

A few guidelines exist to help determine when testing is best done. If a patient has just started a new medication and is experiencing temporary side effects, it is not a good time to evaluate the patient. If a patient is toxic or is approaching a toxic level, it may have significant effects on performance.

Some research over the years has examined the effects of specific psychotropic medications on test performance. Examining specific medications is beyond the scope of this chapter, but there are a few general guidelines. Most studies have shown that the acute symptoms of the disease are more deleterious for cognitive performance than medications for the symptoms if the patient is taking an optimal dose.

Antidepressants have not been found to cause significant adverse effects on test performance in individuals with good clinical response who are not experiencing acute side effects. Generally speaking, neuroleptics have also not been found to cause significant problems on tests of cognitive function to suggest any advantage to stopping medication in an individual who is obtaining clinical benefit. Lithium may cause some modest decrements in upper extremity motor performance, but has not been found to produce changes in neuropsychological test scores that would result in diagnostic or interpretive error.

12. What does it mean when neuropsychological testing and the results of neuroimaging disagree?

Relationships between neurobehavioral measures and neuroimaging techniques have changed dramatically over the past 20 years and likely will continue to, primarily as a result of the evolution of neuroradiologic technology. Furthermore, as the development of neurophysiological measures advances, more opportunities will become available for understanding brain-behavior relationships. For example, research studies using both advanced MRI and neuropsychological testing have increased knowledge about localization of higher cerebral functions in the brain, but such research has also shown how difficult it is to make broad generalizations about localization of function for individual patients.

Therefore, in individual cases, apparent discrepancies or contradictions may exist between neurobehavioral measures and neuroimaging results. These differences may be in either direction (more abnormality in structure than behavior or vice versa). Reasons for this may include:

1. There may be long-standing, probably congenital, structural abnormalities, but the patient has relatively normal neurocognitive functioning because the brain organized with the abnormality already in place.

2. The physiological changes associated with brain lesions identified by computed tomography or magnetic resonance imaging may exceed the boundaries of the structural abnormality.

3. Individual differences in functional brain organization are complex and not yet completely understood.

4. Neurobehavioral measures may be incorrectly interpreted, e.g., interpreting errors on sensory or motor tests resulting from peripheral nervous system injury as central nervous system impairment.

5. Changes at a microscopic level may cause behavioral change, but may not be visible with current imaging technology.

BIBLIOGRAPHY

1. Bigler ED: Frontal lobe damage and neuropsychological assessment. Arch Clin Neuropsychol 3:279–297, 1988.
2. Bigler ED, Yeo RA, Turkheimer E (eds): Neuropsychological Function and Brain Imaging. New York, Plenum Press, 1989.
3. Hill CD, Stoudemire A, Morris R, Matino-Saltzman D, Markwalter HR: Similarities and differences in memory deficits in patients with primary dementia and depression-related cognitive dysfunction. J Neuropsychiatry Clin Neurosci 5:277–282, 1993.
4. Lezak MD: Neuropsychological Assessment, 2nd ed. New York, Oxford University Press, 1983.
5. Newman PJ, Sweet JJ: Depressive disorders. In Puente AE, McCaffrey RJ (eds): Handbook of Neuropsychological Assessment: A Biopsychosocial Perspective. New York, Plenum Press, 1992.
6. Orsillo SM, McCaffrey RJ: Anxiety disorders. In Puente AE, McCaffrey RJ (eds): Handbook of Neuropsychological Assessment: A Biopsychosocial Perspective. New York, Plenum Press, 1992.
7. Reitan RM, Wolfson D: The Halstead-Reitan Neuropsychological Battery: Theory and Interpretation, 2nd ed. Tucson, AZ, Neuropsychology Press, 1993.
8. Sweet JJ, Newman P, Bell B: Significance of depression in clinical neuropsychological assessment. Clin Psychol Rev 12:21–45, 1992.
9. Walker E, Lucas M, Lewine R: Schizophrenic disorders. In Puente AE, McCaffrey RJ (eds): Handbook of Neuropsychological Assessment: A Biopsychosocial Perspective. New York, Plenum Press, 1992.

7. PSYCHIATRIC SYMPTOMS AND PERSONALITY TESTING BY QUESTIONNAIRE

Garry Welch, B.Sc., M.A., Ph.D.

1. What are the potential uses of self-reporting psychiatric and personality tests?

There are many potential clinical and research uses, although it should be emphasized that tests often require a high level of expertise to interpret their scores and profiles. The potential uses include:

- History taking and formulating clinical hypotheses
- Screening and diagnosis of clinical problems and mental disorders
- Determining appropriate referral to specialty services
- Monitoring change and response to treatment interventions
- Conducting research into factors associated with the disorders
- Auditing and assessing clinical services

2. What is the role of reliability in psychiatric and personality tests?

Reliability of measurement is important because it sets an upper limit on the validity, or clinical usefulness, that the measure will likely have when applied to various individuals and in various settings. Unreliable measures cannot be highly valid, and in practical terms, results obtained from them may cloud the true meaning of test scores, thereby undermining clinical decision-making.

3. How does one determine if a given test is reliable?

When considering reliability, the question is whether the measure provides repeatable or reproducible test scores that accurately reflect the patient's true status and that contain little influence from unimportant extraneous factors. For example, if a test is supposed to detect current anxiety state, it will be reliable if it mostly measures current anxiety and does not take into account other factors such as the individual's recall of the answers given the last time the test was administered, or unclear questions in the test or in poorly-worded instructions.

Reliability indices used to describe psychiatric and personality questionnaires range in value from 0 (no reliability) to 1.0 (perfect reliability) and are of two types: (1) the test-retest index that indicates how stable the test scores are over a short period under conditions where the individuals are assumed not to have changed much on the topic of interest, and (2) the internal reliability index, which shows whether the questions are all highly intercorrelated and are therefore likely to be measuring the same thing.

Test-retest reliability is typically measured by the correlation coefficient or (more preferably) the intraclass correlation coefficient (ICC). Test-retest reliability coefficients can be difficult to interpret if they are not high (i.e., around 0.80). Lower reliability values may indicate either that the test is, in fact, unreliable or simply that the individuals tested have changed in status over the period of testing. Test-retest coefficients obtained for known fluctuating variables (e.g., depressed mood or anxious mood) would be expected to be lower than those for a relatively stable personality trait such as extroversion where test-retest reliability may be around 0.90. Internal reliability indices are easier to interpret than test-retest and typically involve the use of Cronbach's alpha index. These should range from 0.70 to 0.80 if the test is to be used to compare groups of people but the upper range should be higher (preferably around 0.90) if the test is to be used to classify individuals. Ideally, both test-retest and internal reliability information should be available for a test. Reliability information obtained from different settings may vary. For example, data gathered in a heterogeneous general population study may not directly apply to a highly selected hospital-based patient population. Typically, reliability coefficients will be somewhat lower in the latter case for technical reasons related to the narrower range of scores obtained.

4. What is meant by the term validity in psychiatric and personality tests?

Although reliability analyses can establish that a test is measuring *something*, in a reproducible fashion, validity analyses can help establish exactly *what* is being measured and whether the test can satisfactorily perform an important clinical task such as early screening for problems, making a diagnosis, monitoring response to treatment, and directing research into the causes of particular disorders. The fundamental question when considering the validity of a test is "Do the test scores have biologic or clinical meaning for the specific task I have in mind and for the particular individuals?" One of the difficulties in assessing validity in psychiatry and psychology is that there is often no absolute standard against which to judge the validity of a test. Although this creates headaches for clinicians and researchers in many branches of medicine, it is a particular problem in mental health, where psychosocial phenomena that can neither be readily observed nor easily described are of interest. Ideally, the validity of psychiatric and personality tests is determined by weighing the evidence from a variety of validity studies that show that the test measures what it was designed to (i.e., its construct validity). In practical terms, validity studies usually involve (1) calculating correlations between the test and other related measures or individual attributes, and (2) looking at the size of differences in mean scores for selected study groups. Terms that describe validity in the literature that are important to understand include *content, predictive, concurrent,* and *discriminant* types of validity. A quick checklist of the main points to consider when evaluating the merits of a measure of psychiatric symptoms or personality traits follows:

Checklist for Reliability and Validity Issues Related to Questionnaires

Reliability
> *Test retest reliability—*
>> Are temporal reliability coefficients around 0.80 over 2-day to 2-week periods?
>> Are values lower for fluctuating variables like mood and higher (around 0.90) for stable variables such as personality traits?
> *Internal reliability—*
>> Are Cronbach alpha values around 0.70–0.80 for group comparisons or around 0.90 for individual screening or classification uses?

Validity
> *Content*
>> Is the breadth of the conceptual domain adequately covered?
>> Is critical content covered?
> *Predictive*
>> Does the test predict future behavior?
> *Convergent*
>> Does test correlate well with existing similar measures?
>> Are similar findings obtained from different sources, e.g., from subject, clinician, or spouse?
> *Discriminant*
>> Do the scores of selected groups differ in their mean as predicted?
>> Are low correlations found with theoretically unrelated variables, or are negative correlations found where these are theoretically expected?
>> For a screening test, does it have 100% sensitivity and high positive-predictive power?
>> Does a measure of treatment response have good responsiveness?

Construct
> This term represents a judgment based on an accumulation of related validity studies made over time that the test measures its intended topic.

5. What is content validity?

It is essentially a subjective judgment based usually on expert consensus and/or a review of the literature that the breadth of the conceptual domain the test is aiming to measure is adequately covered or that the most clinically significant areas of the domain (i.e., critical content) are well covered. Usually if a new psychiatric or personality test appears in the literature it has some practical or theoretical advantage over the older ones. For example, a new test may be briefer and quicker to administer, have better worded questions, or have new questions that reflect recent changes in theory or clinical practice. Or it may be a companion measure to be used as a screening device to replace a longer questionnaire or clinical interview in special situations in which the use of the latter is impractical (e.g., community surveys).

6. What is predictive validity?

This term indicates interest in predicting some important behavior at a point in the future. For example, scores of a screening test of depressive symptoms might be expected to correlate highly with later suicidal behavior or later antidepressant drug use.

7. What does convergent validity show?

It verifies the test correlates highly with measures to which it is thought to be theoretically related. For example, one measure of depression would be expected to have high correlations with other measures of depression. Another approach may be to establish that test scores obtained from different sources are at least moderately correlated, e.g., those from patient, therapist, or family members.

8. What does the term *discriminant validity* establish?

That the test is not correlated with measures to which it is theoretically unrelated, e.g., that depressed scores are not correlated with those measuring intelligence, or that test scores are significantly different for groups theoretically expected to differ beforehand, e.g., depressed patients should score higher than either normal controls or successfully treated patients on a measure of depression that is under scrutiny.

9. Define *responsiveness*.

The term describes the ability of a test to detect true change in patient clinical status over time (usually in the context of treatment). For example, scores for a depression test should be lower on retesting for a depressed patient group improved by a drug treatment or psychotherapy of known efficacy. Deyo et al.[3] provide a good discussion of responsiveness and examples of suitable indices.

10. Which indices are most useful in diagnosis and screening?

Diagnostic and screening discriminant validity relates to the screening and classification of illness. The most useful validity indices in screening and classification of illness (typically they are expressed as percentages) are positive predictive power (PPV), which indicates the proportion of high scorers (using a given cut-off score) on a test who were found to be clinically ill by clinical interview, and sensitivity, which indicates the proportion of truly ill individuals who scored high on the test. For a good screening measure, ideally there will be 100% sensitivity at the recommended cut-off score, to ensure no potential true cases will be missed, and as high a PPV as possible to minimize the number of false positives (high scorers who are in fact not ill) who will be interviewed. Psychiatric and personality measures are rarely used alone to determine diagnosis but are used commonly in screening and as a adjunct to the diagnostic interview.

11. Explain construct validity.

This umbrella or summary term involves judging how well a given test measures the underlying concept that it was intended to. Construct validity is programmatic and requires the gradual accumulation of evidence through a wide range of appropriate validity studies that measure different aspects of the test's validity. It may include information from all the above types of validity plus those from *factor analytic studies*. These statistical studies examine the pattern of correlations among scores for individual questions in a test to determine whether groups of conceptually similar items intercorrelate highly.

12. These guidelines should give reliable results?

Remember, no measure is reliable and valid for all purposes and red flags should be raised if a test is uncritically described as "reliable and valid" in a clinical or research article you have read. Available information on the potential usefulness of a given test should be considered in light of your specific purpose in using it, while considering the characteristics of the patients or subjects to be tested and the setting they are to be drawn from. Also, it should be restated that many psychiatric and personality tests require a high level of training and clinical expertise to accompany their use and that interpretation and appropriate professional help should be sought if appropriate.

13. What is a valid questionnaire to measure depression? What are its potential clinical uses?

The Beck Depression Inventory (BDI) is the most widely used and validated self-report questionnaire for measuring the symptoms of depression. It has 21 questions and is straightforward to administer and score. Information on its reliability and clinical usefulness (and normative data) is available for many different medical, psychiatric, and general population samples to aid the interpretation of a given individual or group BDI score. It has mostly been used to assess severity of depression. It is not recommended as a diagnostic tool although cut-off scores for non-depressed (<10), mildly depressed (10–14), moderately depressed (15–22), and severely depressed (23+) have been previously recommended by the original authors based on validity studies. Among medically ill patient groups, physical symptoms common to depression become problematic when interpreting BDI scores. Among patients with renal failure, for example, a cut-off of 15 best discriminates clinically depressed patients from the non-depressed, although only 40% of individuals scoring above the cut-off of 15 will, in fact, be clinically depressed on subsequent full psychiatric interview. This is because of the presence of common confounding somatic symptoms including fatigue, anorexia, and sleep and bowel dysfunction that result from problems such as elevated blood urea nitrogen levels, acidemia, electrolyte imbalances, and problems with calcium metabolism. The BDI is mostly used to monitor change in the severity of depressive symptoms over time in individuals receiving treatment for depression or who are taking part in research studies of depression.

14. What about one to measure anxiety?

The State Trait Anxiety Inventory is the most widely used and well validated self-report measure of the symptoms of anxiety. It has 20 questions that measure state (i.e., situation-specific) anxiety and 20 that measure trait (i.e., those resulting from enduring personality style) anxiety. The test is simple to administer and score and takes only 10 minutes to complete. The State scale has been widely used in the assessment of current anxiety in general population, psychiatric, and medical settings. As expected, both have good internal reliability and the State scale has lower reported test-retest reliability (0.16 to 0.62) than the Trait scale (0.65–0.82). The State scale correlates well with other similar anxiety measures and is a responsive measure of treatment outcome in clinical trials involving psychotropic drugs, medical procedures, and psychotherapy. Evaluation of potentially confounding somatic State Trait Anxiety Inventory items has yet to be carried out in suitable medical settings.

15. What are the practical uses of the normative data provided for psychiatric and personality tests?

Normative data can be very useful in interpreting individual or group scores because they provide yardsticks against which the clinical or other significance of a given individual or group score can be judged. They are typically presented as mean test scores for selected groups along with the variability of these scores (the standard deviation) and are to be found in test manuals and research papers. Norms may be available for a wide range of groups and the test user must select the most appropriate. Medically- or psychiatrically-ill groups, general population groups, or groups based on specific demographic factors (such as age or sex) are typically provided. To compare the score of an individual with others, it is often useful to transform individual scores to "standard or Z scores" recalculated in standard deviation units. Individuals scoring at the group mean are then converted to a score of 0 and those scoring above or below one standard deviation from the mean converted to a score of 1 and –1 respectively. This is handy because it is expected that 68% of people will always fall within one standard deviation of the mean. For example, if an individual scores 76 on a test and the comparison group has a mean score of 65 and a standard deviation of 8, the individual's new Z score will be 1.4 (i.e., his or her score is 1.4 standard deviations above the group mean). Because some people prefer not to work with negative numbers, the Z-scores are often converted to T-scores so that all values are positive. With T-scores, the group mean and standard deviation are reset to some other, more convenient value, although the relative value of any individual's score is unchanged. For example, in intelligence testing, T-score means and standard deviations are commonly reset from 0 to 1 to 100 and 15, respectively, and in personality testing they are reset to 50 and 10.

16. How is human personality broadly conceptualized today? How can such personality dimensions be measured by questionnaire?

Although this is a complex area with a long history of debate among competing schools of thought about the nature of personality, a broad general acceptance now exists that the recently developed "Five-Factor Model" of personality provides the most comprehensive and accepted global description of human personality available. The model suggests that personality can be best described in general terms by five concepts (with aspect of personality involved in parentheses): (1) neuroticism (emotional), (2) extroversion (interpersonal), (3) openness to experience (experiential), (4) agreeability (attitudinal), and (5) conscientiousness (motivational).

17. What is the Five-Factor Model?

It has been a major recent advance in the field of personality assessment that has begun to help integrate widely varying (and historically conflicting) schools of thought on the nature of personality (e.g., behaviorism, humanism, social learning, cognitive-developmental, and psychoanalysis) and has formed a conceptual basis for organizing the wide array of currently available personality tests. Critics of the Five-Factor Model have noted that some important concepts (such as impulsivity) are not included and that it is essentially atheoretical and descriptive, rather than explanatory. The Five-Factor Model is important in that it promises to provide a broad conceptual framework for the several hundred specific personality factors that have been described to date.

The Five-Factor Model has been mostly closely associated with the 60-item NEO Personality Inventory in general population studies. It is being more widely applied in psychiatry to provide a broad dimensional assessment of personality and to complement the familiar "case/non-case" categorical or diagnostic approach typically used for personality disorders. It also has application in behavioral medicine and industrial psychology.

18. Do others exist?

A wide range of specific personality measures are available to assess more finely grained concepts of personality than those measured in the Five-Factor Model. The more common of these include: the Eysenck Personality Questionnaire, the 16PF, the California Personality Inventory, and the Minnesota Multiphasic Personality Inventory. Typically, such personality measures are used to help generate useful clinical hypotheses, but are not generally good diagnostic tools for psychiatric problems. Patient profiles are commonly generated from test scores and the overall profile pattern is often interpreted rather than simply looking at individual subscale scores. For example, many clinically useful profiles have been suggested using the Minnesota Multiphasic

Personality Inventory subscales and literally thousands of studies have been carried out involving this test and its applications.

19. What are good questionnaires to use in evaluating eating disorders?

Two measures of the symptoms of anorexia nervosa and bulimia nervosa are available to screen for clinical and subclinical eating disorders, to describe fully if eating disorder symptoms are present, and to detect change in symptom status over time. They are also widely used in research to improve understanding of the nature and treatment of eating disorders. The two recommended measures are the Eating Disorder Inventory–2 (EDI–2) and the Bulimia Test–Revised (BULIT–Revised). These are *not* diagnostic measures but are principally useful adjuncts to clinical assessments and decision making:

The EDI–2's 91 questions assess a wide range of behaviors, feelings, and symptoms found in eating disorders. It has three core clinical subscales related to eating and weight and shape concerns and eight more that provide information on general problems often present with eating disorders. The Drive for Thinness, Bulimia, and Body Dissatisfaction subscales are the most important clinically. The Drive for Thinness subscale has been applied with a cut-off score of 14 to identify any potential eating disturbance. The scores for all 11 subscales are presented as individual patient profiles and the overall pattern compared with normative profiles provided in the EDI–2 manual. The EDI–2 subscales are:

Core clinical subscales

1. *Drive for thinness*—excessive fear of weight gain, preoccupation with weight and dieting
2. *Bulimia*—frequent bouts of uncontrollable eating binges and thoughts about binges
3. *Body dissatisfaction*—about body size and shape

General subscales

1. *Ineffectiveness*—feelings of insecurity, worthlessness, and inadequacy
2. *Perfectionism*—high expectations for personal performance and achievement
3. *Interpersonal distrust*—feelings of alienation, avoidance of close relationships
4. *Lack of interoceptive awareness*—inability to identify accurately one's own emotional states and bodily sensations related to eating and hunger
5. *Maturity fears*—desire to retreat or regress to the relative safety and security of childhood
6. *Asceticism*—belief in the virtue of self-discipline, control of bodily urges, and self-denial
7. *Lack of impulse regulation*—a tendency toward impulsivity, self-destructive behavior, and recklessness
8. *Social insecurity*—perceptions of self-doubt and insecurity in social relationships

20. How is the EDI-2 used?

Typically a patient profile is compared with those given for available norms to clarify the nature and severity of the problems. The EDI-2 can be most helpful in providing information to understand the patient, planning treatment, and assessing progress.

21. Compared to the EDI-2, what is the function of the BULIT–Revised?

The BULIT–Revised was designed to screen for bulimia nervosa and to monitor changes in related bulimic symptom severity over time. It is composed of 28 core questions with 8 others used for descriptive purposes but not scored. The BULIT–Revised test includes questions on the nature and frequency of binge eating, loss of control during binges, use of purging behaviors, and dissatisfaction with bodily shape. The internal reliability of the BULIT–Revised is high and has been found to correlate well with related measures. As a community screening measure, Welch and colleagues showed that a cut-off score of 98 was optimal for use among young women (i.e., clinically important bulimia nervosa cases should not be missed using this cut-off score), although many false-positive cases will be included (around 30%) because of technical problems related to the low base rate of bulimia nervosa among females in community samples (i.e., around 2 to 3% prevalence). This problem also relates to tests used to screen for anorexia nervosa. These measures can, however, be very useful in reducing the subsequent interviewing workload where community studies are involved. Also, in the clinical setting individual BULIT–Revised questions and the total score can help in assessment and in monitoring response to treatment.

22. What tests are good options for measuring general psychiatric distress or probable psychiatric caseness by questionnaire?

Two useful tools are the General Health Questionnaire, which is designed for research use in community and non-psychiatric settings, and the Symptom Check List–90, designed for use in psychiatric and medical populations. The General Health Questionnaire comes in short, intermediate, and long versions; the intermediate 30-question version is probably the most commonly used. Its principal use is in identifying probable nonpsychotic psychiatric illness. The General Health Questionnaire is simple to use and score, although it should be cautioned that long-standing patient problems may be missed, because the test asks how the patient feels relative to "usual." The test manual recommends two additional questions that can be added to adjust for this problem ("use of psychiatric drugs" and "history of nervous problems"). The General Health Questionnaire has been found to correlate highly with similar screening measures and the 30-question version is found to have an overall sensitivity of 74% and a specificity of 82% based on a recent review of validity studies to date. Patients with physical health problems may score higher because of the presence of somatic anxiety symptoms in the test.

The other is the Symptom Check List–90, which assesses non-psychotic psychiatric symptoms in nine different symptom areas (somatization, obsessive-compulsion, paranoid ideation, psychoticism, phobic anxiety, depression, anxiety, interpersonal sensitivity, and hostility) and offers a global score related to the intensity of perceived psychological distress and the number of psychological symptoms (Global Severity Index). The nine Symptoms Check List–90 subscales generally have good internal and test-retest reliability, and the Global Severity Index has been found to correlate well with similar measures and have good responsiveness to detect changes in psychological distress. A standardized (T-score) cut-off score of 63 has been suggested for the Global Severity Index to detect probable psychiatric illness. Norms for the General Health Questionnaire and Symptom Check List–90 are available for a range of medical, psychiatric, and general population groups.

23. Are there computer programs available to help score and interpret some of the current psychological tests mentioned here?

Yes, this is a burgeoning field with many new programs coming onto the market each year. Stoloff and Couch provide a recent listing of useful, currently available computer programs to help score and interpret commonly used tests.[7] The measures covered include the BDI, the Spielberger State-Trait Anxiety Inventory, the 16PF, the Minnesota Personality Inventory, and the California Personality Inventory mentioned above.

24. The phrase "quality of life" pops up everywhere. What is it? What measures can be used to assess it?

Health-related quality of life is a complex, patient-centered and dynamic description of the changes in patient functioning and well-being over time, which are related to the patient's illness, treatment, and complications. A general consensus now exists that in its fullest sense, the phrase quality of life encompasses four distinct areas that cover the patient's total experience of illness: (1) physical health and symptoms, (2) functional status and activities of daily living, (3) mental well-being (including existential and spiritual aspects of living), and (4) social health, including social role functioning and social support. This may include the patient's relationship to the medical team and hospital environment.

Quality-of-life measures can be used to compare individual patient profiles with those of a similar patient group or to compare quality of life across different patient groups. These are commonly termed "generic" and include the SF-36, the Sickness Impact Profile, and the Nottingham Health Profile. Another measure of quality of life is the disease-specific. These are tailored to the specific issues of a given illness and can provide greater sensitivity to detect subtle changes in quality of life than more generic measures. Selection of the appropriate generic or specific measures depends on the goal of the specific research or clinical issue.

A consensus exists that patient-focused self-reporting is the preferred mode of assessment of the subjective aspects of quality of life such as psychological and social functioning, not only because self-reporting measures are inexpensive and easy to administer, but also because patient evaluations of quality of life provide the most important information in assessing the patient's perspective on the patient's quality of life. Some potential applications of quality of life measurement include:

1. Screening and monitoring for psychosocial problems in individual patient care
2. Population surveys of perceived health problems for medical audit
3. Outcome measures for use in health services or evaluation research
4. Outcome measures in clinical trials
5. Cost/utility analyses

BIBLIOGRAPHY

1. Bowling A: Measuring Health: A Review of Quality of Life Measurement Scales. Philadelphia, Open University Press, 1991.
2. Costa PT, McCrae RR: The NEO Personality Inventory (Manual). Odessa, FL, Psychological Assessment Resources, 1985.
3. Deyo R, Kiehr P, Patrick DL: Reproducibility and responsiveness of health status measures: Statistics and strategies for evaluation. Controlled Clinical Trials 12:142s–158s, 1991.
4. Garner DM: Eating Disorder Inventory–2 Professional Manual. Odessa, FL, Psychological Assessment Resources, 1991.
5. Patrick D, Deyo R: Generic and disease-specific measures in assessing health status and quality of life. Med Care 27:S217–S232, 1989.
6. Proceedings of the International Conference on the Measurement of Quality of Life as an Outcome in Clinical Trials. Controlled Clinical Trials 12:243s–256s, 1991.
7. Stoloff M, Couch J: Computer Use in Psychology: A Directory of Software, 3rd ed. Washington, DC, American Psychological Association, 1992.
8. Streiner D, Norman GR: Health Measurement Scales: A Practical Guide to Their Development and Use. Oxford, Oxford University Press, 1989.
9. Thelen M, Farmer J, Wonderlich S, Smith M: A revision of the bulimia test—the BULIT–R. Psychological Assessment 3:119–124, 1987.
10. Thompson C: The Instruments of Psychiatric Research. Chichester, 1989.
11. Welch GW, Thompson L, Hall A: The BULIT–R: Its reliability and clinical validity as a screening tool for DSM–III R bulimia nervosa in a female tertiary education population. Int J Eating Dis 14:95–105, 1993.

8. STANDARDIZED PSYCHIATRIC INTERVIEWS

Jacqueline A. Samson, Ph.D

1. When should I use a standardized interview?

Standardized interviews are necessary when collecting data for research or for comparing your own patients with those reported in the psychiatric literature. In addition, a standardized interview may be desirable in everyday clinical practice, because it provides a systematic means of evaluating patients that is less subject to bias or incomplete assessment. In clinical practice, it is easy to spend a great deal of time discussing the problems volunteered by the patient and to fail to ask about other problems that are less apparent but no less important clinically. This is particularly true of symptoms that may be embarrassing to the patient or perceived by the patient as socially unacceptable. Problems with alcohol or drug abuse, sexual compulsions, or symptoms related to trauma are often missed or misdiagnosed for this reason. Learning a standardized interview is a valuable training device, because it enhances understanding of specific syndromes and helps to develop an understanding of the questions most useful in eliciting psychiatric information.

2. How is a standardized interview different from a clinical interview?

In a standardized clinical interview, specific guidelines define the areas of questioning to be covered and the kind of information to be elicited from a patient. The interviewer is expected to cover all of the areas included in the guidelines and to ask for a sufficient amount of detail to complete ratings in each area. The format of the interview is also specified to ensure that the interview is conducted in a comparable fashion by all clinicians both within and across institutions.

3. What is the difference between a fully structured and a semistructured interview format?

A fully structured interview specifies the wording to be used for questions and the order in which they are to be asked. The format is defined and must not be altered by the interviewer in any way. In a semistructured interview, the wording and ordering of questions are specified but may be modified by the interviewer to suit the needs of a particular patient, as long as all areas are covered in the interview. Fully structured interviews provide a high degree of consistency from one interview to another and have been used extensively in epidemiologic studies that involve many raters. Semistructured interviews are less standardized but allow for clarifications and probes that can improve the validity of responses from atypical or severely impaired patients.

4. What kinds of standardized interviews are available?

The two most common types of standardized interviews are interviews to assess psychiatric diagnosis (diagnostic interviews) and interviews to assess the severity of certain types of symptoms at a specific point in time (cross-sectional symptom severity rating scales).

5. What are the most commonly used fully structured diagnostic interviews?

The most commonly used fully structured diagnostic interview is the Diagnostic Interview Schedule (DIS). The DIS was developed for use in large scale epidemiologic surveys15 and is designed for administration by specially trained nonclinicians. The DIS instrument is structured to obtain both lifetime and current diagnoses (within the last year). Questions are organized by symptoms, and patients are asked (1) whether the symptom has ever occurred in their lifetime, and (2) whether the symptom occurred within the last 1-month, 6-month, or 12-month period.

Probes are included for each symptom to determine whether alcohol or drugs were involved, whether the patient sought treatment, and whether there was impairment in occupational or social functioning. Symptoms are coded as present if they are independent of alcohol or drug use and resulted in either treatment or impairment of functioning. Diagnoses are assigned by computer on the basis of algorithms applied to coded interview data.

A modified version of the DIS, called the Composite International Diagnostic Interview (CIDI), was created by the World Health Organization in 1990 to allow for assignment of diagnoses according to the International Classification of Diseases (ICD-10).

Summary of Diagnostic Interviews

INTERVIEW	ACRONYM	DIAGNOSTIC SYSTEM	FORMAT	TYPE OF INTERVIEWER
Schedule for Affective Disorders and Schizophrenia	SADS	Research diagnostic criteria (RDC)	Semistructured	Clinician
Diagnostic Interview Schedule	DIS	DSM–III	Fully structured	Lay person
Structured Clinical Interview for DSM Diagnosis	SCID	DSM–III–R, DSM–IV	Semistructured	Clinician
Composite International Diagnostic Interview	CIDI	DSM–III–R, ICD-10	Fully structured	Lay person

6. What are the most commonly used semistructured diagnostic interviews?

The Schedule for Affective Disorders and Schizophrenia (SADS) interview was developed by Endicott and Spitzer as part of the study sponsored by the National Institute of Mental Health (NIMH) on the psychobiology of depression. The schedule contains 82 scales to assess symptoms of depression, mania, psychosis, and anxiety. Multiple questions are provided for each rating scale, and the interviewer may select from among these questions the phrasings that work best with a particular patient. Supplementary information based on observation, clinical report, or chart review may be incorporated into interview ratings. At the completion of the interview, specific inclusion and exclusion criteria are applied to the symptom ratings and diagnoses are assigned by the rater. The SADS has two parts. Part I documents the symptoms associated with the current episode. Part II documents symptoms during previous episodes of illness. A diagnostic system called the Research Diagnostic Criteria (RDC) was developed for use with the SADS questions. The RDC system and SADS interview were developed before the DSM–III systems (in fact, the DSM–III systems were modeled to a degree on the RDC) but are easily modified to obtain DSM–III or DSM–IV diagnoses.

More recently, Spitzer et al. created the Structured Clinical Interview for DSM–III–R Diagnosis (SCID). Unlike the SADS (which was created for more comprehensive research use), the SCID was specifically developed to obtain an accurate psychiatric diagnosis relatively quickly. Thus, certain questions may be skipped as soon as it becomes apparent that the patient will not meet the necessary diagnostic criteria. Symptoms are scored as absent, present, or subthreshold. Unlike the SADS, current and past diagnoses are assessed in the same interview. This strategy may be modified for patients who have difficulty shifting mental set from present to past and back to present. The questions given in each section follow the diagnostic criteria outlined in DSM–III–R; at the conclusion of each module, it is noted whether or not the patient meets full diagnostic criteria. Versions of the SCID are available with questions worded so as to assume that the patient is currently symptomatic (patient version) and with questions worded with no assumption of present or past patient status (nonpatient version).

7. How do various interviews accommodate the diagnostic changes found in DSM–IV?
Whenever there is a change in the standard system of diagnoses, all of the tools and methodologies for assignment of diagnoses must be updated. Currently, the various interviews are being revised and field-tested for DSM–IV. Although changes in standard systems of diagnoses have the benefit of updating clinical methods to reflect state-of-the-art knowledge about psychopathology, they also create difficulties for researchers in long-term studies and make it difficult to compare results across studies collected at different points in time with different diagnostic systems. Thus, many researchers continue to use the interviews in the original form in order to maintain consistency of data collection over time and across studies.

8. How long does it take to complete the diagnostic interview?
The duration of the interview depends on the amount of psychopathology presented by the patient and the ability of the patient to give a concise history. A completed interview with a good informant who shows a moderate amount of psychopathology (for example, a current episode of major depression, dysthymic disorder and a past episode of panic disorder) requires about $1\frac{1}{2}$ hours.

9. What if the psychiatrist does not have the time to administer the assessment? Do any questionnaires that the patient can fill out provide the same information?
At present there are no widely used self-report questionnaires for assessing psychiatric diagnosis. Valid diagnostic assessment requires a clinician who can interpret signs and symptoms against a standard and consider all the symptoms reported in assigning a differential diagnosis. However, some success has been reported by researchers who created an interactive computer program to assign a diagnosis based on the fully structured method used in the DIS.

In contrast, a wide variety of self-reported questionnaires are available to assess symptom severity. Some of these questionnaires are general and cover a wide variety of symptoms, whereas others are more specifically focused on one symptom dimension, such as depression.

Cross-Sectional Assessments

RATING METHOD	SYMPTOMS (CROSS-SECTIONAL)			FUNCTIONING
	Depression	*Anxiety*	*General*	
Interview	Hamilton Depression Rating Scale	Hamilton Anxiety Rating Scale	Brief Psychiatric Rating Scale (BPRS)	Global Assessment of Functioning (GAF)
	Inventory for Depressive Symptomatology (IDS)			Clinical Global Impression Scale (CGI)
	Montgomery-Asberg Scale			
	Raskin Scale			
Self-report	Beck Depression Inventory	Beck Anxiety Inventory	Symptom Checklist-90 (SCL-90)	Social Adjustment Scale (SAS)
	Inventory for Depressive Symptomatology (IDS-SR)	State-Trait Anxiety Inventory	Profile of Mood States (POMS)	
	Zung Inventory			

10. When should the examiner use a symptom severity rating scale instead of a diagnostic interview?
Symptom severity rating scales are designed to measure the severity of specific symptoms at a particular point in time. They are used to measure symptom severity once a diagnosis has already been made. Typically, symptom assessments are repeated to monitor response to treatment. For

example, to monitor response to an antidepressant drug, a psychiatrist may administer a Hamilton Depression Rating Scale (HDRS), which measures the severity of depressive symptoms, before starting the drug, and then repeat the assessment each time the patient comes in. The initial score is compared with the follow-up scores to determine whether there is a significant improvement in symptoms over time.

11. Assessments of symptoms do not tell me whether or not a person is functioning in the community. Are there any measures to monitor improvement in actual functioning?
Yes. Several simple scoring systems are widely used by clinicians to document functioning. The Global Assessment of Functioning Scale, published by the American Psychiatric Association in 1994, provides descriptions of possible levels of functioning along a continuum ranging from functioning in all areas to persistent inability to maintain personal hygiene. The Clinical Global Impression Scale (CGI), included in the manual of Guy in 1976, asks the clinician to rate the overall severity of the illness compared with all other psychiatric patients. The CGI ratings range from normal, not at all ill (a score of 1) to the most extremely ill patients. In addition, a number of self-reported questionnaires ask patients to assess their own functioning across a number of social roles. The Social Adjustment Scale, developed by Weissman and Bothwell in 1976, has been widely used for this purpose and has published norms for scoring available. One drawback with self-reported instruments is that questions are usually based on the patient's experience of satisfaction with their role performance. Thus, ratings do not directly assess actual functioning against an external standard.

Global Assessment of Functioning (GAF) Scale

Consider psychological, social, and occupational functioning on a hypothetical continuum of mental health–illness. Do not include impairment in functioning due to physical (or environmental) limitations.

Code (**Note:** Use intermediate codes when appropriate, e.g., 45, 68, 72.)

100   **Superior functioning in a wide range of activities, life's problems never seem to get out of hand, is sought out by others because of his or her many positive qualities.**
91   **No symptoms.**

90   **Absent or minimal symptoms** (e.g., mild anxiety before an exam), **good functioning in all areas, interested and involved in a wide range of activities, socially effective, generally satisfied with life, no more than everyday problems or concerns** (e.g., an occasional argument
81   with family members.)

80   **If symptoms are present, they are transient and expectable reactions to psychosocial stressors** (e.g., difficulty concentrating after family argument); **no more than slight impairment in
71   social, occupational, or school functioning** (e.g., temporarily falling behind in schoolwork).

70   **Some mild symptoms** (e.g., depressed mood and mild insomnia) **OR some difficulty in social, occupational, or school functioning** (e.g., occasional truancy, or theft within the household),
61   **but generally functioning pretty well, has some meaningful interpersonal relationships.**

60   **Moderate symptoms** (e.g., flat affect and circumstantial speech, occasional panic attacks) **OR moderate difficulty in social, occupational, or school functioning** (e.g., few friends, conflicts
51   with peers or co-workers).

50   **Serious symptoms** (e.g., suicidal ideation, severe obsessional rituals, frequent shoplifting) **OR any serious impairment in social, occupational, or school functioning** (e.g., no friends,
41   unable to keep a job).

40   **Some impairment in reality testing or communication** (e.g., speech is at times illogical, obscure, or irrelevant) **OR major impairment in several areas, such as work or school, family relations, judgment, thinking, or mood** (e.g., depressed man avoids friends, neglects family, and is unable
31   to work; child frequently beats up younger children, is defiant at home, and is failing at school).

Table continued on following page.

Global Assessment of Functioning (GAF) Scale (Cont.)

30 **Behavior is considerably influenced by delusions or hallucinations OR serious impairment in communication or judgment** (e.g., sometimes incoherent, acts grossly inappropriately, suicidal preoccupation) **OR inability to function in almost all areas** (e.g., stays in bed
21 all day; no job, home, or friends).

20 **Some danger of hurting self or others** (e.g., suicide attempts without clear expectation of death; frequently violent; manic excitement) **OR occasionally fails to maintain minimal personal hygiene** (e.g., smears feces) **OR gross impairment in communication** (e.g., largely in-
11 coherent or mute).

10 **Persistent danger of severely hurting self or others** (e.g., recurrent violence) **OR persistent inability to maintain minimal personal hygiene OR serious suicidal act with clear expecta-
1 tion of death.**

0 Inadequate information.

The rating of overall psychological functioning on a scale of 0–100 was operationalized by Luborsky in the Health-Sickness Rating Scale (Luborsky L: Clinicians' judgments of mental health. Arch Gen Psychiatry 7:407–417, 1962). Spitzer and colleagues developed a revision of the Health-Sickness Rating Scale called the Global Assessment Scale (GAS) (Endicott J, Spitzer RL, Fleiss JL, Cohen J: The global assessment scale: A procedure for measuring overall severity of psychiatric disturbance. Arch Gen Psychiatry 33:766–771, 1976). A modified version of the GAS was included in DSM–III–R as the Global Assessment of Functioning (GAF) Scale.

BIBLIOGRAPHY

1. American Psychiatric Association: Diagnostic and Statistical Manual of Mental Disorders–III. Washington, DC, American Psychiatric Association, 1980.
2. American Psychiatric Association: Diagnostic and Statistical Manual of Mental Disorders–III-R. Washington, DC, American Psychiatric Association, 1987.
3. American Psychiatric Association: Diagnostic and Statistical Manual of Mental Disorders–IV. Washington, DC, American Psychiatric Association, 1994.
4. Beck AT, Brown G, Epstein N, Steer RA: An inventory for measuring clinical anxiety: Psychometric properties. J Consult Clin Psychol 55:893–897, 1988.
5. Beck AT, Ward CH, Mendelson M, et al: An inventory for measuring depression. Arch Gen Psychiatry 4:561–571, 1961.
6. Derogatis LR: SCL-90-R Administration, Scoring and Procedures Manual—II. for the Revised Version. Towson, MD, Clinical Psychometric Research, 1983.
7. Endicott J, Spitzer RL: A diagnostic interview. The Schedule for Affective Disorders and Schizophrenia. Arch Gen Psychiatry 35:837–844, 1978.
8. Guy W: ECDEU Assessment Manual for Psychopharmacology, Revised, 1976. Rockville, MD, DHEW Publication No. (ADM) 76-338, 1976, pp 217–222.
9. Hamilton M: The assessment of anxiety states by rating. Br J Med Psychol 32:50–55, 1959.
10. Hamilton M: The development of a rating scale for primary depressive illness. Br J Soc Clin Psychol 6:278–296, 1967.
11. Lipman RS: Differentiating anxiety and depression in anxiety disorders: Use of rating scales. [description of Raskin and Covi scales]. Psychopharm Bull 18:69–105, 1982.
12. McNair DM, Lorr M, Droppleman LF: Manual for the Profile of Mood States. San Diego, Educational and Industrial Testing Service, 1971.
13. Montgomery SA, Asberg ML: A new depression scale designed to be sensitive to change. Br J Psychiatry 134:382–389, 1979.
14. Overall JE, Gorham DR: The Brief Psychiatric Rating Scale. Psychol Rep 10:799–812, 1962.
15. Robins LN, Helzer JE, Croughan JL, Ratcliff KS: National Institute of Mental Health Diagnostic Interview Schedule: Its history, characteristics and validity. Arch Gen Psychiatry 38:381–389, 1981.
16. Robins LN, Wing J, Wittchen H-U, Helzer JE: The Composite International Diagnostic Interview: An epidemiologic instrument suitable for use in conjunction with different diagnostic systems and in different cultures. Arch Gen Psychiatry 45:1069–1077, 1988.
17. Rush AJ, Giles DE, Schlesser MA, et al: The Inventory for Depressive Symptomatology (IDS): Preliminary findings. Psychiatry Res 18:65–87, 1986.

18. Spielberger CD: Manual for the State-Trait Anxiety Inventory. Palo Alto, CA, Consulting Psychologists Press, 1983.
19. Spitzer RL, Endicott J, Robins E: Research diagnostic criteria. Rationale and reliability. Arch Gen Psychiatry 35:773–782, 1978.
20. Spitzer RL, Williams JBW, Gibbon M, First MB: The structured clinical interview for DSM-III-R (SCID). I: History, rationale and description. Arch Gen Psychiatry 49:624–629, 1992.
21. Weissman MM, Bothwell S: Assessment of social adjustment by patient self-report. Arch Gen Psychiatry 33:1111–1115, 1976.
22. Williams JBW, Gibbon M, First MB, et al: The structured clinical interview for DSM-III-R (SCID). II: Multisite test-retest reliability. Arch Gen Psychiatry 49:630–636, 1992.
23. Wittchen H-U, Robins LN, Cottler LB, et al, and Participants in the Multicentre WHO/ADAMHA Field Trials: Cross-cultural feasibility, reliability and sources of variance in the Composite International Diagnostic Interview (CIDI). Br J Psychiatry 159:645–653, 1991.
24. World Health Organization: Composite International Diagnostic Interview (CIDI). Version 1.0. Geneva, World Health Organization, 1990.
25. Zung WWK: A self-rating depression scale. Arch Gen Psychiatry 12:63–70, 1965.

9. BRAIN IMAGING AND EEG IN PSYCHIATRY

Russell G. Vasile, M.D.

1. What brain imaging techniques are commonly employed in the clinical practice of adult psychiatry?

Important Features of Brain Imaging Modalities

BRAIN IMAGING TECHNIQUE	KEY FEATURES
Computerized tomography (CT)	Useful in the detection of intracranial mass lesions. Particular role in detection of intracranial calcification and skull fracture
Magnetic resonance imaging (MRI)	Coronal, sagittal, and transverse images facilitate detection of subtle lesions including tumors, strokes, and demyelinization. Lesions in the posterior fossa, mid-brain, basal ganglia and brainstem well visualized
Single photon emission computed tomography (SPECT)	Measures regional cerebral blood flow. Useful in the assessment of stroke and in discriminating Alzheimer's disease from multi-infarct dementia
Positron emission tomography (PET)*	Measures localized metabolic activity by measuring regional glucose utilization. A research tool with superior image resolution and data acquisition characteristics
Electroencephalography (EEG)	Key role in the assessment of seizure activity. Provides instantaneous measure of brain electrical activity. Computer-assisted methods facilitate topographic display of data (quantitative EEG, or brain electrical activity mapping, BEAM)

* Because metabolic rates and localized regional blood flow are closely linked in the brain in most circumstances, the results of PET and SPECT are often comparable.

2. What is the clinical role for brain imaging in the assessment of psychiatric patients?
Brain imaging studies are primarily used to exclude organic factors that could be contributing to psychiatric symptomatology. As such, they play a complementary role in the overall clinical assessment of psychiatric patients. Psychiatric symptoms including cognitive dysfunction, mood disturbance, and psychotic manifestations may be caused by occult organic disorders influencing brain function. Imaging studies can detect or exclude these factors.

Brain imaging studies help evaluate a broad range of neuropsychiatric disorders. The structural imaging techniques, CT and MRI, are of value in conditions that manifest tangible anatomic defects. They play an important role in the differential diagnosis of dementia and the detection of space-occupying lesions such as tumors, subdural hematomas, or brain tissue defects secondary to stroke. SPECT scanning can identify characteristic patterns of regional cerebral blood flow in multi-infarct and Alzheimer's dementia; in the early assessment of strokes and cerebrovascular defects, SPECT can provide evidence of defects in cerebrovascular perfusion before they are discernible by MRI or CT scanning. PET scans are far more expensive than SPECT studies and are far less available to clinicians. Although PET studies do not yet have significant clinical applicability, they show great promise as a research tool.

EEG, and quantitative EEG, which assess electrophysiologic activity by providing measures of the amount and location of different brain waveforms, can detect seizure disorders and also contribute to the assessment of dementia. Both these conditions exhibit characteristic patterns on EEG. Toxic states, including drug intoxication or metabolic encephalopathies, also exhibit characteristic patterns on EEG.

Brain Disorders Presenting with Psychiatric Symptoms and Imaging Techniques to Assist Diagnosis

---

Dementia
    MRI (structural assessment of atrophy)
    SPECT (blood flow patterns may identify Alzheimer's disease)
    EEG (characteristic increase in slow-wave activity in dementia)

Tumor
    MRI (anatomic assessment)
    SPECT (useful to assess tumor vascularization)
    EEG (may reveal focal slowing)

Stroke
    MRI and CT (useful after infarction)
    SPECT (may identify early ischemic changes before CT and MRI)
    EEG (identifies extent of functional disruption of electrophysiologic activity)

Parkinson's disease
    MRI (identifies characteristic defects in neuroanatomy)

Temporal lobe epilepsy
    EEG (characteristic abnormal spikes a key to diagnosis)
    SPECT (hyperfusion of seizure focus during seizure, hypoperfusion interictally)

Multiple sclerosis
    MRI (can reveal subtle neuroanatomic defects)

Huntington's disease
    MRI (subtle neuroanatomic defects demonstrable)

AIDS
    SPECT (emerging reports suggest SPECT abnormalities characterized by diffuse focal hypoperfusion)

Toxic metabolic conditions
    EEG (disruption in usual EEG coherence, excessive fast wave activity)

Head Trauma
    CT (excellent to assess bone fracture, and issues related to possible subarachnoid bleeds and other hemorrhagic events)
    MRI (superior resolution of subtle anatomic defects, but CT studies may be easier to obtain in urgent situations)

---

3. What are the most important indications for CT and MRI scanning in psychiatry?

The most important indications are structural lesions resulting from stroke, tumor, subdural hematoma, brain atrophy, or multi-infarct dementia.

There are several reasons to consider the evaluation of brain structures in psychiatric practice:

1. To confirm or rule out structural lesions which may be contributing to psychiatric symptoms. Such lesions require specific management and could possibly be reversible. Examples include subdural hematoma, tumor, or multiple sclerosis.

2. To assess psychiatric symptoms that could in part have a defined neuropathologic basis. For example, confusion in an elderly, depressed patient might be related to multi-infarct dementia, which could be demonstrated by a brain imaging study.

3. To rule out or confirm other diagnostic possibilities that could be contributing to a patient's psychiatric symptoms. For example, to exclude organic pathology in a patient suffering from a conversion disorder.

4. When is MRI better used?
MRI has largely supplanted CT in assessing brain structures. MRI affords significantly superior tissue resolution in which gray and white matter structures can be precisely imaged and differentiated. MRI affords visualization in coronal, sagittal, and transverse planes, and is not limited to the transverse plane as CT is. MRI studies have no radiation risk, making multiple studies feasible. MRI is superior to CT in the study of demyelinating diseases, such as multiple sclerosis. MRI is of particular value in assessing the basal ganglia and periventricular areas of the brain. The posterior fossa of the brain is well imaged by MRI, and is inaccessible to CT because of the presence of bony artifacts. MRI, therefore, affords visualization of the posterior fossa, temporal lobes, cerebellum and brain stem, all regions inaccessible to CT scans. T1-weighted studies afford excellent discrimination between gray-white matter structures, whereas T2-weighted studies afford detection of pathologic lesions in the white matter and basal ganglia secondary to tumors, small infarctions, or demyelinating diseases. MRI is superior to CT in the assessment of brain injury 48–72 hours following trauma, particularly in the evaluation of nonhemorrhagic intracranial injuries.

5. Besides lower cost, does CT have other advantages?
The major strength of CT is its ability to image bone, which is not well imaged by MRI. CT is also superior to MRI in detecting subarachnoid hemorrhage, bone fracture, and in differentiating acute parenchymal hemorrhage from edema. CT is superior to MRI in revealing calcifications and meningeal abnormalities, as well as certain hemorrhagic events. Evaluation is more logistically complex and slower in obtaining an MRI study, and many patients experience a claustrophobic reaction at being placed in the MRI apparatus.

6. What is functional MRI?
This technique uses MRI to measure changes in physiologic variables, including regional cerebral blood volume, and regional oxygen and glucose consumption, and it can be used in experiments involving activation paradigms that measure changes in blood volume in resting and activated states. Functional MRI is an increasingly used research tool, and it promises to play a role in clinical practice in the future.

7. Are there any MRI or CT findings that specifically characterize depression, mania or schizophrenia?
Neither MRI nor CT scanning can be said to demonstrate characteristic neuroanatomic abnormalities diagnostic of schizophrenia or affective illness.

CT scanning is of limited value in the assessment of patients with primary affective illness because of low resolution in the brain and bone artifact obscuring potentially important structures. Some studies found larger ventricles in patients with affective disorders compared with controls. Increased ventricular size was associated with psychotic symptoms, psychomotor retardation, and elevated urinary free-cortisol levels in the depressed patient populations studied.

MRI studies of patients with primary affective disorder have not yielded consistent results. MRI studies of relatively younger bipolar and elderly depressed patients have described "hyperintensities," which appear as bright white areas on MRI studies in the periventricular white matter of younger bipolar and elderly depressed patients. But subcortical hyperintensities have also been described in demented patients and have been associated with hypertension and vascular disease.

MRI research on schizophrenic patients has generated much data on subtle neuroanatomic abnormalities, particularly in ventricular and temporolimbic structures, but no consistent pathognomonic neuroanatomic abnormality can be said to have been demonstrated in schizophrenia.

8. What are the most significant indications for SPECT and PET scanning in psychiatry?
SPECT scanning is clinically useful in assessing regional cerebral blood flow in the acute stages after acute cerebral infarction and in assessing chronic ischemia and incipient infarction. SPECT

can assist in the differential diagnosis of dementia. Recent studies have suggested that Alzheimer's disease can be differentiated from multi-infarct dementia on the basis of the pattern of regional cerebral blood flow in these conditions. The perfusion defects in Alzheimer's disease are almost always bilateral, involve the association cortex, and are most severe in the posterior temporoparietal lobes. The hypoperfusion exhibited in the posterior temporoparietal lobes in Alzheimer's disease is often present in the early phases of the disease, with frontal lobe hypoperfusion a later manifestation. Multi-infarct dementia has a more patchy, diffuse pattern of hypoperfusion with widely scattered focal cerebral perfusion defects. SPECT also may play a role in the localization and assessment of epileptic seizure foci in patients with focal epilepsy. Postical SPECT has been used to identify unilateral temporal foci as regions of increased activity (e.g., increased regional cerebral blood flow) and can be used to confirm the epileptic focus in those patients who have reduced uptake in the same location on interictal SPECT.

SPECT is particularly useful in the acute assessment of blood flow to the brain and is commonly used in neurologic settings to assess stroke patterns. Acute changes in cerebral blood flow may not result in structural defects for several hours; hence structural changes following stroke may be evident only over time.

In focal seizure disorders SPECT images reveal a sharp increase in regional cerebral blood flow during the acute seizure; by contrast, interictally, the seizure focus is commonly hypoperfused relative to normal nonirritable tissue. This helps assess temporal lobe disorders and focal lesions giving rise to complex partial seizures. This use of SPECT may provide, in some circumstances, an alternative to the use of the more invasive depth electroencephalography.

Clinical Indications for SPECT

Differential diagnosis of dementia	Focal epilepsy
Alzheimer's disease versus	Identification of seizure focus
multi-infarct dementia	Brain tumor
Cerebrovascular disease	Assessment of blood supply of tumor
Assessment of infarction	tissue; necrosis of tumor tissue
versus ischemia	versus recurrence

9. How do PET and SPECT work?

Both PET and SPECT use computer-assisted techniques to reconstruct cross-sectional images of radiotracer distributions. A typical reconstruction resolution value for PET is in the range of 4–6 mm, whereas that of SPECT is 6 mm to 8 mm. The commonly used PET radionuclides are ^{15}O, ^{13}N, ^{11}C, and ^{18}F, which have short half-lives ranging from 2 minutes to 2 hours. The radiotracers utilized in SPECT imaging such as ^{99m}technetium have a half-life of 6 hours, whereas ^{123}I has a half-life of 13 hours. SPECT studies can be performed several hours after injection of the radiotracer. The half-life of the particular radionuclide employed in a study is important in that it has an impact on flexibility in study design. A longer half-life radionuclide facilitates studies of longer duration, affording more time for data acquisition as, for example, when utilizing a cognitive activation paradigm such as the Wisconsin Card Sort.

10. Are there any drawbacks to these devices?

The cost of a PET system, which requires a cyclotron for radioisotope production, is 1 to 3 million dollars; that of a SPECT system is 0.3 to 0.6 million dollars. The cost per study for a SPECT ranges from $500 to $1,000. PET studies cost between $1,500–$2,000.

11. Are there any SPECT or PET findings that can specifically characterize psychiatric disorders such as depression, mania, schizophrenia or anxiety disorders?

SPECT scans cannot currently be considered diagnostic of depressive disorders or mania. Several noteworthy SPECT studies have been published demonstrating specific regions of hypoperfusion in depressed patients which resolve upon successful treatment of depression. Most studies have implicated frontal and temporal brain regions as exhibiting hypoperfusion in acute depression, but other brain regions, such as the caudate nucleus, have been implicated as well; the literature does not reveal a consensus "gold standard" finding as yet.

Studies of schizophrenic patients have implicated the frontal lobes as regions of hypoperfusion, specifically in relation to activating tasks such as the Wisconsin Card Sort.

Increased frontal lobe blood flow in obsessive-compulsive disorder has been reported by several investigators, and in a few studies it has been demonstrated to revert to normal levels following treatment with serotonergic antidepressant agents.

PET studies of schizophrenia have generally reported lower metabolic rates in the frontal regions, particularly in response to cognitive tasks designed for frontal lobe activation. Hypofrontality appears to be associated with the negative symptoms of schizophrenia. Temporal lobe abnormalities have also been reported. PET research on obsessive-compulsive disorder has indicated an increase in frontal lobe and basal ganglia metabolism. Several PET studies of major depressive disorder have observed reduction in metabolic rate, particularly in the frontal lobes; this hypofrontality appears to be more marked in bipolar than unipolar patients and in some studies appears to be most prominent in the left lateral frontal region.

Future Applications of PET and SPECT

Neuroreceptor mapping
  Identification of neuroreceptor patterns in primary psychiatric disorders such as depression and schizophrenia

Identification of pathways of normal cerebral function
  Assess pathways of sensory function, including visual and auditory
  Identify sites of affective and cognitive function

Quantification of metabolism in specific brain regions in primary psychiatric disorders
  Analysis of subtypes of affective illness, bipolar versus unipolar depression
  Obsessive compulsive disorder
  Panic disorder

Increase understanding of medical disorders that contribute to psychiatric symptoms
  AIDS dementia
  Chronic fatigue syndrome
  Substance abuse (cocaine)

12. What is the role of EEG and quantitative EEG in psychiatry?

EEG affords a continuous measure of brain electrical activity with a chronologic resolution in milliseconds. Recent advances in computer software technology have given rise to computerized quantitative EEG techniques that provide a color-coded topographic display of EEG data, making it more accessible to visual interpretation. Quantitative EEG or brain electrical activity mapping (BEAM) studies use conventional, standard EEG but organize and display the data in a color-coded fashion that facilitates its visuospatial interpretation.

EEG data consist of the assessment of the amount and spatial location of various EEG frequencies ranging from fast activity (alpha) to slow-wave activity (delta). Additionally, EEG assesses discontinuities in electrical activity characterized by spike and wave formations consistent with seizure activity. Finally, evoked responses to auditory and visual stimulation can be assessed in relation to established norms for visual evoked responses (VER) and auditory evoked responses (AER). Patterns of the amount and location of the various EEG frequencies can be of diagnostic value. For example, an increased amount of topographically diffuse delta activity is commonly encountered in dementia. Drug-induced toxic states are associated with increased alpha activity. The diagnosis of seizure disorder may be established by the characteristic spike and wave formation demonstrated on the EEG. EEG provides instantaneous data and 24-hour EEG studies can now be obtained on an ambulatory basis to facilitate documentation of seizure activity and its correlation to behavioral phenomena.

EEG has been used to assess brain function in a range of settings including dementia, in which slow wave activity is prominent; toxic states, typically characterized by fast activity; and seizure disorders, noteworthy for spike and wave patterns characteristic of seizure activity.

EEG is of particular value in the assessment and differential diagnosis of cognitive dysfunction. Dementia is not uncommonly characterized by the presence of increased slow wave activity. The evaluation of unusual behavioral presentations, which may reflect an occult underlying seizure disorder, represents another potential role for EEG in clinical psychiatry. For example, a patient with marked obsession and quasi-philosophical preoccupations may be exhibiting behaviors consistent with the interictal personality features of patients with temporal lobe dysfunction. EEG could be a critical technique in the diagnostic assessment of such a disorder.

Currently, active research efforts are under way to describe patterns of EEG activity that might distinguish depression from the early stages of dementia. As yet, no definitive EEG characteristics exist which consistently discriminate these disorders.

13. How might brain imaging be used in assessing the patient with cognitive dysfunction?

Brain imaging studies could identify reversible causes of cognitive dysfunction, such as subdural hematoma or meningioma. EEG could be helpful in discriminating between toxic-metabolic states, which could contribute to cognitive dysfunction, and incipient dementia, which would have a different pattern of electrical activity on the EEG. SPECT scanning reveals a typical pattern of blood flow in Alzheimer's dementia and a different pattern in other dementias such as multi-infarct dementia. Transient ischemic disorders and cerebrovascular insufficiency could also be assessed by the SPECT modality.

14. How might brain imaging studies be useful in assessing a patient with depression?

A variety of conditions that cause apathy, lethargy, trouble concentrating, and sadness can be confused with primary depression. Indeed, the concept of "secondary" depression, or depression secondary to a discrete medical cause, is well established. Such secondary depressions could include certain post-stroke depressions, and depression secondary to Parkinson's disease, multiple sclerosis, or other neurologic conditions. Post-stroke depression is particularly common following left anterior frontal lobe infarctions, whether they are cortical or subcortical lesions. Additionally, the differential diagnosis between dementia and depression may be difficult to establish without the data available through brain imaging studies.

MRI and CT reveal structural defects in certain conditions such as stroke; EEG shows a typical pattern in dementia and seizure activity and may also show asymmetries following strokes. SPECT scans may confirm the diagnosis of stroke, dementia, or underlying seizure foci.

Imaging studies may be of particular value in the treatment of the refractory depressed patient or the depressed patient with atypical features in whom the possibility of an occult neuropathologic condition contributing to the depressive disorder should be seriously considered.

15. When might brain imaging studies be indicated for assessing a patient with psychosis?

Several organic conditions may result in psychotic symptoms that could be confused with schizophrenia. Occult frontal or temporal lobe tumor, unusual seizure disorders, or drug-induced psychosis may need to be ruled out in the assessment of psychotic conditions. MRI or CT can assess organic states such as frontal lobe tumors, subdural hematoma, or stroke that could result in unusual behavioral or psychotic manifestations. EEG will be of particular value in excluding toxic-metabolic conditions that could be contributing to psychotic symptoms. SPECT scanning can assess the possibility of cerebrovascular insufficiency as a contributory factor in altered mental status.

16. Which main areas in research in brain imaging could prove clinically relevant in the near future?

The major developments in brain imaging research involve the development of new ligands for specific receptor sites, enabling researchers to assess more precisely neuroreceptor function in specific psychiatric conditions and to evaluate change in receptor function following psychotropic medication treatment. Ligands are currently available through PET and SPECT to assess cholinergic, benzodiazepine, and dopaminergic receptors. Mapping receptor distribution and assessing interaction with pharmacologic probes are becoming increasingly feasible. Additionally, ongoing developments in software technology will increasingly facilitate the integration of anatomic and physiologic techniques through the coregistration of MRI and SPECT images. This will allow precise neuroanatomic superimposition of these different modalities, facilitating more exact localization of pathophysiologic dysfunction in brain disorders.

BIBLIOGRAPHY

1. Abou-Saleh MT (ed): Brain imaging in psychiatry. Br J Psychiatry 157(S9): 1990.
2. Andreasen NC (ed): Brain Imaging: Applications in Psychiatry. Washington, DC, American Psychiatric Press, 1989.
3. Belliveau JW, Kennedy DN Jr, McKinstry RC, et al: Functional mapping of the human visual cortex by magnetic resonance imaging. Science 254(5302):716–719, 1991.
4. Holman BL, Devous MD: Functional brain SPECT: The emergence of a powerful clinical method. J Nucl Med 33:1888–1904, 1992.
5. Holman BL, Johnson KA, Gerada B, Carvalho PA, Satlin A: The scintigraphic appearance of Alzheimer's disease: A prospective study using technetium 99m-HMPAO SPECT. J Nucl Med 33:181–185, 1992.
6. Hughes JR, Wilson WP (eds): EEG and Evoked Potentials in Psychiatry and Behavioral Neurology. Boston, Butterworth, 1983.
7. Gelenberg AJ (ed): Clinical applications of NeuroSPECT in psychiatry. J Clin Psychiatry 53(S):11, 1992.
8. Gelenberg AJ (ed): SPECT imaging in psychiatry: A new look at depression. J Clin Psychiatry 54(S):11, 1993.
9. Grafman J, Tamminga CA: Cortex, IV: Regional cerebral blood flow. Am J Psychiatry 152:163, 1995.
10. Hauser P (ed): Brain Imaging in Affective Disorders. Washington, DC, American Psychiatric Press, 1991.
11. Jeste DV, Lohr JB, Goodwin FK: Neuroanatomical studies of major affective disorders. A review and suggestions for further research. Br J Psychiatry 153:444–459, 1988.
12. Jolles PR, Chapman PR, Alavi A: PET, CT, and MRI in the evaluation of neuropsychiatric disorders: Current applications. J Nucl Med 30:1589–1606, 1989.
13. Maurer AH: Nuclear medicine: SPECT comparisons to PET. Radiol Clin North Am 26(5):1059–1074, 1988.
14. Morris P, Rapoport SI: Neuroimaging and affective disorder in late life: A review. Can J Psychiatry 35(4):347–354, 1990.
15. Oldham JM, Riba MB, Tasman A (eds): Brain imaging. In Review of Psychiatry. Washington, DC, American Psychiatric Association, 1993.

III. Principal Clinical Disorders and Problems

10. SCHIZOPHRENIA AND SCHIZOAFFECTIVE DISORDERS

Herbert T. Nagamoto, M.D.

1. Define schizophrenia.
Schizophrenia is a complex illness characterized by hallucinations, delusions, behavioral disturbances, disrupted social functioning, and associated symptoms in what is usually an otherwise clear sensorium.

2. What are the clinical features of schizophrenia?
Schizophrenia involves at least a 6-month period of continuous signs of the illness. Active symptoms may include:

1. **Delusions**, which are false beliefs that (1) persist despite what most people would accept as evidence to the contrary and (2) are not shared by others in the same culture or subculture.

2. **Hallucinations**, which are perceptions that appear to be real when no such stimulus is actually present. Hallucinations may involve any of the five normal senses, but in schizophrenia they are usually auditory.

3. **Disorganized speech**.

4. **Grossly disorganized or catatonic behavior**. Catatonia, a syndrome characterized by stupor with rigidity or flexibility of the musculature, may alternate with periods of overactivity.

5. **Negative symptoms**, such as (1) affective flattening or decreased emotional reactivity; (2) alogia or poverty of speech; (3) avolition or lack of purposeful action. Usually work performance, social relations, and self-care decrease below the highest previous levels.

Prodromal or residual phases may include social isolation or withdrawal, peculiar behavior, digressive overelaborate speech, odd beliefs such as ideas of reference (thinking that others' words, actions, or expressions are in reference to oneself when this is not the case) or magical thinking, unusual perceptual experiences, or marked lack of initiative, interests, or energy.

Age of onset is usually during adolescence or early adulthood. The course is highly variable but generally involves significant functional impairment.

Violent acts sometimes receive significant attention; no evidence indicates that they are more frequent among schizophrenic than in the general population.

Some schizophrenic patients have various **somatic complaints** as part of their illness, but they also may be medically ill and not complain or incorporate symptoms into their delusional system.

Life expectancy is reduced by death from suicide and other causes. Approximately 40% of schizophrenics attempt suicide at some point in their lifetime, and 15–20% succeed.

3. How common is schizophrenia?
The lifetime incidence of schizophrenia is approximately 1%. This figure is remarkably stable across racial, cultural, and national lines.

4. What medical conditions may induce psychosis and be mistaken for acute schizophrenia?
Psychosis, which is characterized by a disturbance in or loss of contact with reality, may include symptoms of schizophrenia, such as delusions, hallucinations, bizarre behavior, ideas of refer-

ence, paranoia (irrational suspiciousness or false beliefs of persecution), disorganized speech, and illogical thinking. A number of medical conditions may induce psychosis:
  1. Substance abuse and drug toxicity (see question 5)
  2. Space-occupying central nervous system lesions—tumor (especially limbic and pituitary), aneurysm, abscess
  3. Head trauma
  4. Infections—encephalitis, abscess, neurosyphilis
  5. Endocrine disease—thyroid, Cushing's, Addison's, pituitary, parathyroid
  6. Systemic lupus erythematosus and multiple sclerosis
  7. Cerebrovascular disease
  8. Huntington's disease
  9. Parkinson's disease
  10. Migraine headache and temporal arteritis
  11. Pellagra and pernicious anemia
  12. Porphyria
  13. Withdrawal states, including alcohol and benzodiazepines
  14. Delirium and dementia
  15. Sensory deprivation or overstimulation states can induce psychosis, such as psychosis included in the intensive care unit

  5. Which street drugs and prescription medications may induce psychosis?

Street drugs	Prescription drugs
Cocaine	Metronidazole and other antibiotics
Phencyclidine	Antidepressants
Lysergic acid diethyl-	L-dopa
amide (LSD)	Bromocriptine
Mescaline	Amantadine
Psilocybin	Ephedrine
Marijuana	Phenylpropanolamine
Morning glory seeds	Indomethacin and other nonsteroidal antiinflammatory agents
Alcohol	Cimetidine and other antihistamines
	Disulfiram
	Carbamazepine and other anticonvulsants
	Digoxin, propranolol, and other cardiac medications
	Thyroid hormones
	Various medications with strong anticholinergic effects

Routine urine toxicology screens usually monitor for only a limited number of substances.

  6. Which tests should a screening medical work-up of psychosis include?
  1. Complete blood count
  2. Serum electrolytes, glucose, blood urea nitrogen, creatinine, calcium, and phosphate
  3. Liver function tests
  4. Thyroid function tests
  5. VDRL or RPR, HIV antibody test in high-risk patients*
  6. Electrocardiogram
  7. Urinalysis and urine toxicology screen
  8. Chest x-ray
  9. Sleep-deprived EEG
  10. Head CT or MRI scan
  11. Blood levels of therapeutic medications, when appropriate
  12. Lumbar puncture, when appropriate
  * VDRL = Venereal Disease Research Laboratory test, RPR = rapid plasmin reagin test, and HIV = human immunodeficiency virus.

7. How is schizophrenia differentiated from manic-depressive illness and other psychiatric conditions?

The differential diagnosis of schizophrenia and other psychiatric conditions that may manifest psychotic symptoms is difficult and best done from a longitudinal perspective on the course of the illness. Such a differential is crucial, because effective treatments vary depending on the conditions. In **affective disorders** (manic depressive illness and major depression), the duration of psychotic symptoms is relatively brief in relation to the affective symptoms. **Schizophreniform disorder**, by definition, involves the symptoms of schizophrenia with a duration of less than 6 months. Patients with **obsessive-compulsive disorder** may have beliefs that border on delusions but generally recognize that their symptoms are at least somewhat irrational. **Brief reactive psychoses** may be seen in patients with borderline or other personality disorders as well as dissociative disorders. **Posttraumatic stress disorder** may involve visual, auditory, tactile, and olfactory hallucinations during flashbacks. Beliefs or experiences should not be considered delusional or psychotic if they are in the context of a person's religion or culture.

8. What causes schizophrenia?

This question thus far has eluded an answer. A number of factors, however, have been implicated in the pathogenesis of schizophrenia, which is often conceptualized as a group of disorders with common symptoms:

Brain structural studies have failed to find a pathognomonic lesion in schizophrenia but have consistently found a number of abnormalities. CT, MRI, and postmortem studies have shown decreased volume and density in limbic and frontal areas in schizophrenic patients. Some of these findings have been corroborated by changes in regional cerebral blood flow and positron emission tomographic (PET) studies.

Multiple neurochemical changes also have been implicated in schizophrenia. It has been long noted that an excess in dopaminergic activity in the central nervous system is central to the development of schizophrenic symptoms. Compelling data also implicate norepinephrine and serotinin systems. With the advent of clozapine, the prototypic atypical antipsychotic, it has been hypothesized that interactions between these systems may be crucial in the pathogenesis of schizophrenia.

Neurophysiological changes have been shown through various neuropsychologic and physiologic measures.

Schizophrenic patients have shown abnormal informational processing on such measures as the Continuous Performance Test. They also have shown abnormal sensory processing on such measures as skin conductance habituation, backward masking, smooth pursuit eye movements, prepulse inhibition of acoustic startle, and evoked potentials, such as P300, CNV, P1, and failure to decrement the P50 auditory response in a conditioning-testing paradigm.

Endocrine factors have long been suspected. Females tend to develop schizophrenia later and often have less severe symptoms than males. In males, the onset of schizophrenia is often during puberty. Changes in prolactin, melatonin, and thyroid function have been found in schizophrenia.

Viral and immune factors have also been implicated. Although the search for a causative virus in schizophrenia has thus far been unfruitful, various factors point to this possibility. For example, a number of immune changes have been found, including IgA, IgG, and IgM. Furthermore, a larger than expected number of schizophrenic patients are born in late winter and early spring, leading to the hypothesis that perinatal viral infections may be involved in causing schizophrenia.

Factors Implicated in the Etiology of Schizophrenia

1. Genetic factors (see question 9)	5. Endocrine factors
2. Brain structural changes	6. Viral and immune factors
3. Neurochemical changes	7. Psychosocial factors
4. Neurophysiological changes	

Psychosocial factors are no longer felt to be causative in schizophrenia but clearly play a role in the course of the illness.

9. What is the role of genetics in schizophrenia?

Genetic factors play a significant role but are not sufficient alone to account for the development of schizophrenia. Compelling data have come from family studies. In the general population, the lifetime risk of developing schizophrenia is approximately 1%. A child born with one schizophrenic parent has about a 14% chance of developing schizophrenia. This risk rises to approximately 25% if both parents are schizophrenic. Another approach has looked at siblings with varying degrees of genetic similarity. Nontwin siblings of a schizophrenic patient have about an 8% chance of developing schizophrenia. For nonidentical (dizygotic) twins, if one twin is schizophrenic, approximately 10% of the other twins develop schizophrenia. This risk, or concordance rate, rises to 40–50% in identical (monozygotic) twins. Although such data support a strong role for genetics in the etiology of schizophrenia, they also clearly show that other factors play a significant role in determining who does and does not develop schizophrenia.

10. What are the treatments for schizophrenia?

Antipsychotic or neuroleptic medications are the cornerstone of the treatment of schizophrenia (see chapter 48). Inpatient treatment in a therapeutic milieu may be crucial in early and acute phases of schizophrenia. Residential treatment settings, group homes, and day hospital programs may help patients to remain outside the hospital. Supportive individual and group psychotherapy may help patients to understand and come to terms with their illness and need for treatment, to identify factors that influence symptoms, and to develop strategies to deal more effectively with the illness. Family therapy sessions also may help families of schizophrenic patients to understand the illness and to help the patient. Families may have a negative impact if they are high in expressed emotion, hypercritical, or overtly hostile toward the patient. Schizophrenic patients often have extremely poor social skills. Social skills training has been shown to be highly effective in helping to improve quality of life. Vocational rehabilitation helps some stabilized patients to return to more productive roles in society.

11. What is schizoaffective disorder?

Schizoaffective disorder has been defined in numerous ways, but essentially it is an illness that combines symptoms of schizophrenia with a major affective disorder, i.e., major depression or manic-depressive illness.

12. How is schizoaffective disorder different from schizophrenia or manic-depressive illness?

In schizophrenia, the total duration of the affective syndrome has been brief relative to the total duration of psychotic disturbance. In manic-depressive illness, delusions and hallucinations primarily occur during periods of mood instability and do not occur longer than 2 weeks without prominent mood symptoms. Whereas some authors argue that schizophrenia and affective illnesses are separate biologic entities, others argue that they exist on a continuum, with schizoaffective disorders at their interface. It is important, however, to make as clear a diagnosis as possible, because the cornerstones of treatment for schizophrenia are neuroleptic medications, whereas mood stabilizers (lithium, carbamazepine, valproate) and antidepressants are crucial in treating affective disorders.

13. Does significant depression rule out schizophrenia?

Although the diagnosis of schizophrenia emphasizes that psychotic symptoms predominate over mood symptoms, schizophrenic patients may suffer significant depression, which strongly contributes to their increased suicide risk. Increased suicide risk may extend even after an episode of depression resolves and may result from the patient's inability to come to terms with the debilitating effects of schizophrenia. Pharmacologic treatment of depression in schizophrenia is somewhat controversial, because antidepressants apparently reduce the efficacy of antipsychotic medications in acutely ill schizophrenic patients. On the other hand, adjunctive antidepressant medications have been shown to be effective in the acute maintenance treatment of depression in schizophrenic and schizoaffective patients.

BIBLIOGRAPHY

1. American Psychiatric Association: Diagnostic and Statistical Manual of Mental Disorders, 4th ed. Washington, DC, American Psychiatric Association, 1994.
2. Braff DL: Information processing and attention dysfunctions in schizophrenia. Schizophr Bull 19:233–259, 1993.
3. DeLisi LE (ed): Depression in Schizophrenia. Washington, DC, American Psychiatric Press, 1990.
4. Freedman R, Waldo M, Bickford-Wimer P, Nagamoto H: Elementary neuronal dysfunctions in schizophrenia. Schizophr Res 4:233–243, 1991.
5. Kaplan HI, Sadock BJ (eds): Comprehensive Textbook of Psychiatry, 6th ed. Baltimore, Williams & Wilkins, 1995.
6. Marsh L, Suddath RL, Higgins N, Weinberger DR: Medial temporal lobe structures in schizophrenia: Relationship of size to duration of illness. Schizophr Res 11:225–238, 1994.
7. Siris SG, Bermanzohn PC, Mason SE, Shuwall MA: Maintenance imipramine therapy for secondary depression in schizophrenia: A controlled trial. Arch Gen Psychiatry 51:109–115, 1994.
8. Weinberger DR (ed): Schizophrenia. In Tasman A, Goldfinger SM (eds): American Psychiatric Press Review of Psychiatry, vol 10. Washington, DC, American Psychiatric Press, 1991, pp 5–136.

11. PARANOID DISORDERS

Theo C. Manschreck, M.D., M.P.H.

1. What are paranoid disorders?

The term paranoid disorders refers to a variety of conditions characterized by delusions and related behavior. One of the earliest described of these disorders was paranoia, now called delusional disorder, a set of conditions of unknown cause whose cardinal psychopathologic feature is the delusion. Paranoia is actually uncommon; other forms are seen frequently.

There are two broad categories of paranoid disorders:

Disorders with known causes (medical and substance disorders)

Idiopathic disorders

Delusional disorder

Paranoid personality disorder

Shared psychotic disorder

Atypical psychosis (psychotic disorders not otherwise specified)

Schizophrenia and schizophreniform disorder

Mood (psychotic forms of mania and depression) disorder

Schizoaffective disorder

2. What is the origin and meaning of the term paranoid?

The concept of paranoia has a long and confusing history in psychiatry. The Greeks used the term *paranoia* (meaning beside one's self) to designate a symptom that we would regard now as a nonspecific and general feature of many mental disorders. The term was not used for almost 2,000 years until it was revived by Karl Kahlbaum, who in 1863 identified a disorder he called paranoia. He described this condition as "a form of partial insanity, which, throughout the course of the disease, principally affected the sphere of the intellect." Emil Kraepelin, a contemporary of Kahlbaum, was influenced by these observations. He retained the concept of paranoia as a separate disorder in his groundbreaking classification of mental illnesses. In recent years *paranoid* has referred to a multitude of behaviors. Some mistakenly regard ordinary suspiciousness as paranoid, and others have tended to use the term to refer to persecutory delusions. It has also been used to characterize grandiose, litigious, hostile, jealous, and even angry behavior regardless of the fact that these behaviors may all be within the normal spectrum. The key principles for understanding the current meaning of paranoid are:

1. It is a clinical construct used to describe various subjective and objective features of behavior which are deemed to be psychopathologic. It is the interpretation that these features are abnormal based on evidence accumulated from patients and other informants that allows these features to be regarded as psychopathologic. This judgment requires some humility and care. It is supported by the presence of the features listed in the table below and their occurrence as part of a behavior pattern which is extreme, intense, based on false assertions, inappropriate, disturbing to others, and possibly bizarre or dangerous. Often the patient is convinced and resolute in his or her belief; counter evidence and argument fail to persuade the patient.

2. It refers to no specific condition. For example, to identify paranoid features does not determine that a schizophrenic condition is present.

Features of Paranoid Disorders

Objective Features

Anger	Hate	Obstinacy
Critical, accusatory behavior	Hostility	Resentment
Defensiveness	Humorlessness	Seclusiveness
Fragile self-esteem	Hypersensitivity	Secretiveness
Grandiosity or excessive self-importance	Inordinate attention to small details	Self-righteousness
		Sullenness
Grievance collection	Irritability, quick annoyance	Suspiciousness
Guardedness, evasiveness	Litigiousness (letter writing, complaints, legal action)	Violence, aggressiveness

Subjective Features*

Delusions of self-reference, persecution, grandeur, infidelity, love, jealousy, imposture, infestation, disfigurement, and disease

* Part of private mental experience. The patient often discloses these features during the clinical interview, but may not do so, even with specific questioning.

3. How common are paranoid conditions?

Paranoid features are among the most common and serious manifestations of psychopathology. They occur in a wide variety of psychiatric and medical illnesses and are, perhaps, the most frequently encountered symptoms of severe psychopathology. However, the frequency of some of the idiopathic conditions remains less clear. These conditions may be uncommon (delusional disorder) or, in some cases, rare (shared psychotic disorder). The exact incidence of organic delusional syndrome (medical and substance disorders) is presumed to be common; atypical psychosis, because of its lack of specificity, is difficult to estimate. The essential strategy in evaluating conditions in which paranoid features are present is a competent and thorough differential diagnosis.

4. What is the etiology of paranoid disorders?

The etiology of paranoid disorders is largely unknown except, of course, in those cases where an organic factor can be isolated. Paranoid features, including the types of delusions that are encountered in delusional disorder, occur in a large number of medical and psychiatric conditions. Many theories exist about the origin of delusions, but evidence to support them is limited.

5. Is there a neuropathology for the paranoid disorders?

Except for those conditions in which a specific organic factor can be identified, the prospects of determining a specific neuropathology or brain pathology to correlate with the psychopathology of the delusional experience is more hope than reality. Nevertheless, there are clues based on various observations from neuropsychiatric studies that suggest where we might find neuropathologic evidence. For example, patients who have severe cortical disorders, such as Alzheimer's disease, tend to experience simple and transient persecutory delusions. Delusions of a more systematized, elaborate, and complex character tend to be more chronic and resistant to treatment and have been associated with subcortical neurologic conditions that generally produce greater cognitive impairment than the typical idiopathic disorders.

6. What are the clinical features of paranoid disorders?

The core feature is delusions. In delusional disorder, it is the presence of persistent, non-bizarre delusions not explained by other psychotic disorders. In this presentation the delusion may emerge gradually and become chronic, and sometimes be associated with a precipitating event. Behavioral, emotional, and cognitive responses are generally appropriate, and neither mood disorders nor schizophrenic illness are present.

7. What is delusional disorder?

In recent years delusional disorder has become a better recognized form of paranoid presentation. The term *delusional disorder* refers to a condition of unknown cause whose chief feature is a non-bizarre delusion present for at least 1 month. The diagnosis of delusional disorder corresponds closely to an older concept, paranoia, as formulated by Emil Kraepelin and others over a century ago. There are several types of such delusions, and the predominant type is identified to make the diagnosis. Minimal deterioration in personality or function and the relative absence of other psychopathologic symptoms have been considered important evidence for distinguishing this disorder from schizophrenia and other psychotic conditions.

Delusional Disorder (DSM–IV)*

A. Non-bizarre delusion(s) (i.e., involving situations that occur in real life, such as being followed, poisoned, infected, loved at a distance, being deceived by spouse or lover, or having a disease), of at least 1 month's duration.

B. The symptom criteria for schizophrenia have never been met. Note: Tactile and olfactory hallucinations may be present in delusional disorder if they are related to the delusional theme.

C. Apart from the impact of the delusion(s) or its ramifications, functioning is not markedly impaired and behavior is not obviously odd or bizarre.

D. If mood episodes have occurred concurrently with delusions, their total duration has been brief relative to the duration of the delusional periods.

E. The disturbance is not caused by the direct physiologic effects of a substance (e.g., a drug of abuse or a medication) or a general medical condition.

* Reprinted with permission from the Diagnostic and Statistical Manual of Mental Disorders, 4th ed. Copyright 1994 American Psychiatric Association.

8. What is a non-bizarre delusion?

Non-bizarre means that the delusion concerns situations that can occur and are possible in real life, such as being followed, having a disease, being secretly in love, and the like.

9. What are the types of delusional disorder?

There are five main types and two additional residual ones: **(1) Erotomanic, (2) Grandiose, (3) Jealous, (4) Persecutory, (5) Somatic, and Mixed and Unspecified.**

In the erotomanic the predominant theme of the delusion is that a person, usually of higher status, is in love with the subject; in the grandiose type the theme is one of inflated worth, power, knowledge, identity, or special relationship to a deity or important famous person; in the jealous type the theme is that one's sexual partner is unfaithful; in the persecutory type the theme is that someone to whom one is close is being malevolently treated in some way; in the somatic type the theme is that the person has some physical defect, disorder, or disease; in the mixed type more than one of the above types are present but no one theme is predominant; and in the unspecified type the delusions do not fit into any of the categories.

10. Why is it difficult to recognize delusional disorder?

Delusional disorder is at best uncommon: many clinicians have probably encountered one or two cases, but many have not. It is difficult to recognize because one of its hallmarks is an absence, or modest occurrence, of psychopathology other than delusions. Such patients, if they are patients at all, are in all likelihood misdiagnosed, perhaps as having mild cases of schizophrenia. Because they may seek out internists, dermatologists, lawyers, or the police, they may never be diagnosed at all.

11. What is the most common type of delusional disorder?

Persecutory, which is also the classic form of the condition. Such individuals frequently are highly litigious and their delusions are often highly systematized (elaborate and detailed).

12. What characteristic features does the jealous type have?
This type, sometimes referred to using eponyms such as the Othello syndrome or conjugal paranoia, is common and associated with dangerousness. Jealousy is a powerful emotion. Individuals
with this delusion may resort to assault, homicide, even suicide in response to their delusional
concerns about a lover's unfaithfulness. It generally affects males, often with no history of psychiatric difficulty. The delusions may appear suddenly and serve to "explain" a host of remote
and recent events involving the spouse's fidelity. This type is particularly difficult to treat, often
diminishing only upon separation, divorce, or death of the spouse.

13. What is morbid jealousy or pathologic jealousy?
Jealousy is often a symptom in other disorders where it may be referred to by these terms.
Because it is a symptom, it may derive from several possible disorders such as epilepsy, mood
disorder, schizophrenia, or substance abuse.

14. What is another name for the erotomanic type, and what features characterize it?
The erotomanic type, also called De Clerambault's syndrome, when the symptom occurs in other
disorders such as schizophrenia, is the delusion of secret love, usually from an individual of
higher social standing. Although this may occur in both sexes, it more usually is found in females. Such patients usually pester, and possibly harass, the object of their love with letters,
phone calls, or unexpected visits. The delusion usually concerns a more "spiritual union" or romantic love, rather than sexual attraction.

15. What behavior might a patient with the grandiose type of delusional disorder exhibit?
These patients suffer from megalomania. Such patients are inclined to join cults, preach on the
street corner, proselytize their beliefs, or attempt to associate with popular or eminent individuals.

**16. What are the characteristics of and other names for the somatic type of delusional dis-
order?**
Patients with this type of disorder seek out professional attention for diseases they believe they
have. When individual tests fail to detect their "diseases," they often move on to other physicians,
unable to respond to reassurance and the evidence collected in their evaluations. There are several patterns: (1) patients concerned about parasites or insect infestation; (2) patients convinced
that their body, nose, face, or hair has been altered; and (3) patients concerned that they emit foul
bodily odors. Patients with such disturbances are more likely to seek help from dermatologists,
exterminators, plastic surgeons, and dentists than psychiatrists. These conditions differ from
simple hypochondriasis because of the degree of reality impairment associated with them. Other
names: monosymptomatic hypochondriac psychosis, monodelusional psychosis, delusional para-
sitosis, delusion of infestation, and epidermozoophobia.

17. What is organic delusional syndrome?
Organic delusional syndrome or disorder refers to delusional illness for which a specific etiology
can be determined. It is a DSM-III term that has been replaced in DSM-IV by psychotic disorders
due to a general medical condition or substance-induced psychotic disorder. In general, many
conditions can be the source of such delusional disorders. These are conditions which arise from
infectious, neurologic, substance or toxicologic factors, metabolic, or even genetic or chromoso-
mal sources. They have been described in both case reports and other observations for many
years. For the clinician, of course, it is important to be aware of the most common causes, so that
these can be identified and diagnosed rapidly.

18. What are the most common sources of organic delusional disorder?
The most common forms of organic delusional disorder result from substance intoxication and
withdrawal. Among the most common of these are alcohol, sympathomimetic or over-the-counter
stimulant drugs and antihistamines, steroids, cocaine, marijuana and phencyclidine.

Common Causes of Delusions

Conditions Due to a General Medical Condition or Substance
  Alcohol abuse
  Drug abuse (especially CNS stimulants)
  Iatrogenic: anticholinergic poisoning, steroid poisoning, "diet-pills," sedative-hypnotic
    withdrawal
  Delirium
  Dementia
  Other neurologic sources: Human immunodeficiency virus syndromes, brain tumors,
    epileptic disorder, especially complex partial seizure disorder
Idiopathic Conditions
  Mood disorders (mania and psychotic depression)
  Schizophrenia and schizoaffective disorder
  Obsessive compulsive disorder
  Somatoform disorders

---

19. What are the features of organic delusional syndrome?

Organic delusional syndrome's essential feature is prominent delusions resulting from a specific organic factor. The diagnosis of this condition is not made if the delusions occur in the context of difficulties in the maintenance of attention, orientation, or confusion, as in *delirium.* The nature of the delusions is variable and, to some extent, depends on the etiology of the disorder. Persecutory delusions are probably the most common type. Amphetamine use, as well as that of cocaine and other stimulants, has been associated with the development of this disorder. But there are sources of organic delusional syndrome that are not related to substance abuse. It has been found in temporal lobe epilepsy, as an interictal syndrome often indistinguishable from schizophrenia; in cases of Huntington's disease; and cerebral lesions of the right hemisphere have also resulted in this disorder. Hallucinations may be present, but they are usually not a prominent characteristic. The associated features are important and include mild cognitive impairment, the presence of varied associated symptoms, many of them found in schizophrenia, such as perplexity, unusual dress and behavior, abnormalities of psychomotor activity, unusual speech, and dysphoric mood. In contrast to delusional disorder in which impairment is frequently not present or is modest, these conditions are associated with impairments in social, cognitive, and occupational functioning.

20. What is shared psychotic disorder?

Also called induced paranoid disorder, *folie à deux,* double insanity, and other terms, it was first described by Lasegue and Falret in 1877. It is believed to be rare, but accurate incidence and prevalence figures are not available. The literature consists almost entirely of single case reports. The delusion involved is characterized by its transfer from one individual to another. Both persons may have been intimately associated for a long time and typically live in relative social isolation from other people. In its most common form the individual who first has the delusion is often chronically ill and typically is the influential member of a close relationship with a more suggestible person who then becomes the induced psychotic disorder patient. It is usually the latter who is less clever, more gullible, submissive, passive, and lower in self-esteem. Old age, low intelligence, impairment of sensory function, alcohol abuse, and cerebrovascular disease have been among the factors that have been associated with this peculiar disorder. A genetic predisposition to idiopathic psychosis has been suggested as a possible risk factor.

There is some question as to whether such people are truly delusional or merely highly impressionable. Frequently, there is passive acceptance of the delusional beliefs of the dominant person, until they are separated, at which point the unusual belief may remit spontaneously. The criteria for the diagnosis require that a psychotic disorder not be present before onset of the induced delusion.

21. What is paranoid personality disorder?

Paranoid personality disorder is a nonpsychotic condition involving a marked change in the personality traits as the individual becomes a young adult. These traits include a pervasive and unwanted tendency to interpret the actions of other people as demeaning or threatening. This threat can be indicated by several behaviors including the expectation of being exploited, the questioning of the loyalty or trust of friends or associates, the reading of hidden meanings into benign remarks or events, the bearing of grudges, the lack of forgiveness for insults or slights, the reluctance to confide in others because of fear that the information will be used against the person, a tendency to be easily slighted and quick to react with anger, intense changes in mood, and a questioning of the fidelity of spouses or sexual partners. Little is actually known about this disorder's prevalence, association with familial transmission patterns, and predispositions. Its relationship to schizophrenia and even to other paranoid disorders is also unclear. It is an interesting clinical phenomenon about which we need considerably more information.

22. What is Capgras syndrome?

Capgras and Reboul-Lachaux first described in 1923 a syndrome consisting of the delusion that doubles of important or significant others and of oneself exist. For example, the patient may claim that his or her spouse has been replaced by an impostor. The syndrome is not related to hallucinations, simple misrecognition, or illusions. It is a delusion. In 1983 Berson summarized 133 cases of this syndrome as reported in the literature. His conclusions were that the disorder appears in both men and women, over a wide range of age, and with a wide range of other mental disorders. The most common diagnosis in such cases has generally been schizophrenia (about 60%); 23% of patients identified with this disorder suffered from diagnosable brain disorder.

23. What are the issues in differential diagnosis of paranoid disorders?

Obviously differential diagnosis is the most important process in the evaluation of patients with paranoid disorders. Most of these disorders are, at the very least, uncommon, and they are idiopathic. In addition, they have features characteristic of many medical and psychiatric conditions. Diagnosis of paranoid disorders requires the exclusion of other conditions and the matching of the features of a particular case to the appropriate criteria. The first step is to recognize, characterize, and judge as pathologic those features that are identified as possibly paranoid. This involves being sensitive to the range of subjective and objective characteristics frequently found in paranoid conditions. Because of the patients' unwillingness to reveal themselves in the process of the interview or to cooperate with clinical investigation, this step is critical, as well as difficult. Careful interviewing of the patient and other informants is usually the basis for determining that the behavior is psychopathologic. Having determined that a paranoid condition is present, the clinician should then evaluate premorbid characteristics, the course of the disease, associated symptoms, and so on. Important in this process is the discovery of confusion, perceptual disturbances, mood and motor disturbances, signs of physical illness, or confusing symptoms that may suggest different causes for paranoid features. In general, isolated acute symptoms of paranoid behavior are often present in early stages or medical conditions.

The final diagnosis in cases where paranoid features are prominent should be made following a complete medical and psychiatric history with special attention to alcohol and drug use. A thorough physical examination includes neurologic and mental status exams and appropriate laboratory studies—particularly serologic, toxic, endocrinologic and microbiologic features—as well as radiographic and electroencephalographic investigations. Where possible, CT and possibly MRI studies should be performed to identify structural brain disease (e.g., a tumor, or multi-infarct dementia) associated with psychopathologic changes.

24. What are the most important conditions to consider in the differential diagnosis?

Certain conditions exist with delusional features that, because of their seriousness or frequency, should be routinely considered in a differential diagnosis, as they are the most likely sources of delusional presentations. Delusions arise in connection with a number of **organic diseases** and syndromes. Frequently, they have in common a disturbance of perception, especially of visual or auditory functioning. Drug intoxications are particularly relevant; abused drugs and even prescribed drugs, such as steroids and L-dopa, have been known to cause delusional syndromes, often without cognitive impairment. Among elderly people, dementia should be considered whenever paranoid features occur. Mental status exams should uncover the characteristic cognitive changes that do not generally occur in delusional disorder. Delirium, for example, has a fluctuating course, with confusion, memory impairment, and transient delusions that contrast with the persistence of delusions in most idiopathic paranoid disorders.

Another major source of delusional presentations is **schizophrenia,** in which delusions may be a presenting feature. This diagnosis should be considered when the delusions are bizarre, when affect is blunted or incongruent with thinking, where thought disorder, if present, is pervasive, and where role functioning is impaired. Paranoid schizophrenic patients may have somewhat less bizarre delusions than patients with other types of delusions; however, their role functioning is impaired, and auditory hallucinations are often present and prominent, unlike most paranoid disorders.

Third are **mood disorders,** in particular depression and mania. Profound changes in mood suggest depression. In paranoid disorders, mood may be depressed, but the change is not usually so overwhelming nor pervasive as in depression. Delusions in depression are frequently related to the mood of depression, the so-called mood congruent delusions. The key is to consider the associated psychopathologic features, in that depression refers to a group of signs and symptoms such as changes in appetite, sleep, libido, concentration, decisiveness, interest, and energy. Depression is often cyclical and may be associated with a positive family history. Manic delusions are often grandiose and, therefore, to some extent mood-congruent. They usually occur during severe stages of mania and are relatively easy to recognize as part of the manic syndrome. Marked instability of mood, often intensely euphoric or irritable, reduced need for sleep, increased energy, lack of inhibition, and increased activity levels should distinguish this from other forms of paranoid disorder.

25. Name other conditions that should be considered in the differential.

Other personality disorder—paranoid features can occur in schizoid and schizotypal personality disorders as well as in paranoid personality disorders. The decisive distinction with most of the other paranoid disorders is the presence of clear-cut delusions, often hallucinations and other psychotic features.

Obsessive-compulsive disorders—Delusions and hallucinations are usually but not consistently absent in these disorders. Fears, rituals, rumination, and preoccupation are generally more pervasive and more likely to influence functioning than in delusional or paranoid disorders.

Somatoform disorders—Body dysmorphic disorder may be difficult to distinguish. The degree of conviction about imagined disfigurement may be helpful in making this distinction. Other psychopathologic features are more likely to be present in somatoform disorders as well. Hypochondriasis may present with some difficulty. The patient almost always retains, however, some degree of uncertainty about their health concerns.

26. What principles apply to the differential diagnosis of elderly paranoid patients?

Disorders associated with aging—In the elderly the differential diagnosis is, if anything, even broader. Although it is possible for idiopathic paranoid disorders *to begin* late in life, the likelihood is low. On the other hand, there is a high risk for paranoid features *to recur* in depression, schizophrenia, and as a result of organic factors. The sudden onset of paranoid features should be considered a sign of medical illness, possibly cerebrovascular disease, and an acute onset may be a harbinger of acute organic delusional syndrome. The incidence of many medical illnesses associated with paranoid features increases with age. Other sources of increased risk for paranoid disturbance among older individuals include a lack of stimulating company, physical illness, aging itself, and reductions in sensory functioning, such as visual acuity and hearing. Each of these should be considered in the evaluation of the patient.

27. What is the treatment for paranoid disorders?

No set treatment guidelines apply to all cases of paranoid disorders. Each of the conditions is sufficiently different to require separate approaches. Let us consider first paranoid personality disorder, which, in addition to being uncommon, is unlikely to come to the attention of clinicians. Such patients may, because of depressive symptomatology or anxiety, eventually fall into the care of psychiatric professionals. But generally speaking, these patients maintain an arm's-length distance from any health care, and specifically psychiatric, facility. Symptomatic therapies and supportive counseling are frequently attempted in such cases. Success is, at best, modest.

Organic delusional syndrome, on the other hand, may be treatable so long as the treatment focuses on the underlying organic factor that initiated and perpetuated the delusional presentation. Obviously, this could include substance abuse, where removal of the initiating factor may result in a rapid improvement in the patient's mental state. Often such patients also require treatment with antipsychotic medication (e.g., risperidone, haloperidol), which may also be effective in reducing the agitation, suspiciousness, and even the delusional thinking associated with these conditions. But if the original initiating factor remains present, the prognosis of such cases is likely to be poor unless symptomatic treatment is continued. With progressive disorders, such treatment may only serve to delay more severe deterioration in behavior.

28. Is delusional disorder treatable?

Delusional disorder is a condition that *may* be treatable. Because of the condition's very nature, the patient may have difficulty admitting a psychiatric illness exists, and may not seek care. Observations have, however, suggested that psychotherapy, medication, and even hospitalization may be important components of the care of such individuals. Patients with delusional disorders may have a refractory condition in which the delusion will not remit with these interventions. Psychotherapy creates a therapeutic alliance with such patients, which may allow them to deal with whatever stressors and concerns contribute to the overall impairment associated with the delusional experience. For example, if the patient is dysphoric and finds it difficult to work, a chance to share some of those concerns with a sympathetic clinician may provide considerable relief. Medications have been promoted recently, but the data concerning their use is limited. Certainly there is value in considering an antipsychotic in a case where a delusion is present. Delusion is, after all, a major symptom of psychosis, and it stands to reason that an antipsychotic agent might have some role in treatment. In practice, however, the success of such interventions as well as other somatic treatment is meager. In recent years hypochondriacal delusions of the somatic type have been reported to respond to pimozide, a potent dopamine blocking agent and antipsychotic medication. These observations have been based on a small series of cases and are uncontrolled. The use of antidepressants has also been promoted by some individuals who have treated patients with delusional disorder. Again, the observation is that patients who have dysphoric mood in association with presence of the delusions may respond nicely.

Hospitalization is recommended in circumstances in which the patient's behavior has become dangerous or self-destructive. Hospitalization may be a satisfactory temporary solution, allowing the patient to be confronted with the impact of the behavior and the need for greater restraint.

29. Is there treatment for shared psychotic disorder?

This is a condition about which little is known concerning treatment. Observations have had a tantalizing quality in suggesting, for example, that separation of the two parties may lead to the diminution of the delusion in the induced psychotic partner. The observation is that with divorce, death, or some other form of separation, the induced party often begins to experience a reduction in delusional thinking, sometimes to the point where the patient can no longer be considered delusional. Apart from this, there are no systematic controlled observations about intervention in the literature.

30. And therapy for atypical psychosis?

Patients who have these conditions must be dealt with individually, identifying the symptoms that constitute the basis for their complaint. Where that is a specific, or particularly prominent, delusional form of thinking, one would need to address it possibly with antipsychotic medications. Again, very little systematic literature is available for this condition, and general guidelines are not possible.

BIBLIOGRAPHY

1. American Psychiatric Association: Diagnostic and Statistical Manual of Mental Disorders, 4th ed (DSM–IV). Washington, DC, American Psychiatric Association, 1994.
2. Berson RJ: Capgras syndrome. Am J Psychiatry 140:969–978, 1983.
3. Cummings JL: Psychosis in neurologic disease: Neurobiology and pathogenesis. Neuropsychiatry, Neuropsychology, and Behavioral Neurology 5:144–150, 1992.
4. Gawin FH, Ellinwood E: Cocaine and other stimulants. N Engl J Med 318:1173–1182, 1988.
5. Kraepelin E: Manic Depressive Insanity and Paranoia. Edinburgh, Livingstone Press, 1921.
6. Krakowski M, Volavka J, Brizer D: Psychopathology and violence: A review of literature. Compr Psychiatry 27:131–148, 1986.
7. Manschreck TC, Petri M: The paranoid syndrome. Lancet 2:251–253, 1978.
8. Manschreck TC: Delusional disorder and shared psychotic disorder. In Kaplan H, Sadock B (eds): Comprehensive Textbook of Psychiatry, 6th ed. Baltimore, Williams & Wilkins, 1995.
9. Manschreck TC: Pathogenesis of delusions. Psychiatr Clin North Am 18:213–230, 1995.
10. Manschreck TC: The assessment of paranoid features. Compr Psychiatry 20(4):370–377, 1979.
11. McAllister T: Neuropsychiatric aspects of delusions. Psychiatr Ann 22:269–277, 1992.
12. Munro A: Psychiatric disorders characterized by delusions: Treatment in relation to specific types. Psychiatr Ann 22:232–240, 1992.
13. Opler LA, Feinberg SS: The role of pimozide in clinical psychiatry: A review. J Clin Psychiatry 52:221–233, 1991.
14. Stoudemire A, Riether A: Evaluation and treatment of paranoid syndromes in the elderly. Gen Hosp Psychiatry 9:267–274, 1987.
15. Webb W: Paranoid conditions seen in psychiatric medicine. Psychiatr Med 8:37–48, 1990.

12. BIPOLAR DISORDERS

Marshall R. Thomas, M.D.

1. What is bipolar disorder? How is it different from manic-depressive illness?
Bipolar disorder encompasses a heterogeneous group of disorders characterized by cyclical disturbances in mood, cognition, and behavior. The diagnosis requires a history of mania for at least 1 week or hypomania for at least 4 days. Bipolar I disorder refers to patients who have had at least one episode of mania, whereas bipolar II disorder refers to patients with a history of hypomania and major depressive episodes. Cyclothymia refers to patients with chronic (at least 2 years) mood swings that fluctuate between hypomania and minor but not major depression.

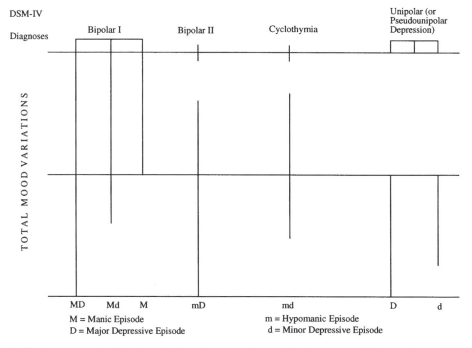

Modified from Goodwin F, Jamison K: Manic-Depressive Illness. New York, Oxford University Press, 1990.

In 1921 the German psychiatrist Emil Kraepelin introduced the term manic-depressive insanity, which included patients with recurrent unipolar depression as well as bipolar disorder and distinguished both groups from schizophrenia, which he termed dementia praecox. Kraepelin emphasized the similarities in course and outcome between patients with highly recurrent mood disorders, regardless of polarity. In 1962 Leonard introduced the term bipolar and emphasized differences between unipolar and bipolar patients.

Many researchers argue that modern adherence to Leonard's bipolar/unipolar dichotomy, although clarifying certain issues, has caused clinicians to overlook the similarities between bipolar and many unipolar patients, who share a common pattern of recurrence, remission, and exacerbation. The modern concept of bipolar spectrum disorder encompasses patients with bipolar I and II disorders, cyclothymia, hyperthymia (chronic hypomania), and pseudounipolar depression. Pseudounipolar depressives are patients with a highly recurrent unipolar illness, a positive family history for bipolar disorder, and a positive therapeutic response to antibipolar treatments.

2. Describe the epidemiology of bipolar disorder.

The lifetime risk for bipolar I disorder is 0.6–0.9% in industrialized nations, with no apparent gender differences; unipolar depression, however, is twice as common in women as it is in men. Differing criteria for what constitutes hypomania have made it difficult to determine the prevalence of bipolar II and cyclothymic disorders. Bipolar II disorder is probably at least as common as bipolar I, and the lifetime prevalence of cyclothymia is estimated at 0.4–1.0%. Over the last 50 years, all mood disorders have increased in prevalence, with an earlier age of onset in each successive generation—a phenomenon referred to as the "cohort effect."

Family studies find that if one parent has a major affective disorder the risk to the offspring is 25–30%, whereas if both parents have an affective disorder the risk to the offspring may be as high as 50–75%. Suicide is common in untreated bipolar disorder; 25–50% of patients attempt suicide at least once. Seasonal variations exist; depression is more common in the spring (March through May) and autumn (September through November), whereas mania is more common in the summer. The peak incidence of suicide occurs in May, with a second peak in October.

3. How does one recognize mania?

Manic states range in severity from milder hypomania to psychotic or delirious manic states. The symptomatology evolves as the episode becomes more severe. The mood in mania may be elated or euphoric, but as severity increases the mood is more likely to become irritable, labile, and dysphoric. Thoughts may race; as mania progresses, thinking becomes disorganized, expansive, and grandiose. Behavior increases from early physical hyperactivity, pressured speech, and decreased need for sleep to later manifestations of hypersexuality, increased impulsivity, and risk taking.

Manic Episode: Diagnostic Criteria

Distinct period of elevated, expansive, or irritable mood
• At least 1 week
• Or hospitalized
Three of the following; 4 if mood only irritable
• Inflated self esteem or grandiosity   • Distractibility
• Decreased need for sleep   • Increased activity
• Pressured speech   • Excessive involvement in pleasurable activities
• Flight of ideas or thoughts racing   with high risk of painful consequences
Marked impairment, psychosis, or hospitalization
Not due to direct effect of substance or medical condition

From American Psychiatric Association: Diagnostic and Statistical Manual of Mental Disorders, 4th ed. Washington, DC, American Psychiatric Association, 1994, with permission.

Hypomanic Episode: Diagnostic Criteria

Distinct period of elevated, expansive, or irritable mood (at least 4 days)
Three additional symptoms; 4 if mood only irritable
Unequivocal change in functioning
Change observable by others
Episode not severe enough to cause:
• Marked impairment
• Hospitalization
• Psychosis
Not due to direct effects of a substance or general medical condition

From American Psychiatric Association: Diagnostic and Statistical Manual of Mental Disorders, 4th ed. Washington, DC, American Psychiatric Association, 1994, with permission.

4. What is a "mixed state"?

A mixed state is diagnosed when the patient simultaneously meets criteria for mania and major depression. Mixed states are common, occurring in approximately 40% of manic patients. Mixed states are sometimes difficult to distinguish from or are misdiagnosed as agitated depressions and borderline conditions. Mixed states are more common in patients with substance abuse and neurologic disorders (e.g., head injury) and are associated with increased suicidality, chronicity, and poorer response to lithium.

5. What is the clinical significance of bipolar II disorder?

Bipolar II (BP II) disorder is diagnosed in patients with episodes of hypomania interspersed with episodes of major depression. Clinically, patients usually present during periods of depression. Often the diagnosis is not clear, because both hypomania and depression may be associated with irritability and the psychomotor symptoms of hypomania may be subtle. BP II disorder is more common in women. Age of onset and psychomotor features appear to be intermediate between bipolar I and unipolar populations. BP II tends to run in families (breeds true) and patients who present as BP II tend to stay in the same category; they have subsequent episodes of hypomania but not mania.

Bipolar II disorder should not be viewed as a minor form of BP I, because psychosocial morbidity, substance abuse, and suicide attempts are at least as common in BP II. What constitutes the best treatment course for patients with BP needs further study. Patients with BP II show a predominance of depression, but antidepressant treatments may induce rapid cycling and mixed states, as they do in BP I disorder. Patients with BP II also may be biologically heterogeneous. For example, severe environmental stressors such as prolonged abuse or neglect may cause forms of mood disregulation that phenotypically resemble BP II (referred to as *bipolar II phenocopy*) in patients without family histories of affective disorders.

6. How does one distinguish bipolar from unipolar depression?

About 10–20% of hospital first admissions for depression later develop a bipolar disorder. Careful scrutiny of the patient's history for episodes of mania or hypomania may help to make the diagnosis in some cases. The clinical course of bipolar depression is characterized by premorbid cyclothymic temperament, recurrences, as well as early-age, rapid, and postpartum onsets. Symptomatically bipolar depressives are more likely to demonstrate psychosis, hypersomnia, anergia (low energy), and severe shut-down depressions that are immobilizing. Bipolar depressives are also more likely to have family histories of bipolar disorder and familial loading for affective disorders in general. In the absence of a premorbid history of mania, hypomania, or cyclothymia, no single associated finding is pathognomonic for bipolar disorder, but clusters of such factors make the diagnosis more likely.

7. Describe the course of illness issues in bipolar disorder.

In the past there has been a tendency to underestimate the rate of recurrence and to overestimate the age of onset of bipolar disorder. Many bipolar adolescents are misdiagnosed as conduct-disordered or schizophrenic, because they may demonstrate labile mood, abnormal thinking, and disturbed behavior several years before their first recognizable major affective episode. For bipolar patients, the mean age of first impairment due to psychiatric symptoms is 18.7 years; the mean age of first treatment is 22 years; and the mean age of first hospitalization is 25.8 years. The lag between age of first impairment and age of first treatment is cause for concern in light of data suggesting that early intervention and treatment may prevent the development of a more malignant course of illness.

Duration of episodes usually remains constant throughout the course of illness, whereas the free interval between episodes shortens with each successive episode. The rate of cycling increases with each successive episode. The average free interval between the first and second episode is 5 years, but by the fourth episode cycles are occurring at least yearly. Although duration of episodes demonstrates interindividual variability, the average untreated manic episode lasts 4 months and the average depressive episode 6–9 months. Manic episodes often begin abruptly over hours to days. Bipolar depressions usually take weeks to develop, but they still have a more rapid onset than unipolar depression.

Approximately 20% of bipolar patients demonstrate rapid cycling. Rapid cycling is more common in women, patients with BP II, and patients who have received antidepressant treatments. Rapid cyclers may have a poorer response to lithium and a higher rate of hypothyroidism.

In clinical cohorts, another 20% of bipolar patients have a chronic course with no free interval between episodes. A history of chronicity, substance abuse, and mixed states is associated with poorer outcome.

8. Describe the relationship between stress and onset of affective episodes in bipolar disorder.
A number of factors make it difficult to study the role of stress in the onset of affective episodes. At times it is difficult to sort out whether stress has led to an episode or whether the prodromal symptoms of an episode have led to the stress. Investigations suggest that stressors are statistically more likely to be associated with the onset of episodes early in the course of illness. This finding, along with the finding of increasing cycling, have suggested that the illness may kindle itself and become increasingly endogenous over time. In kindling, a model borrowed from neurology, a subthreshold stimulus applied at a regular interval over time becomes capable of inducing seizure activity.

Interpersonal and work difficulties are common precipitants associated with mood destabilization. Sleep reduction may be a final common pathway that leads to mania in a variety of situations, including stress-induced sleep disruption, parturition, and travel. There is also a high rate of bipolarity in patients whose moods demonstrate seasonal variation.

9. List medical conditions that may cause, mimic, or exacerbate bipolar disorder.
Organic factors may cause or exacerbate both mania and depression. The DSM-IV provides a separate diagnostic category for organically derived mood disorders: mood disorder due to . . . [indicate the general medical condition]. Historically, the term "secondary mania" has been used to designate manic states that arise from neurologic, endocrinologic, metabolic, infectious, or other medical conditions. Many organic factors may contribute to depression or mania individually, but few can engender a true bipolar syndrome with cycling between two states.

Organic Causes of Bipolar Mood Syndromes

Drugs	Isoniazid, steroids, disulfiram
Neurologic factors	Multiple sclerosis, closed head injury, CNS tumors, epilepsy, Huntington's disease, cerebrovascular accident
Metabolic factors	Thyroid disorders, postoperative states, adrenal disorders, vitamin B12 deficiency, electrolyte abnormalities
Infection	AIDS dementia, neurosyphilis, influenza

Modified from Goodwin F, Jamison K: Manic-Depressive Illness. New York, Oxford University Press, 1990.

Patients with an organic affective disorder are less likely to have a positive family history and may respond to treatment of the underlying condition. Other organic affective syndromes, such as those associated with brain trauma and multiple sclerosis, are not reversible but benefit from antibipolar treatments. Patients with a genetic predisposition to bipolarity may have a lower threshold for developing organic affective syndromes secondary to organic stressors.

10. What psychiatric conditions are commonly comorbid with bipolar disorder?
Bipolar disorder is the axis I disorder most likely to be associated with comorbid substance abuse or dependence; 60% of bipolar patients demonstrate abuse or dependence in one form or another. A study by the National Institutes of Mental Health (NIMH) found that 46% of bipolar patients

abused or were dependent on alcohol and 41% abused or were dependent on marijuana, cocaine, opiates, barbiturates, or hallucinogens. All forms of substance abuse are more common in manic or mixed phases of the illness. Comorbid substance abuse is associated with significantly poorer outcomes and increased rates of suicide.

Anxiety symptoms, axis II disorders, and certain psychotic conditions are found more commonly in patients with bipolar disorder. During mixed manic states and depressive episodes, bipolar patients may experience extreme anxiety that may remit with control of the affective disorder. Some bipolar patients may appear character-disordered (borderline or narcissistic), because their mood disorder is inadequately treated, whereas others demonstrate a comorbid axis II diagnosis in the absence of mood disregulation. Up to 50% of bipolar patients have psychotic symptoms such as delusions or hallucinations at some point in the course of their illness. The presence of psychotic symptoms only during periods of prominent mood disturbance distinguishes psychotic affective disorders from schizophrenia and schizoaffective disorder, in which psychotic symptoms exist outside of periods of mood disturbance.

11. What are the advantages and disadvantages of using lithium in the treatment of bipolar disorder?
Lithium has been in clinical use for over 40 years. It remains the only drug approved by the Food and Drug Administration for the treatment of bipolar mania and the prevention of bipolar recurrence. Lithium appears to be highly effective for mild manic symptoms and classic euphoric mania. Although lithium is less effective in treating bipolar depression, approximately 50% of bipolar patients with mild-to-moderate depression respond to treatment if given enough time. Lithium appears more effective in treating patients with mania-depression-interval (MDI) as opposed to depression-mania-interval (DMI) sequences. One distinct advantage of lithium for some patients is the fact that its standard preparations are significantly less expensive than other antimanic drugs.

Despite lithium's remarkable efficacy in euphoric mania, 30–50% of bipolar patients either are unable to tolerate or fail to respond to lithium. Even for patients who benefit the rate of response is slow: 10–14 days for mania and 4–8 weeks for depression. Gastrointestinal distress, cognitive dullness, polyuria, and tremor represent common acute effects. Weight gain is a common cause of discontinuation over the long term; 25% of patients gain 10 pounds or more. Approximately 10% of patients develop hypothyroidism. Elderly patients with compromised renal function require careful dosage adjustment. Patients with mixed states, severe mania, psychosis, substance abuse, and a history of neurologic insults are less likely to respond to lithium monotherapy.

12. What are the advantages and disadvantages of using anticonvulsants in the treatment of bipolar disorder?
Although lithium is considered by most clinicians to be the first-line drug in the treatment of mania and bipolar mood cycling, many patients either are unable to tolerate or fail to respond to lithium. As a result, in the last 15–20 years, there has been increasing interest in the use of anticonvulsants, particularly valproic acid and carbamazepine, to treat bipolar mood disorders. Controlled trials have demonstrated the efficacy of both drugs in acute mania, and some studies (of valproate in particular) have suggested a more rapid onset of antimanic action compared with lithium. Fewer studies of long-term prophylactic efficacy exist, and controlled studies are difficult to perform because of ethical concerns about the use of placebo in this population. Studies of anticonvulsants in depression find them less useful than lithium and antidepressants in treating depressed mood, although some bipolar depressives, especially those with mixed states and rapid cycling, may respond well.

The disadvantages of these agents are mainly related to side effects. Valproic acid is usually well tolerated, and rapid loading at 500 mg 3 times/day can be accomplished in hospital settings for many acutely agitated patients. Carbamazepine is more difficult to dose and requires a more gradual upward titration. Carbamazepine also autoinduces its own metabolism and heteroinduces the metabolism of other drugs. As a result, careful drug level monitoring is required, and other drugs, such as antipsychotics and birth control pills, may be rendered less effective unless dosage adjustments are made.

13. How does stage of illness affect treatment strategy in bipolar disorder?

The treatment strategy in bipolar disorder depends on the current stage of the illness, dimensional assessment of the illness, and knowledge of past treatment. The treatment of acute mania (described in chapter 49) includes the use of antimanic drugs and depending on the severity of illness adjunctive agents such as sedative-hypnotics, benzodiazepines, and antipsychotic agents. The treatment of acute depression (discussed in more detail in the controversies section below) is complicated in bipolar patients by the need to minimize the use of antidepressant agents. Because bipolar disorder is almost always recurrent, preventive treatment with antibipolar agents is usually indicated, especially once the patient has had two or more episodes. The high rate of suicide attempts in all phases of illness dictates an ongoing assessment of safety issues throughout the course of treatment.

CONTROVERSIES

14. What is the treatment for bipolar depression?

Issue. All antidepressants appear capable of inducing mania, mixed states, and mood cycling, thus worsening the long-term course of the illness.

Discussion. Patients with mild-to-moderate bipolar depression may respond to antimanic agents such as lithium alone, although there is often a significant lag time of up to 8 weeks before a full antidepressant response. Tricyclic antidepressants (TCAs) probably should be avoided, because they may be more likely than other antidepressants to induce cycling and also appear to be marginally effective in the treatment of bipolar depression. Preliminary reports suggested that bupropion decreased cycling in some bipolar patients, but subsequent reports find that it too can induce mania at least in some patients. Recent data suggest that selective serotonin reuptake inhibitors (SSRIs), such as fluoxetine, sertraline, and paroxetine, may be less likely to induce mania and hypomania than TCAs and monoamine oxidase inhibitors (MAOIs). MAOIs, on the other hand, appear to be particularly effective in patients with anergic depressions or atypical symptoms (mood reactivity, hypersomnia, hyperphagia, leaden fatigue, and rejection sensitivity), many of whom may be bipolar.

Currently most clinicians attempt to treat mild-to-moderate bipolar depression without an antidepressant. If an antidepressant is required, a short-acting SSRI (sertraline or paroxetine) or bupropion is the first choice. If these are ineffective, an MAOI or electroconvulsive therapy (ECT) may be used. Patients with rapid cycling depressions or mixed states of mania and concurrent depression require cessation of antidepressant agents and treatment with anticonvulsant combination strategies.

15. Describe the neurochemical hypotheses of bipolar disorder.

Issue. Classical models of bipolar disorder have focused on neurotransmitter systems and their interactions with one another. Investigations into noradrenergic, serotonergic, cholinergic, dopaminergic, and GABAergic activity in bipolar patients and the effects of antibipolar treatments on these systems have yielded inconsistent results.

Discussion. Although neurotransmitters are of central importance, neurotransmitter balance models have been unable to explain the clinical heterogeneity of bipolar disorder and phenomena such as mixed states, rapid cycling, and episode switching (rapid transitions from depression to mania or vice versa). Recent research has focused on G-protein activity and intracellular second-messenger systems. Elevated G-protein and intracellular calcium signals have been found in bipolar patients. These changes may lead to overactivity or inhibition of cell systems, depending on the degree of signal hyperactivity and other variables within the cell. Antibipolar treatments such as lithium, carbamazepine, and ECT have been shown to attenuate such overactive cell processes.

BIBLIOGRAPHY

1. American Psychiatric Association: Diagnostic and Statistical Manual of Mental Disorders, 4th ed. Washington, DC, American Psychiatric Association, 1994.
2. Clayton PJ: Bipolar illness. In Winokur G, Clayton PJ (eds): The Medical Basis of Psychiatry, 2nd ed. Philadelphia, W.B. Saunders, 1994, p 47.
3. Goodwin F, Jamison K: Manic-Depressive Illness. New York, Oxford University Press, 1990.
4. McElroy S, et al: Clinical and research implications for the diagnosis of dysphoric and mixed mania or hypomania. Am J Psychiatry 149:1633, 1992.
5. McElroy S, et al: Valproate in the treatment of bipolar disorder: Literature review and clinical guidelines. J Clin Psychopharmacol 12(Suppl):42, 1992.
6. Simpson SG, Folstein SE, Meyers DA, et al: Bipolar II: The most common bipolar phenotype? Am J Psychiatry 150(6):986, 1993.
7. Wehr T: Sleep-loss as a possible mediator of diverse causes of mania. Br J Psychiatry 159:576, 1991.
8. Zornberg G, Pope H: Treatment of depression in bipolar disorder: New directions for research. J Clin Psychopharmacol 13(6):397, 1993.
9. Altshuler L, et al: Antidepressant-induced mania and cycle acceleration: A controversy revisited. Am J Psychiatry 152(8):1130, 1995.

13. DEPRESSIVE DISORDERS

Lawson R. Wulsin, M.D.

1. What are the seven secrets of depression?
Depression is (1) common, (2) often missed, (3) not hard to diagnose if you look for it, (4) often severe, (5) often recurrent, (6) costly, and (7) highly treatable. These facts are "secrets" in the sense that they are not well understood by the American public or by many physicians.

Depression is among the five most common disorders seen in a primary physician's office. Unrecognized and untreated depression has been publicly acknowledged as a major public health problem in the United States for the past 15 years. As many as half of the cases of depressive disorders go unrecognized by the patient or the doctor, and among those recognized most will remain untreated. The reasons for such neglect include stigma, misunderstandings about the seriousness and treatability of depression, and preferential attention by patient and doctor to somatic complaints.

The disability caused by depressive disorders rivals that of coronary artery disease and is greater than the disability resulting from chronic lung disease or arthritis, according to the Medical Outcomes Study. The cost of depressive disorders in terms of treatment, work missed, and loss of function approximates $16 billion annually in the U.S. Depression is associated with 80% of suicides. Yet it is highly treatable, with 80% of patients responding to antidepressant therapy, psychotherapy, or both, when treated by qualified professionals. The cost of diagnosis and treatment is small, relative to other common severe medical disorders, whereas the cost of *not* treating a depressive disorder is great.

2. What does the term "depressive disorders" include?
The DSM–IV diagnoses listed below are implied by the term depressive disorders:
- Major depressive disorder, single episode
- Major depressive disorder, recurrent
- Dysthymic disorder
- Depressive disorder not otherwise specified
- Adjustment disorder with depressed mood
- Mood disorder due to general medical condition
- Substance-induced mood disorder

Although major depressive disorder, particularly when recurrent, is the most severe of these depressive disorder subtypes, dysthymic disorder, or dysthymia, may be more common in primary care settings; dysthymia is also associated with significant morbidity and deserves treatment.

3. List the criteria for diagnosing a major depressive episode.
1. At least five of the following criteria for the same 2-week period (including at least one of the first two):

Criteria for a Major Depressive Episode

• Depressed mood	• Fatigue, loss of energy
• Loss of pleasure or interest	• Increased sense of worthlessness or guilt
• Significant weight (appetite) loss or gain	• Decreased concentration
• Insomnia or hypersomnia	• Recurrent morbid thoughts or suicidal
• Agitation or retardation	ideation

Reprinted with permission from the Diagnostic and Stastical Manual of Mental Disorders, 4th ed. Copyright 1994 American Psychiatric Association.

74

2. Not due to substance abuse, medical illness, or bereavement
3. Significant distress or impairment of functioning
4. Not due to medication or general medical condition
5. Not better accounted for by bereavement

Guidelines for application of these criteria are useful and easily available in the mood disorders module of *Prime MD, the Structured Clinical Interview for DSM–III–R,* and the pocket-sized *Diagnosing DSM–IV Psychiatric Disorders in the Primary Care Setting.* These guidelines provide questions that best assess whether the patient meets a given criterion, and provide directions on how to score the patient's responses when information is either ambiguous or insufficient.

Specifiers describe the severity, the current phase of the disease (remission, recurrence), and some salient features such as seasonal pattern or rapid cycling.

4. What is the difference between major depression and dysthymia?

Dysthymia requires only three of the nine criteria listed in question 3 and over a longer period of time (2 years). It may be a primary disorder, but it is often secondary to chronic medical problems (e.g., constant pain, cancer) or psychiatric illness (recurrent major depression, schizophrenia). Depressive disorder not otherwise specified (NOS) includes minor depression (a few symptoms for less than the 2 years of dysthymia) and recurrent brief depression (severe episodes which last less than 2 weeks).

5. How common is major depression?

The point prevalence in Western industrialized nations is 2.3 to 3.2% for men, and 4.5 to 9.3% for women. The lifetime risk is 7 to 12% for men, 20 to 25% for women. In primary care settings 6 to 10% of patients have current major depression. These figures make major depression as common in primary care practices as upper respiratory tract infections and hypertension.

6. How serious an illness is major depression?

Major depression is as serious as diabetes or heart disease. In a recent study of 11,242 primary care outpatients,[12] the "poor functioning uniquely associated with depressive symptoms, with or without depressive disorder, was comparable with or worse than that uniquely associated with eight major chronic medical conditions (such as advanced heart disease, diabetes, gastrointestinal disorders, back problems, arthritis)." This study and others suggest that the depressive disorders (not only major depression, but dysthymia and depressive symptoms) are associated with poor physical and social functioning. Depression increases mortality significantly through suicide, accidents, and exacerbation of medical illness.

7. What percentage of the medically ill have a depressive disorder?

Rates vary depending on the measures used to assess depression and the population studied. Rates rise with severity of medical illness, so that hospitalized patients have higher rates (20 to 33%) of depression than primary care clinic patients (5 to 20%). The depressed person often initially presents a somatic complaint (pain, insomnia, or fatigue), and the diagnosis of depression is often missed by either patient or clinician. Recent studies estimate that only half of the people with recognized major depression get any treatment, primarily because of under-recognition of the disorder, of the effectiveness of treatment, and of the high costs of not treating depression.

Although no single intervention has improved recognition and treatment of depression, a combination of efforts results in good treatment outcomes by primary care physicians: physician training, patient education, convenient mechanisms for screening at-risk patients, convenient methods for establishing a diagnosis of depression, well-tolerated effective antidepressants, short-term psychotherapy focused on depression recovery and prevention, convenient methods for monitoring response to treatment, and access to consultation for complicated cases. Until 15 years ago, these resources were not available to most physicians, but today most primary care physicians can get access to these resources at minimal cost.

8. What are some easy bedside measures for evaluating depression?

The Beck Depression Inventory is a 21-item self-report questionnaire that patients usually find easy to understand and complete in 5 minutes. Scoring and interpretation are simple, providing a tool for screening and monitoring progress. Another self-report questionnaire commonly used in primary care settings is the General Health Questionnaire. Clinician rating scales, such as the Hamilton Depression Rating Scale, require specific training in the administration and scoring but can be easily learned through a structured interview guide. The best translation of the DSM–IV criteria into conversational English that is precise and clear can be found in the modules for major depression and dysthymia of the *Prime MD, Structured Clinical Interview for DSM–III–R* or in *Diagnosing DSM–IV Psychiatric Disorders in the Primary Care Setting*.

9. How do you diagnose depression?

After the index of suspicion for depressive disorders is raised by the history, physical examination, mental status exam, or response to a screening measure, the clinician should then proceed to interview the patient carefully to establish which criteria the patient meets for any of the depressive disorders. Ask about duration, persistence, and severity of each symptom. Collaborative sources, such as relatives and past records, will help when the patient's responses are ambiguous, insufficient, or distorted by depression. Include your own observations when assessing the patient's agitation, energy level, concentration, and hopelessness.

Because the vegetative signs of depression may also be caused by medical illnesses and medications, the diagnosis of depression in the medically ill should not rest solely on the presence of such factors as fatigue, insomnia, and anorexia. Look also for the cognitive and affective criteria such as poor concentration, a sense of hopelessness or worthlessness, depressed mood, and anhedonia. When in doubt about the overlap between medical illness and depression (Is the anergia and retardation caused by cancer and pain medications or depression?), it is usually preferable to treat a suspected depression in a medically ill person to relieve the suffering from depression and to reduce the exacerbations of the medical illness caused by the depression.

10. What is the effect of depression on medical illness?

Depressive disorders complicate the course of medical illness with a variety of possible mechanisms: magnifying pain, impairing adherence to regimens, decreasing social supports, and dysregulating humoral and immunologic systems. Untreated depression has been shown to increase rates of death dramatically in nursing home patients and in patients with myocardial infarctions. Depressed patients with chronic medical conditions show significantly more disability than non-depressed patients, thus making it equivalent to bearing the burden of two independent diseases.

11. What percentage of depressed patients commit suicide? What percentage try?

About 15% of depressed patients commit suicide. About 10 times as many make suicidal acts. Depressive disorders are associated with about 80% of suicidal events. Other factors that increase the risk of suicide for the depressed person include alcohol and drug abuse, panic disorder and other states of intense anxiety, family history of suicide, medical illness, hopelessness, few social supports, recent personal loss, and unemployment. Treatment of the factors which contribute to suicide risk dramatically reduces both the immediate and chronic risks.

12. After the first episode, how likely is a patient to have a second major depressive episode?

More than 50% of those who have a first major depressive episode will have a recurrence. Untreated episodes in general last 6 to 24 months, with two thirds achieving a spontaneous full recovery. Risk factors for recurrences include incomplete recovery, previous recurrences, a strong family history of recurrent affective disorders, and a history of "double depression," i.e., major depression superimposed on dysthymia (AHCPR 1993).[1]

13. What are the important subtypes of major depression?

1. With psychotic features (This subtype requires treatment with an antipsychotic medication as well as an antidepressant. It generally represents a more severe form of major depression warranting aggressive treatment and prevention.)

2. With seasonal pattern (This subtype requires at least two episodes of major depression at the same season in successive years. Clear seasonal patterns allow some predictability and preventive treatment with phototherapy, or antidepressants in combination with psychotherapy.)

3. With melancholia (Severe vegetative signs of anergia, insomnia, and anorexia with diurnal worsening in the morning. These signs of melancholia are often the first to respond to antidepressant trials, with cognitive and affective signs following.)

4. With atypical features (In contrast to melancholia, this subtype features overeating, oversleeping, weight gain, and overreactive moods. It often responds better to monoamine oxidase inhibitors than to tricyclics.)

5. With postpartum onset (This subtype has a 10 to 15% prevalence within 6 months after delivery of the child. A previous episode of depression or bipolar disorder may justify preventive treatment at time of the next delivery.)

These subtypes are often described as specifiers in listing the formal diagnosis of major depression. They are important in some cases for their implications for treatment (e.g., with psychotic features), in others simply for research purposes, and in some cases for prevention (e.g., with seasonal pattern, with post-partum onset).

14. What is the best biologic marker of major depression?

There are no good (cheap, easy, accurate) biologic markers for any of the depressive disorders. The most accurate diagnostic marker of major depression is the following profile on sleep electroencephalography: decreased total sleep, increased sleep latency, decreased rapid eye movement (REM) latency, increased REM density, and decreased stage 4 sleep. However, the sleep EEG is not yet a practical tool for the diagnosis of depression in primary care settings. The key to diagnosis is a careful depression history and the mental status exam.

15. Describe the differential diagnosis of a major depressive episode.

The differential diagnosis of a major depressive episode should include at least the following:
- Mood disorder resulting from a medical condition
- Substance-induced mood disorder
- Dementia
- Bipolar disorder
- Attention deficit/hyperactivity disorder (ADHD)
- Adjustment disorder with depressed mood
- Bereavement
- Sad mood

Attribution of a depressive disorder to a medical disorder depends on the timing of the two disorders, the severity of the medical disorder, and sometimes, the patient's eventual response to treatment of the underlying medical disorder. The same applies to substance-induced mood disorders.

Dementia's extensive overlap of symptoms with depression has led to the term **pseudo-dementia** for depression in elderly people who appear demented but who do respond to antidepressants. The onset of depression is generally faster than dementia and accompanied by more cognitive and affective distress (guilt, hopelessness, and poor concentration that improves transiently with extreme effort).

Diagnosis of the depressive phase of bipolar disorder rests on a history of mania or hypomania, or sometimes on identifying a mixed state of simultaneous depressed and manic symptoms.

Attention deficit/hyperactivity disorder (ADHD) can be complicated by a secondary depression or present some symptoms of depression (poor concentration, restlessness, insomnia, or sense of worthlessness). School history and course of illness as well as response to treatment clarify this differential diagnosis. Adjustment disorder and bereavement are temporally linked to identifiable events with specified durations, beyond which these diagnoses may evolve into major depression.

The common experience of sad mood is not by itself sufficient for any diagnosis, and it lifts within hours or days. On the other hand, clusters of depressive symptoms which last 10 but not 14 days, and are sometimes severe, will not qualify for major depressive disorder but should be diagnosed depressive disorder NOS and should, in most cases, be treated as if a major depressive disorder.

16. What are the options for treating a major depressive episode?
Every patient who receives the diagnosis of major depression should learn to understand the options for treatment. They consist of antidepressant medications, psychotherapy, electroconvulsive therapy, or some combination of these. A substantial body of research has established the efficacy of each of these methods of treatment. Furthermore, with systematic trials of treatment by qualified clinicians, 80 to 90% of people with major depression will recover.

No set guidelines exist for an adequate trial of psychotherapy, but 1 hour a week for 20 weeks is a substantial trial if the therapy is focused on managing the depression (e.g., cognitive therapy for depression, or interpersonal therapy for depression). Significant symptom relief often occurs within 4 to 6 weeks.

For antidepressants 4 to 6 weeks on a therapeutic level of an antidepressant is an adequate trial. The antidepressants for which the level/response relationship has been well studied include imipramine, desipramine, amitriptyline, and nortriptyline. For selective serotonin reuptake inhibitors (fluoxetine, sertraline, paroxetine), an adequate trial is 4 to 6 weeks on 20 mg/day of fluoxetine or its equivalent, for most patients with major depression.

17. When is a person considered "refractory" to antidepressants?
Failure of two or more adequate trials may suggest refractoriness to those medications. However, close scrutiny of most drug failures reveals inadequate trials, intolerance of side effects, or complicating medical or psychosocial factors. Further carefully selected therapy trials usually result in recovery.

18. When should a depressed person be referred to a psychiatrist?
The primary care physician should refer patients with depressive disorders to psychiatrists in the following situations:
- Suicidal risk
- Need for hospitalization
- Failure of an adequate antidepressant trial
- Complicated medical or psychiatric comorbidity
- Suspected need for combined medication and psychotherapy
- Evaluation for pharmacotherapy

The psychiatrist may manage the acute episode and refer the patient back to the primary care physician for maintenance treatment. Alternatively, the two clinicians may choose to work collaboratively with patients who have complicated medical and psychiatric comorbidity.

BIBLIOGRAPHY

1. Agency for Health Care Policy and Research: Depression in Primary Care. Rockville, Maryland, U.S. Department of Health and Human Services, 1993.
2. American Psychiatric Association: Diagnostic and Statistical Manual IV. Washington, DC, American Psychiatric Association, 1994.
3. Beck AT: Depression Inventory. Philadelphia, Center for Cognitive Therapy, 1978.
4. Eisenberg L: Treating depression and anxiety in primary care. N Engl J Med 326:1080–1084, 1992.
5. Frasure-Smith N, Lesperance F, Talajic M: Depression following myocardial infarction: Impact on 6-month survival. JAMA 270:1819–1825, 1993.

6. Goldberg DP, Hillier VF: A scaled version of the General Health Questionnaire. Psychol Med 9:139–145, 1979.
7. Kaplan HI, Sadock BJ (eds): Comprehensive Textbook of Psychiatry, 6th ed. Baltimore, Williams & Wilkins, 1995.
8. Katon W: Depression: Relationship to somatization and chronic medical illness. J Clin Psychiatry 45:4–11, 1984.
9. Regier DA, Hirschfeld RMA, Goodwin FK, et al: The NIMH depression awareness, recognition, and treatment program: Structure, aims, and scientific basis. Am J Psychiatry 145:1351–1357, 1988.
10. Rovner BW, German PS, Clark R, et al: Depression and mortality in nursing homes. JAMA 265:993–996, 1991.
11. Schulberg HC, Burns BJ: Mental disorders in primary care: Epidemiologic, diagnostic, and treatment research directions. Gen Hosp Psychiatry 10:79–87, 1988.
12. Spitzer RL, Williams JBW, Kroenke K, et al: Utility of a new procedure for diagnosing mental disorders in primary care: The PRIME-MD 1000 Study. JAMA 272:1749–1756, 1994.
13. Spitzer RL, Williams JBW, Gibbon M, First M: Structured Clinical Interview for DSM-IIIR–Non-patient version (SCID-NP, version 1.0). Washington, DC, American Psychiatric Press, 1990.
14. Wells KB, Stewart A, Hays RD, et al: The functioning and well-being of depressed patients: Results from the Medical Outcomes Study. JAMA 262:914–919, 1989.
15. Williams J: A structured interview guide for the Hamilton Depression Rating Scale. Arch Gen Psychiatry 45:742–747, 1988.
16. Zimmerman M: Diagnosing DSM-IV Psychiatric Disorders in the Primary Care Setting. Philadelphia, Psychiatric Press Products, 1994.

14. PANIC ATTACKS AND PANIC DISORDER

Jon A. Bell, M.D.

1. What is a panic attack?

A panic attack is characterized by the rapid onset of fear, terror, or discomfort accompanied by at least 4 of the following:

- Palpitations, rapid heart rate
- Sweating
- Trembling or shaking
- Shortness of breath or difficulty in breathing
- Choking or difficulty in swallowing
- Chest pain or pressure
- Nausea, inability to control bowels

- Dizziness, lightheadedness
- Numbness, tingling
- Hot flashes or chills
- Feelings of unreality or depersonalization (i.e., not connected to environment or to one's body)
- Fear of dying (e.g., of a heart attack)
- Fear of going crazy or losing control

In a panic attack 4 or more of these 13 symptoms reach peak intensity in 10 minutes or less. In most cases a panic attack is readily distinguished from anxiety by its intensity and rapid, powerful onset. A panic attack is often overpowering or overwhelming. The individual experiences intense fear and feels that he or she may die, lose control, or go crazy. A strong urge to flee or escape the situation is usually reported.

2. What causes panic attacks?

To evaluate a person who has had one or more panic attacks, it is essential to establish the circumstances under which the attacks occur. In some individuals panic attacks occur unexpectedly, for no apparent reason (e.g., while watching television or waiting in line at the post office). Others have panic attacks only when they encounter specific anxiety-provoking situations, such as a crowd, an enclosed space, or distance from home. Some individuals have both spontaneous and situation-specific attacks. Most clinicians and researchers agree that the relationship between a panic attack and a specific trigger is a learned response. Spontaneous or unexpected attacks have been explained as a disturbance in the alarm or rapid response systems of the central nervous system (i.e., a fight-or-flight response with no trigger or external danger). Some argue that subtle but important triggers (e.g., feelings of breathlessness) play a key role in the genesis of "spontaneous" panic attacks.

3. What is the differential diagnosis for panic attacks?

PSYCHIATRIC DISORDERS	MEDICAL DISORDERS
Panic disorder	Hyperthyroidism
Social phobia	Hyperparathyroidism
Specific phobia	Pheochromocytoma
Obsessive compulsive disorder	Vestibular dysfunction
Posttraumatic stress disorder	Seizure disorders
Major depression	Cardiac arrhythmias
Substance intoxication (e.g., stimulants)	Medication toxicity (e.g., beta antagonists)
Substance withdrawal (e.g., benzodiazepines or alcohol)	

4. Describe the medical evaluation of a patient with panic attacks.

A detailed history is the most important step in the medical evaluation of panic attacks. The patient who has had panic attacks often focuses on particular symptoms, such as rapid heart beat and chest pain or dizziness and sweating, to the exclusion of relevant concurrent symptoms, circumstances of attack(s), rapidity of onset, and duration of attack. What initially sounds like a cardiac event or a stroke may be a recognizable panic attack as further history is obtained about the circumstances and progression of symptoms.

Even with a detailed history it may not be possible to determine whether a cardiac arrhythmia is present or whether the patient has hyperthyroidism. A focused physical assessment and disease-specific set of laboratory tests often are necessary (e.g., serum levels of thyroid-stimulating hormone [TSH] or cardiac monitoring for arrhythmias).

A common feature of anxious patients is fear of illness. Limited laboratory testing and education about panic attacks or panic disorder are sufficient to reassure most patients. A few, however, are extremely difficult to reassure and request or seek additional and unnecessary lab tests such as brain-imaging (CT scan or MRI). It is sometimes necessary to perform tests or procedures to reassure the patient and to engage him or her in treatment. Without engagement the patient who fears serious illness will seek another doctor to find out "what is really wrong."

5. What are the features of panic disorder?

Panic attacks are symptoms that may be caused by various factors. As many as 10% of the general population have reported single or infrequent panic attacks that do not seem to be due to a specific or clinically significant psychiatric or medical disorder. Panic disorder is a syndrome. People with panic disorder have recurrent, unexpected panic attacks—often more than 1 attack/week. The attacks are accompanied by 1 month or more of persistent concern about having additional attacks, worry about the significance of the attack (e.g., heart disease or fear of losing control) or significant changes in behavior (e.g., reduced physical activity because of provoking symptoms). For some patients with panic disorder the predominant characteristic is recurrent panic attacks. Others are plagued by concern or dread about having more attacks, so-called anticipatory anxiety. Attacks may occur infrequently, but the dread is always present. Some patients have few major attacks (full-blown panic attacks) but many minor attacks (with fewer than 4 associated symptoms). When panic attacks have occurred in certain situations, patients begin to associate such situations with panic attacks. Understandably, they do not want to have more attacks. The solution appears to be to avoid such situations. Hence, patients become phobic and begin to avoid situations from which escape may be difficult or in which they cannot rapidly obtain help with panic symptoms. This phobia, called agoraphobia, limits or restricts activities. The agoraphobic patient may need a companion to perform everyday functions such as driving or grocery shopping or may be unable to go outside a narrowly defined geographic area. In its most severe forms agoraphobia limits a person to his or her home.

6. Who suffers from panic disorder?

Panic disorder has been diagnosed in children as young as 8 years old. Many patients have their first panic attack in adolescence. Most people with panic disorder have the fully developed syndrome, including recurrent panic attacks, anticipatory anxiety, and phobic avoidance (agoraphobia) by the age of 30. Panic disorder develops in persons over 30 years old. New-onset cases are unusual after 40 years of age, but a few people in their 50s and 60s have developed panic disorder. One should be more suspicious of medical illness (such as thyroid disorder) symptoms that mimic panic attacks when the patient is older than 40–50 years.

Studies of both community and clinical populations consistently find that women are approximately twice as likely as men to suffer from panic disorder. The typical patient with panic disorder is a young woman with alarming physical symptoms and a high level of fear and concern about her physical well-being. Regardless of gender, most patients seek assistance from a medical provider such as a primary care physician or an emergency department physician.

In the general population the lifetime prevalence for panic disorder is 5% for women and 2% for men. In clinical populations (people seen in health care facilities) the proportion of patients with panic disorder is higher. Studies of primary care patients report that 6–8% have panic disorder. Studies in cardiology practices—a natural place to seek assessment for people who experience overwhelming episodes that suggest cardiac disease—report that up to 14% of patients have panic disorder.

7. What other psychiatric problems or disorders may be associated with panic disorder?
Various associated conditions have been identified in patients with panic disorder. One of the most common is depression. Patients with panic disorder have both acutely severe episodes (major depression) and chronic struggles with depression (dysthymia). Rates for major depression range as high as 50% or more over the course of panic disorder. Functioning already impaired by panic disorder usually deteriorates further as depression develops. Success in battling symptoms of panic disorder is lost as the despair and pessimism of depression develop. It is essential to inquire specifically about depressive symptoms in all patients with panic disorder; if found, depression should be treated aggressively.

Many people who suffer excessive anxiety, including panic disorder, have discovered that alcohol relieves some of their symptoms. Alcohol is used to reduce generalized feelings of anxiety and to block episodes of panic. When alcohol is consumed, many patients with panic also have described a reduction in phobic symptoms. For some people with intense, recurrent, disruptive symptoms, alcohol use becomes a form of self-treatment. Unfortunately, this treatment carries considerable risks. Because tolerance develops with regular use, the amount of alcohol needed to achieve the same degree of symptom alleviation increases from 2 or 3 to 5 or 6 drinks. With repeated exposure to increasing amounts of alcohol, physical dependence develops. Based on studies of patients seeking treatment for alcohol abuse and dependence, as many as 15% have an anxiety disorder.

Another common problem for patients with panic disorder is a second anxiety disorder, such as obsessive compulsive disorder or social phobia. The same type of learning in response to fear-provoking thoughts or situations and to intense symptoms occurs in panic disorder and other anxiety disorders. Patients with social phobia develop patterns of anxious behavior and avoidance similar to patterns seen in patients with panic disorder. Physiologic characteristics also may be shared with anxiety disorders.

8. Is panic disorder inherited?
Studies of the families of patients with panic disorder confirm a familial link. The lifetime prevalence of panic disorder in the general population is 3–4%. In the families of patients with panic disorder rates are 3–6 times higher. The increased prevalence in blood relatives of patients with panic disorder may be due to genetic factors, but such factors have not been identified. Learning also clearly plays a role. The child who grows up around a parent with panic disorder learns an array of anxious and fear-driven behaviors by modeling the parent. Studies of women with panic disorder and their children confirm that the children suffer from anxiety disorder (e.g., separation anxiety disorder or panic disorder) at rates higher than other children.

9. What alterations in central nervous system functioning are present in panic disorder?
Investigations in the 1960s established that panic attacks may be provoked in patients with panic disorder by intravenous infusion of sodium lactate. The same infusion had no effect in people without panic disorder. Although subsequent experiments established that lactate, the byproduct of heavy muscular exertion, does not cause panic disorder, an important insight was gained; panic attacks are associated with physiologic differences.

Subsequent studies with modern imaging technologies (e.g., positron emission tomography) have established that three brain areas function differently in individuals with panic disorder. The locus ceruleus nuclei, paired noradrenergic cell bodies in the pons, are the alarm center from which a panic attack erupts. Temporal lobe structures (e.g., amygdala) are responsible for strong emotions such as fear. Frontal cortical areas are probably involved in avoidant behavioral strategies. A lactate infusion in patients with panic disorder activates these areas of the brain. When a successfully treated patient has the same infusion, the areas are no longer activated.

10. How is panic disorder treated?
Panic disorder can be treated with medications alone, cognitive behavioral treatment (CBT) alone, or a combination of the two modalities. Medications are effective in reducing the frequency and intensity of panic attacks but have not proved effective in reducing anticipatory anxiety or phobic avoidance. On the other hand, CBT has been shown to be effective in treating all aspects of panic disorder. Therefore, treatment for most patients should include CBT strategies.

Medications shown to be effective in reducing the frequency and intensity of panic attacks include alprazolam, clonazepam, imipramine, desipramine, and phenelzine. Medications are effective when taken on a regular schedule and on a daily basis. Anecdotal reports and open-label studies suggest that selective serotonin reuptake inhibitors (SSRIs), such as fluoxetine, sertraline, or fluvoxamine, may be therapeutic.

CBT begins with a detailed analysis of anxious behaviors (thoughts, physical sensations, actions, emotions). Relaxation skills are taught to the patient, who then practices such skills on a daily basis. Distorted and catastrophic patterns of thinking are examined and challenged to reduce anticipatory anxiety. Finally, exposure to anxiety-provoking stimuli (e.g., crowds or exertion) helps to overcome phobic avoidance. An effective course of CBT takes 15–20 sessions for most patients.

BIBLIOGRAPHY

1. American Psychiatry Association: Diagnostic and Statistical Manual of Mental Disorders, 4th ed. Washington, DC, American Psychiatric Association, 1994.
2. Ballenger JC, et al: Medication discontinuation in panic disorder. J Can Psychiatry 54(Suppl):15–21; discussion, 22–24, 1993.
3. Barlow DH, Craske MG: Mastery of Your Anxiety and Panic II. Albany, NY, Graywind Publications, 1994.
4. Cox BJ, et al: Suicidal ideation and suicide attempts in panic disorder and social phobia. Am J Psychiatry 151:882–887, 1994.
5. Eaton WW, et al: Panic and panic disorder in the United States. Am J Psychiatry 151:413–420, 1994.
6. Keller MB, et al: Course and outcome in panic disorder. Prog Neuropsychopharmacol Biol Psychiatry 17:551–570, 1993.
7. Reckels K, et al: Maintenance drug treatment of panic disorder: II. Short and long-term outcome after drug taper. Arch Gen Psychiatry 50:61–68, 1993.
8. Roy-Byrne PP, et al: Psychopharmacologic treatment of panic, generalized anxiety disorder, and social phobia. Psychiatr Clin North Am 16:719–735, 1993.
9. Schweizer E, et al: Maintenance drug treatment of panic disorder: I. Results of a placebo-controlled comparison of alprazolam and imipramine. Arch Gen Psychiatry 50:51–60, 1993.
10. Shear MK, et al: Cognitive behavioral treatment compared with nonprescriptive treatment of panic disorder. Arch Gen Psychiatry 51:395–401, 1994.
11. Sheehan DV: The Anxiety Disease. New York, Bantam, 1986.
12. Tesar GE, et al: Recognition and management of panic disorder. Adv Intern Med 38:123–149, 1993.

15. SOCIAL PHOBIA AND SPECIFIC PHOBIAS

Jon A. Bell, M.D.

1. Define phobia.

Phobia is an excessive and persistent fear in a specific situation (e.g., crowds) or of clearly identifiable objects (e.g., snakes) that is out of proportion to the inherent danger. The fear cannot be
explained or reasoned away. Phobic individuals feel no voluntary control of their fear and avoid
the situation or object to control the fear. Anxiety is experienced when phobic individuals come
in contact or imagine contact with the situation or object.

2. List situations or objects that commonly provoke phobic reactions.

Animals or insects: dogs, snakes, spiders
Environmental: water, heights, storms
Blood-injury: seeing blood, venipuncture, medical procedures
Situational: closed spaces, flying, bridges, tunnels
Social: interactions, performances

3. When does a phobic reaction become a psychiatric problem?

Fear and avoidance of a situation or object do not mean that a person has a phobic disorder. For
example, a 65-year-old woman who fears and avoids dogs will function well and experience little
anxiety if she has no cause to be in contact with dogs. When her 8-year-old grandson gets a dog,
she no longer can easily avoid dogs. She experiences anxiety whenever she visits her grandson
and her relationships with her family are disrupted. Now she has a **specific phobia** of dogs, because avoidance, anxious anticipation, and distress interfere with important relationships,
whereas before she was only afraid of dogs. Fear of flying becomes a phobic disorder when a job
promotion forces a businesswoman to travel frequently to other cities and causes unrelenting
anxiety. Fear of medical procedures becomes a phobia when a dental infection requires aggressive treatment and the phobic individual cannot go to a dentist because he is too anxious and
frightened. A 35-year-old man who dreads public speaking and speaking in groups cannot advance to the next level in his occupation because his is overwhelmed by anxiety and avoids public
scrutiny at all costs. He suffers from **social phobia**. Common to all situations in which fears
become phobias (phobic disorders) are the elements of dysfunction (interpersonal or occupational) and significant anxiety and distress.

4. Are phobias common psychiatric problems?

Researchers in the epidemiology of psychiatric disorders have been surprised by how prevalent
phobias are in the general population. A recently published study of the prevalence of psychiatric
disorders in the general population reported that 6.6% of men and 9.1% of women were diagnosed as having social phobia during the past 12 months (overall average for adults = 7.9%).
When respondents were asked about social phobias at any time in their lives, the rate increased to
11.1% of men and 15.5% of women (overall average for adults = 13.3%). Specific phobias were
diagnosed in 4.4% (12-month interval) and 6.7% (lifetime) of men and 13.2% (12-month interval) and 15.7% (lifetime of women (overall averages for adults = 8.8% [12-month interval] and
11.3% [lifetime]). The only disorders more prevalent than specific and social phobias were major
depression (17.1%, lifetime) and alcohol dependence (14.1%, lifetime).

5. Do phobias begin in childhood?

Almost all children have irrational fears of commonly encountered situations or objects, such
as darkness, heights, insects or spiders, closed spaces, animals (e.g., dogs), and storms. Most

children outgrow such fears or, to be more precise, do not develop enduring fears that under the right circumstances may become phobias. A child who is confined in a toy chest by a playful, if not mean, older sibling learns from such an experience to be frightened by closed spaces from which escape is not possible. Anxiety surges when the prospect of being trapped seems possible. Although the child in this example appears to have moved closer to developing **claustrophobia** because of a specific event, not all phobias can be traced to clearcut incidents that reinforced fears. More common is a gradual, insidious growth of discomfort and fear for no obvious reason to the point that they become intense and disruptive enough to be called a phobia. Phobias of animals or insects usually begin in childhood as do phobias of environmental events and phobias of situations such as tunnels or bridges. Phobias of situations also develop in adults, e.g., a phobia of flying after a turbulent and frightening flight. Social phobias often develop by adolescence, sometimes after a significant episode of social embarrassment. However, many people with social phobias report a general feeling of discomfort in many social situations for as long as they can remember.

6. When do people with phobic disorders seek help?
Most phobic individuals rely on avoidance to manage anxiety. They find ways to live within limitations imposed by fears, often so successfully that they experience little anxiety. If they are successful, they have no need to seek help. When they are forced to go beyond their limitations, anxiety rises and they may seek treatment. A 38-year-old man who is phobic of flying is forced to deal with his phobia when he wants to take his children to Disneyland and his family wants to fly to California. Then he asks his primary care provider or a mental health professional for help. When phobias are publicly discussed in newspapers or magazines and on radio and television talk shows, phobic individuals learn more about their problem and available treatment. They usually feel shame and embarrassment about being so frightened of something that does not cause fear in most people; hence compelling external pressures are often necessary to motivate them to seek treatment. One study found that people with more than one specific phobia and panic attacks in response to the phobic situation were more likely to seek treatment than people with only one specific phobia and less intense anxiety. Intense anxiety, family pressure, and/or public education efforts help people with phobic disorders to overcome their embarrassment.

7. What routine questions could be asked to help identify people with phobic disorders?
Most health care and mental health care providers do not routinely ask patients about fears, although anxiety and fearfulness are common problems. Routine questions about fears identify some people with phobic disorders who otherwise may not reveal their difficulties. To screen for social phobia, one can ask whether a person has experienced fear of discomfort while doing things in front of other people. To screen for specific phobias, one can ask whether a person has been afraid of animals, insects, heights, blood, closed spaces, or other situations. Follow-up questioning about the intensity of the fear and activities disrupted by the fear help to determine whether a phobia is present.

8. What are the characteristics of social phobia?
People with social phobia become markedly and persistently fearful of interactive or performance situations in which they are exposed to the scrutiny of others. They fear that they will act in ways that will be embarrassing or humiliating, including becoming highly anxious. Performance situations that are often feared include public speaking, public performance (e.g., music or theater), eating in public, and writing in public (e.g., signing a check or credit card receipt). Interactive situations that are often feared include talking on the telephone, speaking to a stranger (e.g., to ask for directions), social gatherings, dating, speaking to store clerks, and speaking to authority figures (e.g., an employer or police officer). Encounters with the feared situation trigger excessive and unreasonable fear and anxiety, which interfere with functioning and cause

distress. Work or social activities are adversely affected. A pattern of avoidance and isolation often develops to reduce anxiety. Many people with social phobia avoid job assignments or even occupations (e.g., teaching or the law) to avert episodes of anxiety and embarrassment. Some people have one specific fear, but most have more than one social phobia. People with generalized social phobia fear most social situations. Alcohol is often used, at times in problematic proportions, to reduce anxiety in interactive situations. There appears to be a familial pattern for social phobia.

9. What is the differential diagnosis of phobias?

Although there is some difference between social phobia and specific phobias, the primary differential diagnosis of phobias includes the following: panic disorder with agoraphobia, other phobias, major depressive disorder, delusional (paranoid) disorder, obsessive compulsive disorder, posttraumatic disorder, hypochondriasis, eating disorders (anorexia and bulimia), and schizophrenia.

Panic disorder is differentiated by a history of panic attacks that are more pervasive (not situation-specific) and the historical onset of panic symptoms prior to avoidant behavior. People with depressive illness may be avoidant and experience panic attacks or anxiety, but they are avoidant because of apathy, loss of interest in social involvement, loss of energy, and low self-esteem. Depressed people also have a cluster of other symptoms typical of depression (see chapter 13). People with avoidant behavior due to unfounded persecutory fears may have delusional disorder or schizophrenia. In obsessive compulsive disorder fear and avoidance (e.g., of dirt or contamination) are driven by the content of obsessional thinking. In posttraumatic stress disorder fearful and avoidant behavior follows a severe stressor (e.g., plane crash, rape). Hypochondriasis requires a conviction that one is ill. Eating disorders have phobic and obsessive compulsive features, but the focus is on distorted body image and eating-related activities.

10. What medications are useful in the treatment of phobias?

Research into medication treatment of phobias has not been extensive. Recent studies of drug treatment of social phobia have shown that the monoamine oxidase inhibitor (MAOI) phenelzine and the benzodiazepine clonazepam are effective in reducing anticipatory anxiety, avoidance, and anxiety during exposure to the feared situation. Doses of phenelzine are standard—a total daily amount of 45–90 mg. Dose increases may need to be titrated slowly because of hypotension and stimulation of anxiety, and a special diet is required. Doses of clonazepam are usually 0.5–1.0 mg twice per day. The beta blocker propranolol may reduce anxiety during public performance. A dose of propranolol (10–40 mg) is taken 30–60 minutes before the performance. Situational use of benzodiazepines has been effective for some phobias, e.g., lorazepam, 0.5–1.0 mg, 1 hour or so before an airline trip, or diazepam, 5–10 mg, before a dental procedure in a person with a phobia of blood injury. Specific serotonin reuptake inhibitors (e.g., fluoxetine, sertraline) have shown promise in treating social phobia.

11. What other treatments are available?

Patterns of anxious behavior are learned. Cognitive-behavioral therapy (CBT) can be used to break anxious patterns and thereby treat phobias. After the patterns of anxious behavior are detailed and analyzed, the patient learns relaxation skills to reduce anxiety in phobic situations. A strategy for exposing the patient to stimuli that evoke anxiety develops as patterns are identified. For example, people who are claustrophobic may tolerate even a small space as long as an open door provides an avenue of escape. They may tolerate a closet but become highly anxious if the door to a spacious meeting room is closed. Having them first imagine and then experience being in a room with the door closed exposes them to a phobic stimulus and induces anxiety. Repeated exposures, often paired with anxiety-reducing (relaxation) techniques such as abdominal breathing, lessen the intensity of anxiety when they are in a room with the door closed. Within just a few weeks fear and anxiety are substantially reduced.

12. Do individuals with social or specific phobias overcome them?

Most people with social or specific phobias do not receive treatment. Some "succeed" by avoiding phobic situations but suffer the price imposed by limitations. Some challenge the phobic stimulus and through exposure overcome the phobia. Results are good for patients treated with CBT or medications; as many as 70–80% improve with treatment. Follow-up studies have concluded that people who receive CBT continue to deal with fear and anxiety successfully more often then people who have been treated only with medication. Without improvement, demoralization and depression often develop. For some, treatment is not sought until depression has become a secondary problem.

BIBLIOGRAPHY

1. American Psychiatric Association: Diagnostic and Statistical Manual of Mental Disorders, 4th ed. Washington, DC, American Psychiatric Association, 1994.
2. Davidson JR, Hughes DC, George LK, et al: The boundary of social phobia: Exploring the threshold. Arch Gen Psychiatry 51:975–983, 1994.
3. Greist JH: The diagnosis of social phobia. J Clin Psychiatry 56(Suppl 5):5–12, 1995.
4. Jefferson JW: Social phobia: A pharmacologic treatment overview. J Clin Psychiatry 56(Suppl 5):18–24, 1995.
5. Kessler RC, McGonagle KA, Zhao S, et al: Lifetime and 12-month prevalence of DSM-III-R psychiatric disorders in the United States: Results from the National Comorbidity Study. Arch Gen Psychiatry 51:8–19, 1994.
6. Liebowitz MR, Gorman JM, Fyer AJ, et al: Social phobia: Review of a neglected anxiety disorder. Arch Gen Psychiatry 42:729–736, 1985.
7. Marks IM: Fears, Phobias, and Rituals: Panic, Anxiety, and Their Disorders. New York, Oxford University Press, 1987.
8. Marks IM: Advances in behavioral-cognitive therapy of social phobia. J Clin Psychiatry 56(Suppl 5):25–31, 1995.

16. GENERALIZED ANXIETY DISORDER

Jon A. Bell, M.D.

1. What distinguishes generalized anxiety disorder (GAD) from normal anxiety?
Everyone experiences anxiety as a normal reaction in everyday life. New and stressful events evoke normal anxiety characterized by apprehension or worry and physical feelings of arousal and activation. Normal anxiety is clearly related to particular situations, such as starting a new job, meeting new people, or taking an important examination. People with generalized anxiety disorder worry excessively, often about matters for which they have no realistic reasons to worry. Worrying becomes the primary attitude or response in daily life. For such individuals anxiety and worry are too intense, out of proportion to circumstances, and disruptive of everyday functioning.

2. Describe the clinical features of GAD.
Most people suffering from GAD have experienced excessive anxiety and worry for at least 6 months. They find it difficult, if not impossible, to control their worries. When they feel anxious or worried, they also experience at least 3 of the following symptoms: restlessness, easy fatigability, difficulty in concentrating, irritability, muscle tension, and disturbed sleep. The combination of anxiety, worry, and associated symptoms causes distress for the affected individual and usually interferes with social or occupational functioning. Worrisome thoughts interfere with attending to activities at hand. Routine life circumstances, such as job or family responsibilities, or minor daily tasks, such as domestic chores, are sources of worry. Irritability adversely affects interpersonal interactions. Sleep disturbances cause fatigue and often increase the overall level of anxiety. Work performance is compromised by difficulty in concentrating.

3. How common is GAD?
GAD has been identified in children and adolescents. It was formerly called overanxious disorder of childhood but is now referred to as generalized anxiety disorder. The prevalence of GAD before 20 years of age has not been established, but more than one-half of adults who seek treatment for GAD report that symptoms of anxiety started before they reached 20 years of age. About 60% of individuals diagnosed with GAD are female. The overall lifetime prevalence for GAD is about 5% (3–4% for men, 6–7% for women). Studies have demonstrated a clear familial or heritable pattern. No specific predisposing characteristics of life events have been identified in studies of GAD.

4. What other conditions feature excessive worrying and high levels of anxiety?
A worried, anxious state of mind is not unique to GAD. People with panic disorder may worry excessively about having another panic attack, whereas people with social phobia worry about public embarrassment or humiliation. Anorexic patients worry about gaining weight, obsessive compulsive patients about germs and contamination, and hypochondriacs about life-threatening illness. Depressed individuals ruminate about problems that they feel they handled inadequately. People with worries that are clearly related to another disorder (panic disorder, obsessive compulsive disorder) do not have GAD.

5. Which comorbid psychiatric disorders occur in persons with GAD?
Many individuals with GAD experience somatic symptoms such as cold and clammy hands, dry mouth, nausea, loss of appetite, sweating, diarrhea, urinary frequency, headaches, and difficulty in swallowing. Such symptoms are also commonly seen in somatoform disorders. Some patients have both GAD and somatoform disorder. Both acutely severe and chronic depression frequently develop in patients with GAD. Other anxiety disorders, such as panic disorder, social phobia,

specific phobias, or obsessive compulsive disorder, are also common. Substance-related disorders, including nicotine dependence, alcohol abuse or dependence, sedative-hypnotic abuse or dependence, and benzodiazepine abuse or dependence often accompany GAD.

6. What medical factors contribute to GAD?

Medical Factors that May Cause Anxiety

Pulmonary diseases	Toxic conditions
Chronic obstructive lung disease	Akathisia
Asthma	Drug side effects
Pulmonary emboli	Withdrawal syndromes (alcohol, sedatives)
Neurologic diseases	Drug intoxication (stimulants, cocaine)
Strokes	Caffeine
Infections	Cardiovascular diseases
Mass lesions	Mitral valve prolapse
Epilepsy (especially temporal lobe)	Coronary artery disease
Closed head injury	Paroxysmal atrial tachycardia
Endocrine disorders	
Hypo- or hyperthyroidism	
Hypo- or hyperparathyroidism	
Diabetes mellitus	
Hypoglycemia	
Pheochromocytoma	
Carcinoid syndrome	

7. What kind of medical care do individuals with GAD seek?

Almost all persons with GAD begin their quest for relief in the office of a primary care provider. They do not usually begin by identifying themselves as worriers who feel too anxious. Instead, they focus on a specific associated symptom, such as getting tired too easily, difficulty in sleeping, or gastrointestinal upset. They usually have made no connection between their worries and their presenting complaints or are reluctant to propose any connection. The physician first investigates the presenting complaint(s), then searches for other contributing factors. A prudent medical evaluation includes a detailed history with special attention to the duration and recurrence of symptoms. People with GAD often have had years of symptoms and difficulties. Such a history should prompt the evaluator to consider and then inquire about anxiety and worry. Laboratory testing should be specific and focused on complaints and possible illnesses. For example, a patient complaining about fatigue who has also gained weight and has cold intolerance should have thyroid function tests. Soon it is clear that the patient has no serious physical illness and that anxiety is a clinically significant problem. Although some patients accept anxiety as an explanation, others are reluctant or reject the diagnosis. Patients who reject the diagnosis of anxiety often seek other opinions and treatment recommendations more compatible with their beliefs that they have medical rather than psychiatric symptoms. Mental health providers usually see patients with GAD after referral from primary care providers.

8. How is GAD treated?

The symptoms of GAD may be relieved by changes in lifestyle, stress reduction, relaxation therapies, cognitive behavioral therapy, and medication. Symptom reduction or relief usually is achieved within a few weeks to a few months, depending on treatment strategies. Changes in lifestyle and stress reduction begin with an examination of daily patterns and habits that can enhance feelings of mastery and control or diminish feelings of tension and anxiety. Most individuals find a reasonable amount of structure and predictability to be useful, because they contribute to feelings of control. Regular vigorous exercise helps to reduce tension and promotes calm and relaxation. Alcohol and caffeine often cause "wired" or anxious symptoms; limiting their use may help one to feel calmer and more in control. Adaptive techniques for dealing with conflict or confrontation may promote feelings of mastery and control. Relaxation therapies emphasize the acquisition of skills that allow the patient to feel relaxed. Relaxation training in the doctor's office is combined with practice at home, often with aids such as audiotapes. Cognitive behavioral therapy addresses detailed patterns of anxious thinking and behavior with relaxation techniques and concerted efforts to modify distorted patterns of catastrophic thinking. Cycles of anxious behavior are broken, and more adaptive approaches to anxiety-provoking situations develop during treatment. Medications are often effective in reducing symptoms. Studies confirm that benzodiazepines, tricyclic antidepressants, and buspirone are reasonable options. Benzodiazepines provide quick relief; patients usually report improvement in 1 week. Tricyclic antidepressants (e.g., imipramine) and buspirone must be taken for a few (at least 3–4) weeks before relief is achieved. The various approaches for treating GAD can be used singly or in combination. Patients must be highly motivated and persistent in their efforts to make behavioral changes. Medications require only compliance with instructions about dosages.

9. Describe the use of benzodiazepines for GAD.
Any anxiolytic benzodiazepine can be used to treat GAD. Selection of a specific benzodiazepine may be based on preference of prescriber and patient, cost, patient's health, elimination half-life, and/or metabolic factors. Older patients, patients with liver disease, and patients in poor general health may suffer toxic effects of benzodiazepines with long elimination half-lives (e.g., diazepam and chlordiazepoxide) or two-step metabolism (e.g., clorazepate and alprazolam) because of accumulation. Safer drugs for such patients are lorazepam and oxazepam, which are short elimination half-life benzodiazepines metabolized by the single step of conjugation with glucuronic acid.

Commonly Used Benzodiazepines and Therapeutic Dosing Range

DRUG	THERAPEUTIC DOSING RANGE (MG)
Chlordiazepoxide	15–40
Diazepam	5–40
Clorazepate	15–60
Oxazepam	10–120
Alprazolam	1–4
Lorazepam	1–6
Clonazepam	0.5–3

Initial doses are usually lower than final effective doses. Titration to a therapeutic dose may take 1–2 weeks. The side effect that usually governs the rate at which the dose is raised is sedation. Relief of anxiety usually starts the first week of treatment. It is imperative to explain and discuss the risk of physical dependence. Whenever a regular daily dose of a benzodiazepine, even in the therapeutic dosing range, is taken for 1 month or longer, the person is at risk for developing dependence. Dependence is usually evident when the dose is reduced or medication is stopped; patients dependent on a benzodiazepine develop withdrawal symptoms. Informing patients about the risk of dependence allows them to make an informed choice about the risks and benefits of treatment. Problems with dependence may be reduced if the use of benzodiazepine is time-limited. For example, it is prudent to stipulate that treatment with lorazepam or clonazepam will last for no more than 2 months to minimize drug exposure. Lifestyle changes and stress reduction may be pursued during the 2 months of medication. Although some patients with GAD take benzodiazepines chronically, every effort should be made to limit use to pulses or intervals of treatment paired with other strategies.

10. Describe the use of buspirone and tricyclic antidepressants for GAD.
Neither buspirone nor tricyclic antidepressants (e.g., imipramine) provide rapid relief of worry and anxiety; however, in most cases both are effective within 4 weeks. Buspirone is

well tolerated by most patients in initial doses of 5 mg 3 times/day. The dose should be raised to 10 mg 3 times/day within 2 weeks. Most patients respond to this dose. Patients who do not tolerate buspirone complain of dizziness, insomnia, nervousness, drowsiness, nausea, headaches, and fatigue.

Imipramine is effective at a dose of 100–150 mg/day (somewhat lower than the dose used to treat depression). It is necessary to start at 25 mg/day and to titrate as tolerated to a therapeutic level. Usual tricyclic side effects—dry mouth, constipation, postural lightheadedness, drowsiness, activation—may complicate treatment. In one study imipramine was found to be superior to benzodiazepines because it relieved the dysphoric mood of patients with GAD, whereas benzodiazepine did not. Other newer antidepressants, such as selective serotonin reuptake inhibitors (e.g., fluoxetine), may be effective for treating GAD.

11. What long-term follow-up is helpful for patients with GAD?

Effective treatment begins with education of patients about their condition. The signs and symptoms of GAD and associated conditions (e.g., depression or chronic bowel symptoms) should be thoroughly discussed and explained. A model that emphasizes production of symptoms by overactivity in the nervous system is useful for some patients. Others can embrace the concept that excessive worry leads to symptoms. Identifying a model for understanding illness with each patient shapes both acute treatment and long-term follow-up. During the course of acute treatment, effective interventions are established that can be applied on an ongoing basis and during subsequent episodes of disruptive anxiety. Daily relaxation exercises (e.g., yoga or meditation) or frequent vigorous exercise (e.g., bicycling or swimming) may help to prevent recurrent symptoms. Strategies that reduce concern and worry serve the same function. GAD is not cured by treatment, but it does become manageable. Long-term strategies should focus on preventing and managing symptoms and treating recurrence aggressively with therapy and/or medication. The primary provider plays a supportive role and responds when more aggressive treatment is required. Providers must avoid pejorative attitudes that attack the patient's sense of integrity (e.g., "It's all in your head, not a real illness"). Instead, acceptance of the patient's legitimate symptoms and concerns (GAD is a medical illness) enhances compliance with treatment, decreases the need for unnecessary lab tests, diminishes doctor shopping, and improves treatment outcome.

BIBLIOGRAPHY

1. American Psychiatric Association: Diagnostic and Statistical Manual of Mental Disorders, 4th ed. Washington, DC, American Psychiatric Association, 1994.
2. Brauman-Mintzer O, et al: Psychiatric comorbidity in patients with generalized anxiety disorder. Am J Psychiatry 150:1216–1218, 1993.
3. Brown TA, et al: The empirical basis of generalized anxiety disorder. Am J Psychiatry 151:1272–1280, 1994.
4. Craske MG, Barlow DH, O'Leary T: Mastery of Your Anxiety and Worry. Albany, NY, Graywind Publications, 1992.
5. Durham RC, et al: Psychological treatment of generalized anxiety disorder. A review of the clinical significance of results in outcome studies since 1980. Br J Psychiatry 163:19–26, 1993.
6. Hoelin-Saric R, et al: Differential effects of alprazolam and imipramine in generalized anxiety disorder: Somatic versus psychic symptoms. J Clin Psychiatry 49:293–301, 1988.
7. Rickels K, et al: Long-term treatment of anxiety and risk of withdrawal: Prospective comparison of clorazepate and buspirone. Arch Gen Psychiatry 45:444–450, 1988.
8. Rickels K, et al: Antidepressants for the treatment of generalized anxiety disorder. A placebo-controlled comparison of imipramine, trazodone, and diazepam. Arch Gen Psychiatry 50:884–895, 1993.
9. Roy-Byrne PP, et al: Psychopharmacologic treatment of panic, generalized anxiety disorder, and social phobia. Psychiatr Clin North Am 16:719–735, 1993.
10. Shader RI, et al: Use of benzodiazepines in anxiety disorders. N Engl J Med 328:1398–1405, 1993.

17. OBSESSIVE COMPULSIVE DISORDERS

Richard L. O'Sullivan, M.D., and Michael A. Jenike, M.D.

1. Define obsessive compulsive disorder.

Obsessive compulsive disorder (OCD) is classified in DSM–IV as an anxiety disorder manifested by either obsessions and/or compulsions that cause significant distress or dysfunction in social or personal areas. Obsessions are **thoughts** and are defined as "recurrent, persistent ideas, images, or impulses that are a significant source of distress or interfere with social or role functioning." Compulsions are **behaviors** or **mental acts** that are "repetitive, purposeful, and intentional and performed in response to an obsession or according to certain rules or in a stereotypical fashion." The thoughts or behaviors cause distress, are resisted at least initially, do not form part of a psychosis, and are recognized as senseless. **Anxiety** is a central feature of OCD, and the repetitive behaviors or mental acts are often a means to neutralize the distress associated with obsessions.

2. Define obsessive compulsive personality disorder.

Obsessive compulsive personality disorder (OCPD) may be misdiagnosed as OCD or comorbid with OCD. OCPD tends to be a chronic, pervasive condition embodying several traits, such as obsessive attention to detail, inflexibility, and perfectionism. Such characteristics differ from but may be confused with the compulsive rituals found in OCD. Obsessive compulsive personality disorder may be distinguished from OCD by the lack of obsessions, compulsions, rituals, and severe anxiety that are common to OCD. The cognitions and behaviors common to OCD are typically very disturbing, or dystonic, to the patient, whereas the personality traits of OCPD tend not to be dystonic. The symptoms of OCD frequently wax and wane in intensity, whereas OCPD traits are relatively enduring.

Obsessive Compulsive Disorder vs. Obsessive Compulsive Personality Disorder*

OBSESSIVE COMPULSIVE DISORDER	OBSESSIVE COMPULSIVE PERSONALITY DISORDER
Either obsessions or compulsions	A pervasive pattern of perfectionism and inflexibility, beginning by early adulthood, present in various contexts and:
Obsessions	
Recurrent and persistent ideas, thoughts, impulses, or images that are experienced as intrusive and senseless and cause marked anxiety or distress.	*At least 4 of 8*
	Preoccupation with details, rules, lists, order, organization and schedules.
Thoughts, impulses are not simply excessive worries about problems.	Perfectionism that interferes with task completion.
Person attempts to ignore or suppress such thoughts or to neutralize them.	Excessive devotion to work and productivity to the exclusion of leisure activities and friendships.
Person recognizes that the obsessions are the product of his or her own mind.	Overconscientious, scrupulous, and inflexible about matters of morality, ethics, or values.
Compulsions	Unable to discard worn-out or worthless objects even when they have no sentimental value.
Repetitive behaviors or mental acts peformed in response to an obsession or rigidly applied rules.	Unreasonable insistence that others submit to his or her way of doing things.
Behavior is designed to neutralize or prevent distress or some dreaded event or situation but are excessive or not realistically connected with what they are meant to neutralize.	Miserly spending style toward self and others; money is viewed as something to be hoarded.
	Rigidity and stubbornness.

Table continued on following page.

Obsessive Compulsive Disorder vs. Obsessive Compulsive Personality Disorder* (Cont.)

OBSESSIVE COMPULSIVE DISORDER	OBSESSIVE COMPULSIVE PERSONALITY DISORDER
Compulsions (Cont.)	
Person recognizes his or her behavior is excessive or unreasonable (except children).	
Obsessions/compulsions cause marked distress, are time-consuming (more than 1 hr/day), or significantly interfere with the person's normal routine.	
If another axis I disorder is present, the content of the obsessions or compulsions is not restricted to it.	
Disturbance is not due to the direct physiologic effects of a substance or general medical condition.	

* DSM-IV criteria.
Reprinted with permission from the Diagnostic and Statistical Manual of Mental Disorders, 4th ed. Copyright 1994 American Psychiatric Association.

3. How is obsessive compulsive personality disorder treated?

Care should be taken to differentiate OCD from OCPD because treatments differ. Little evidence suggests that behavioral or pharmacologic treatments, which are effective for OCD, are useful in treating OCPD. Traditional psychodynamic psychotherapy is often the treatment of choice for OCPD and may be helpful over the long term, but controlled data about effective treatments for OCPD are lacking.

4. When do everyday habits or idiosyncrasies cross the line to become OCD or require treatment?

Habits, idiosyncrasies, and compulsiveness are common human behaviors. Thoughts or behaviors become maladaptive or may require treatment when they are sufficiently distressing or so time-consuming that they interfere with functioning.

5. Is OCD a common problem?

OCD is a common problem, affecting 1–3% of populations in cross-cultural studies. It may begin at any age but most commonly becomes evident in early adulthood. Childhood cases are more common in boys than girls, but overall in adults the disorder is more common in women. The clinical presentation in childhood and late-onset cases is generally similar to adult presentations but may require more diagnostic acumen for practitioners not familiar with OCD. For example, a child who is a slow learner because he or she has to keep rereading a sentence (a form of checking) may be misdiagnosed as having a primary learning problem instead of OCD. Another example is a child who appears to have a bladder problem because of frequent trips to the bathroom, when in fact contamination obsessions drive the child to wash his hands compulsively. In older patients, anxious preoccupations with physical symptoms, sometimes misinterpreted as "ruminations," may actually be obsessions.

6. When does OCD start? How can it be recognized?

Obsessive compulsive behaviors usually have existed for many years before they come to professional attention. Onset of symptoms is generally gradual but is occasionally abrupt. The mean age of onset is approximately 22 years. OCD may start as intrusive thoughts that seem odd and frightening, such as violent images that enter the mind. Such images are distressing and are resisted, at least initially. In addition, the thoughts do not feel as though they are voluntarily created but rather as though they are intruding into consciousness. OCD also may begin as repetitive ritualized behaviors that need to be done in the same way over and over. Frequently patients show more than one obsession or compulsion, and these may change over time.

Common obsessions include contamination, aggression, bodily fears, concerns about safety or harm, and need for exactness, completeness, or symmetry. Compulsions frequently include checking, washing, repeating, counting, collecting, and hoarding. Compulsions are usually paired with obsessions. Performance of a compulsion may temporarily relieve some of the anxiety generated by an obsession. For example, after shaking hands or touching doorknobs, a person with contamination obsessions may need to wash the hands repeatedly until he or she feels clean and the anxiety associated with the obsession lessens, at least temporarily. If a person has concerns about safety or harm to others, he or she may need to recheck that nothing terrible has happened; for example, by repeatedly calling people or checking behind the car to see that no one has been run over. Such behaviors can be extremely time-consuming, sometimes taking up much of a person's day, and may have a severe, deleterious impact on functioning of the individual and family.

Although OCD may start at any time, a particularly important clinical problem is the development of postpartum OCD, which may be acute and severe in onset and easily confused or dismissed as normal anxieties of motherhood. In addition, severe or bizarre obsessions may be misdiagnosed as psychotic symptoms, particularly in people with a psychotic disorder. Attention should be paid to the potential for misdiagnosis in this population as well.

7. What are current theories about the pathophysiology of OCD?

Whereas early literature referred first to demons, then to psychodynamic influences as the genesis of OCD, growing evidence suggests a neurobiologic basis. Family studies suggest that at least some forms of OCD have a familial predisposition. Neuropsychological assessments of groups of patients with OCD demonstrate abnormalities. Structural and functional neuroimaging studies implicate basal ganglia structures, especially the striatum, as well as orbitofrontal hyperactivity in the pathophysiology of OCD. A failure of brain development has been suggested by the findings of increased gray matter and decreased white matter in OCD patients compared with normal controls. The role of environmental influences in the development and expression of OCD is not clear.

8. What disorders are possibly related to OCD?

Several disorders bear some similarities to OCD and are commonly considered within a spectrum of OCD disorders:

Trichotillomania (compulsive or repetitive hair pulling)

Body dysmorphic disorder (obsession with an imagined or exaggerated perception of a defect in appearance)

Tourette's syndrome (motor and vocal tics)

Globus hystericus (episodic fear of choking and inability to breath, often with sensation of a lump in the throat)

Compulsive skin picking or nail biting

Bowel and bladder obsessions

Olfactory reference syndrome

9. How does one screen for OCD and related disorders?

Patients are frequently secretive about symptoms because of shame about their obsessions and compulsions. Thus they are often reluctant to disclose what to them may seem to be disturbed and embarrassing thoughts and behaviors. The degree of shame, coupled with a reluctance to discuss symptoms, often results in misdiagnosis or undertreatment of the full range of suffering. Thus the first step is to ask screening questions in **every** initial evaluation. Patients may have symptoms of more than one disorder, such as both OCD and trichotillomania, or body dysmorphic disorder and skin picking. They may not realize that the conditions are treatable.

Screening Questions for Obsessive Compulsive and Related Disorders

1. Do you have thoughts, ideas, or mental images that come into your mind that you cannot seem to get rid of?
2. Are these thoughts troubling to you in some way—do they make you anxious or upset?
3. Are there any behaviors or habits that you do over and over that seem excessive or unusual?
4. Is your life negatively affected by an inflexible need to do things "just right" or in a ritualized, repetitive way?
5. Do you find that you tend to collect things excessively or have trouble throwing things out so that your home becomes cluttered?
6. Do you find yourself touching, rubbing, or picking at parts of your body repeatedly?
7. Do you ever pull out your hair?
8. Are there any aspects of your appearance that you find yourself troubled by or preoccupied with?
9. Have others commented on behaviors or actions you perform that seem unusual or excessive to them or to yourself?

10. How often is psychosis associated with OCD?
Although patients frequently report that they feel "crazy" as a result of symptoms, frank psychosis, delusions, and hallucinations are relatively uncommon in patients with OCD. If psychosis is present, it generally should not be considered as part of OCD, and other diagnoses or comorbid conditions should be considered. However, some people with body dysmorphic disorder are preoccupied with the perception of a defect to delusional proportions, and some patients with olfactory reference syndrome have delusional perceptions of odor.

11. How is OCD misdiagnosed?
OCD may be misdiagnosed as a psychotic disorder, depression, or other anxiety disorder. OCD may also be underdiagnosed when it occurs in people with developmental disorders, mental retardation, or Tourette's syndrome. The differential diagnosis should include such disorders. Neuroleptic medications have been used incorrectly to treat OCD when obsessions are misdiagnosed as psychotic symptoms or schizophrenia. Misdiagnosis generally occurs because the clinician has not inquired about the full range of symptoms that may be present in OCD, has considered "spectrum" disorders to be typical OCD, or has mistaken OCD symptoms as part of another disorder. Diagnosis may be complicated by the reluctance of some patients to disclose fully their range of symptoms, particularly with obsessions that are sexual or violent in nature, related to bodily function, or blasphemous. Although patients are often fearful that they may act on their obsessions, it is important to reassure them that it is extremely rare for patients to act upon obsessive thoughts.

12. Does routine brain imaging have a role in OCD?
Although research applications of neuroimaging have shown structural and functional brain abnormalities in people with OCD, clinical brain imaging is generally not indicated, with a few exceptions. Because obsessive compulsive symptoms may occur as a result of various illnesses, new onset of OCD symptoms in patients over age 55 may be an indication for a magnetic resonance imaging or computed tomography scan of the brain to assist in the differential diagnosis and to rule out other pathology. In atypical patients or patients with systemic autoimmune, inflammatory, vascular, or neoplastic diseases in which brain lesions also may arise, neuroimaging of the brain may be indicated. If cognitive difficulties or focal neurologic abnormalities exist, neurologic consultation and brain imaging also may be indicated.

13. How does one begin treatment for OCD?
After the diagnosis is made, the patient should be educated about the disorder. Options for behavioral and medication treatment should be reviewed. Social supports, such as self-help groups for patients and families, should be considered. Education may include several excellent

patient-oriented books. A treatment plan that considers the relative benefits of pharmacologic and behavioral interventions is typically made on a case-by-case basis. The severity or types of symptoms, as well as the resources and motivation of the patient, may be important factors in treatment planning.

14. What are effective treatments for obsessive compulsive disorder?

Clinical experience and research support two primary modes of treatment for OCD: behavioral and pharmacologic. The majority of patients report a significant improvement in symptoms with these treatment modalities. Inadequate empirical support justifies the use of psychodynamic psychotherapy as treatment for OCD. Patients with OCD, however, may have other problems that respond to psychotherapy. In addition, patients with early onset OCD may benefit from psychotherapy, because they are likely to have missed a number of developmental milestones. Psychoeducational support groups may be helpful for patients with OCD and also for their families. Excellent sources of information about local resources include the following:

Obsessive Compulsive Foundation. PO Box 70, Milford, CN 06460 (203-878-5669).

Trichotillomania Learning Center (TLC). 1215 Mission St., Suite 2, Santa Cruz, CA (408-457-1004).

Tourette Syndrome Association, Inc. 42-40 Bell Blvd., Bayside NY 11361-2874 (718-224-2999).

Anxiety Disorders Association of America. 6000 Executive Blvd., Suite 513, Rockville, MD 20852 (301-231-8368).

15. What are the components of behavior treatment for OCD?

Behavior therapy is generally effective for checking and washing rituals. Behavior therapy is symptom-focused and goal-directed and may be accomplished in as few as a dozen sessions, depending on symptom severity. Motivation and compliance are important factors in success. Behavior therapy typically begins with a behavioral analysis, identifying the various target behaviors and associated cognitions that are problematic. The environmental context for the behaviors is identified, with recognition of internal and external cues and reinforcers important in symptoms maintenance. Primary treatment for compulsive rituals consists of exposure and response prevention. Such techniques involve a graded progressive exposure to the anxiety-inducing stimulus with prevention of the associated ritualistic response. Behavior therapy is less effective for patients with obsessions and no rituals. Thought-stopping has been used with limited success. Results vary, but behavior therapy is overall an effective treatment; many patients maintain their response over extended periods. Virtually all patients should be offered a course of behavior therapy.

16. What are the first-line medications for OCD treatment?

A number of medications have demonstrated efficacy in treating OCD. All are potent serotonin reuptake inhibitors (SRIs) and effective antidepressants: clomipramine (Anafranil), fluoxetine (Prozac), sertraline (Zoloft), paroxetine (Paxil), and fluvoxamine (Luvox). Although chemically distinct, they have similar efficacy in treating patients with OCD. Patients may vary in tolerance or response to each agent. The medications also differ in pharmacokinetics, side effects, and interactions. It is believed that their antiobsessional effects result in part from blocking serotonin reuptake. It is still unclear, however, exactly how serotonin fits into the pathophysiology of OCD. Initial drug choice should be an SRI, and if the first choice is not successful or if side effects limit use, the other agents, including clomipramine, should be tried. Patients who do not respond to one medication may benefit from another in the same class. Dosage may be increased as tolerated to the upper end of recommended doses, and a trial usually should last for 10 weeks before medication is changed or augmentation strategies are begun. Response times vary. Rare patients report a quick reduction in symptoms, but maximal response may take several months. Tolerance and side effects are important factors in choice of agent, because pharmacotherapy for OCD may be long-term for some patients.

17. Should behavior therapy or medications be started first? Should they be started together?

Absolute guidelines for when to begin which type of treatment are lacking, but some general principles may help to guide clinical decision making. In general, medications should be avoided as a first-line treatment in children or pregnant women, until the patient has not responded to behavioral therapy and the severity of the illness dictates pharmacotherapy. Medications have been successfully used in the elderly as well as in patients with other serious medical problems, but care should be exercised about side effects and interactions. Patients in our clinic frequently have combined medication and behavioral therapy. The two treatments complement each other. Some patients have great success with medications or behavioral therapy alone. Patients with significant comorbid DSM–IV axis I or II illnesses, poor motivation or compliance, chaotic social situations, or only obsessions tend to do poorly in behavior therapy alone. Behavioral therapy for compulsive rituals yields improvement in about two-thirds of patients, with lasting gains over several years of follow-up. Treatment with SRIs alone generally result in moderate improvement of patients.

18. How does one gauge response to OCD treatment?

The Yale-Brown Obsessive Compulsive Scale (YBOCS) is a quick and simple clinician-administered scale that gives reliable ratings of symptom severity for obsessions and compulsions. In addition, assessment of anxiety and depressive symptoms with self-report instruments is useful. Clinical global assessments of severity and improvement are also frequently used. Treatment refractoriness may be defined as less than 25% decrease in OCD symptoms on the YBOCS or persistent significant symptoms despite adequate trials of first-line behavioral therapy or medications. It is rare that patients have complete resolution of symptoms, but the great majority get considerable relief. Strategies for pharmacologic approaches to the approximately 20% of patients who are refractory to standard treatments are shown below.

Pharmacologic Strategies for Obsessive Compulsive Disorder

AGENT	DOSE	DURATION
First-line: SRIs		
Clomipramine	Up to 250 mg/d	> 10 wk
Fluoxetine	Up to 80 mg/d	> 10 wk
Fluvoxamine	Up to 300 mg/d	> 10 wk
Sertraline	Up to 200 mg/d	> 10 wk
Paroxetine	40 to 60 mg/d	> 10 wk
Augmentation		
Clonazepam	Up to 5 mg/d	> 4 wk
Neuroleptics		
Pimozide	Up to 3 mg/d	> 4 wk
Buspirone	Up to 60 mg/d	> 8 wk
Alternative Monotherapy		
Clonazepam	Up to 5 mg/d	> 4 wk
Phenelzine	Up to 90 mg/d	> 10 wk
Tranylcypromine	Up to 60 mg/d	> 10 wk
Buspirone	Up to 60 mg/d	> 6 wk

Adapted from Jenike MA, Rauch SL: Managing the patient with treatment-resistant obsessive compulsive disorder: Current strategies. J Clin Psychiatry 55 (Suppl):11–17, 1994.

19. What conditions frequently coexist with OCD? How does this affect treatment planning and response?

Common comorbid conditions include major depression, simple and social phobia, eating disorders, substance abuse, panic disorder, and Tourette's syndrome. Comorbid axis I conditions may need to be treated first, concomitantly, or after treatment of OCD, depending on the relative clinical severity of the comorbid condition. Avoidant and dependent personality disorders are among the most common in OCD probands. Schizotypal, borderline, and avoidant personality disorders may negatively affect response to pharmacotherapy. Conversely, patients who appear to have a personality disorder while they have significant OCD symptoms may no longer meet criteria for a personality disorder once their OCD is effectively treated.

20. What is the relationship between OCD and Tourette's syndrome?
Symptoms in OCD and Tourette's syndrome may overlap; Tourette's patients frequently have OCD symptoms, and tics are common in OCD patients. Family and genetic studies and other current evidence suggest a common pathophysiology with a different phenotypic expression in some forms of Tourette's syndrome and OCD. Treatment of OCD comorbid with Tourette's syndrome generally requires neuroleptics (or clonidine) and an SRI. Behavioral therapy for tics is not highly successful overall but may be useful for compulsive rituals. The clinical and phenomenologic overlap between OCD and spectrum disorders is an exciting area of current research.

21. What is the role of neurosurgery in treatment of OCD?
Severe, disabling, treatment-refractory OCD symptoms have been successfully treated with various neurosurgical procedures, including frontal leucotomy, limbic leucotomy, anterior capsulotomy, and cingulotomy. Such procedures are reserved for patients who have failed extensive trials of behavioral and pharmacologic interventions and are literally disabled and dysfunctional as a result of OCD. Risks are those associated with any neurosurgical procedure, including infection, seizure, and potential loss of normal functioning. Neurosurgery should be considered after everything else has failed.

22. How long does OCD last? Is treatment lifelong?
OCD tends to be a chronic disorder. There may be episodic or continuous forms, and in occasional patients acute episodes do not recur. Duration of active treatment varies. Some patients have chronic low levels of symptoms by which they are not severely affected except at times of increased stress or when a concomitant axis I disorder, such as depression, occurs. At such times, patient may benefit from periodic use of medication or booster sessions of behavioral therapy. Development of behavioral skills is important in helping to keep symptoms and interference as low as possible. Some patients may require only relatively short-term use of medications (6–12 months), whereas others may need to be on medications for an extended period. Current research is attempting to determine which patients may need long-term treatment.

BIBLIOGRAPHY

 1. American Psychiatric Association: Diagnostic and Statistical Manual of Mental Disorders, 4th ed. Washington, DC, American Psychiatric Association, 1994.
 2. Baer L: Getting Control: Overcoming Your Obsessions and Compulsions. Boston, Little Brown, 1991.
 3. Baer L, Jenike MA, Black DW, et al: Effect of axis II diagnoses on treatment outcome with clomipramine in 55 patients with obsessive-compulsive disorder. Arch Gen Psychiatry 49:862–865, 1992.
 4. Baer L, Rauch SL, Ballantine T, et al: Cingulotomy for intractable obsessive-compulsive disorder. Arch Gen Psychiatry 52:384–392, 1995.
 5. Baxter LR: Neuroimaging studies of obsessive compulsive disorder. Psychiatr Clin North Am 15:871–884, 1992.
 6. Black DW, Noyes R, Goldstein RB, Blum N: A family study of obsessive compulsive disorder. Arch Gen Psychiatry 49:362–368, 1992.
 7. Breiter HCR, Filipek PA, Kennedy DN, et al: Retrocallosal white matter abnormalities in patients with obsessive compulsive disorder. Arch Gen Psychiatry 51:663–664, 1994.
 8. Goodman WK, Price LH, Rasmussen SA, et al: The Yale-Brown Obsessive Compulsive Scale. II: Validity. Arch Gen Psychiatry 46:1012–1016, 1989.
 9. Greist JH, Jefferson JW, Kobak KA, et al: Efficacy and tolerability of serotonin transport inhibitors in obsessive-compulsive disorder: Meta-analysis. Arch Gen Psychiatry 52:53–60, 1995.
10. Insel TR, Winslow JT: Neurobiology of obsessive compulsive disorder. Psychiatr Clin North Am 15:813–824, 1992.

11. Jenike MA, Baer L, Minichiello WE (eds): Obsessive-Compulsive Disorders: Theory and Management, 2nd ed. Chicago, Mosby-Year Book, 1990.

12. Jenike MA, Baer L, Ballantine T, et al: Cingulotomy for refractory obsessive-compulsive disorder. Arch Gen Psychiatry 48:548–555, 1991.

13. Jenike MA, Rauch SL: Managing the patient with treatment-resistant obsessive compulsive disorder: Current strategies. J Clin Psychiatry 55(Suppl):11–17, 1994.

14. King RA, Riddle MA, Goodman WK: Psychopharmacology of obsessive-compulsive disorder in Tourette syndrome. In Chase TN, Friedhoff AJ, Cohen DJ (eds): Advances in Neurology, Vol. 58. New York, Raven, 1992, pp 283–294.

15. McElroy SL, Phillips KA, Keck PE, et al: Body dysmorphic disorder: Does it have a psychotic subtype? J Clin Psychiatry 54:389–395, 1993.

16. Minichiello WA, O'Sullivan RL, Osgood-Hynes D, Baer L: Trichotillomania: Clinical aspects and treatment strategies. Harv Rev Psychiatry 1:336–344, 1994.

17. Orloff LM, Battle MA, Baer L, et al: Long-term follow-up of 85 patients with obsessive-compulsive disorder. Am J Psychiatry 151:441–442, 1994.

18. Pauls DL, Towbin KE, Leckman JF, et al: Gilles de la Tourette's syndrome and obsessive compulsive disorder: Evidence supporting a genetic relationship. Arch Gen Psychiatry 43:1180–1182, 1986.

19. Phillips KA: Body dysmorphic disorder: The distress of imagined ugliness. Am J Psychiatry 148:1138–1149, 1991.

20. Pitman RK, Green RC, Jenike MA, Mesulam MM: Clinical comparison of Tourette's disorder and obsessive-compulsive disorder. Am J Psychiatry 144:1166–1171, 1987.

21. Rapoport JL: The Boy Who Couldn't Stop Washing. New York, E.P. Dutton, 1989.

22. Ricciardi JN, Baer L, Jenike MA, et al: Changes in DSM-III-R axis II diagnoses following treatment of obsessive-compulsive disorder. Am J Psychiatry 149:829–831, 1992.

18. POSTTRAUMATIC STRESS DISORDER

Marita J. Keeling, M.D.

1. What are the essential characteristics of posttraumatic stress disorder (PTSD)?

The person with PTSD must have been exposed to an event involving death, serious injury, or threat to physical integrity of self or others and evoking a response of intense fear, helplessness, or horror. Such events may include military combat, violent personal assault, severe automobile accidents, or life-threatening illness. PTSD also may result from witnessing such events or learning that a loved one has experienced such events.

In patients with PTSD the response lasts longer than 1 month and consists of persistent reexperiencing of the event, persistent avoidance of associated stimuli, and persistent symptoms of increased arousal. Persistent reexperiencing may include intrusive recollections of the event, dreams, flashbacks, and intense distress or physiologic reactivity with exposure to reminders of the event. Persistent avoidance may include avoiding thoughts, feelings, or other reminders of the event, partial amnesia, diminished involvement in usual activities or relationships, restricted emotions, and a sense of a foreshortened future. Persistent symptoms of increased arousal may include sleep disturbance, irritability, difficulty in concentrating, hypervigilance, and exaggerated startle response. In addition the distress must be significant enough to cause impairment in social, occupational, or other functioning. There are three types of PTSD:
- Acute—duration of symptoms is less than 3 months
- Chronic—duration of symptoms is greater than 3 months
- Delayed—onset of symptoms is at least 6 months after the stressor

2. Describe the historical development of understanding of PTSD and limitations of the diagnostic criteria.

In the 19th century *railway spine* was diagnosed in patients whose world view had been shattered by traumatic experiences. The term reflected the cultural view that an actual physical disruption of the nervous system had occurred. After World Wars I and II people who had been exposed to combat sometimes suffered from a constellation of symptoms variously termed *shell-shock, battle fatigue,* or *traumatic or war neurosis.* The original edition of the American Psychiatric Association's Diagnostic and Statistical Manual (DSM) in 1952 included *gross stress reaction,* which referred to combat as one possible type of stress. DSM-II in 1968 changed the diagnosis to *transient situational disturbances.* DSM-III (1980) first used the term PTSD to describe a characteristic constellation of symptoms following "a recognizable stressor that would evoke symptoms of significant distress in almost everyone." DSM-IIIR in 1987 broadened the definition of traumatic event to include events "outside the range of usual human experience and that would be markedly distressing to anyone." DSM-IV again restricted the concept to experiences that threaten physical integrity.

3. List associated features of PTSD.
- Survivor guilt (e.g., why did I survive when other, better people died?)
- Impaired relationships, which may extend to marital problems, sexual dysfunctions, divorce, loss of job
- Impaired capacity to regulate and tolerate feelings
- Self-destructive and impulsive behavior
- Dissociative symptoms
- Somatic complaints
- Personality change (e.g., becoming angrier, more aloof)
- Change in world view or belief system

- Feelings of ineffectiveness, shame, despair, hopelessness, permanent damage, hostility, or constant fear of danger
- Social withdrawal

4. Discuss comorbid diagnoses.

Comorbid diagnoses are quite common. In a study of firefighters who had been exposed to a natural disaster, only 23% of those who developed PTSD did not have another diagnosis. In addition, comorbidity appeared to be a good predictor of the development of chronicity. Clearly it is important to identify and treat concurrent psychiatric illness. Depressive symptoms and disorders are probably the most common coexisting symptoms and conditions. Anxiety disorders, phobias, obsessive compulsive disorder, somatization, eating disorders, and substance-related disorders also may occur. Although these and other disorders are commonly observed in the context of treatment for PTSD, studies are limited in terms of assessing whether they preceded or followed the onset of PTSD.

5. How does PTSD differ in children and adults?

Children may experience generalized dreams (e.g., monsters, being chased) rather than trauma-specific dream content. Instead of having intrusive thoughts or flashbacks, they may show repetitive play with themes of the traumatic event or demonstrate compulsive reenactment of the event. Such play or reenactment may be quite deleterious in and of itself. For example, sexualized traumatic play or reenactment by children who have been sexually abused may traumatize other children and adults and result in impaired social relationships and school problems as well as problems with identity development. Certainly some children who have been sexually abused may link sexuality and aggression and develop perpetrating behavior (even in early childhood) and numerous sexual dysfunctions in later life. Reenacting the trauma (e.g., hitchhiking with strangers after a kidnapping) places the child at great personal risk of further trauma. (In adulthood a revictimization syndrome or "sitting-duck syndrome" may be seen.) In general, because of their limited capacity to express events and emotions in words, children's behavior must be carefully observed for indications of persistent reexperiencing, persistent avoidance, and hyperarousal. Self-destructive behavior, such as biting and headbanging, are common.

Children also have been observed to develop **omen formation**, in which they report that some omen that they chose to ignore preceded the traumatic event. It is thought that many such symptoms are the child's attempt to regain a sense of control. Children are also more likely to experience somatic symptoms, again probably because of limitations in expressing thoughts and feelings. The frequency and degree of development of psychogenic amnesia are unclear.

The physiologic hyperarousal that children experience may interfere with learning, concentration, and memory. Children may be diagnosed with attention deficit disorder. In addition, they may lose recently acquired maturational achievements and show regression (e.g., inability to maintain toilet training or tolerate separation from parents). The use of dissociation to compartmentalize memories and feelings is thought by many to be the precursor to development of serious dissociative disorders in later life. Emotional numbing is thought to interfere with normal development and the capacity to fantasize and therefore plan for the future. In addition, the loss of awareness of emotional feelings may result in an inability to distinguish between emotions and somatic symptoms and lead to the development of adults with alexithymia (i.e., the inability to describe or identify emotional states) or somatization disorders. Recent studies also demonstrate a strong link between adults with borderline personality disorder and childhood sexual trauma. This finding may relate to arrested cognitive and emotional development caused by early response to traumatic events.

6. Describe the typical course of PTSD.

PTSD may develop in early childhood or at any later time. Onset may be immediate or delayed, sometimes occurring many years after the traumatic event. Complete recovery occurs within 3 months in about one-half of people. For many others it is a waxing and waning illness with considerable variability in the relative predominance of symptoms. Often people shift from periods in which avoidant symptoms are predominant to periods in which persistent reexperiencing is more noticeable. Patients typically first seek psychotherapeutic treatment during a phase of reexperiencing (nightmares, flashbacks, intense anxiety), although coexisting depression and suicidal impulses are also common presentations. PTSD complicated by comorbid disorders (whether preexisting or secondary) may have particularly complex, dangerous, and treatment-resistant courses; hospitalization for safety or stabilization may be necessary. Sometimes the term **posttraumatic personality disorder** is used to emphasize the enduring nature of characteristic maladaptive patterns of thinking and behaving and poor response to treatment.

Exposure to reminder stimuli may cause a relapse of the illness even after many months or years of remission. Anniversary dates often result in an exacerbation of symptoms, even when patients are unaware of thinking about the traumatic experience. Sometimes the events that trigger the first occurrence or reappearance of symptoms seem minor to others (e.g., hearing firecrackers on the Fourth of July for a Vietnam veteran or watching the movie *The Burning Bed*, which deals with rape and wife-battering, for a rape survivor).

7. What is the differential diagnosis?

Acute stress disorder is the diagnosis used when the symptoms have not lasted for as long as a month. **Adjustment disorder** is diagnosed if the stressor was not life-threatening or symptoms last for less than 1 month or do not meet full criteria for PTSD. If the stress was the death of a loved one, the diagnosis is **bereavement**.

Many of the symptoms of avoidance also may be seen in depressive disorders, and **major depression** is the most common coexisting disorder. Avoidance is also seen in **phobic disorders**. Symptoms of hyperarousal may occur in **anxiety disorders**. Intrusive thinking occurs in **obsessive compulsive disorder**. Flashbacks must be differentiated from hallucinations or other perceptual disturbances that may occur in any of the psychotic disorders, including **delirium, dementia**, and **substance-induced disorders**. Flashbacks and amnesia are considered dissociative symptoms by many practitioners, who thus consider PTSD a type of dissociative disorder; other practitioners consider **dissociative disorders** to be forms of PTSD (with the general assumption that childhood trauma was the original cause). Some patients with PTSD may be diagnosed with **antisocial personality** disorder (e.g., Vietnam veterans who demonstrate substance abuse, episodes of rage, and value conflicts). In **malingering** (feigning a psychiatric disorder) avoidance of punishment (e.g., in criminal settings) or financial gain (e.g., lawsuits, disability benefits) may be the motivation. Unconscious creation or exacerbation of symptoms may occur in individuals who achieve secondary gains such as obtaining approval, emotional contact, or a sense of belonging from those around them.

Persistent PTSD presents with symptom patterns that overlap with those of **borderline personality disorder**. Indeed they may coexist in patients with early childhood sexual trauma.

8. What risk factors may increase the severity of symptoms?

There are surprisingly few clear data about risk factors, probably because (1) a number of sociocultural factors (e.g., culture, gender, socioeconomic status) may influence the outcome and (2) the specific stressor may affect the specific type of symptoms. For example, many practitioners believe that PTSD caused by sexual trauma is quite different from the response of survivors to a fire or a volcano. Because symptoms remain trauma-specific, they vary with the nature of the trauma. For example, a rape survivor may have difficulties in sexual and interpersonal relations, whereas survivors of natural disasters may avoid fire or specific geographical areas.

In general, the greater the severity, duration, and proximity of the individual to the traumatic event, the greater the likelihood of developing PTSD. One problem in assessing risk factors is the fact that most studies focus on only one subgroup of survivors (e.g., Vietnamese boat refugees in Norway, American Vietnam war veterans, rape victims, school children who witnessed a shooting). It is difficult to determine, therefore, the significance of factors such as cultural background, sex, and age, in causing variation in patterns. The prevalence of PTSD may be extremely high (e.g., 93% of Laotian hill people refugees and as many as 50% of combat veterans), but the figures vary considerably, depending on how exposure is measured.

In some instances, observation of traumatic events (e.g., watching people die in a fire) results in more symptoms than actual injury. This phenomenon is thought to be related to survivor guilt. **Previous exposure** to traumatic events, such as prolonged child abuse, may sensitize individuals to later events (i.e., the straw that broke the camel's back). **Lack of social support systems** or community cohesion appears to increase symptoms. Symptoms also may increase and/or persist with additional adversity related to the initial event (e.g., legal proceedings after a rape or divorce after the death of a child). In effect, the result is continuous trauma. **Previous psychiatric disturbance** also may increase the likelihood of developing PTSD.

Interpersonal sensitivity, somatic symptoms, aggressive feelings and actions, avoidance, subjective experience of suffering, high level of dissociative symptoms immediately after the trauma, and preexisting depression are implicated in severity of symptoms. When physical injuries or pain are involved with the original trauma, chronic pain syndromes may develop in which the perception of pain far outweighs the objective findings (e.g., chronic pelvic pain in women with a history of rape).

However, it is not necessary to have predisposing factors to develop PTSD, especially when the stressor is extreme.

9. Describe a typical course of psychotherapeutic treatment.

There is no such thing as a typical course of treatment. An eclectic range of treatments and combinations has been used, including psychodynamic psychotherapy, cognitive-behavioral therapy, desensitization with learned relaxation, group therapy, hypnosis, narcosynthesis, and pharmacotherapy. A central goal of treatment is to provide the patient with a reparative sense of regaining control, which helps to restructure a new and hopefully constructive world view and directly combats the feelings of helplessness and loss of control, which are the essence of traumatic experience. The traumatized individual feels that his or her concept of the world and role within it has been irretrievably shattered and that the sense of safety or personal power cannot be regained. In order to recover, the traumatized individual must make the **identity shift** from victim to survivor to thriver (i.e., one who can healthily enjoy life again and no longer has a primary identification associated with trauma).

In acute settings safety must be provided first (e.g., battered women's shelters), and basic needs for medical care, food, shelter, and clothing must be met. Early identification of the disorder and education of patients so that they understand what to expect and have a framework for understanding their response are thought to reduce the patient's experience of being "crazy" and the tendency to feel intense self-blame. Explaining that aggressive thoughts or actions are a common response to feeling out of control may reduce dangerous responses.

Most agree that chronic PTSD may result in an extended course of illness and may be crippling; therefore, early treatment must be provided wherever possible. It is also generally thought that providing the opportunity to describe the traumatic experience as fully as possible in words is helpful. One of the few controlled studies of rape survivors found that both prolonged exposure (i.e., having the patient relive the experience over and over again in imagination in the context of a safe setting) and stress inoculation training (i.e., training the patient to relax and to develop various coping mechanisms) were effective forms of treatment; prolonged exposure, however, was the most successful.

Sexual dysfunctions may require specific sex therapy. Often couple or family therapy is indicated for patients with interpersonal problems. Group psychotherapy may be particularly helpful, because survivors experience a sense of belonging, discover that their symptoms are "normal" in a traumatized population, maintain social contacts, share coping strategies, and talk about their feelings in a safe setting. Outdoor experiences of physical and emotional mastery, such as those offered by Outward Bound for victims of trauma, may be extremely helpful. Self-defense programs for victims of muggings and rape may likewise facilitate redevelopment of a sense of security.

It is critically important to treat coexisting disorders such as alcohol abuse. Individuals who abuse alcohol or other substances have a poorer prognosis for recovery and also develop related sequelae. Generally, substance abuse must be treated before PTSD. Care must be taken in prescribing potentially addictive medications, because iatrogenic substance dependence may occur quite easily.

Common symptoms of PTSD may interfere with treatment. For example, avoidance symptoms may result in a patient who appears to be noncompliant and uncooperative. Especially if the trauma involved human perpetration, the patient may demonstrate high levels of distrust. Strategies should be developed to reduce the risk of dropping out of treatment.

Because it is intensely distressing to hear about the traumas of their patients, a secondary PTSD may develop in health care providers. In attempting to protect himself or herself from such emotional stress, it is easy for the physician to blame the victim. Providers must guard against this response while attempting to maintain a warm, supportive, and educational stance with frequent repetitions of reassurance and information.

Overall, however, it is difficult to treat the 50% of survivors who do not recover within the first 3 months. As a consequence, practitioners constantly look for new forms of treatment. Eye-movement desensitization and reprocessing is a recently developed treatment that many practitioners believe to be particularly promising. Induction of rapid eye movements in the patient is combined with attempts to restructure cognitive distortions. In ego state therapy the practitioner assists the patient (often through hypnosis) to picture unconscious ego states such as "inner children" to facilitate a dialog between the primary conscious state and unconscious states. This technique may allow further exploration of unconscious conflicts and needs and enable a kind of "internal family therapy" that resolves such conflicts and meets needs in a healthy way.

10. What medications may be useful in the treatment of PTSD?

Pharmacologic treatment is notoriously variable and limited, depending on the patient. Generally, medications that are known to be effective in prominent syndromes (such as depression or anxiety) are the logical starting point. Often physicians prescribe a long series of trials of different medications with limited or no obvious benefit to the patient. It is not unusual to find unusual combinations of medications, which frequently reflect the desperation of the patient.

A common pitfall is to change medications too rapidly without reaching adequate doses or trial periods, because the patient reports ongoing, intense feelings or complains of side effects. The practitioner should empathize with the patient about how difficult it is to wait and/or to tolerate side effects while providing information and reassurance. Some practitioners advocate that patients should have an unusual amount of control of choice and decision-making and believe that the psychological benefits of regaining a greater sense of control over their lives outweighs the consequent limitations of medication. This approach is controversial.

Agents that reduce autonomic arousal, such as clonidine, beta-adrenergic blockers, and benzodiazepines, have proved helpful, although no controlled studies exist. Virtually all other classes of psychotropic agents, including tricyclic antidepressants, monoamine oxidase inhibitors, lithium carbonate, carbamazepine, and neuroleptics, have been tried, but virtually no controlled studies exist. Recent studies indicate that selective serotonin reuptake inhibitors may be particularly useful.

11. Discuss the neurobiologic implications of research in PTSD.

Current research in PTSD is fascinating. Studies of nonhuman primates as well as humans have shown many **neurochemical effects** of stress—including effects on catecholamine, cortisol, serotonin, and endogenous opioid responses—that may lead to more effective pharmacologic treatments.

Developmental effects also have been observed. Early disruptions of social attachment bonds in studies of nonhuman primates have clearly demonstrated that early trauma reduces the long-term capacity to cope well with later social disruptions and to modulate physiologic arousal. Clinical observations of the effects of child abuse and other disruptions in humans are consistent with such findings. Children have higher than normal levels of catecholamines long after the traumatic event has passed. Obviously, such findings suggest that pharmacologic and other interventions that may prevent long-term sequelae must be developed and put into practice as quickly as possible.

Although people often demonstrate emotional avoidance or constriction in their attempts to cope with environmental stress after trauma, physiologically their bodies continue to react with **autonomic arousal** (e.g., catecholamine flooding, as if life-threatening conditions still exist). The normal function of autonomic arousal to alert the individual and to stimulate a suitable fight/flight reaction is lost; people can no longer rely on body cues to interpret levels of danger. This phenomenon also results in a loss of affect modulation; people experience intense feelings of fear, anger, or anxiety, even when the stimulation is minor (e.g., an authority figure speaks in a tone of annoyance). There are no shades of gray in PTSD; everything (physiologically, emotionally, and cognitively) becomes all or nothing. This problem must be addressed in psychotherapy to retrain individuals to assess and modify their responses to ongoing life experiences.

Nonspecific **central nervous system abnormalities** and neurologic "soft signs" have been observed in survivors of trauma. Positron emission tomography has shown differential blood flow to regions of the brain, particularly the hippocampus. People subjected to a stimulus resembling the original trauma, even many years later, produce endogenous opioids and analgesia that is reversible with naloxone. Opioid production may play a role in psychic numbing. In addition, sound evidence suggests that endogenous opioid changes in the CNS play a direct role in the development of self-mutilation behaviors when survivors of trauma accidentally discover that injury produces a profound calming reaction. The temporal lobe, which plays a major role in memory storage, is also implicated in PTSD. The locus ceruleus may play a role in flashbacks and traumatic nightmares.

As in many areas of medicine, most research to date has been laboratory-based and focused on Western men. Future research must focus on possible sex-related differences and cross-cultural differences in how cognitive reconstruction may modify belief systems and perceptions and therefore alter biochemical responses. More clinical studies are necessary to determine accuracy and practical applications of research data.

CONTROVERSIES

12. Does DSM-IV offer adequate criteria for the diagnosis of PTSD?

Despite general agreement on types of symptoms of PTSD, a major controversy is how to define the nature of a traumatic event. As indicated above, DSM-IV requires that the event involve actual or threatened death or serious injury or threat to the physical integrity of self or others. In addition, the response must involve intense fear, helplessness, or horror. However, individual or cultural factors, including personality and prior life experiences, may affect response to an experience that many may consider relatively minor.

One example is sexual harassment or sexual relationships in a usually proscribed setting (e.g., between priest and parishioner, patient and physician). Such situations rarely include a threat to physical integrity, and yet individuals may otherwise meet all criteria listed in DSM-IV. Failed adoption, miscarriage, and a spouse's affair have resulted in a syndrome indistinguishable from PTSD. Yet by DSM-IV guidelines, such individuals must be diagnosed with another disorder. Although it is laudable to limit the definition of PTSD so that it does not become so general that it loses meaning, some individuals may remain untreated because they do not meet the formal criteria. Practitioners and researchers have different opinions about such issues, and they are likely to remain controversial for some time.

In addition, some patients probably would be treated most effectively if diagnosed with PTSD, but for various reasons the diagnosis may not be considered. This problem is especially likely in delayed PTSD. For example, the survivor of a rape that occurred many years earlier may not mention the rape to the evaluator because of her need to avoid painful feelings, or a Vietnam veteran may demonstrate only symptoms of avoidance at evaluation, although other symptoms may ebb and flow or present occasionally, depending on responses to reminder stimuli. Such patients may not receive the treatment they require because the correct diagnosis has not been made.

13. What is the likelihood of complete amnesia?
The issue of amnesia for aspects of the traumatic event is another controversial topic. It is generally agreed that partial amnesia can and does occur. However, there is considerable disagreement about the possibility of complete amnesia for an event or series of events, such as childhood sexual abuse. Clearly, if amnesia for past traumatic events is extensive and complete, the diagnosis may be missed, because the patient cannot report the stressor.

14. What is the appropriate role of early identification and education?
The concept of early identification and education at first glance does not appear to be controversial. Despite its simplicity, however, it has become controversial in the treatment of sexual abuse, particularly when adults are thought to present with delayed PTSD due to childhood trauma. The difficulty is that overzealous therapists may overdiagnose PTSD, assume that symptoms are caused by sexual abuse, use overinclusive and nonspecific lists of "common symptoms," and encourage the development of symptoms in patients who were not in fact abused. Therapists who advocate immediate identification and education point out that many victims of abuse may repress memories (to what degree this may occur is also controversial) or deny their experiences to avoid emotional pain and therefore may go without necessary treatment if the therapist does not raise the possibility of PTSD and sexual trauma. Such variable viewpoints have become crystallized in the current debate about false memory syndrome (see chapter 82).

15. What is the appropriate role of hypnosis in recovering suppressed memories?
A related area of controversy is the use of hypnosis to enhance memories of the traumatic experiences. Individual practitioners frequently report that they are certain that the "memories" recovered are accurate and that vivid reexperiencing of the trauma is helpful in working through and recovery. However, research indicates that it is not possible to determine whether hypnotically enhanced memories are accurate or confabulated without obtaining outside corroboration. Thus a major current concern is the possibility that both patients and therapists will believe in experiences that did not occur.

BIBLIOGRAPHY
1. Courtois CA: Adult survivors of sexual abuse. Prim Care 20:433–445, 1993.
2. Davidson JRT, Foa EB (eds): Posttraumatic Stress Disorder. DSM-IV and Beyond. Washington, DC, American Psychiatric Press, 1992.
3. Epstein RS: Posttraumatic stress disorder: A review of diagnostic and treatment issues. Psychiatr Ann 19:556–563, 1989.
4. Herman JL: Trauma and Recovery. New York, Harper-Collins, 1992.
5. Kluft RP (ed): Incest-related Syndromes of Adult Psychopathology. Washington, DC, American Psychiatric Press, 1990.
6. Pynoos RS (ed): Posttraumatic stress disorder. In Oldham JM, Riba MB, Tasman A (eds): Review of Psychiatry, vol 12. Washington, DC, American Psychiatric Press, 1993.
7. Reiker PP, Carmen EH: The victim-to-patient process: The discomfirmation and transformation of abuse. Am J Orthopsychiatry 56:360–370, 1986.
8. Saigh PA: The behavioral treatment of child and adolescent posttraumatic stress disorder. Adv Behav Res Ther 14:247, 1992.
9. Scrignar CB: Post-traumatic Stress Disorder: Diagnosis, Treatment, and Legal Issues, 2nd ed. New Orleans, Bruno Press, 1988.
10. Sugarman A (ed): Victims of Abuse. The Emotional Impact of Child and Adult Trauma. Madison, International University Press, 1993.
11. Terr LC: Psychic trauma in children and adolescents. Psychiatr Clin North Am 8:815–835, 1985.
12. Van der Kolk BA: Psychological Trauma. Washington, DC, American Psychiatric Press, 1987.
13. Van der Kolk BA, Fisler RE: The biologic basis of posttraumatic stress disorder. Prim Care 20:417–431, 1993.

19. PSYCHOACTIVE SUBSTANCE USE DISORDERS: OVERVIEW, DEFINITIONS, AND COMMONALITIES

Jane A. Kennedy, D.O.

1. Define psychoactive substance use disorder, addiction, and dependence.

Terms used to define substance use disorders are varied and confusing. For the most part, loss of control, compulsion to use, and continued use despite adverse consequences are indicative of **psychoactive substance use disorder.** To many, the term **addiction** implies the psychological compulsion to use a substance whereas the term **dependence** implies the physiologic components of withdrawal or tolerance.

However, the Diagnostic and Statistical Manual Fourth Edition (DSM–IV), of the American Psychiatric Association expands the definition of dependence. For a diagnosis of psychoactive substance dependence, three or more criteria, which may or may not include physiologic tolerance or withdrawal, must be met. Other criteria include persistent efforts to cut down or stop use; using more or for a longer time than intended; filling one's time with drug or alcohol activities, such as intoxication or drug procurement; giving up important life activities, such as work or family; and continued use despite knowledge that it will cause or worsen physical or psychological problems.

For a diagnosis of psychoactive substance use disorder, only one criterion is needed: repeated failure to fulfill significant role obligations; recurrent use in physically hazardous situations, such as driving when intoxicated; repeated substance-related legal problems; or continued substance use despite related social or interpersonal problems. For both abuse and dependence, such maladaptive behaviors must have a duration of at least 1 month. A diagnosis of dependence suggests a more serious condition.

2. Does addiction run in families?

Yes. The risk of addiction is 3–4 times higher for children of substance abusers than for children of non-substance abusers. The cause may be genetic, environmental, or a combination of factors. Familial patterns have been studied primarily in alcoholic families. Twin studies reveal a higher concordance of alcoholism in monozygotic than dizygotic twins, and adoption studies show that twins raised apart have a similar increase in prevalence of alcoholism, whether raised in non-alcoholic or alcoholic families. However, because the concordance in monozygotic twins is not 100%, environmental factors may play an equally important part in the development of alcoholism.

3. How should a physician ask about drug and alcohol problems?

Most patients with alcohol or drug problems are fearful of negative reactions from their physician if they tell the truth. The physician should start by asking questions about tobacco, alcohol, and marijuana in a matter-of-fact, nonjudgmental manner. Questions should address how much (not whether) the patient drinks, blackouts, drunk driving, and whether *the patient* thinks that he or she ever drinks more than he or she should. Similar questions should be asked about each category of drugs, including routes of administration.

Several screening questionnaires have been found to be useful in primary care. The Michigan Alcohol Screening Test (MAST) has 25 questions to be answered by the patient but may be too lengthy in the primary care setting. The CAGE questionnaire is easier to use for taking a history. It consists of four questions.

1. Have you tried to **C**ut down on alcohol?
2. Have you been **A**nnoyed when someone criticized your drinking?
3. Have you felt **G**uilty about your drinking?
4. Have you used alcohol as an **E**ye-opener by having a drink in the morning?

Two or more positive answers suggest alcohol problems with high sensitivity and specificity. The physician may substitute or add the word drug to get a similar screen of drug problems.

4. What is the relationship between substance use disorders and psychiatric illnesses?

Dual diagnosis of substance use disorder and psychiatric illness is a complex issue. In primary substance use disorders, chronic use may induce psychiatric symptoms; for example, psychosis from stimulants or hallucinogens or depression from alcohol dependence. In substance use disorders secondary to psychiatric illnesses, patients may self-treat their symptoms; for example, alcohol may be used to relieve anxiety or to decrease manic symptoms. In addition, patients may have independent syndromes of substance abuse and major mental illness.

The diagnosis of comorbid psychiatric and substance use disorders is significant, and the reported prevalences may depend on the populations surveyed. In the general population, 27% have a diagnosis of substance abuse or dependence at some time during their lifetime. On the other hand, nearly half of patients with schizophrenia had a substance use disorder, and substance abuse or dependence was found in 84% of patients with antisocial personality disorder. Substance abuse or dependence was seen in 24% of patients with anxiety disorders and 32% of patients with affective disorders; in patients with bipolar illness, the prevalence of substance use disorder was 56%. In addition, comorbid substance use disorders are seen in approximately 90% of prisoners who have schizophrenia, bipolar disorder, or antisocial personality disorder. About 50% of patients admitted to public psychiatric hospitals and 40–50% of hospitalized medical patients have comorbid substance abuse or dependence.

It is best to wait 3–6 weeks after a patient becomes abstinent before diagnosing a psychiatric disorder; often the symptoms of depression, anxiety, or psychosis disappear as the patient clears of substance abuse. However, in patients with a definite history of psychiatric disorder before onset of substance abuse or during periods of abstinence, treatment can be initiated immediately.

5. Does treatment work?

Yes, but no one treatment works for all patients. Some people stop alcohol use without formal treatment or with brief interventions, such as advice from their physician. Many types of formal treatment modalities are discussed in the following chapters about specific substances. In general, substance use disorders are chronic and relapsing; the treatment goal is to decrease the frequency and duration of relapses as well as morbidity and mortality. Like other chronic diseases such as hypertension or diabetes, the aim is management rather than cure.

Stopping the substance use must be the primary goal. In the early phases of treatment, patients need external controls, such as urine or breath monitoring, behavioral contracting, and involvement of family or employer to help them stop. Once the patient is abstinent, the focus is prevention of relapse, which includes reducing accessibility of the substance, identifying stimuli that may trigger cravings, understanding feelings, and developing coping responses and improved social skills. Relapse is high during the first year of treatment, but as periods of abstinence lengthen, the likelihood of relapse decreases. Ongoing treatment should involve a biopsychosocial model, attending to health and psychiatric problems as well as marital, occupational, legal, financial, and social functioning. For any substance use disorder, a worse prognosis is associated with unemployment, lack of social support system, and presence of psychopathology, especially antisocial personality disorder.

6. Is inpatient treatment better than outpatient treatment?

The long-term benefit of inpatient hospitalization vs. outpatient treatment has not been documented. Patients with complicated medical or psychiatric problems, severe withdrawal, suicidality, or risk of seizure require inpatient treatment, but extended hospital stays have not been associated with increased long-term abstinence.

7. Should patients be completely abstinent? Or can they learn to control their use?
At this time little evidence suggests that controlled use can be achieved; abstinence should be the goal. Some patients want to abstain from their drug of abuse but use other substances in moderation; this practice is a potential trigger of relapse. Not infrequently, patients switch substances (quit heroin and become dependent on alcohol) or develop a second dependence (continue alcohol and add benzodiazepines).

8. Should all patients attend a self-help group?
Self-help groups may be extremely beneficial. Alcoholics Anonymous (AA), Narcotics Anonymous (NA), Cocaine Anonymous (CA), Rational Recovery (RR), or other such groups provide structure and support, decrease stigma, and offer hope as patients see others recover. However, outcome research shows that the drop-out rate in the first year of AA attendance is high (50–75%) and that although AA is helpful to those who stay, others may need to seek professional treatment. Self-help programs can be used in combination with professional treatment.

9. What is a therapeutic community?
Therapeutic community (TC) refers to residential, long-term (6–12 months) treatment usually with gradual re-entry into society. In general, the approach is based on milieu therapy and highly confrontive, with strict limits and structure. Graduates of the programs often become staff members, having increased their level of responsibility as they progressed through the program. The drop-out rate in the first few months of treatment is high (75–80%), but graduates have improved outcome in terms of drug use, crime, and employment.

10. Should family members be included in alcohol or drug treatment?
Behavior associated with substance use disorders significantly affects family members, who may participate indirectly or directly in maladaptive patterns. They should be included in the patient's treatment, both for themselves and to help monitor and provide external control for the patient. Part of relapse prevention should be an agreement that the spouse will contact the treatment provider if concern develops about relapse.

BIBLIOGRAPHY

1. American Psychiatric Association: Diagnostic and Statistical Manual of Mental Disorders, 4th ed. Washington, DC, American Psychiatric Association, 1994.
2. Arif A, Westemeyer J: Manual of Drug and Alcohol Abuse. New York, Plenum, 1988.
3. Ciraulo DA, Shader RI: Clinical Manual of Chemical Dependence. Washington, DC, American Psychiatric Press, 1991.
4. Galanter M, Kleber HD: Textbook of Substance Abuse Treatment. Washington, DC, American Psychiatric Press, 1994.
5. Institute of Medicine: Broadening the Base of Treatment for Alcohol Problems. Washington, DC, National Academy Press, 1990.
6. Kessler RC, McGonagle KA, Zhao S, et al: Lifetime and 12-month prevalence of DSM-III-R psychiatric disorders in the United States. Arch Gen Psychiatry 51:8–19, 1994.
7. Lowinson JH, Ruiz P, Millman RB, Langrod JG: Substance Abuse: A Comprehensive Textbook. Baltimore, Williams & Wilkins, 1992.
8. Milhorn HT Jr: Chemical Dependence: Diagnosis, Treatment, and Prevention. New York, Springer-Verlag, 1990.
9. Miller NS: Comprehensive Handbook of Drug and Alcohol Addiction. New York, Marcel Dekker, 1991.
10. Regier DA, Farmer ME, Rae DS, et al: Comorbidity of mental disorders with alcohol and other drugs. JAMA 264:2511–2518, 1990.

20. ALCOHOL USE DISORDERS

Jane A. Kennedy, D.O.

1. Who drinks alcohol?
About 75% of the population in the United States drinks, and about 23% reported alcohol abuse or dependence in the National Comorbidity Survey reported in 1994. Men are 2–3 times more likely than women to be problem drinkers, although women may hide their drinking more frequently.

2. Does alcoholism run in families?
Good evidence suggests a genetic link, and the strongest vulnerability appears to be for sons of alcoholic fathers. Several studies, including twin and adoption studies, show that children of alcoholics are about 4 times more likely to develop alcohol problems. Specific biologic abnormalities have been noted, such as decreased brain-wave reactivity (P300, a measure of visual evoked response) in children of alcoholics and decreased intensity of reaction to alcohol in sons of alcoholics.

3. What are the signs and symptoms of alcohol intoxication?
A person intoxicated by alcohol may have ataxia, slurred speech, mood lability, decreased concentration and memory, poor judgment, facial flushing, enlarged pupils, and nystagmus. Although alcohol initially has a stimulant effect, increasing levels result in depression of respiration, reflexes, blood pressure, and body temperature, potentially followed by stupor, coma, and death.

Blood alcohol levels are measured in grams percent (g%) or grams per 100 milliliters (mg/dl); in most states drivers are said to be "impaired" at levels of 0.05 g% (50 mg/dl) and "under the influence" at levels of 0.1 g% (100 mg/dl). Lack of intoxication at a level of 100 mg/dl is evidence of tolerance, and alcohol dependence disorder should be suspected.

4. What are the usual symptoms and time course of alcohol withdrawal?
In someone dependent on alcohol, stopping or suddenly decreasing the amount of alcohol intake may result in withdrawal symptoms, which reflect central nervous system (CNS) and autonomic hyperactivity. Symptoms begin to appear in 4–24 hours, usually peak at 36–48 hours, and subside in about 5 days. Symptoms typically are in proportion to duration of drinking, but the presence of medical illness may increase the severity.

Mild withdrawal may manifest as insomnia, irritability, anxiety, and mild gastrointestinal problems that start a few hours after stopping alcohol and last up to 48 hours. Symptoms may progress first to tremor, sweating, tachycardia, elevated blood pressure, nausea, vomiting, and diarrhea and then to fever, hallucinations, delusions, confusion, agitation, and grand mal seizures. Hallucinations may appear within 24–96 hours and may be auditory, tactile, or visual (most common). Delirium tremens (DTs) usually appears between 24 and 72 hours and may have a mortality rate of 5–15%; this syndrome which is characterized by extreme agitation, delirium, psychosis (delusions and hallucinations), and fever, may last up to 5 days.

5. What about alcohol withdrawal seizures?
Alcohol withdrawal seizures ("rum fits") most often occur 6–48 hours after stopping or reducing alcohol and may occur in 5–10% of patients in alcohol withdrawal. The seizures generally stop within 6–12 hours; they may be multiple and are usually grand mal. If a patient has a past history of alcohol withdrawal seizures, the risk of recurrence is increased 10-fold.

Because < 5% of alcohol withdrawal seizures are focal, other causes, such as subdural hematoma, should be evaluated. Seizures that occur beyond 48 hours may be due to causes such as withdrawal from sedatives. Many alcoholics have chronic obstructive pulmonary disease (COPD), and seizures may be related to theophylline toxicity. Seizures also may be caused by metabolic disorders such as hypoglycemia or hypomagnesemia, which are not uncommon in alcoholics.

6. What is the treatment of alcohol withdrawal?
Removal of alcohol leads to a state of hyperexcitability. Most patients are able to withdraw without medication, but patients with moderate-to-severe symptoms are best treated with a sedative. Overall, the benzodiazepines have been found to be the most useful and the most practical. The long-acting benzodiazepines, such as chlordiazepoxide, diazepam, or chlorazepate, are used in decreasing doses to prevent seizure and to decrease the other symptoms of hyperexcitability. For patients with severe liver disease, who may encounter problems with accumulation of long-acting benzodiazepines and their metabolites, oxazepam is recommended because of its lack of active metabolites and its independence of liver metabolism. Oxazepam and lorazepam may be given intramuscularly, whereas other benzodiazepines are poorly absorbed with intramuscular administration.

Many other agents have been examined for treatment of alcohol withdrawal with various success:
- Alpha$_2$ adrenergic agonists: clonidine and lofexidine reduce noradrenergic symptoms but have no anticonvulsant effects and may cause hypotension.
- Antipsychotics: Haldol in low doses may be useful in patients with hallucinations and agitation that do not respond to benzodiazepines but should not be used alone. Antipsychotics do not prevent seizures and may lower seizure threshold. Thorazine, which may cause severe hypotension and lower seizure threshold, should not be used.
- Barbiturates: effective anticonvulsants but narrow therapeutic index and greater tendency to induce respiratory depression.
- Carbamazepine: an anticonvulsant with many side-effects and thus no advantage over benzodiazepines.
- Ethanol: contraindicated because of toxicity and potential to cause high fluid load.
- Propranolol: contraindicated because it does not prevent seizures, may obscure withdrawal signs, and is contraindicated in various conditions seen in chronic alcoholics, such as lung diseases with bronchospasm, congestive heart failure, hypotension, and insulin-dependent diabetes.
- Valproic acid: found by one controlled study to be ineffective and to cause considerable side effects.

7. What is the treatment of alcohol withdrawal seizures?
Benzodiazepines should be used for the treatment of withdrawal seizures—most commonly, the long-acting drugs such as chlordiazepoxide, diazepam, or chlorazepate. Some clinicians avoid the use of diazepam, because it may cause euphoria. For elderly patients or patients with compromised liver function, short-acting benzodiazepines, such as oxazepam or lorazepam, avoid accumulation of metabolites and may be administered parenterally.

8. Do patients need phenytoin for prophylaxis of alcohol withdrawal seizures?
Little evidence supports the use of phenytoin for the treatment or prophylaxis of alcohol withdrawal seizures unless the patient has a preexisting seizure disorder.

9. What is Wernicke-Korsakoff syndrome?
Wernicke's disease, or Wernicke's encephalopathy, is characterized by confusion and drowsiness, ataxia, and ocular disturbances (usually due to weakness or paralysis of the sixth cranial nerve), including nystagmus. Wernicke's syndrome may have acute onset or develop slowly over 1 week

or so. Korsakoff's psychosis is a state of amnesia that usually follows Wernicke's syndrome; patients have anterograde amnesia (inability to retain new memories, even their physician's name) and possibly retrograde amnesia (inability to recall the past). Otherwise they appear alert, responsive, and normal and may try to cover their memory problem by fabricating answers or "confabulating." In the string test, which has been used in diagnosis of Korsakoff's psychosis, the physician asks the patient to take an imaginary string in his or her hands, and the patient complies, as though the string were real.

Treatment with thiamine may reverse the ocular abnormalities and ataxia almost completely, but the confusion and amnestic problems may not respond as well. Rapid treatment of Wernicke's syndrome may prevent the onset of Korsakoff's psychosis; if treatment is delayed, the patient may become demented and unable to care for him- or herself. Thus Wernicke's encephalopathy is a medical emergency.

10. When is thiamine needed?

Chronic alcoholics are often malnourished. Thiamine deficiency is common and may cause Wernicke-Korsakoff syndrome. The treatment is immediate administration of thiamine, 100 mg intramuscularly, followed by 100 mg intramuscularly or orally for the next 2 days. Because administration of glucose may deplete already deficient B-vitamins, thiamine should be given before glucose is administered.

11. What are the medical complications of chronic alcohol use?

Gastrointestinal complications. Gastrointestinal problems include gastritis, peptic and gastric ulcer, esophagitis, esophageal varices, alcoholic hepatitis, cirrhosis, and pancreatitis. Except for cirrhosis, these conditions are often reversible with abstinence from alcohol. Although a minority of alcoholics (15–20%) develop cirrhosis, the majority of patients with cirrhosis are alcoholics (50–80%).

Neurologic complications. As stated above, Wernicke-Korsakoff syndrome is a medical emergency. Hepatic encephalopathy may occur because the liver is no longer able to metabolize and detoxify substances. Asterixis, or "liver flap," appears late; early symptoms include confusion, agitation, and personality changes. Peripheral neuropathy is usually symmetrical and in the lower extremities. With prolonged drinking, alcohol dementia may occur with memory defects and difficulty with abstract thinking and new learning. Cerebellar degeneration, which causes a wide-spread gait, may be associated with Wernicke-Korsakoff syndrome. Stopping alcohol intake and vitamin treatment may improve these conditions.

Cardiovascular complications. Hypertension is associated with excessive alcohol intake, and patients who continue to drink heavily may not respond as well to antihypertensive medication. With abstinence, many patients become normotensive. Alcoholic cardiomyopathy has a fairly nonspecific presentation, and the diagnosis is usually based on the alcohol history; it should be suspected in patients under age 50 who present with heart failure. Alcohol ingestion and alcohol withdrawal cause sinus tachycardia.

Pulmonary complications. Alcoholics show increased incidence of tuberculosis and bacterial pneumonias; in addition, aspiration pneumonia may occur with vomiting and altered levels of consciousness. Because at least 90% of alcoholics are smokers, the incidence of bronchitis, emphysema, and chronic obstructive pulmonary disease is increased.

Hematologic complications. Macrocytosis (enlarged red blood cells) is an early laboratory manifestation of chronic alcoholism. It may be caused by folate deficiency or the direct toxicity of alcohol (unrelated to vitamin depletion). Iron deficiency anemia may occur in alcoholics because of chronic gastrointestinal bleeding, but the associated low mean corpuscular volume may be hidden by concurrent macrocytosis. Alcohol impairs the production and function of white blood cells, both neutrophils and lymphocytes, and increases the risk of infection. Blood platelet production also may be suppressed, and platelet function may be impaired. In addition, splenic enlargement secondary to liver disease may cause thrombocytopenia through increased sequestration of platelets.

Endocrine complications. Alcohol suppresses testosterone levels in men by effects on the pituitary gland and the testicle, and impaired metabolism of estrogen by the liver increases estrogen levels. Both events may result in signs of feminization, such as gynecomastia and feminine fat distribution; decreased libido; testicular atrophy; and impotence. Women experience menstrual irregularities, ranging from cessation of menses to excessive bleeding.

12. Is smoking associated with drinking?
At the minimum, 80–90% of alcoholics are regular and often heavy smokers. Some of the medical complications of alcoholism may be caused by cigarette smoking, and increased mortality also may be due to complications from smoking. A higher rate of alcoholism should be expected in smoking populations, such as patients with chronic obstructive pulmonary disease.

13. How can the physician detect alcohol problems in patients?
The history and physical exam of a patient reveal a great deal. Certainly the diagnosis of alcoholism abuse or dependence must be pursued in a patient who shows withdrawal symptoms such as tremors and diaphoresis or who is intoxicated and smells of alcohol. Symptoms of medical conditions associated with excessive alcohol use, such as diarrhea, anemia, or impotence, also should suggest the diagnosis. Patients have been known to receive an extensive work-up for diarrhea caused by alcohol withdrawal, because the physician did not ask about drinking. The physician should ask about alcohol intake without being accusatory; problem drinkers will be honest if they do not feel threatened.

14. What physical findings are common in chronic heavy drinkers?

Flushed facies	Dilated superficial veins on the abdomen
Parotid gland enlargement	Right upper quadrant tenderness
Gynecomastia in men	Hepatomegaly
Spider angiomata	Muscle wasting or tenderness
Abdominal distension from ascites	Paresthesias in feet and calves
Abnormal gait due to cerebellar degeneration	

15. Can laboratory tests diagnose alcohol abuse and dependence?
Verbal questioning is more sensitive than laboratory tests for detecting alcohol problems; no one test can prove their presence. Several tests evaluated together, however, are sometimes useful, although often in the later stages of disease. The gamma-glutamyltransferase (GGT) test has been used most commonly; although not specific (many other factors may cause increased GGT), abnormally high values are seen in most chronic alcoholics. An elevated mean corpuscular volume (MCV) may be a sign of chronic heavy alcohol consumption and is thought to be a direct effect of alcohol on bone marrow or folate metabolism; again, an elevated MCV may have many other causes. Aspartate aminotransferase (AST, SGOT) and alanine aminotransferase (ALT, SGPT) are nonspecific indicators of hepatic damage but are frequently elevated in alcoholic liver disease; an ALT/AST ratio of > 2 is especially suspicious. Other blood tests found to be elevated with chronic alcohol intake are alkaline phosphatase, high-density lipoprotein cholesterol (HDL), and uric acid. It is best to look at laboratory markers in combination; the more tests that are elevated, the more likely the patient will be a heavy drinker. The carbohydrate-deficient transferrin (CDT) test, which is being evaluated as a state marker for alcoholism, appears promising.

16. What is fetal alcohol syndrome?
The fetus is affected by maternal alcohol intake, probably in a dose-dependent manner. The minimal safe amount of alcohol that will not cause fetal problems is unknown, but certainly the likelihood of fetal alcohol syndrome (FAS) increases with increasing amounts of alcohol intake. The early weeks of the first trimester are thought to be the time of greatest vulnerability. Infants with FAS are smaller, may have mental retardation, and have characteristic facial features, such as no philtrum (ridge) between the nose and upper lip, thin upper lip, low-set ears, and short palpebral

fissures. Cigarette smoking, malnutrition, and drug use may be complicating factors in the spectrum of clinical problems seen in these infants.

17. Are there any useful pharmacologic approaches in the treatment of alcohol abuse and dependence after withdrawal.

Disulfiram (Antabuse) has been used as a deterrent to drinking; it inhibits aldehyde dehydrogenase, which breaks down acetaldehyde, a metabolite of alcohol. If a patient drinks while taking disulfiram, the increased level of acetaldehyde causes flushing, throbbing, headache, nausea, vomiting, tachycardia, hypotension, and hyperventilation; rarely, cardiovascular collapse and death may occur. A large study showed marginal efficacy of disulfiram, but patients were not monitored. Results are improved if the patient is required to take the disulfiram under observation.

Naltrexone, an opioid blocker, has been approved for use in the treatment of alcohol problems; it decreases craving, and reduces likelihood of continued drinking if the patient relapses. Because the reinforcing property of alcohol seems to be attenuated for some drinkers, naltrexone is helpful as an adjunct to treatment of alcohol dependence. No studies have reported the use of naltrexone beyond 12 weeks.

BIBLIOGRAPHY

1. Brewer C: Combining pharmacological antagonists and behavioral psychotherapy in treating addictions. Br J Psychiatry 157:34–40, 1990.
2. Fuller RF, Branchey L, Brightwell DR, et al: Disulfiram treatment of alcoholism: A Veterans Administration cooperative study. JAMA 256:1449–1455, 1986.
3. O'Malley SS, Jaffe AJ, Chang G, et al: Naltrexone and coping skills therapy for alcohol dependence. Arch Gen Psychiatry 49:881–887, 1992.
4. Stibler H: Carbohydrate-deficient transferrin in serum: A new marker of potentially harmful alcohol consumption reviewed. Clin Chem 37:2029–2037, 1991.
5. Volpicelli JR, Alterman AJ, Hayashida M, O'Brien CP: Naltrexone in the treatment of alcohol dependence. Arch Gen Psychiatry 49:876–880, 1992.

21. OPIOID USE DISORDERS

Jane A. Kennedy, D.O.

1. What are opioids?

Opioids include naturally occurring substances such as opium and morphine, semisynthetic drugs such as heroin and hydromorphone, and totally synthetic drugs such as methadone or meperidine. These substances act at specific opioid receptors in the brain and the body, as do the endogenous opioids (endorphins, enkephalins, and dynorphins).

2. Who uses opioids?

Opioid users are sometimes divided into heroin addicts and prescription opioid abusers ("medical addicts"). Less than 1% of the U.S. population is dependent on heroin, and around 100,000 people are in methadone maintenance treatment. Prescription drug abusers are frequently patients with real or fabricated pain, or health professionals with access to medications by prescription or diversion.

3. Describe the signs and symptoms of opioid intoxication.

Soon after injecting heroin, the person may vomit because of activation of the chemoreceptor trigger zone in the medulla; for the heroin user, this reaction often indicates "good" heroin. Feeling sedation, warmth, and euphoria ("flush and rush"), the user "nods," with the head dropping toward the chest. Speech may be slurred, and attention and memory are impaired. The pupils are pinpoint, and the users may scratch as they nod because of histamine release. The feeling of warmth is probably due to peripheral vasodilation, and hypotension may occur; respiratory depression and suppression of the cough reflex are centrally mediated.

4. What other effects are seen with use of opioids?

Analgesia due to reduced perception of and reaction to pain is common; tolerance to analgesic doses of opioids has been shown experimentally to develop within 48–72 hours. Constipation, sweating, and decreased libido may be chronic side effects of opioid use, but no evidence suggests organ damage from long-term use of opioids. Derangement of the neuroendocrine system may result from chronic opioid administration, but it has been shown that neuroendocrine and immune function improve in patients on methadone maintenance. Smooth muscle constriction may cause urinary retention and biliary colic.

High doses of meperidine and of propoxyphene are associated with a stimulantlike effect that may include seizures and pupillary dilation; such effects seem to be caused by nor-metabolites. Use of meperidine in the presence of monoamine oxidase (MAO) inhibitors may cause hypertensive crisis.

5. What about tolerance with opioids?

Tolerance to euphoria, sedation, respiratory depression, vomiting, and analgesia occurs with regular use, and increased amounts of the drug are needed to create the same effect; however, there is little or no tolerance to constipation or miosis. Exceptions include patients on methadone maintenance, who do not become tolerant to long-term doses once they have been stabilized, and many patients with chronic malignant and nonmalignant pain, who maintain analgesia at a constant dose without development of tolerance. It is possible for patients to build tolerance over time to extremely high doses of opioids that would cause death in nontolerant people.

As with alcohol, tolerance dissipates quickly with abstinence but increases rapidly with reintroduction of the drug, obtaining levels of past tolerance within days rather than years (which were required for its development).

6. What happens with overdose of opioids?

The main effect of overdose is respiratory depression, which is the most common cause of death. Patients are usually comatose, cyanotic, and hypotensive with pinpoint pupils, although pupils may dilate as hypoxia occurs. Pulmonary edema is frequently associated with overdose of heroin and seizures with overdose of meperidine.

7. How is overdose treated?

Opioid overdose is treated with injection of naloxone. In the presence of long-acting opioids such as methadone, repeated doses of naloxone are needed.

8. What are the complications of opioid use?

With injection of opioids, infections such as HIV, hepatitis, endocarditis, osteomyelitis, meningitis, septicemia, and abscesses, may result from unsterile conditions and needle sharing. Patients using acetaminophen or aspirin in high quantity over time are at risk of hepatic and renal toxicity; gastric irritation also may result from use of aspirin compounds. Two-thirds of heroin addicts have abnormal liver enzymes (which often normalize in methadone treatment), and one-third to one-half are positive for hepatitis B. Tuberculosis is more common in heroin addicts than in the general population.

9. What are symptoms of withdrawal from opioids?

Early symptoms	Intermediate symptoms
Myalgia	Sweats
Nausea	Fever
Rhinorrhea	Chills
Lacrimation	Piloerection ("cold turkey")
Increased production	Insomnia or restless sleep
of phlegm	Muscle spasms, often in lower limbs ("kicking")
Yawning	Bone pain (often in thighs)
Late symptoms	**At any stage**
Vomiting	Dilated pupils
Diarrhea	Anxiety
Hypertension	Irritability
Tachycardia	
Hyperventilation	

Opioid withdrawal has been described as a severe flulike syndrome, and addicts use the term "sick" to mean withdrawal. With short-acting opioids, withdrawal starts 6–24 hours after the last dose, peaks in 1–3 days, and subsides in about 5–7 days. With longer-acting drugs such as methadone or l-alpha acetyl methadol (LAAM), withdrawal starts after 1–3 days, peaks at 3–6 days, and may take 2 weeks to subside completely. Although withdrawal from the long-acting drugs may be less severe, the longer duration makes it seem worse to many addicts.

A syndrome of prolonged low-grade withdrawal (protracted abstinence syndrome) is described by many addicts, especially if they have stopped the drug abruptly; it may last weeks to months and is characterized by dysphoria, low energy, chronic sleep disturbance, and chronic constipating disturbance.

10. Describe the treatment for opioid withdrawal.

Opioid withdrawal does not cause seizures and is not life-threatening, although addicts may feel that it is. Addicts usually treat withdrawal with more opioid drugs; if they are not available, alcohol, barbiturates, or benzodiazepines may be used for sedation. Because cross-tolerance with such drugs is incomplete, the most effective way to alleviate opioid withdrawal is with an opioid drug; methadone is most commonly used, but there are several alternatives. Relapse rates after detoxification are high; below are suggestions for short-term detoxification, although patients need longer-term treatment to maintain abstinence.

Methadone. Treatment of opioid withdrawal with opioids requires a special license. Methadone may be used for short-term (days) detoxification in hospitalized patients as well as long-term detoxification (up to 6 months) in licensed treatment programs. It is hard to know the extent of a patient's addiction by self-report during withdrawal; the patient may exaggerate because of fear that the physician will not help at all. Generally the first dose should not exceed 20–30 mg, and the total dose on the first day should not exceed 40 mg. Because methadone has an average half-life of 24 hours, doses accumulate during the first five days, risking overdose without careful titration. For short-term withdrawal in the hospital, patients usually can be stabilized on 40 mg and tapered by 10–20% per day.

Clonidine. Because opioids suppress the adrenergic neurons in the locus ceruleus, withdrawal causes increased beta-adrenergic activity; clonidine, an alpha$_2$-adrenergic agonist used as an antihypertensive agent, suppresses some symptoms of withdrawal and provides some sedation. Usually the need for clonidine follows the same curve as the withdrawal symptoms; maximal doses for outpatients should not exceed 1.2 mg/day, usually prescribed as 0.1–0.2 mg every 3–4 hours. Hypotension may occur, and patients should be monitored after the first dose and daily; the hypotensive effect makes clonidine less useful for women, who generally have a lower baseline blood pressure than men.

Buprenorphine. Buprenorphine is not yet available in the U.S. except as a parenteral analgesic, but ongoing studies suggest its usefulness for opioid withdrawal as well as for maintenance treatment. It is a partial mu agonist, with a long-acting (24 hours) effect similar to that of methadone. It has several advantages over methadone: withdrawal from buprenorphine is mild and short-lived, risk of overdose is low, and induction on naltrexone is more rapid. Cocaine use was decreased with buprenorphine in uncontrolled studies in primates and humans, but this finding was not replicated in a controlled study.

11. What is methadone maintenance treatment?

Although the most researched approach in the field, methadone maintenance treatment remains "controversial." It has been shown repeatedly to decrease morbidity and mortality, to reduce crime, and to improve health and social functioning for opioid addicts. In addition, alternatives to methadone treatment have not shown equal success. However, because it does not fit the "abstinence" philosophy in the treatment field, opioid maintenance treatment remains stigmatized and underused.

Methadone maintenance may be used only in specially licensed treatment programs. Federal regulations require that physiologic evidence of opioid dependence must be demonstrated before starting a patient on methadone; if a patient in seen in the emergency department or hospital, withdrawal symptoms must be carefully documented. Research has clearly shown that retention in treatment is improved and illicit opioid use is decreased if patient doses are stabilized at > 60 mg/day, with an optimal range of 60–100 mg.

LAAM, a long-acting synthetic opioid, has recently been released for use in licensed treatment programs. It is taken every other day, thus reducing the need for "take-home" doses of medication.

12. What complications or problems are associated with methadone maintenance treatment?

The most common side effects are constipation and sweating, but patients also may have problems with decreased libido, weight gain, fluid retention, and sexual dysfunction. Medications that induce liver enzymes may interfere with methadone metabolism; the most common examples are rifampin, carbamazepine, and dilantin. Valproic acid does not interfere with methadone dose. Agonist-antagonist drugs such as Stadol, Talwin, or Nubain should not be prescribed for patients on methadone; the antagonists cause an abstinence syndrome.

13. How long should a patient stay on methadone maintenance?

Research has demonstrated that the longer a patient stays in methadone treatment, the better the prognosis and the less the risk of HIV infection. For some patients treatment may last 1 year; for others it may be life-long. Recent research showed that 80% of patients relapsed in the first year off methadone; because of the risk of HIV infection now associated with relapse, most patients are not encouraged to withdraw from methadone. "Medical maintenance" clinics have been developed to manage stable, long-term patients who receive monthly supplies of methadone at a doctor's office, similar to treatment of hypertension or other medical problems; they are monitored for drug use and diversion by random urine tests and random calls to bring in remaining medication for counting.

14. Should methadone maintenance be used to treat pregnant opioid addicts?

The fetus is highly affected by going in and out of withdrawal as the mother uses short-acting opioids, and the mother is less likely to obtain prenatal care; both factors result in more complications of pregnancy and lower birth weights. Methadone maintenance is strongly indicated for the pregnant opioid addict; healthier infants are born.

Methadone doses should be high enough to keep the mother from using opioid drugs (to avoid both drug effect and risk of HIV for the fetus) but as low as possible to decrease withdrawal for the infant. Mothers already on methadone may want to decrease their dose, with slow tapering at 1–2 mg/week. Tapering is done most safely during the second trimester. Although there is no risk of seizure in adults who withdraw from opioids, it is a risk with infants who should be closely monitored for withdrawal symptoms and treated with phenobarbital or paregoric if they occur.

15. Describe the treatment of pain in methadone maintenance patients.

Most methadone-maintained patients develop tolerance to its analgesic effects. For injuries and surgical procedures, patients need their regular methadone dose for opioid dependence treatment, and whatever short-acting analgesics are usually prescribed for other patients undergoing the same procedure.

Patients with chronic pain sometimes get long-term analgesia from methadone, as may patients with chronic pain and addiction problems. Few controlled studies have examined this issue in a systematic manner, but patients with chronic pain often end up in methadone treatment clinics.

16. What is the role of naltrexone?

Naltrexone is an oral, long-acting opioid receptor antagonist that has been shown to be a successful, nonopioid treatment in certain populations. It works by blocking the opioid receptors; thus if a person tries to get high, the effect is blocked. Naltrexone has been shown to be quite successful in treating health professionals who may have easy access to opioids on the job, and it is often recommended for opioid addicts who have been incarcerated and are returning to areas where opioids are again accessible.

Patients cannot have any opioids in their system when starting naltrexone; otherwise, the drug precipitates an abstinence syndrome that may last over 24 hours. For many opioid addicts, this is the biggest difficulty with starting naltrexone; they must abstain from short-acting opioids for 5–7 days and from long-acting opioids for 10–14 days. Many patients withdraw from opioids using clonidine during this period; then they are given an injection of naloxone before starting the oral, long-acting antagonist to be sure that opioids are no longer present. The naltrexone dose is 50 mg/day, but it may be given 3 times/week, e.g., 100 mg, 100 mg, and 150 mg every Monday, Wednesday, and Friday, respectively. This regimen allows monitoring without requiring daily attendance; usually half doses (50–50–100) are given in the first week.

BIBLIOGRAPHY

1. Ball JC, Lange WR, Myers CP, Friedman SR: Reducing the risk of AIDS through methadone maintenance treatment. J Health Soc Behav 29:214–226, 1988.
2. Gerstein DR: The effectiveness of drug treatment. Res Publ Assoc Res Nerv Ment Dis 70:253–273, 1988.
3. Novick DM, Pascarelli EF, Joseph H: Methadone maintenance patients in general medical practice. JAMA 259:3299–3302, 1988.
4. Romac DR: Safety of prolonged, high-dose infusion of naloxone hydrochloride for severe methadone overdose. Clin Pharmacol 5:251–254, 1986.

22. SEDATIVE-HYPNOTIC USE DISORDERS

Jane A. Kennedy, D.O.

1. What drugs are considered sedative-hypnotics?

Sedative-hypnotic drugs include the barbiturates, barbiturate-like drugs, and benzodiazepines. They are a diverse group of synthetic drugs with clear medical uses and may be prescribed as anxiolytics (tranquilizers), hypnotics (to induce sleep), anticonvulsant medications, and muscle relaxants. Short-acting and long-acting forms are available; all have the potential for abuse. Most are taken orally, but some may also be injected intramuscularly or intravenously. Sedative-hypnotics are extensively prescribed in the United States. Barbiturates were introduced in 1903 but for the most part have been replaced by the benzodiazepines, which were introduced in 1960.

2. Who abuses sedative-hypnotics?

Sedative-hypnotics are abused by both street addicts and patients with prescription drug abuse. Street addicts may use them as adjuvants to boost the effect of drugs such as opioids, to take the edge off stimulants, or to help manage drug or alcohol withdrawal. Prescription addicts may use the drugs alone, seeking sedation or euphoria, but usually combine them with other substances. Community surveys estimate that about 5% of the general population have used sedative-hypnotics for nonmedical purposes; prevalence is markedly greater in certain populations, such as patients on methadone maintenance.

3. How may the physician recognize sedative-hypnotic intoxication?

Barbiturate and benzodiazepine intoxication appears similar to alcohol intoxication without the odor of alcohol on the breath. Signs and symptoms are sedation, impaired psychomotor performance, slurred speech, ataxia, nystagmus, poor memory and concentration, and labile emotions.

4. Are sedative-hypnotics lethal in overdose?

Benzodiazepines, when used alone, are remarkably safe in overdose, whereas barbiturates are quite dangerous. Barbiturates or benzodiazepines in combination with other central nervous system depressants may cause death via respiratory depression or hypotensive shock. Profound and protracted coma may be seen with glutethimide (Doriden), a sedative sometimes abused in combination with Tylenol #4 ("Dors and Fours").

5. Does use of sedative-hypnotics result in physiologic dependence, tolerance, or withdrawal?

With regular use of high doses of sedatives, **dependence** occurs after about 1 month. However, development of dependence on benzodiazepines in lower, therapeutic doses is controversial. It is now thought that dependence may occur with daily use of therapeutic doses, usually after 2–4 months, but only in a subset of patients. Low-dose dependence is primarily a withdrawal syndrome; most patients taking a therapeutic regimen do not require increasing doses for continued efficacy.

Tolerance to the sedation and the mood effects of sedative-hypnotics may lead to ingestion of larger and more frequent doses to achieve the desired psychoactive effects. Because tolerance does not occur to respiratory depression, overdoses of barbiturates may be lethal. When benzodiazepines are taken alone, remarkably high doses are tolerated; however, toxicity is significantly enhanced when other depressants are added. Most addicts are aware of the relative safety of benzodiazepines compared with barbiturates; thus barbiturate dependence is infrequent.

Withdrawal syndromes may be severe and life-threatening; the onset varies from hours to days, according to the half-life of the drug. Signs and symptoms include tachycardia, tremor,

restlessness and insomnia, diaphoresis, nausea, vomiting, anxiety and agitation, transient hallucinations, and grand mal seizure. The clinical symptoms of withdrawal from either high-dose
barbiturates or benzodiazepines are similar. Less severe withdrawal may be seen with discontinuation of lower (therapeutic) doses of benzodiazepines, but the severity may be increased with the
shorter-acting, more potent benzodiazepines.

6. Does regular use of sedative-hypnotics cause medical problems?

Unlike alcohol, sedative-hypnotics rarely cause direct organ toxicity. Paraldehyde and chloral hydrate, rapid-acting hypnotics, may be irritating to the throat and gastric mucosa, when taken
orally or cause necrosis if injected intramuscularly.

7. Are Quaaludes still abused?

Methaqualone was removed from the market in the U.S. around 1980, but it is still available on
the street in certain regions. Marketed originally as a "nonaddictive" sedative, it was widely
abused, produced dependence, and was associated with lethal overdose as well as serious withdrawal syndromes. Unusual overdose symptoms include muscular hypertonicity, shivering, myoclonus, seizures, and excessive salivation and bronchial secretions, which may compromise the
airway. Methaqualone was falsely rumored to be an aphrodisiac; abusers felt a pleasant high
along with contentment.

8. Are muscle relaxants addictive?

Muscle relaxants may be abused, usually for their sedative properties. Grand mal seizures have
been seen in patients who abruptly discontinue carisoprodol (Soma), because a metabolite of
Soma is meprobamate, a barbiturate.

9. What is the treatment for sedative-hypnotic withdrawal?

Some patients who take prescribed lower doses become physiologically dependent without abusing the drug for psychoactive effects. This problem is not seen as an addiction, and the drug can
be tapered over several weeks on an outpatient basis, with careful monitoring and patient-physician communication.

Patients who abuse a sedative-hypnotic should be stabilized on an oral, long-acting barbiturate, such as phenobarbital, or benzodiazepine, such as chlorazepate (Tranxene). After stabilization, the dose is tapered. Optimally, the withdrawal should be planned ahead of time and
performed in the hospital. This approach allows supervision of the patient in case of intoxication
or severe withdrawal symptoms, such as seizure, and prevents the patient from using other drugs
or alcohol during withdrawal. Hospitalization is not always possible, and sometimes benzodiazepine detoxification is accomplished on an outpatient basis with strict monitoring. Patients
must be well-motivated or have strong contingent consequences; they should be seen on a daily
basis and receive medication daily. Risk of seizure or other medical complications should be
minimal. Whenever possible, one should avoid using the abused substance for the taper, because
craving and other conditioned behaviors may create difficulties.

The amount of the abused drug should be converted to an equivalent amount of the long-acting
sedative. This conversion, however, may be difficult, because one must rely on self-report and consider concurrent use of other drugs and alcohol. The pentobarbital challenge test determines the
degree of tolerance to a standard dose of a short-acting barbiturate, and the results may be converted
to an equivalent dosage of the long-acting substitute to be used for the taper. In patients taking high
doses of methadone, caution is advised; a pentobarbital challenge may produce severe sedation.

BIBLIOGRAPHY

1. Perry PJ, Alexander B: Sedative/hypnotic dependence: Patient stabilization, tolerance testing,. and with-
    drawal. Drug Intell Clin Pharm 20:532–537, 1986.
2. Seivewright N, Dougal W: Withdrawal symptoms from high dose benzodiazepines in poly drug abusers.
    Drug Alcohol Depend 32:15–23, 1993.

23. COCAINE AND AMPHETAMINE USE DISORDERS

Jane A. Kennedy, D.O.

1. Who uses cocaine and amphetamine?

Cocaine use in the United States has escalated dramatically since the early 1970s when about 5 million had tried the drug at least once compared with about 40 million in the late 1980s. Cocaine is most commonly used by persons aged 18–30. Recent indicators suggest a drop in cocaine use among casual, recreational users but sustained or increased prevalence among hardcore users.

Amphetamine use is highest among 18–25 year olds; in some parts of the country it is highly associated with motorcycle gang members. Since tightened regulation of prescription amphetamine in the late 1970s, only about 25% of abused amphetamine is prescription drug; the other 75% is illicitly manufactured.

2. Do cocaine and amphetamine have the same effect?

In recent years attention has focused on cocaine dependence, because its use is more widespread than use of amphetamines. Both drugs, however, increase the central action of dopamine and both the central and peripheral action of norepinephrine. In theory, they should be quite similar in effect, but most users have a distinct preference for either cocaine or amphetamine. Both drugs are quite reinforcing. Animals will self-administer stimulants continuously until they die, forsaking food and water, suffering repeated seizures and exhaustion; for many humans, similar effects have been seen.

3. What forms are available? What are the routes of administration?

Amphetamine is available in oral prescription medication as dextroamphetamine and methamphetamine; it is also manufactured illicitly as powder or crystallized ("ice") methamphetamine. Cocaine hydrochloride is obtainable pharmaceutically for use as a local anesthetic; it is available illicitly in either powder or crystallized ("rock" or "crack") forms.

Cocaine and amphetamines are snorted, injected, and smoked; amphetamines also may be taken orally. "Crack" is the smokable form of cocaine, and "ice" is the smokable form of amphetamine. Smoking is the most rapid route of delivery to the brain and thus the most reinforcing; however, dependence may occur with all routes of administration. A stimulant and a depressant injected together, most frequently cocaine and heroin, is called a "speedball."

4. Do stimulants have approved medical uses?

Cocaine hydrochloride is used as a local anesthetic; use of amphetamines such as dexedrine or methylphenidate has been limited to treatment of attention deficit hyperactivity disorder, narcolepsy, and resistant depression.

5. What are the signs and symptoms of stimulant intoxication?

The most common signs and symptoms are enlarged pupils, tachycardia, hypertension, and hyperreflexia; the user feels euphoric, energetic, talkative, alert, and grandiose, with decreased appetite and need for sleep. Some people, however, may feel anxious, agitated, tense, and dysphoric, and others may feel calmed, slowed down, and focused. Stomach cramps, nausea, vomiting, and diarrhea may occur. Many users clench and grind their teeth.

Higher doses and more chronic use frequently lead to psychosis, usually with a paranoid quality. Reactions may range from "tweaking," a sense of hypervigilance and fearfulness (small noises may be interpreted as police outside the door), to overt psychosis with auditory and visual hallucinations, ideas of reference, and full-blown delusions.

Stimulants often induce stereotypic behaviors such as repetitive counting or cleaning, prolonged sexual activity, or picking at the skin ("cocaine bugs") due to formication (a sensation of insects crawling on the skin).

6. What is the duration of effect from cocaine and amphetamine?
Cocaine's rapid, short-lived "rush" of 15–20 minutes contrasts with the sustained effect of amphetamine, which may last for hours. The high associated with "ice" (smokable amphetamine) may last up to 48 hours and may be associated with prolonged psychosis and aggression.

7. Does tolerance occur?
Tolerance occurs to euphoria, wakefulness, anorexia, and possibly to convulsant and cardiovascular effects; users may increase frequency of dosing intervals and quantities as they try to reproduce the euphoria.

8. Discuss the complications of stimulant use.
Sympathomimetic responses include decreased gastrointestinal motility, bladder stimulation resulting in painful urination, tachycardia with tachyarrhythmias, hypertension (hypotension also has been reported), and fever. Increased stimulation of the central nervous system may cause seizure. Other complications include cardiac ischemia, coronary artery constriction with angina or myocardial infarction, stroke, and cardiac or respiratory arrest. Cerebral and renal vasculitis are more common with amphetamines.

Although psychosis usually clears within days of stopping stimulant use, in some instances the psychosis persists, or the user develops a sustained sensitivity to its recurrence, even with small doses of amphetamine or cocaine. Panic disorder also may be precipitated by cocaine and persist even after use is discontinued. Bipolar patients may become manic with use of stimulants.

Other complications depend on route of administration. Intravenous use is associated with transmission of the human immunodeficiency virus (HIV), hepatitis, and endocarditis. Nosebleeds, nasal septum irritation or perforation, and sinusitis may result from nasal insufflation, and pulmonary complications such as cough, bronchitis, and pneumothorax may result from smoking. In addition, marked weight loss and malnutrition may occur during a "run," when many users go for days without eating. Use of sedatives to help with insomnia and "crashing" may create a secondary drug dependence.

Sexual promiscuity, due either to increased sexual interest or to exchanging sex for money or drugs, may put the user at high risk for sexually transmitted diseases, especially HIV infection.

9. What happens with overdose?
Death may occur from seizures, severe fever, cerebrovascular hemorrhage, or cardiovascular arrest. Treatment of overdose is supportive; seizures respond to diazepam, and psychosis may require antipsychotic medication.

10. Is there a stimulant withdrawal syndrome?
Many users experience only fatigue and exhaustion, and sleep for 12–24 hours. For others, dysphoria may be severe and associated with suicidal ideation. Increased appetite, insomnia, vivid dreams, and psychomotor retardation or agitation also may be seen. Some users experience protracted depression, which may respond to antidepressants.

Treatment of withdrawal, especially the reemergence of craving for the drug, has been attempted with the use of dopamine agonists such as bromocriptine or amantadine; open studies looked promising, but controlled trials have reported marginal results or have not supported their efficacy. Similarly, amino acid precursors of catecholamines have not proved to be useful.

11. What are the effects of stimulant use in pregnancy?

Vasoconstrictive properties of stimulants lead to decreased blood flow to the placenta and thus decreased oxygen delivery to the fetus. At the very least, infants have low birth weights; children also have been reported to have central nervous system hyperactivity in the first year of life, with irritability, jumpiness, hyperreflexia, and decreased attention spans. The incidence of abruptio placentae, premature delivery, sudden infant death syndrome, and cerebral hemorrhage is increased. Lower IQ levels were found in 4-year-old children exposed to amphetamines in utero.

12. What are the pharmacologic treatments of cocaine dependence?

Multiple medications have been tried without success; open trials frequently appear promising, but controlled studies show no efficacy. Desipramine, which appeared to increase abstinence from cocaine in controlled trials, has not shown the same effectiveness in repeat studies. Carbamazepine also appeared promising in open trials but did not hold up under randomized, controlled conditions. Buproprion, fluoxetine, flupenthixol, imipramine, levodopa/carbidopa, maprotiline, and trazodone also have been tried without effect. Buprenorphine, an opiate agonist-antagonist, was found to decrease cocaine use in methadone maintenance patients, but a controlled study did not replicate this finding.

13. What other treatments are useful for cocaine?

The most successful approach has been behavioral contracting with positive reinforcement for negative urine screens. Compared with patients randomized to 12-step group treatment, retention was significantly better (58% vs. 11%), as was abstinence (42% vs. 5%).[2] More frequent contact (at least twice weekly) has been associated with improved outcome, and Kang et al. showed that once weekly therapy was ineffective, whether it was group, family, or individual psychotherapy.

BIBLIOGRAPHY

1. Delaney-Black V, Roumell N, Shankaran S, Bedard M: Maternal cocaine use and infant outcomes [abstract]. Pediatr Res 25:242A, 1990.
2. Higgins S, Budney AJ, Bickel WK, Foerg FE, Donham R, Badger MS: Incentives improve outcome in outpatient behavioral treatment of cocaine dependence. Arch Gen Psychiatry 51:568–576, 1994.
3. Kang S-Y, Kleinman PH, Woody GE, et al: Outcomes for cocaine abusers after once-a-week psychosocial therapy. Am J Psychiatry 148:630–635, 1991.
4. Weddington WW, Brown BS, Haertzen CA, et al: Comparison of amantadine and desipramine combined with psychotherapy for treatment of cocaine dependence. Am J Drug Alcohol Abuse 17:137–152, 1991.

24. MARIJUANA, HALLUCINOGENS, PHENCYCLIDINE, AND INHALANTS

Jane A. Kennedy, D.O.

1. What is marijuana?

Marijuana is obtained from the cut and dried upper leaves, flowers, and stems of the cannabis plant; its main psychoactive ingredient is delta-9 tetrahydrocannabinol (THC). The potency of THC in marijuna cigarettes varies greatly (1–15% but has increased 15–30-fold since the 1970s). Hashish is obtained from dried resin secreted on the flowering tops (10–20% THC), and hashish oil is extracted with the use of organic solvents (15–30% THC).

2. Who uses marijuana?

Marijuana, the most widely used illicit drug in the U.S., is often said to be a gateway drug for teens, but it also has been used socially for many years by adults. About one-third of the U.S. population has used marijuana, and in the age range of 18–25 years, about 60% have used it at least once.

3. How is marijuana taken?

Marijuana usually is prepared from dried leaves and flowers and smoked as a cigarette or in a pipe, although in some parts of the world it is taken in tea. It also may be eaten orally, commonly in brownies; the euphoria is less intense but longer lasting. Because extracts are not water-soluble, marijuana is not used intravenously.

4. What are the psychological and physical effects of marijuana?

A person may feel euphoric, and giddy, with uncontrollable laughter, talkative, or sedated; sensory perceptions may be enhanced. Short-term memory, attention span, and judgment are impaired; difficulty with abstract thinking and time distortion also occur. Anxiety, panic, paranoia, and dysphoria may result, and daily users may have chronic depression, irritability, and lethargy. Cannabis-induced psychosis has been reported but may be secondary to underlying psychotic disorder. "Red eyes" or conjunctival injection are a good clue of recent marijuana use. Common physical symptoms are increased heart rate, increased appetite, and dry mouth. Motor performance may be impaired for up to 10 hours after use. The effect of smoking marijuana peaks within 10–30 minutes, and intoxication may last several hours, depending on the dose. The effect of oral ingestion peaks within 45–60 minutes.

5. What are the medical consequences of marijuana use?

Decreases in sperm count, testosterone levels, and luteinizing hormone (LH) have been reported. Pulmonary complications, such as chronic cough, bronchitis, and chronic obstructive pulmonary disease (COPD), are seen; however, because most marijuana smokers are also cigarette smokers, it is difficult to lay blame on marijuana. The carcinogens in cigarettes are also present in marijuana but in increased amounts; thus the risk for malignancy may be increased.

6. What are the medical uses for THC?

THC has been used to treat glaucoma (by lowering intraocular pressure), nausea and vomiting caused by chemotherapy, weight loss problems in patients with acquired immunodeficiency syndrome, and muscle spasm in multiple sclerosis. In general, THC has not been shown to be more efficacious than available prescription medications, and many patients do not like the psychoactive effect.

7. Is tolerance or withdrawal associated with marijuana?

Most chronic users report tolerance to the euphoric effects and a need for increased frequency or increased amount of marijuana to get the same effect. A withdrawal reaction has been reported with chronic use of very high doses, but it is rare and is not listed as a diagnosis in DSM–IV.

8. How long does THC stay in the urine?

THC is fat-soluble and is excreted slowly. Casual users may have a positive urine screen for 5–10 days and chronic users for up to 30 days.

9. What is the amotivational syndrome?

The amotivational syndrome has been described in several countries and several age groups of marijuana users, but in the U.S. it has been applied mainly to adolescents. Symptoms are apathy, disinterest, fatigue, and decrease in goal-directed activities. The syndrome has not been well researched and may not exist.

10. Is marijuana a gateway drug that leads to other drug use?

A study of young men in Manhattan noted that of those who had not smoked marijuana, < 1% progressed to cocaine or heroin, whereas of those who were heavy marijuana users (> 1000 times), 82% used cocaine and 33% used heroin. It is unlikely that marijuana causes further drug use, but it may expose the young users to drug experience, risk-taking behavior, and people who use other drugs.

11. What are hallucinogens?

Hallucinogens are said to produce sensory hallucinations without causing delirium or cognitive impairment; the hallucinations may be auditory, visual, olfactory, tactile, or gustatory. Often what is actually experienced is an illusion (distortion of an actual sensory perception) rather than a hallucination.

12. What is LSD?

Lysergic acid diethylamide (LSD) or "acid" is a synthetic hallucinogen.

13. Who uses LSD?

Data from the 1991 household survey revealed that about 8% of the population had used LSD or phencyclidine (PCP) at least once in their lifetime, 1.4% in the last year, and 0.3% in the past month. Recent use was most common in 18–25 year olds. Whites were twice as likely to use either drug as African-Americans, and 1989 data from emergency departments revealed that over half of the LSD-related emergency visits were adolescents age 10–19 years.

14. How is LSD taken?

LSD is usually taken orally, although it may be absorbed through the skin, dropped in the eyes, or injected intravenously.

15. What are the intoxication effects of LSD?

Onset of effects begins in about 30 minutes, peaks at 2–3 hours and lasts about 8–12 hours. Effects are dose-related. Perceptual and psychic changes occur, although the person usually recognizes that such changes are drug-induced. Effects may include depersonalization and derealization, a dreamlike state, illusions (melting face), synesthesias ("hearing" a color), intensification of sound and color, and prolonged afterimages. A person feels excitation, distorted sense of time, peacefulness, or delusions, such as being able to fly. Hallucinations are often visual geometric figures; auditory hallucinations are rare. "Bad trips," which include anxiety, fear of insanity, suicidal depression, and panic attacks, may occur in anyone (even people who have "good trips"); injuries may occur from delusional behavior, such as trying to fly.

Physical symptoms such as dizziness, weakness, motor restlessness, or nausea may occur initially, along with stimulantlike signs such as increased blood pressure and heart rate, fever, and dilated pupils. Sweating, tremors, incoordination, hyperreflexia, and blurred vision also may be present.

16. Is tolerance or withdrawal associated with LSD?
Tolerance to euphoria and perceptual experiences occurs rapidly (within a few days) with daily use, and most users report that they must wait several days between "trips" because of tolerance. Cross-tolerance exists with mescaline and psilocybin, but not with PCP. A withdrawal syndrome has not been identified, and animal studies show that LSD is not a highly reinforcing drug. Users rarely report compulsion or loss of control with LSD.

17. What are "flashbacks"?
Called hallucinogen persisting perception disorder in DSM–IV, flashbacks are transient, distressful reexperiencing of hallucinogenic effects during abstinence. Usually the flashback is a visual distortion (illusion) or actual hallucination, such as shadows, colored or geometric objects, macropsia or micropsia, intensified color, halos, or afterimages; it is generally unpleasant and frightening. Flashbacks usually stop after several months of abstinence but may last for years in some patients.

18. What are the adverse effects of LSD?
Overdose has not been a problem, but patients may present to the emergency department with a "bad trip" (agitation and fear) or with injuries secondary to impaired judgment or delusions, such as trying to fly out of a second story window. Bad trips are usually treated with a quiet room, low sensory stimulation, and "talking down" with support and reassurance. A benzodiazepine may be useful, especially with extreme anxiety and panic.

A prolonged psychotic state may be associated with hallucinogens such as LSD and PCP, as well as with stimulants and even cannabis. Whether this state is drug-induced or an unmasking of preexisting psychotic illness remains controversial; sometimes it responds to antipsychotic medication. Persistent auditory or visual hallucinations also may respond to carbamazepine.

19. What other hallucinogens are abused?
Similar symptoms and problems are seen with other hallucinogens; many have both amphetamine and hallucinogenic actions. Morning glory seeds and Hawaiian baby woodrose contain LSD derivatives, and the spices nutmeg and mace contain a substance related to methylene dioxyamphetamine (MDA). Mescaline from the peyote cactus, psilocybin from Mexican mushrooms ("magic mushrooms"), and bufotenin from toad skin are other natural hallucinogens.

20. What is "ecstasy"?
3,4-Methylene dimethylamphetamine (MDMA) is a synthetic substance called ecstasy, E, XTC, or Adam. Along with other "designer drugs," ecstasy has been popular at "raves," which are all-night dances in large warehouses with high-tech music and videos. MDMA may be taken as a pill or suppository, snorted as powder, or injected intravenously. Physically it has amphetamine-like effects; psychoactive effects include feelings of euphoria, spirituality, personal insight, and desire for intimacy. Fatal overdose has occurred as well as severe psychotic reactions, and animal studies suggest direct toxicity to serotonergic neurons.

21. What is phencyclidine?
Phencyclidine (PCP), also called angel dust, sherm, or embalming fluid, was synthesized for use as a general anesthetic in the 1950s but was discontinued because of side effects such as delirium, agitation, hallucinations, and psychotic reactions. It was also used as an anesthetic for animals (thus the street names animal or horse tranquilizer), but this use also has been discontinued.

22. Who uses PCP?
PCP is most commonly used in large cities such as Los Angeles, St. Louis, New York, and Washington, DC. It is most popular with black or Hispanic men in their 20s.

23. How is PCP used? What are its effects?
Most frequently cigarettes (tobacco, marijuana, mint, oregano) are dipped in PCP and smoked, but PCP also may be taken orally, intravenously, or by nasal insufflation. Physical symptoms include elevation in blood pressure and body temperature, muscle rigidity, decreased pain sensation, and dilated pupils with both horizontal and vertical nystagmus. The psychoactive effect is euphoria and sometimes aggressive behavior. "Bad trips" are best treated with diazepam or neuroleptics with low anticholinergic profiles; restraints should be avoided because rhabdomyolysis has been reported.

24. What is ketamine?
Ketamine is a dissociative anesthetic that is used medically; it is a derivative of PCP with similar chemical structure and activity. Ketamine is occasionally abused, usually by health professionals with easy access.

25. What are inhalants?
Volatile substances such as gasoline, glue, spray paint, solvents, and lighter fluids are inhaled ("sniffed, huffed"); they are inexpensive, easily accessible, and legal.

26. Who uses inhalants?
About 20% of high school seniors in the U.S. have tried inhalants, and increasing numbers of children age 9–12 have been reported to experiment with their use. Although inhalant abusers are usually under 20 years old, emergency department visits among people 26 years and older have increased to 38% of total visits for inhalants. Whites, Native Americans, and Hispanics tend to use inhalants more than African Americans, and users are predominantly male. Although many inhalant users are experimenters or polysubstance abusers, a recent study showed that inhalant abusers were more than 5 times more likely to become intravenous drug users than non-inhalant users.

27. What are the effects of inhalants?
A rapid-onset (seconds to minutes) and short-lived euphoria occurs with inhalation of volatile substances. The user feels excitement, disinhibition, light-headedness, and confusion. Hallucinations may occur as well as nausea, vomiting, headache, and blurred vision. There may be a rash around the nose and mouth, and the person's clothes, skin, or breath may smell of solvents.

28. What are the complications of inhalants?
Risk of sudden death due to cardiac arrhythmia, laryngospasm or asphyxiation
Neurologic damage (in chronic users), with abnormal electroencephalogram, cerebellar degeneration, intellectual impairment, and dementia
Impaired motor responses
Memory loss
Renal and hepatic toxicity
Bone marrow suppression
Pulmonary complications (chemical pneumonitis and emphysema in chronic users)

29. Describe the treatment for abuse of marijuna, hallucinogens, PCP, or inhalants.
Treatments have not been well studied. Users rarely seek treatment on their own and are usually under court order. Currently, little knowledge is available to guide treatment of these drug disorders. Many patients are young, and family participation is strongly encouraged. Most treatment

approaches have aimed at achieving abstinence through support, limit-setting, and reinforcement techniques; relapse prevention includes decreasing availability and acceptability of drug use.

BIBLIOGRAPHY

1. Crowley TJ: Learning and unlearning abuse in the real world: Clinical treatment and public policy. NIDA Research Monograph No. 84. Washington. DC, U.S. Government Printing Office, 1988, pp 100–121.
2. Clayton RR, Voss HL: Young men and drugs in Manhattan: A causal analysis. NIDA Research Monograph No. 39. Washington, DC, U.S. Government Printing Office, 1981.
3. Dinwiddie SH: Abuse of inhalants: A review. Addiction 89:925–939, 1994.
4. Millman RB, Sbriglio R: Patterns of use and psychopathology in chronic marijuana users. Psychiatr Clin North Am 9:533–545, 1986.
5. Schutz CG, Chilcoat HD, Anthony JC: The association between sniffing inhalants and injecting drugs. Compr Psychiatry 35:99–105, 1994.
6. Solowij N: Ecstasy (3,4-methylenedioxymethamphetamine. Curr Opin Psychiatry 6:411–415, 1993.
7. Steele TD, McCann UD, Ricaurte GA: 3,4-Methylenedioxymethamphetamine (MDMA, "Ecstasy"): Pharmacology and toxicology in animals and humans. Addiction 89:539–551, 1994.

25. DUAL DIAGNOSIS: SUBSTANCE ABUSE AND PSYCHIATRIC ILLNESS

S. Tziporah Cohen, M.D., and Alan M. Jacobson, M.D.

1. What is dual diagnosis?
The term dual diagnosis is used to describe patients who have both a substance use disorder and another major psychiatric disorder. Examples include a cocaine-dependent patient with panic disorder and an alcoholic patient with major depression. The term is used to highlight the difference between such patients and patients with a single diagnosis; patients with a dual diagnosis have special needs in terms of diagnosis and treatment. Although the term dual diagnosis refers to all patients with concomitant diagnoses of substance abuse and other psychiatric illness, the population is highly heterogeneous. Both of the patients mentioned above, for example, have dual diagnoses, but their disorders may require very different treatments.

2. Is dual diagnosis common?
Yes. Dual diagnosis is extremely common and often unrecognized. Of patients with a substance use disorder, approximately 50% have at least one other psychiatric disorder, most commonly a mood or anxiety disorder. Conversely, almost 30% of patients with other psychiatric disorders also have a history of substance abuse.

3. Why is it important to determine whether a patient has both a substance use and another psychiatric disorder?
The importance of identifying substance abuse in a patient with a psychiatric disorder cannot be overstated. In general, patients with a dual diagnosis have higher morbidity, lower likelihood for initial treatment success, higher relapse rates, increased rates of hospitalization, and decreased adherence to treatment. They also are at increased risk for suicide. The presence of substance abuse also may make diagnosis of both disorders more complicated. For treatment of either disorder to be successful, both must be identified and treated individually.

4. Do certain psychiatric conditions tend to be seen with substance abuse?
Many studies have shown specific associations between certain psychiatric disorders and substance abuse. For example, antisocial personality disorder is highly correlated with substance abuse. In one extensive study, 84% of individuals with antisocial personality disorder also had a history of substance abuse. Mood disorders also are commonly associated with substance abuse; in the same study, 32% of individuals with a diagnosis of mood disorder were also substance abusers. In addition, specific psychiatric disorders are associated with specific drugs of abuse, such as bipolar disorder with alcohol and panic disorder with sedatives and hypnotics.

5. What is the cause of dual diagnosis?
Many mechanisms have been proposed to explain the occurrence of a substance use disorder and another psychiatric illness in the same individual, but no evidence suggests that any one mechanism is the only possible explanation.

  1. **Psychopathology may serve as a risk factor for addictive disorders or may affect the course of an addictive disorder.** For example, a 32-year-old woman with a severe social phobia found that alcohol relieved her anxiety enough to allow her to function at her job. With repeated use, however, she became dependent on alcohol. Withdrawal symptoms led to more anxiety, which led to more drinking, and eventually she developed full-blown alcohol addiction. A second example is a 26-year-old male alcoholic with bipolar disorder who had periods of abstinence for

as long as 6 months. However, each time he entered a manic episode, he stopped going to Alcoholics Anonymous meetings and began drinking again.

2. **There may be familial (genetic) links between certain psychiatric disorders and substance use disorders.** For example, a 40-year-old man with a history of alcoholism was diagnosed with major depression. Family history showed that his mother had been dependent on alcohol in her early thirties and had recently had a depressive episode. His maternal grandmother also had a history of depression. His maternal uncle had been an alcoholic and committed suicide at age 38. The patient's sister had been diagnosed with major depression in college.

3. **Psychiatric symptoms may develop in the course of chronic intoxication with an abused substance.** For example, a 55-year-old man who had been smoking marijuana almost daily for several years developed depressive symptoms as well as paranoid ideation. The symptoms disappeared when he stopped using marijuana.

4. **Psychiatric disorders may emerge as a consequence of substance use and persist after remission.** For example, a 30-year-old woman with no history of psychiatric illness began using cocaine. After almost a year of use, she began having occasional panic attacks when high. After several more months, the attacks occurred in between cocaine highs. Years later, despite having been drug-free for 6 months, the panic attacks continued. They were successfully treated with imipramine.

5. **The occurrence of both disorders in the same individual is pure coincidence.** Because both mental illness and substance abuse are highly prevalent in the general population, an individual may have both a substance use disorder and a psychiatric disorder by chance, just as one individual may have both asthma and migraine headaches.

6. What is the self-medication hypothesis?

The self-medication hypothesis holds that substance abuse occurs when an individual attempts to self-medicate his or her psychiatric symptoms. This hypothesis is based on a small group of drug abusers and has not been validated experimentally. The theory holds that patients do not abuse drugs randomly; rather, they discover a drug that relieves painful feelings and thereby serves as a coping mechanism. Repetitive use of the drug as self-medication eventually may lead to dependence. Even after treatment of the psychiatric disorder, the addiction may persist, and require independent treatment. For example, a 24-year-old man, who describes himself as having been depressed all of his life, tried heroin at a party and said that for the first time he felt relief from emotional distress. Soon he was using heroin daily and needed increasing amounts to get the same relief.

7. Can certain psychiatric symptoms be confused with withdrawal symptoms or intoxication?

Absolutely. Many psychiatric symptoms can be caused by substance use or withdrawal. Depressive symptoms, such as insomnia, decreased libido, anhedonia, and suicidality are often seen with chronic alcoholism and marijuana use and may be indistinguishable from a major depressive episode. Manic symptoms, such as euphoria, inflated self-esteem, and decreased need for sleep, may occur during cocaine intoxication. Withdrawal from certain drugs also may cause psychiatric symptoms, such as the hallucinations associated with delirium tremens or the psychomotor agitation associated with sedative withdrawal.

Psychiatric Symptoms Associated with Substance Abuse

SUBSTANCE	PSYCHIATRIC SYMPTOMS DURING INTOXICATION	PSYCHIATRIC SYMPTOMS DURING WITHDRAWAL
Alcohol	Anxiety, depression, sudden mood changes, paranoia, suicidality, memory loss	Hallucinations (delirium tremens, alcohol hallucinosis), anxiety, insomnia, psychomotor agitation

Table continued on following page.

Psychiatric Symptoms Associated with Substance Abuse (Cont.)

SUBSTANCE	PSYCHIATRIC SYMPTOMS DURING INTOXICATION	PSYCHIATRIC SYMPTOMS DURING WITHDRAWAL
Cocaine	Mania, acute paranoid ideation, panic attacks	Depression, anhedonia, anxiety
Stimulants	Mania, paranoia, nightmares	Dysphoria, psychomotor retardation, irritability, guilt, suicidality
Inhalants	Anxiety, personality changes	Anxiety, depression
Cannabis	Anxiety, paranoid ideation, suicidality	
Opioids	Panic reactions, lethargy	Depression
Depressants	Depression, anxiety, paranoia, psychosis	Insomnia, irritability, psychomotor agitation
Hallucinogens	Hallucinations, paranoia, depersonalization, confusion	Flashbacks (may occur years after last use)

8. Can substance abuse *cause* mental illness?

Substance abuse may induce other psychiatric disorders that persist even after drug use is discontinued. For example, some cocaine abusers develop panic attacks. Initially the attacks occur solely during cocaine intoxication, but with time they may occur between cocaine highs and even persist after complete cessation of drug use. The attacks often can be treated successfully with imipramine or other treatments for panic disorder. Certain hallucinogens, such as lysergic acid diethylamide (LSD), may cause perceptual disturbances or visual hallucinations that continue for years after last use. The term **posthallucinogen perceptual disorder** has been coined to describe the occurrence of such disturbances, traditionally called flashbacks. Substance abuse also may exacerbate another already present but unrecognized psychiatric disorder. In this case the substance abuse does not cause the other disorder but rather makes it clinically apparent.

9. How can one tell whether a patient's psychiatric symptoms are caused by substance abuse?

Timing, timing, timing! Because drug intoxication can mimic many psychiatric symptoms and disorders and thus confound diagnosis, it is crucial to assess mental illness only after a period of abstinence. How long the drug-free period must last before an accurate psychiatric diagnosis can be made depends on both the drug and the suspected disorder. Generally it is recommended that the patient be drug-free for 2–4 weeks before concluding that another psychiatric disorder is present. A good history, from both the patient and family members, is crucial to understanding the clinical picture. A good history or prior familiarity with the patient may also help to sort out confusing symptoms and to make diagnoses with a shorter waiting period.

10. Do patients with a dual diagnosis need special treatment?

Yes and no. The most important issue is the need to treat *both* disorders. Treatment that minimizes the importance of either diagnosis results in unnecessarily high rates of relapse. Patients need to be educated about both diagnoses and how they interact.

Several treatment settings and methods are available to treat the substance-abusing psychiatric patient. Inpatient hospitalization may take place in a dual-diagnosis treatment unit, a substance abuse treatment unit, or a psychiatric treatment unit. Dual-diagnosis units are the ideal setting, but they are not always available. Patients can be adequately treated in other settings, provided that the clinicians involved in their care are knowledgeable about their special needs. Outpatient programs are becoming more common and may involve intensive treatment that includes medication management, support groups, psychotherapy, self-help groups, and social services.

11. What is the role of psychotropic medications?

Pharmacotherapy is not only appropriate in certain patients with dual diagnoses; it is often necessary (as in some patients with psychiatric illness alone). Medications generally are directed toward the coexisting psychiatric disorder. However, several issues need special attention. Many drugs of abuse interact with psychotropic medications. Abused substances may increase or decrease the metabolism of certain medications via the induction of hepatic enzymes or a change in plasma protein binding. They can either lower or raise plasma levels, resulting in decreased efficacy or dangerous side effects. Such interactions must be taken into consideration in prescribing medications for a substance-abusing patient or a patient with substance-abusing potential. Certain medications, such as benzodiazepines, are addictive in and of themselves, and their potential for abuse in patients with substance abuse histories is increased. Although such medications are often necessary, clinicians should prescribe the least habit-forming option that is efficacious. For example, a patient with panic disorder may be treated with a tricyclic antidepressant rather than an anxiolytic, which has a higher addictive potential.

Interactions Between Drugs of Abuse and Psychotropic Medications

DRUG OF ABUSE	THERAPEUTIC AGENT	POSSIBLE INTERACTIONS
Alcohol	Disulfiram (Antabuse)	Produces flushing, hypotension, nausea, tachycardia; fatal reactions possible
	MAO inhibitors	Impaired hepatic metabolism of tyramine in some beverages produces dangerous, possibly fatal hypertension
	Tricyclic antidepressants	Additive CNS impairment
	Antipsychotics	Increased CNS impairment on psychomotor skills, judgment, and behavior; possible increased risk of akithesia and dystonia
	Anticonvulsants	Chronic alcohol use results in induction of hepatic microsomal enzymes, reducing phenytoin levels; possible seizure risk
Barbiturates	Tricyclic antidepressants	Reduced efficacy of tricyclics; may potentiate respiratory depression
	MAO inhibitors	Inhibited barbiturate metabolism, prolonging intoxication
	Antipsychotics	Induced hepatic microsomal enzymes may reduce chlorpromazine levels
	Anticonvulsants	Valproic acid increases phenobarbital levels and toxicity; induced hepatic microsomal enzymes may reduce carbamazepine levels and unpredictable phenytoin levels
Benzodiazepines	Disulfiram	Enhanced benzodiazepine effects (oxazepam and lorazepam not affected)
	MAO inhibitors	Rare reports of edema with chlordiazepoxide
Opiates	MAO inhibitors	Meperidine may produce severe excitation, diaphoresis, rigidity, hyper/hypotension, coma, and death
	Antipsychotics	Hypotension and excessive CNS depression possible with meperidine and chlorpromazine

Table continued on following page.

Interactions Between Drugs of Abuse and Psychotropic Medications (Cont.)

DRUG OF ABUSE	THERAPEUTIC AGENT	POSSIBLE INTERACTIONS
Opiates *(Cont.)*	Anticonvulsants	Propoxyphene increases carbamazepine levels with risk of toxicity; methadone metabolism may be increased by carbamazepine or phenytoin, causing withdrawal
Stimulants	MAO inhibitors	Hyperpyrexia, severe hypertension, death when used with cocaine or amphetamines
	Antipsychotics	Cocaine and amphetamines may cause delusions and hallucinations of chronic psychoses to break through antipsychotics

MAO = monoamine oxidase, CNS = central nervous system.
Adapted from Gastfriend DR: Pharmacotherapy of psychiatric syndromes with comorbid chemical dependence. J Addict Dis 12(3):155–170, 1993, with permission.

12. Does any evidence suggest that psychotherapy is helpful in treating patients with a dual diagnosis?
Psychotherapy, particularly supportive-expressive or cognitive-behavioral models, has been shown to be useful in treating patients with substance use disorders and psychiatric illness, although its efficacy depends on the specific psychiatric disorder and the drug of abuse. Patients with comorbid mood and anxiety disorders tend to benefit from psychotherapy more than patients with personality disorders. In general, psychotherapy provides support for continued abstinence as well as adherence to medication regimens. It also addresses underlying emotional states, such as depression or anxiety, that may contribute to the maintenance of substance abuse.

13. What is the role of self-help groups, such as Alcoholics Anonymous or Narcotics Anonymous?
Twelve-step groups such as Alcoholics Anonymous, Cocaine Anonymous, and Narcotics Anonymous are known to contribute successfully to the maintenance of abstinence in substance-abusing patients. Although they may be helpful for patients with dual diagnoses, they do not address issues specific to this population, such as use of psychotropic medications or difficulties in living with mental illness. Self-help groups especially for patients with a dual diagnosis may better address such concerns, but because of the heterogeneity of the population, patients may not feel that they have much in common with other participants. For some patients, however, such groups are invaluable tools, and participation should be encouraged on an individual basis.

BIBLIOGRAPHY

1. Abraham HD, Aldridge AM: Adverse consequences of lysergic acid diethylamide. Addiction 88:1327–1334, 1993.
2. Bell CM, Khantzian EJ: Drug use and addiction as self medication: A psychodynamic perspective. In Gold MS, Slaby AE: Dual Diagnosis and Substance Abuse. New York, Marcel Dekker, 1991, pp 185–203.
3. Cohen ST: Substance abuse and mental illness. In Friedman L, et al: Sourcebook of Substance Abuse and Addiction. Baltimore, Williams & Wilkins, 1996.
4. Dackis CA, Gold MS: Psychopathology resulting from substance abuse. In Gold MS, Slaby AE: Dual Diagnosis and Substance Abuse. New York, Marcel Dekker, 1991, pp 205–220.
5. Giannini AJ, Collins GB: Substance abuse and thought disorders. In Gold MS, Slaby AE: Dual Diagnosis and Substance Abuse. New York, Marcel Dekker, 1991, pp 57–93.
6. Khantzian EJ: The self-medication hypothesis of addictive disorders: Focus on heroin and cocaine dependence. American Journal of Psychiatry 142:1259, 1985.
7. Meyer RE: How to understand the relationship between psychopathology and addictive disorders: Another example of the chicken and the egg. In Meyer RE: Psychopathology and Addictive Disorders. New York, Guilford Press, 1986, pp 3–15.

8. Mirin SM, Weiss RD, Griffin ML, Michael JL: Psychopathology in drug abusers and their families. Compr Psychiatry 32:36, 1991.

9. Norris CR, Extein IL: Diagnosing dual diagnosis patients. In Gold MS, Slaby AE: Dual Diagnosis and Substance Abuse. New York, Marcel Dekker, 1991, pp 159–184.

10. Regier DA, Farmer ME, Rae DS, et al: Comorbidity of mental disorders with alcohol and other drug abuse: Results from the epidemiologic catchment area study. JAMA 264:2511, 1990.

11. Slaby AE: Dual diagnosis: Fact or fiction? In Gold MS, Slaby AE: Dual Diagnosis in Substance Abuse. New York, Marcel Dekker, 1991, pp 3–27.

12. Weiss RD, Mirin SM: The dual diagnosis alcoholic: Evaluation and treatment. Psychiatr Ann 19:261–265, 1989.

13. Weiss RD, Collins DA: Substance abuse and psychiatric illness. Am J Addict 1:93, 1992.

14. Weiss RD, Mirin SM, Frances RJ: The myth of the typical dual-diagnosis patient. Hosp Community Psychiatry 43:107, 1992.

26. DISSOCIATIVE IDENTITY DISORDER (MULTIPLE PERSONALITY DISORDER) AND OTHER DISSOCIATIVE DISORDERS

Marita J. Keeling, M.D.

1. What is dissociative identity disorder?

In DSM–IV the term dissociative identity disorder replaces the term multiple personality disorder, which was used in DSM–IIIR. To fit the diagnosis, the patient must demonstrate the presence of two or more distinct identities (each with its own relatively enduring pattern of perceiving, relating to, and thinking about the environment and itself). At least two of these personality or ego states recurrently take control of the person's behavior. DSM–IV adds a third criterion: the patient must be unable to recall important personal information to a degree that is too extensive to be explained by ordinary forgetfulness. In addition, medical conditions or substance abuse, which may cause dissociative symptoms, must be ruled out.

The problem lies in the inability to integrate various aspects of identity, memory, and consciousness. However, the first major controversy in an extraordinarily controversial diagnosis is the fact that a significant number of practitioners believe that the disorder does not exist or, if it does, is extremely rare. In their opinion, most, if not all, instances, are created iatrogenically by the combination of a biased therapist and a highly suggestible patient who is willing to "create" personalities for secondary gain such as approval, companionship, or avoidance of responsibility. In contrast, other practitioners believe that the disorder is underdiagnosed, with an incidence as high as 4% among psychiatric inpatients, and should be viewed on a continuum from normal experiences of dissociation to development of several hundred personalities or "personality fragments." Such practitioners believe that only a small number of "classic" multiple personalities meet DSM–IV criteria but that underdiagnosis results in less than optimal forms of therapy for numerous patients.

The issue of prevalence is further complicated by the trendiness of the diagnosis, widespread publicity in the media of dramatic examples, and grass-roots organizations of patients who believe that they have the disorder. Most practitioners agree that many self-diagnosed as well as formally diagnosed patients do not in fact have multiple personality but meet other needs by behaving as if they do.

The female-to-male ratio is 9:1. This ratio has been thought to reflect the increased likelihood of sexual abuse of female children, but sociocultural and other factors may play a role.

2. What sort of personalities do people with dissociative identity disorder have?

Although hundreds of personalities have been reported by patients diagnosed with dissociative identity disorder, a total of 10–20 is most common. Typically personalities are organized by occupation or dominant interest (e.g., cook, worker, student, sexually active personality) age (different ages sometimes are thought to relate to ages at which specific traumatic events occurred), and emotion (e.g., anger, sadness, calmness). Personalities may be of any age, sex, or ethnic background. They also may be fantastic (e.g., fairy or wizard), spiritual (e.g., angel or demon), nonhuman (e.g., monster or dog), or partial (e.g., head without body). It is probably most useful for the physician to conceptualize the development of personality states as the patient's attempt to express emotions and conflicts and to determine the function of a particular ego state. For example, a demon may embody a deep-seated sense of being evil; a dog, the idea of unconditional love; a sorcerer, the wish to solve problems and defeat enemies with magic; and a bodiless head, the denial of physical reality and therefore of physical pain or limitations.

Personalities have different experiences of the presence of one another. Some report awareness of all of the others (termed coconsciousness), and some are amnesic for most of the others.
Often a helper personality (internal self helper [ISH]) performs a controlling and coordinating
function. Protector personalities may behave dangerously. Practitioners disagree about the nature
of the primary, host, or presenting personality, which some believe is the true identity and others
view as merely another ego state. Personalities may be seen by one another and may hear each
other speak (in a hallucinatory fashion). They frequently demonstrate different types of handwriting and different styles of language, drawing, and other activities. Personalities may demonstrate
intense dislike for one another, argue, and even attempt internal homicide (i.e., suicide) on the
grounds that they are trying to get rid of a troublesome person.

3. What causes multiple personality?

Until recently it was thought that severe childhood trauma, particularly extensive sexual abuse,
was the cause of multiple personality. DSM–IIIR states that "several studies indicate that in
nearly all cases, the disorder has been preceded by abuse (often sexual) or another form of severe
emotional trauma in childhood." It was believed that the development of dissociated personality
states was the child's best response to trauma. For example, a physically abused child may create
an alterego (perhaps initially perceived as an imaginary companion) who can "take the abuse."
The primary personality can use denial and say, "I'm not the bad girl, so and so was bad, and she
gets punished." This response enables the child to maintain a loving connection with the abuser
(often a parent) and to continue relatively normal development in some areas of life, such as academic achievement.

However, such reports of severe abuse have led to another area of controversy. In recent
years many patients diagnosed with dissociative identity disorder have claimed unusual forms of
abuse, such as multigenerational intrafamilial satanic rituals or politically based programming in
secret military experiments. Although many practitioners believe such reports, virtually no hard
evidence validates such experiences, and their increasing frequency has led to comments such as,
"If the number of babies reported by our patients had been sacrificed, the Eastern seaboard would
have been depopulated!" As a consequence, many practitioners question the entire process of
memory formation in such patients, even the occurrence of relatively common forms of abuse
(such as child sexual abuse and incest).

Thus, it is not known what causes dissociative identity disorder or predisposes individuals to
its development. A genetic capacity for extensive dissociative abilities appears to be necessary.

4. Describe some effects of the widespread publicity about dissociative identity disorder.

Prominent public examples have played a role in what some consider a backlash against adults
who were abused as children. Adult children have successfully sued parents for child abuse
after recovering repressed memories. Prominent and flamboyant public figures have declared
their backgrounds of abuse. Some criminal figures have used a diagnosis of multiple personality disorder as a defense in murder trials. Many of these examples have aroused public outrage.
The False Memory Syndrome Foundation consists primarily of friends and relatives of patients
with dissociative identity disorder who say that they have been accused unjustly of horrible
abuse. The foundation actively promotes dissemination of information about the inaccuracy of
memory.

Of course, actual perpetrators of abuse would be unlikely to admit to illegal or immoral practices. Many practitioners are now afraid that individuals who in fact were abused as children will
become even more afraid to reveal the truth and therefore will not receive much needed treatment. The current stance taken by the American Psychiatric Association is that *physicians should
neither believe nor disbelieve unsubstantiated reports of abuse from their clients.* This is an attempt to find some sort of middle ground. The controversy creates considerable difficulty in
forming a successful and useful therapeutic relationship.

Patients with dissociative identity disorder are also unusual in that, unlike most patients
with psychiatric disorders, they are often willing to speak up publicly about their symptoms and

experiences. In part this willingness appears to be related to their convictions that the disorder was caused by abuse in early childhood and that the politically correct stance is to stand up fiercely for the rights of children. Others believe that the popularity of the diagnosis is related to avoidance of responsibility for dysfunctional and even antisocial patterns of behavior. Practitioners tend to become polarized into diametrically opposed camps on such issues. It is most likely that a middle ground is correct, i.e., individuals may have had traumatic experiences that predisposed them to the development of dissociative symptoms and they may use such symptoms as coping mechanisms, albeit dysfunctional ones, in later life.

5. What is dissociation?

The term dissociation directly describes the "dis-association" of cognitive functions. For example, individuals may dissociate memory from consciousness and experience amnesia (or "lost time" in the common parlance of dissociative identity disorder) for recent or remote events. Dissociation is probably akin to the psychoanalytic concept of repression. Motor functions may be dissociated from awareness in sleep-walking or automatic behavior such as driving while daydreaming. The experience of physical pain may be dissociated from awareness; thus people have the capacity to induce analgesia. Lamaze training teaches pregnant women to use dissociation to manage labor and delivery more comfortably. Indian fakirs who drag heavy objects attached to hooks that pierce their skin also use dissociative techniques. Hypnosis deliberately induces dissociative states in individuals for various purposes, such as induction of analgesia. Biofeedback is a dissociative technique that enables people to develop greater control over physiologic processes. Intense concentration for study or sports is a self-induced dissociative state that enables people to screen out distracting stimuli and to focus more effectively.

Obviously most of the above dissociative experiences are "normal," that is, common. Indeed, the capacity to dissociate is a natural human ability with a probable genetic basis. Only about 5% of the population has the capacity to attain an extremely deep trance in which they experience unusual phenomena, such as experiencing negative hallucinations (that is, being unable to see objects in front of them) or developing physical evidence of burns caused by fantasy alone. Probably most patients with dissociative identity disorder are in this 5% of the population.

In dissociative states people experience an alteration in logic and thinking. In normal waking states adults generally have logical, linear, and complex thought patterns. In "trance logic" people experience time distortion, nonlinear thought, simple language, increased creativity, intense emotions, and magical and paradoxical thinking patterns. Such differences are similar to the differences described between left and right brain thinking and may reflect shifts in brain functioning.

Individuals in dissociative states are also highly suggestible. This trait may be one of the bases for some of the problems that arise in treatment of patients with dissociative identity disorder who by definition are in dissociated states a great deal of the time. In the right circumstances such patients may come to believe irrational or bizarre ideas that originated in an external suggestion. Such ideas can be maintained because of the capacity to hold coexisting sets of beliefs that are mutually exclusive. For example, "I am a 26-year-old white woman, and I am also a crying 3-year-old and a 6-foot tall dangerous black male." People may be particularly susceptible to absorbing ideas in hypnotic trances, and it has been observed that, after introduction of an idea during hypnosis, people may tenaciously hold onto the belief that the idea was theirs.

6. Name three other dissociative disorders.

1. **Dissociative amnesia** is characterized by one or more episodes of inability to recall important information (usually of a traumatic or stressful nature) that cannot be explained by ordinary forgetfulness. Dissociative amnesia is typically caused by acute psychological traumas. Amnestic symptoms also may be caused by psychoactive substances and medical conditions (e.g., partial complex seizures) or occur in the course of other major disorders such as dissociative identity disorder, posttraumatic stress disorder (PTSD), or borderline personality disorder. Care must be taken in making the diagnosis when the memory loss is thought to be related to childhood trauma.

2. **Dissociative fugue** is diagnosed when a patient suddenly and unexpectedly travels away from home, is unable to remember his or her past, and also experiences confusion about his or her identity or even assumes a new identity. Dissociative identity disorder, PTSD, borderline personality disorder, psychoactive substance use, medical conditions (e.g., partial complex seizures), and malingering may lead to fugue states.

3. **Depersonalization disorder** is diagnosed when patients report feeling detached from their mental processes or body (e.g., feeling as if they are in a dream). Reality testing (i.e., patients accurately report who they are and what is going on around them) remains intact, but the disorder results in significant distress or impairment in functioning. As with the amnesia and fugue states, posttraumatic stress disorder, borderline personality disorder, dissociative identity disorder, and medically related conditions must be considered in the differential diagnosis.

7. Describe the typical course of dissociative identity disorder.
Dissociative identity disorder may present in childhood, adolescence, or adulthood. Some believe that it is especially underdiagnosed in childhood and that prompt identification and treatment are important to facilitate normal identity development. It has been reported that diagnosis is generally made only after 6–7 years of psychiatric treatment. Whether this delay is due to secrecy (developed to protect the patient from abuse), lack of awareness on the part of the treater, or iatrogenic origin is, of course, controversial.

When the disorder has been diagnosed, the course fluctuates. People may have activity of alter personality states continuously or episodically for many years. Dissociative identity disorder is diagnosed less in adults over age 40, but it is unclear whether the disorder has a natural tendency to remit with age or whether practitioners focus on different age groups.

8. Discuss comorbid diagnoses and associated features.
Symptoms of **PTSD** are common, including nightmares, flashbacks, and startle responses. Many practitioners consider that dissociative identity disorder is a form of PTSD, but the problem of whether or not child abuse in fact occurred confuses the issue. **Borderline personality disorder** has been found to coexist in over 80% of patients with dissociative identity disorder. Self-destructive behavior, such as self-mutilation, impulsivity, and intense and fluctuating emotions and relationships, are common in patients with borderline pathology. Depressive disorders, anxiety disorders, substance abuse, sexual dysfunction, eating disorders, and sleep disorders are common. In addition, somatization (e.g., headaches, irritable bowel syndrome, chronic pain syndromes) and conversion reactions may be present.

9. What is the differential diagnosis?
Surprise—another area of controversy! Visual and auditory hallucinations suggest the diagnosis of a psychotic disorder, and rapid shifts of personality states and moods suggest a bipolar disorder with rapid cycling, but these distinctions may be difficult to make. Furthermore, the extent to which a physician is wedded to the idea that dissociative identity disorder *does or does not exist*, often dictates the diagnosis.

At least in some instances dissociative identity disorder can be faked (e.g., by actors under experimental conditions) so effectively that even experienced practitioners are fooled. Clearcut dissociative symptoms, sudden shifts in identity states, reversible amnesia, high scores on scales of dissociation, and increased susceptibility to hypnosis may help to support the diagnosis. Special care needs to be taken with diagnosis in criminal settings or when financial gain is an issue. Corroboration of preexisting dissociative symptomatology (e.g., reports from friends or family, notebooks with different types of handwriting) may be necessary to distinguish dissociative identity disorder from malingering, factitious disorder (with help-seeking behavior), or personality disorders.

Complex partial seizures should be distinguished from dissociative identity disorder, although the two disorders may occur simultaneously. Psychoactive substances can produce dissociative phenomena. Dissociative identity disorder should be diagnosed in preference to one of the other dissociative disorders if symptoms overlap.

10. Describe a typical course of psychotherapeutic treatment.

The approaches to treatment of dissociative identity disorder are wide-ranging and often controversial. Certainly patients with this disorder are complex and often difficult to treat, particularly when they have numerous coexisting disorders. Because research and clinical experience are scant and because patients often have been so dangerous and/or suicidal that there appears to be little to lose, many therapists have justified quite unusual treatments that normally would not be acceptable in other psychiatric disorders. Unusual treatments include very high dosages and unusual combinations of medications (e.g., high doses of multiple benzodiazepines, stimulants, antidepressants, and anticonvulsive agents); long-term hospitalizations (of 1 year or more); focus on uncovering and working through traumatic memories by means of hypnosis and guided imagery; and reparenting approaches, with hugging, child-like alter egos, childlike play, and use of stuffed toys and baby foods. Unfortunately, none of these approaches has proved effective. High-dose and combined medications cause complications such as toxicity and substance dependence; long hospitalizations and regressive approaches foster greater and greater dependency on the therapist and promote loss of functioning that may be disabling; and hugging and other boundary-crossing behavior have resulted in serious violations of the patient-therapist relationship. These consequences, in combination with the rapidly increasing prominence of managed care in the insurance market, have led to reconsideration of such treatment approaches.

Most therapists now use a **goal-oriented, problem-solving, cognitive-behavioral, limit-seeking approach**, with minimal hospitalization and avoidance of techniques that promote regression. **Hypnosis** is still widely used to uncover traumatic material and to facilitate integration and switching of personalities so that conflicts and internal "group therapy" can be more easily explored. Many practitioners still feel that **abreacting** (i.e., intensely reliving) a traumatic experience is necessary to work through memories (i.e., to integrate memory, cognitions, and emotions so that the patient can let go of the trauma). Of course, this concept is of limited value when the therapist questions whether the trauma occurred at all. The therapist should adhere to basic principles of psychotherapy, and any technique that may cause clinically significant or obvious problems in patients with other diagnoses should be used with caution.

When multiple personality disorder was first recognized, the logical goal appeared to be integration of the different personalities. Various techniques to encourage this goal (e.g., hypnotic imagery) have been attempted with varying degrees of success. Some people still believe that identity integration is the only acceptable outcome for completed therapy. Others believe that functional integration (i.e., cooperative functioning) among alter personalities is sufficient if the person can lead a healthy, happy life with reasonable ability to work and conduct relationships. Generally speaking, identity integration occurs spontaneously when functional integration is achieved.

Some practitioners believe that it is necessary to "map the system," that is, to identify the various personalities, their functions, sources (presumed to be traumatic), and conflicts. Others observe that the more the therapist explores the different personalities, the more they seem to be created; in this context, it is easy to lose sight of the person's real-life difficulties (such as marital problems). Probably the most useful approach is to balance empathic attempts to understand and share the person's inner experience with therapy focused on here-and-now problems, consequences of dysfunctional behavior, and goals for real life.

The process of successful therapy with an outcome of functional behavior often takes 5–10 years. Unfortunately, successful outcomes are still quite unusual. Many patients change therapists frequently, become disabled, and suffer consequences of other disorders (such as substance abuse or depression). There are no adequate outcome studies to date.

Treatment of coexisting psychiatric disorders, especially substance abuse and personality disorders, is essential.

Group therapy may or may not be effective. Participation may reduce the patient's sense of isolation and provide a safe place to discuss traumatic material that patients without dissociative identity disorder cannot tolerate, to study interpersonal relationships, to develop more functional interactions, and to learn more about coping mechanisms. However, members of groups also may develop intense pathologic transferences to one another and to therapists, compete for attention by striving to be the sickest, and otherwise reinforce identity fragmentation and dysfunctional behavior. **Couples therapy** and **family therapy** often may be needed to assist with dysfunctional interactions such as unconscious reinforcement or enabling of dysfunctional behavior on the part of significant others, who perceive their behavior as kind and supportive.

Adjunctive forms of therapy such as art therapy, journal therapy, music therapy, movement therapy, massage therapy, "body work," holistic medications, and spiritual approaches (e.g., exorcism and various rituals) have also been used. The wide range of types of therapy probably reflects the identity fragmentation of the patient and the desperation of health care providers who work with such difficult patients. Their utility remains clouded.

11. What major pitfalls does the physician face?
It is difficult to explain why many highly regarded psychiatrists and other therapists appear to have lost sight of basic principles in working with patients with dissociative identity disorder. It is difficult for the therapist to understand the internal experience of having multiple personalities without becoming overwhelmed. The patient's experience is something like the following: "If I believe that it is not me who is responsible for my actions but an 'other' (within this experience of perceiving myself as a 'group') I may feel truly helpless and out of control." Many patients with dissociative identity disorder feel that they can do nothing to prevent self-mutilation, rage, antisocial behavior, or suicide attempts. They also may discover quite quickly that people around them are fascinated by the peculiarities of their experience and that it is easy to get away with generally unacceptable behavior (e.g., alcohol abuse, sexual indiscretions) by pleading lack of awareness or directing the interest of others toward gory and bizarre traumatic material. Although occasionally this pattern may be conscious (e.g., to avoid responsibility for a major crime), in most cases it is probably unconscious. Patients with dissociative identity disorder are not "bad," although many practitioners may become extremely angry and frustrated and feel victimized by their patients. Physicians may then express their anger by emotional abandonment, emotional abuse, and occasionally physical abuse of the patient.

It is difficult for a therapist to maintain a balance of empathy with the patient's personal perception of multiple identity and helplessness while maintaining a realistic recognition that the patient must accept the predictable consequences of his or her behavior, whether or not he or she feels in control. Therapists, especially those with little experience in working with patients with severe personality disorders, frequently come to believe that such patients are truly helpless. It is only a small step for the therapist to begin to feel personally responsible for rescuing the patient and keeping him or her alive. The therapist may begin to spend inordinate amounts of time providing telephone therapy, managing finances, allowing the patient to stay in his or her home, and/or "falling in love" with the patient because he or she is so "special." It is important to be aware of such intense countertransference responses and to seek consultation and supervision quickly.

It is helpful to keep firmly in mind that most patients with dissociative identity disorder also meet the criteria for borderline personality disorder. The much larger body of data and clinical experience related to this disorder provide useful guidelines when crises occur.

12. What medications can be useful in the treatment of dissociative identity disorder?
Because of the lack of controlled studies, the use of medication for patients with dissociative identity disorder varies from none at all (because of limited success as well as the assumption that symptoms are related to psychological conflicts) to complex medication regimens. Antidepressants, antianxiety agents, and neuroleptics are used most commonly. Carbamazepine has been reported to be useful in reducing episodic violence. Lithium is sometimes helpful for regulating "switching" of personality states, which is akin to mood swings, as are propranolol and other beta-adrenergic blockers. Medication for treatment of coexisting disorders, such as major depression, bipolar disorder, psychosis, or anxiety, also should be used.

13. Discuss some of the neurobiologic research in the field of dissociative identity disorder.
There have long been anecdotal reports of remarkable behaviors in patients with dissociative identity disorder. For example, different personalities have reportedly demonstrated differences in EEG tracings, responses to medication or psychoactive substances, allergic reactions, and perception of pain. Many of the reported differences involve subjective experiences, such as vision and hearing, and therefore may be psychological perceptions consistent with the experiences of being many different people. Hard scientific data related to measurable neurophysiological changes are lacking. However, an increasing number of small studies are being performed. Unfortunately, virtually all are flawed by poor methodology or have not been published; in addition, the results are contradictory. Nevertheless there is some indication of variation in (1) cerebral blood flow (particularly perfusion of the temporal lobe); (2) EEG patterns (especially alpha waves), visual evoked potentials, and brain electrical activity mapping; and (3) galvanic skin responses between different personality states or before and after integration. Evidence also suggests the presence of thyroid and other neuroendocrine abnormalities in patients with multiple personality disorder. At this point in time no conclusions can be drawn other than that more research with controlled double-blind studies is needed.

14. Is any aspect of dissociative identity disorder *not* controversial?
No.

BIBLIOGRAPHY

1. Bloch JP: Assessment and Treatment of Multiple Personality and Dissociative Disorders. Sarasota, Professional Resource Press, 1991.
2. Braun BG (ed): Treatment of Multiple Personality Disorder. Washington, DC, American Psychiatric Press, 1986.
3. Beahrs JO: Dissociative identity disorder: Adaptive deception of self and others. Bull Am Acad Psychiatry Law 22:223–237, 1994.
4. Ganaway GK: Historical versus narrative truth: Clarifying the role of exogenous trauma in the etiology of MPD and its variants. Dissociation 11:205–220, 1989.
5. Miller SD, Triggiano PJ: The psychophysiological investigation of multiple personality disorder: Review and update. Am J Clin Hypnosis 35:47–61, 1992.
6. North CS, Ryall JM, Ricci DA, Wetzel RD: Multiple Personalities, Multiple Disorders: Psychiatric Classification and Media Influence. New York, Oxford University Press, 1993.
7. Putnam FW, Guroff JJ, Silverman EK, et al: The clinical phenomenology of multiple personality disorder: Review of 100 recent cases. J Clin Psychiatry 47:285–293, 1986.
8. Putnam FW: Diagnosis and Treatment of Multiple Personality Disorder. New York, Guilford Press, 1989.
9. Spiegel D (ed): Dissociation, Culture, Mind and Body. Washington, DC, American Psychiatric Press, 1994.
10. Young WC: Sadistic ritual abuse: An overview in detection and management. Prim Care 20:447–458, 1993.

27. SEXUAL DISORDERS AND SEXUALITY

Harold P. Martin, M.D.

1. Name the three categories of sexual disorders.
Paraphilias
Gender identity disorders
Sexual dysfunction

2. What are paraphilias?
Paraphilia is defined by DSM–IV as a disorder in which a person experiences "recurrent, intense sexually arousing fantasies, urges, or behavior involving (1) nonhuman objects, (2) the suffering or humiliation of oneself or one's partner, or (3) children or non-consenting adults."

Patients may not be able to become sexually aroused unless involved with a paraphilia or may have an obsessive need to engage in the paraphiliac fantasy or behavior. According to DSM–IV, impairment in social or occupational functioning or significant emotional distress is necessary for a diagnosis. However, even if patients are comfortable with their paraphilia and have no apparent impairment of job or social life, the diagnosis can be made if the paraphiliacal behavior is obligatory for sexual arousal or recurrent, persistent, and obsessive. Behaviors may result in social or legal ramifications (e.g., pedophilia, exhibitionism). Indeed, for many paraphiliacs, the only emotional distress is the fear of discovery, legal punishment, or disapproval by persons they care about. Types of paraphilias include:

1. **Exhibitionism**: sexual arousal from exposing one's genitals to strangers.
2. **Fetishism**: use of nonliving objects—usually clothes—that the patient may hold, rub, smell, for sexual arousal.
3. **Transvestic fetishism**: cross-dressing, which usually is seen in heterosexual men, who find cross-dressing sexually arousing.
4. **Pedophilia**: fantasies, urges, or behaviors involving sexual activity with children.
5. **Voyeurism**: observing unsuspecting persons unclothed or involved in sex.
6. **Sexual sadism**: sexual arousal from inflicting suffering (physical or psychological on others).
7. **Sexual masochism**: sexual arousal from being hurt, humiliated, threatened, or made to suffer in some other way.
8. **Frotteurism**: touching or rubbing against a nonconsenting person.

The paraphilias are found almost exclusively in men. The difference between these and normal variations in sexual practices lies in the obligatory nature of the acts or thoughts or the recurring, unrelenting need for such behaviors with less and less interest in usual sexual behaviors.

3. Define gender identity disorder.
Gender identity disorder is a condition wherein a person experiences a strong, persistent desire to be of the opposite sex or insists that he or she is in actuality of the opposite sex. Patients experience persistent, strong discomfort in their assigned sex. Physical examination is essential to rule out the rare instances of intersex conditions (e.g., congenital ambiguous genitalia, hypogonadism, androgen insensitivity syndrome) and may require lab studies such as testosterone/estrogen blood levels or karyotyping for sex chromosomes.

This disorder is difficult to diagnose or understand in children. It is not a situation wherein girls act like tomboys or boys seem sissylike. It is a situation wherein a child wants to be of the opposite sex. Even then, ambivalence about sexual identity in childhood usually disappears in adulthood. Many homosexual men report feeling different from other boys when they were young but never wanted to be girls; rather, they found no interest in the stereotyped sexual roles of boys.

Depression, anxiety, substance abuse, and personality disorder are common comorbid conditions. Suicide attempts are not uncommon. Psychotherapy may be especially helpful when difficulties in interpersonal relationships, social isolation, or impaired self-esteem are paramount. A small percentage of patients seek sex-change surgery.

It is essential to differentiate this disorder from homosexuality. Homosexuality involves a sexual orientation to people of the same sex, not a wish for a man to become a woman or a woman to become a man. Sexuality includes sexual **identity**, sexual **roles**, and sexual **orientation** or choice. When individuals have different views on sexual roles or different sexual orientation, they are not considered pathologic or disordered. Only gender identity problems are considered a psychiatric disorder.

4. What are the sexual dysfunctions?
Sexual dysfunction refers to problems in sexual desire, sexual arousal, sexual orgasm, or pain with sexual activity.

Sexual desire disorders include hypoactive sexual desire and sexual aversion disorder.

Sexual arousal disorders include both female arousal disorder and male erectile disorders, both of which involve difficulties in becoming sexually aroused even if sexual desire is present and normal.

Orgasmic disorders include female and male orgasmic disorders, e.g., difficulties in having orgasms or premature ejaculation in men.

Dyspareunia or **vaginismus** are disorders involving pain with sexual intercourse and may plague female patients.

The final categories are **substance-induced sexual dysfunctions**, and **sexual dysfunction due to a medical condition**, which underline the fact that sexual dysfunction may be caused by either biologic or psychologic causes.

5. What types of questions about sexual functioning should be asked of all adult patients during a review of systems?
More important than specific questions is inclusion of questions about sexual functioning in a review of systems. Examples of questions include the following:
1. Are you currently sexually active? If so, with males, females, or both? With just one person or more than one person?
2. Do you have questions or concerns about your sexual life?
3. Do you use birth control? What and how do you use it?
4. Have you ever had a sexually transmitted disease?
5. Has your medical problem affected your sexual functioning?
6. For male patients the clinician may add:
    Do you have problems getting or keeping an erection?
    Do you have any problem with having an orgasm?
7. For female patients the clinician may add:
    Do you have any problems having orgasms?
    Do you have any problem becoming physically aroused?
    Do you have any problem with pain or discomfort during intercourse?

Such questions need to be asked because sexual dysfunction is a common side effect of many medications and a not uncommon symptom of many medical conditions (e.g., diabetes, hypothyroidism, hypertension). If clinicians ask about sexual functioning, the chance of diagnosing a sexual problem increases by at least 10-fold.

Many physicians fail to ask screening questions about sexual function because they are uncomfortable. Yet they ask personal questions about other organ systems, such as bowel movements, menstrual periods, and alcohol intake. In addition, physicians may be afraid that they may find a sexual problem and not know what to do.

6. How common are sexual disorders or concerns?

At least 30% of people have either a sexual dysfunction or a concern about their sexual life. A recent survey of over 1200 men in Massachusetts aged 40–70 years found that 50% had mild-to-severe impotence. About one-third of sexual dysfunctions are caused by biologic factors, another one-third by psychological factors, and the final one-third by both biologic and psychologic factors. More patients have concerns about their sexuality without having a true sexual dysfunction.

7. What are common sexual concerns of men?

Most common is concern over the size of the penis, followed by worry about whether they are adequate lovers. Rarely do such concerns reflect a true disorder. Men also commonly voice dissatisfaction with the frequency or types of sexual contact with their spouse. The common sexual dysfunctions include inability to get an erection when one wants it, inability to maintain the erection long enough for intercourse, and reaching orgasm too quickly or conversely taking too long to ejaculate.

8. What are women's concerns?

The most common concern of women revolves around orgasms, e.g., inability to achieve orgasms or not having orgasms with intercourse. The second most common area of concern is related to normalcy of sexual activities. Examples include whether it is permissible to have sex during menstruation; whether married people masturbate; or whether it is sick to have fantasies about someone other than one's partner during intercourse. Finally, as with men, women voice concerns about tension between themselves and their spouse or mate, such as differences in how frequently they have sex and what kind of sexual behavior each wants or does not want.

9. Why may a woman not have orgasms with sexual intercourse?

Twenty to thirty percent of normal women do not have orgasms with intercourse. This is not a disorder or dysfunction but reflects inadequate clitoral stimulation during intercourse. Direct stimulation of the clitoral area—before, during, or after intercourse—may be required for such women to have orgasms. Manual or oral stimulation before vaginal containment or manual stimulation of the clitoris during intercourse may solve the problem. The woman may need more genital stimulation before intercourse than she has received. It is important for the woman to know that this variant of sexual response is normal and that many women require more than just intercourse for orgasm.

10. What is the difference between global and situational sexual disorders?

A global problem occurs in any setting, with any partner, and during masturbation. It is not related to time of day, type of sexual activity, or other variables. A situational problem, in contrast, occurs only with a certain person, situation, place, or time.

Situational sexual dysfunctions are almost always psychological in etiology and are often relatively easy to treat. Global sexual dysfunctions may be either biologic or psychological in origin but are much more likely to be biologic and are often more difficult to treat.

11. What types of medications commonly cause sexual dysfunction?

The most common group are the psychotropic drugs. Antidepressants may interfere with desire, arousal, or orgasm. Selective serotonin reuptake inhibitors (SSRIs) have about a 30% incidence of sexual side effects. Antipsychotic drugs and lithium commonly cause sexual problems, although not as frequently as the SSRIs. Much less often sexual side effects occur with benzodiazepines, valproate, or carbamazepine. Indeed, sexual side effects are one of the most common reasons that patients stop taking psychotropic drugs.

Other medications frequently implicated for causing sexual side effects include antihistamines, alpha- or beta-adrenergic blockers, cimetidine, HIV drugs, chemotherapy, tamoxifen, digitalis, and steroids. When sexual problems are present, it is wise to check the side effects of all medications that the patient is taking.

12. What drug causes the most sexual dysfunction?

Alcohol. Although alcohol loosens sexual inhibitions in a few people, much more often the opposite effect occurs and sexual function deteriorates. Even 1 or 2 drinks or beers may interfere with sexual desire or arousal. Illicit street drugs also may interfere with sexual function, including cocaine, amphetamines, hallucinogens, narcotics, and marijuana.

13. What medical disorders commonly affect sexual functioning?

Any disease that affects the **circulation** may interfere with sexual arousal, including diabetes, hypertension, and atherosclerosis. Any disease that results in **neuropathy**, such as alcoholism, multiple sclerosis, or diabetes, may affect arousal and/or orgasm. **Injury, irradiation**, and **retroperitoneal surgery** may interfere with neuronal and vascular supply to the genitals and diminish or destroy arousal capability. Serious diseases that tax **energy**, such as congestive heart failure, chronic obstructive pulmonary disease, cancer, HIV with wasting, or chronic infections, diminish desire and arousal. **Depression** typically interferes with sexual desire; **mania** classically increases desire or interest; and **anxiety** may interfere with performance, primarily arousal. **Endocrinopathy** also may be a problem (e.g., thyroid disease, low testosterone or estrogen levels, prolactinemia, adrenal insufficiency).

14. When the patient complains of a sexual dysfunction, what should the clinician do next?

A complete history and physical exam are essential, keeping in mind the medications and medical problems noted above.

A detailed sexual history needs to be obtained, noting when the problem started, whether it is global or situational, what the patient thinks is the cause, and what the patient has tried to remedy the problem.

Ideally the doctor should talk to the patient's partner. The partner usually views the sexual problem quite differently, giving quite discordant data. This interview also may clarify whether the partner is supportive or whether the problem is primarily an interpersonal conflict playing out as a sexual symptom.

When a biologic basis seems likely or possible, screening laboratory tests should include the following:

Complete blood count	Urinalysis
Liver function tests	Creatinine or blood urea nitrogen
Thyroid screen	Testosterone level in males
Prolactin level	Estrogen level in females

15. After a history, physical exam, and normal screening tests, what next?

Men should be referred to a urologist interested in sexual dysfunction. More sophisticated work-up of endocrine function, genital circulation, and a nocturnal tumescence test may be indicated.

Women should be referred to an endocrinologist or gynecologist with a particular interest in sexual dysfunction. This is not always easy to find. Endocrine integrity needs to be evaluated in greater detail.

Both **men and women** benefit from a psychiatric evaluation. Patients with a biologic cause of sexual dysfunction often have a secondary psychological reaction to sexual inadequacy that needs treatment and support.

16. What psychiatric disorders commonly interfere with sexual function?

Depression has as one of its hallmarks a lack of interest in activities that one used to enjoy. Sex is one of the most common activities in which the depressed patient has lost interest. Furthermore, anhedonia, or lack of pleasure in all activities, is a second common symptom of depression.

Anxiety disorders probably interfere with sexual function as commonly as depression. Increased anxiety interferes with normal function of the parasympathetic nervous system, which is required for sexual arousal.

Posttraumatic stress disorder can be accompanied by sexual dysfunction—decreased desire, decreased arousal, or aversion to sexuality, especially when the trauma was sexual in nature (such as rape or sexual abuse).

Many psychological bases for sexual dysfunction are not technically disorders or psychiatric diseases. Learned inhibition regarding sexuality and one's body is common. Sometimes decreased interest in sex or difficulties with arousal are the ways of expressing anger at one's mate. People who are ashamed of their body or feel unattractive may avoid sexuality. Patients may be afraid to have sex after myocardial infarction or stroke. Sexual disinterest not uncommonly starts during pregnancy or shortly after a child is born—for either the mother or father—and usually requires psychiatric treatment.

17. What is performance anxiety?

The classic patient with performance anxiety is the man whose anxiety about getting or maintaining an erection or having an orgasm causes the very problem about which he is so anxious. His sympathetic nervous system is so revved up from thinking and worrying that it prevents adequate sexual performance. The key to treatment is to get the patient to stop worrying, thinking, and becoming anxious about his anticipated sexual prowess or inadequacy and just to let it happen.

Women also may have performance anxiety. They may be anxious about whether they will become aroused, have an orgasm, or please their partner or whether the sexual experience will be unpleasant. The same principles apply in treatment.

18. What is the role of the primary care physician (PCP) in treating sexual problems?

The answer varies with the interest and comfort of the physician. The first principle of treatment is education of the patient, an important function for primary care physicians. Over 50% of the questions, concerns, or dysfunctions that patients have about their sex lives can be adequately answered or helped by the PCP. The PCP can answer questions about sex, prescribe bibliotherapy, and allay anxieties of most patients.

When the problem is due to medications, the PCP may change dosages or medications, advise the patient about side effects, and possibly suggest means of physical intimacy other than intercourse when the offending medication cannot be safely stopped. The PCP is in an ideal position to recommend changes in alcohol intake. Some patients find that if they refrain from alcoholic drinks until after sex, their desire, arousal, and general performance are greatly improved.

When the basis for the sexual problem seems to be marital or relationship discord, referral to a mental health professional is in order. Both depression and anxiety are frequently treated by primary care physicians. However, medication may not be enough, especially in anxiety disorders. The PCP also may need to talk to the couple about their concerns, give them reading materials about sex, and provide basic education and support. Referral to a psychiatrist may be required if this approach is not enough. In summary, the PCP can treat many if not most sexual problems that their patients present to them. At any time, however, it is perfectly appropriate to refer the patient or couple to a psychotherapist who has experience and interest in treating sexual problems.

19. Do any medications improve sexual function?

When a medical problem causes sexual difficulties, treatment of the underlying disorder usually also treats the sexual dysfunction. Adjusting medications is discussed above.

Yohimbine has been used to increase sexual desire. Although some clinicians swear by it, most controlled studies find that it is only slightly better than placebo.

SSRIs have been used to help men who have premature ejaculation. This approach basically capitalizes on a common side effect of SSRIs—marked delay in ejaculation. Most other medications tried for improving sexual function are experimental, anecdotal, or unstudied.

20. If a medical disorder prevents sexual arousal, what can be done to help?
A therapist can help the couple to find means of sexual fulfillment without intercourse (e.g., cuddling, manual or oral stimulation of genitals, sensate focus). The therapist may need to help the patient and partner deal with the loss of usual sexual behaviors.

   If the man cannot become aroused, one should consider procedures such as the vacuum pump, injections such as papaverine, or penile implants. Urologic consultation is essential. For women appropriate types of artificial lubrication may be prescribed.

21. Briefly discuss sexual development from birth to school age.
Infants are very much into exploring their bodies. They discover and explore feet, hands, ears, and genitals. They find that touching their genitals is a pleasant experience. This discovery may upset parents who may label such behavior as masturbation rather than exploration.

   From 2–5 years of age children are interested in their genital anatomy and how it differs from people of the opposite gender. They are also quite interested in sexual roles, e.g., how males and females are similar and different in terms of games they play, what they enjoy, ways they talk. It is important to answer children's questions with accurate and simple explanations. Although it may be embarrassing at times, it is quite important to handle children's curiosity about sexuality in a matter-of-fact way, without heightening the feeling that the whole subject of sexuality is taboo.

22. What are children's concerns about puberty?
Children are concerned whether they experience the physical changes of puberty later or earlier than their peers. Girls are especially self-conscious about breast development, because it seems so obvious to others. Being like other children is the key: not to be too tall or too short, not to develop too soon or too late. Girls may be terrorized by their first menstrual period (especially if it occurs without prior discussion and appropriate information), worrying that they are bleeding to death or sick or that other people can smell or sense that they are having the "curse." A boy's first nocturnal emission may be frightening, because the boy may think that he has wet the bed or that something is terribly wrong. Anticipatory education from parents or physician helps to reduce such anxieties.

   Children engage in sexual intercourse at increasingly younger ages. At a minimum the PCP has a role in discussing birth control, sexually transmitted diseases, and safe sex. PCPs should ask about sexual behavior in children from 10–12 years of age.

   Adolescence is a time when defining one's identity is a key task. Adolescents typically try out different roles and identities and often provoke their parents. The PCP needs to be sensitive to adolescents (and their parents) who are unsure about sexual orientation, sexual attractiveness, and how to negotiate the whole world of sex and relationships. Counseling adolescents often involves listening with respect to their concerns and reassuring them.

23. Where do children get information about sex?
Most sexual information comes from friends and peers, not from parents, school, or books. Hence, their early sexual education is unreliable and often includes misinformation. PCPs provide a tremendous service by encouraging parents to give information about sex to their children. They also may be an important source of information about sex, sexual behavior, and sexual concerns.

24. Is it true that most people over 70 years old do not have sex?
No. Frequency of sexual intercourse decreases, but most couples, if unfettered by medical disease, continue to have intercourse 2–4 times a month. Self-stimulation also continues in senior citizens.

25. What changes in sexual functioning occur with aging?
There is no abrupt change in sexual functioning. Changes in sexual ability start when people are in their 40s. In men the changes include:

- A need for more physical stimulation of the penis to induce erection
- Slower, less firm erection
- Longer time to reach orgasm
- Decreased force of ejaculation
- Longer time to get an erection after orgasm
- Fewer spontaneous erections
- Erections that come and go even during intercourse

26. Why do such changes occur?
Such changes typically are due to less efficient blood supply to the genitals, wearing out of venous valves, pain from the vicissitudes of age, slower neuronal reflexes, and perhaps decreased testosterone. In addition, for psychological reasons a man may feel that he can or should no longer be as sexually active as in his youth.

27. How may sex improve with increasing age?
There are obvious advantages in taking longer to reach orgasm, taking more time for mutual caressing, and not feeling the need to have an orgasm. Sometimes inhibitions lessen with age, and less fear of pregnancy is a plus for men and women.

28. What common changes in women's sexuality occur with increasing age?
- Decreased vaginal lubrication and thinning of vaginal mucosa occur after menopause; for this reason, estrogen replacement should be considered. Local vaginal lubricants, including estrogen, may be helpful.
- Sexual arousal occurs more slowly.
- Irritation of the urethra is more common.
- Sex may be more pleasurable without concern for pregnancy or the need to use birth control; orgasm may be easier to achieve.

29. What may help with changes associated with aging?
The most essential aid is information and education. It is quite helpful for people to know what is happening to their bodies and why. Older patients should be reassured that sex does not have to disappear from their life.

Lubricants, estrogen replacement, and Kegel exercises should be discussed if not recommended to women after 50 years of age.

Older couples benefit from practical suggestions and advice to prevent changes in sexual function from discouraging an active sex life. The importance of spending more time in caressing, including genital stimulation needs to be stressed. Men need to know that even with a 50–75% erection vaginal containment is possible. Intercourse can be quite enjoyable even if the man does not have an orgasm. Men may view the ability to go longer before ejaculation as an asset rather than a liability.

30. Is "use it or lose it" concept valid?
Despite the lack of good scientific data, most sex therapists are convinced that the longer a person goes without sex, the more difficult it is to resume sexual behavior. When one's partner is unable to engage in intercourse or if one's partner leaves or dies, sexual self-stimulation with some regularity is of value to keep the apparatus in good working order.

31. What are Kegel exercises?
The person volitionally and repeatedly tightens the muscles of the perineum for 3–4 minutes. The clinician may describe the exercise as the muscle tightening that holds in urine, bowel movements, or flatulence. Doing these exercises a few times a day helps to keep the muscle tone of the perineum taut and more satisfactory for both partners during sex. This exercise is valuable for both men and women.

32. What is safe sex?

Safe sex is the concept of having sex without fear of contracting a sexual disease from one's partner. In fact, there is only one method of truly safe sex—complete abstinence from sexual contact with another person. Other safe-sex practices are ways to decrease the risk of contracting a disease, but it is important to note that none is 100% safe. Nonetheless, decreasing the odds of disease transmission is especially important for people having sex with strangers or multiple partners, people at high risk of carrying sexually transmitted disease, or people with new partners whose past or current sexual history is unknown.

The underlying concept is to avoid contact with bodily fluids of the other person—especially genital fluids or blood. The use of a condom is essential, whether vaginal, anal, or oral sex is practiced. Condoms should be lubricated with a water-soluble lubricant; oil-based lubricants increase the risk of breakage. Using nonoxynol-9 or other spermicides with the condom may provide additional safety. Because heat or rough treatment may ruin condoms, patients should be advised not to carry them in a wallet or the glove box of a car.

Low-risk behaviors for transmission of sexually transmitted diseases include mutual masturbation or dry kissing.

Low-to-moderate risk behaviors include fellatio without climax, cunnilingus or anilingus, and vaginal or anal intercourse with condoms.

High-risk behaviors include anal or vaginal intercourse without a condom, sharing sex toys, fisting, or any sexual behavior that may damage mucosal linings or draw blood.

Pamphlets with information about safe sexual practices should be openly available in the primary physician's office. Patients should not have to request them; they should be able to pick them up discreetly.

33. Why is sex such a crucial issue for physicians to know about and deal with?

Physicians are consulted when organs are not functioning properly—eyes, lungs, kidneys, bowels. Patients should feel just as comfortable in talking with a physician when their genitals do not function properly; they should be able to get help and support from physicians when their sex life is not satisfactory.

Problems with sexuality not infrequently lead to divorce. Certainly they cause tremendous psychological pain and distress. There simply are not many people to whom patients can talk about sexual concerns. PCPs should make clear that they will listen and be interested in the patient's sexual concerns and offer information, suggestions, support, and, when needed, referral for solution.

BIBLIOGRAPHY

1. Anderson et al: Use of a "permission giving" patient checklist in identification of social and sexual problems. Henry Ford Hosp Med J 34:267–269, 1986.
2. Barbach L: For Yourself: The Fulfillment of Female Sexuality. New York, Doubleday, 1976.
3. Barbach L: For Each Other: Sharing Sexual Intimacy. New York, Doubleday, 1982.
4. Feldman et al: Impotence and its medical and psychosocial correlates: Results of the Massachusetts Male Aging Study. J Urol 151:54–61, 1994.
5. Heiman, Lopiccolo, Lopiccolo: Becoming Orgasmic: A Sexual Growth Program for Women. New York, Prentice-Hall, 1976.
6. Kaplan H: The New Sex Therapy. New York, Bruner/Mazel, 1974.
7. Krane et al: Impotence. N Engl J Med 1648–1649, 1989.
8. Levine S: Sexual Life: A Clinician's Guide. New York, Plenum Press, 1992.
9. McIlvenna T: The Complete Guide to Safe Sex. Specific Press, 1987.
10. Meyer JK: Clinical Management of Sexual Disorders. Baltimore, Williams & Wilkins, 1976.
11. Rosenthal S: Sex Over 40. New York, St. Martin's Press, 1987.
12. Russell: Sex and couples therapy: A method of treatment to enhance physical and emotional intimacy. Journal Sex & Marital Therapy 16:111, 1990.
13. Schiavi et al: Healthy aging and male sexual function. Am J Psychiatry 147:766–771, 1990.

28. EATING DISORDERS

Andrew W. Brotman, M.D.

1. What are the criteria for the diagnosis of anorexia nervosa?
Individuals meet criteria for the diagnosis of anorexia nervosa (AN) if: (a) they refuse to maintain a body weight at or above minimally normal weight for age and height (within 85% of expected), (b) they have an intense fear of becoming fat, (c) they have a disturbed body image, and (d) in post-menarcheal females, have amenorrhea. The DSM-IV will include two subtypes of anorexia nervosa, the restricting type, and the binge eating/purging type. Restricters engage in neither binge eating nor purging, but the other type of anorectic alternates binge eating or purging with food restriction.

2. What are the clinical and demographic characteristics of patients with anorexia nervosa?
The prevalence of AN is approximately 0.5% of the female population. Females comprise 90% of sufferers of this disorder. The age of onset seems to be bimodal, occurring either in the prepubertal period or else in the late teens; the age ranges generally between 12 and 30. Patients with AN are by definition cachectic, and the percentage who meet criteria for major depression may exceed 50%. Although suicide attempts and substance abuse involved in this condition are relatively rare, the mortality rate can exceed 10%, usually because of an arrhythmia secondary to hypokalemia and low weight. Exercise can be common and ritualistic in this disorder and the course of illness may be chronic. At a 5 to 10 year follow-up, the remission rate is only 40%. An additional 35% of patients may achieve 85% of their ideal weight but still have an abnormal relationship with food, and 25% have chronic anorexia nervosa.

3. What are the physical findings and medical complications of anorexia nervosa?
Signs and symptoms of AN typically include the presence of lanugo, dry skin, emaciation, cold intolerance, hair loss, sunken eyes, bradycardia, hypotension, edema, and hypothermia. Cardiovascular, hematologic, gastrointestinal, renal, metabolic, skeletal and endocrine changes are listed in the table below.

Medical Complications

Cardiovascular
- EKG (low voltage, ST depression, T-wave inversions)
- Bradycardia, arrhythmia
- Hypotension
- Congestive heart failure (secondary to refeeding)
- Mitral valve prolapse

Hematologic—mild pancytopenia

Gastrointestinal
- Decreased motility
- Elevated liver function tests and amylase
- Acute vascular compression of the duodenum

Renal
- Elevated blood urea nitrogen levels
- Partial diabetes insipidus
- Stones

Skeletal—osteoporosis

Endocrine
- Decreased T_3
- Increased reverse T_3

4. What are the clinical criteria for hospitalization of these patients?

Studies do not discuss this issue and therefore the decision to hospitalize remains arbitrary. Nonetheless, particularly low or unstable vital signs, severe metabolic abnormalities, persistent weight loss despite adequate outpatient treatment, cardiac arrhythmias, severe depression, severe suicide risk, unremitting comorbid substance abuse, or general treatment resistance would be reasons sufficient to hospitalize. The threshold for hospitalizing younger people who have not finished growing may be somewhat lower than in older individuals so that their growth will not be permanently affected.

The goals of hospitalization include nutritional rehabilitation, biologic, social, and psychological therapy, family evaluation, and multidisciplinary assessment and treatment. In anorexia nervosa, the main goal of treatment is weight restoration; in bulimia nervosa it is control of binging and purging. A variety of protocols are in effect at various inpatient sites, but outcome studies do not convince that one type of therapy is clearly better than another.

5. What is it like to talk to a patient with anorexia nervosa?

The anorectic can be alert and cheerful, or sad and withdrawn, depending on the stage of the illness. Patients with anorexia are not particularly hyperactive, but toward the end of the illness they *can* become hypoactive. They can have substantial mood swings, demonstrate rigidity of thinking, and can be controlling and manipulative. Major defense mechanisms include denial of their illness and intellectualization. Their thinking can be black-and-white or good versus bad without the capacity to integrate the two. Anorectics are frequently mistrustful of others, strive for perfection, have obsessive-compulsive personalities, a constricted affect, and are therefore socially isolated. They are, by and large, hyposexual.

6. Describe pharmacologic strategies for treating anorexia nervosa.

Unfortunately, no medication has consistently outperformed placebo for the treatment of anorexia nervosa. Controlled trials of medication have had modestly positive results with the serotonin antagonist cyproheptadine and with the antidepressant amitriptyline. However, both of those medications in other studies have had either equivocal or clinically insignificant results. Other controlled trials which have not achieved clinically positive results include clomipramine, lithium, thiothixene, pimozide, sulpride, THC and naloxone. At this point, several pharmacologic strategies may be a useful adjunct to psychotherapy. Antianxiety agents can in some cases be used before meals to help the anorectic carry out a behavioral plan which includes a certain caloric intake. This is generally a time-limited strategy. Antidepressants, particularly the serotonin reuptake inhibitors and certain tricyclics, can be useful, particularly in the anorectic with depression, prominent neurovegetative signs, severe anxiety, obsessive compulsive disorder, or who is otherwise resisting treatment. The desired effects are weight gain, increased interest in eating, decreased anxiety and depression, decreased obsessional thoughts, and a increased willingness for treatment. Antipsychotics are not commonly used in anorexia nervosa unless comorbid psychosis is also present. Antipsychotic drugs are sometimes used for the anorectic with extraordinary anxiety and inability to eat, when antianxiety agents are ineffective. There have been several case reports on the use of electroconvulsive therapy but the evidence is anecdotal.

7. What are the criteria for the diagnosis of bulimia nervosa?

The diagnosis of bulimia nervosa (BN) requires recurrent episodes of binge eating defined as the rapid consumption of a large amount of food in a reasonably short period of time, usually less than 2 hours. One of the hallmarks of the disorder is that there is a fear of not being able to stop eating when the binge is in progress. Individuals regularly engage in some sort of purging behavior such as self-induced vomiting or laxative abuse, but they may use severe dieting or fasting to counteract the binge. The binge-eating episodes need to occurr at least twice weekly for 3 months, and there must be an accompanying over-concern with body shape and weight.

Patients can meet criteria for both AN and BN. There are other eating disorders that are "not otherwise specified," but which may be unusual. For example, some individuals eat normal meals but self-induce vomiting after meals in order to control weight. In this case, they do not binge, so they do not meet criteria for BN, and they are of normal weight, so they do not meet criteria for AN, but they do engage in unusual eating behaviors.

8. What are the clinical characteristics for bulimia nervosa?
The prevalence rate for BN is approximately 0.6 to 0.8% in women, with up to an 8% lifetime prevalence. As with AN, it is predominantly a disorder of women in a 9:1 ratio. The age of onset tends to be in the late teens with ages ranging from 12 to 40. Weight is usually normal but individuals can engage in ritualistic exercise, fasting, or purging behaviors including self-induced vomiting, laxative abuse, and the use of ipecac and diuretics. Suicide attempts are relatively common, as is substance abuse, particularly of stimulant drugs such as cocaine and amphetamines. The course of this disorder tends to be chronic and is characterized by multiple relapses.

9. What are the physical findings and medical complications of bulimia nervosa?
Signs and symptoms of BN include dizziness, hypotension, parotidomegaly, dental problems, and abrasions of the knuckles caused by biting down on them during self-induced vomiting. Most medical complications of bulimia nervosa are secondary to chronic vomiting or laxative abuse. These include:
1. Fluid and electrolytes: K decreased, CL decreased, dehydration, alkalosis.
2. Gastrointestinal: sore throat, esophagitis, Mallory-Weiss tears, parotidomegaly, cathartic colon, constipation.
3. Dental: caries, enamel loss.

10. What is it like to talk to a patient with bulimia nervosa?
There may be very few outward signs of an eating disorder in the bulimic. They may be superficially sociable and perceived by others as being strong and giving. Unfortunately, they frequently have low self-esteem, conflicts with intimacy, feel misunderstood, and have difficulty managing anger. They may suffer from mood swings and by definition are preoccupied with control over eating. Questions should be asked about other impulsive behaviors, including stealing, substance abuse, and suicide attempts.

11. Describe the pharmacotherapy for bulimia nervosa.
The predominant treatment for BN is the use of antidepressants. Several antidepressants have been shown in controlled studies to be superior to placebo for the treatment of binge eating and purging. These medications include imipramine, phenelzine, amitriptyline, desipramine, isocarboxazid, trazodone, and fluoxetine. A trial of bupropion was also positive but is not approved for the treatment of BN because of associated seizures.

Comorbid depression is *not* necessary for the use of an antidepressant. Medications are generally given in a manner and dose similar to treating someone for depression. Abstinence is not usually the outcome of a trial of antidepressants, but a significant diminution in binge eating and purging is common. Generally, pharmacotherapy is given in the context of an overall psychotherapeutic relationship with the eating disorder patient.

12. What is binge-eating disorder?
Binge-eating disorder is a new diagnostic category which is essentially a subtype of obesity. Most individuals with this disorder are obese, but have recurrent episodes of binge eating with associated loss of control. They have significant distress about this and struggle against it. The binges occur at least twice a week for a 6-month period, and the individual does not meet criteria for bulimia nervosa. Most people with this disorder have dieted repeatedly. Binge eaters tend to have more disrupted lives than other obese individuals of the same weight. The prevalence of the disorder in weight loss clinic samples is about 30%, in non-patient samples, it is less than 5%. Unlike AN and BN, which are predominantly disorders of women, the female to male ratio for binge eating disorder is 1.5 to 1.

13. Should treatment for obese individuals with binge-eating disorder be any different than for other obese individuals?

It is unclear whether obese persons who eat in binges have a different response to treatment. Some early indications suggest that the use of cognitive behavioral treatment directed toward the binge, and possibly the use of antidepressants, such as desipramine or fluoxetine, may result in improved outcome. The diagnosis of binge-eating disorder and implications for treatment await validation.

14. What is the essential medical work-up for anorexia, bulimia, and/or binge-eating disorder?

Generally these disorders do not require a "million dollar work-up." They tend to be apparent on clinical exam and a psychiatric interview. Anorexia nervosa is an inherently public disorder on the basis of obvious cachexia. Bulimia nervosa can be difficult to diagnosis if the patient is secretive about it, and no definitive medical tests exist to make the diagnosis, although amylase levels may be increased, and potassium levels decreased with chronic vomiting. Individuals with binge-eating disorder tend to be obese and are generally forthright about their behavior. Routine laboratory work, including CBC, electrolytes, liver function, fasting blood sugar, and thyroid function tests is useful. Other tests should be individualized depending on the patient's presenting complaint.

The formal differential diagnosis for AN and BN can include a variety of conditions such as colitis, enteritis, thyroid diseases, diabetes, ulcers, hypothalamic tumors, and seizure disorders. Psychiatric comorbidity can include depression, obsessive-compulsive disorder, anxiety, substance abuse, bipolar disorder, and psychotic disorders.

15. What is the etiology of eating disorders?

No definitive etiology has been documented, but theories abound. The most prominent ones are as follows:

A **sociocultural** theory suggests that the pressure to be thin as promoted by the media and societal values can lead to AN and BN. In these societies, patients with eating disorders usually have a weight phobia, which has been conceptualized by some theorists as a way to avoid postpubertal conflicts.

Cognitive behavioral practitioners believe that distorted cognitions and learned behaviors lead to eating disorders.

Psychodynamic theorists suggest that there may be a "developmental arrest" leading to eating disorders, and a significant comorbidity of personality disorders.

Biochemical theories are also prominent. One line of evidence revolves around the comorbidity of major depressive disorder with eating disorders. Approximately half of all anorectics have concurrent major depressive disorder and greater than half of bulimics have concurrent major depressive disorder. In many cases, onset of depression precedes onset of the eating disorder. This may suggest a similar etiology between the development of eating disorders and depression. Some clinicians view eating disorders similarly to other addictive behaviors and treat them as they would alcoholism or substance abuse. An alteration of neurotransmitters may be present in these disorders although definitive proof is lacking. Some evidence exists that decreased cerebrospinal fluid norepinephrine and decreased methoxyhydroxyphenylglycol may be associated with AN. Decreased brain serotonin and impaired secretion of cholecystokinin in response to a meal may be associated with BN. Other researchers believe that hypothalamic dysfunction may be a cause of or perhaps a result of eating disorders.

Familial disturbances have been widely cited as a potential etiology for both AN and BN. A familial aggregation seems to exist in AN but it is unclear whether this is hereditary or environmental.

Feminist psychology theorists believe that the pressure to be a "super woman," particularly in Western industrialized society, predisposes women to eating disorders. There have been no explanations for the preponderance of women suffering from these disorders as potent as the feminist and sociocultural views.

Dietary factors, in and of themselves, including excessive dieting, predispose to AN and BN as does a past history of obesity or a family history of obesity.

Other etiologic factors including childhood sexual abuse, comorbid diabetes mellitus, participation in weight-restrictive sports, participation in high-achieving occupations, and other factors have been researched with varied results.

My own view is that eating disorders are a heterogeneous group of conditions which are, in a minority of cases, subsets of other psychiatric disorders such as depression, anxiety, or obsessive-compulsive disorder. In most cases, they may begin as a diet, as an attempt to match a culturally defined physical shape, or as a means of control, but soon take on a life of their own. They become almost addictive in quality, and are then employed as a response to all types of emotions.

16. What kinds of treatments are available for eating disorders?

Many theoretical approaches have been used for the treatment of eating disorders. Most of the evidence focuses on shorter-term, more easily measured treatments such as cognitive behavioral, interpersonal, and pharmacologic interventions. **Cognitive behavioral** treatments have been a useful intervention for both AN and BN. Theoretically, the approach is to unlearn distorted thinking, normalize eating habits, and eliminate purging through a structured treatment whose goal is unequivocally symptom control. Manuals have been written on the use of this treatment for eating disorders. **Interpersonal psychotherapy** is also a short-term treatment that has been codified in a manual that focuses on here-and-now relationships and has demonstrated success with people with depression and eating disorders. **Psychodynamic treatment** is still probably the most used approach, with the theory being that underlying conflicts may need to be resolved in order to reduce the symptoms of eating disorders. **Family therapy** is particularly successful with young anorectics who continue to live with their families and do not have chronic illness. **Nutritional counseling** is geared toward education and advice about calories and food groups. **Pharmacotherapy** has been found particularly useful in treating BN and may have a role in AN as well. **Ongoing medical care,** and more intensive programs such as day hospital programs, intensive outpatient programs, evening programs, and halfway houses are all used to treat selected individuals with eating disorders.

I have found it quite useful to begin with a treatment contract and a cognitive-behavioral approach. Adjunct use of medication is frequently helpful and, after eating behavior stabilizes to some degree, psychodynamic treatment may be indicated.

17. Is it useful to have a "treatment contract" with an eating disorder patient?

This is somewhat controversial. Some practitioners will continue to see an eating disorder patient on an outpatient basis irrespective of the patient's clinical condition, whereas others set up treatment parameters which are rather strict. Many practitioners find it useful to have parameters beyond which outpatient treatment is no longer possible and hospitalization or some other intervention becomes necessary. Targets include reaching minimally acceptable weight levels on an outpatient basis, maintaining potassium levels, reducing levels of laxative abuse, continuing proper use of medication, determining the status of medical conditions, and lowering the level of suicidality. The agreement between the patient and clinician is that if these levels are not maintained, hospitalization will take place. This can be negotiated explicitly at the beginning of treatment. A review of this plan with patients and potentially their families can decrease later conflict and help to minimize the dilemma of whether or not to hospitalize.

18. Has managed care had an impact on the treatment of eating disorder patients?

It certainly has. The goal of hospitalization for a patient with AN has traditionally been weight restoration. However, the length of time it takes to get to within 90% of ideal body weight can be substantial. Generally, one cannot gain more than 3 or 4 pounds a week (and this is at the high end of the scale); so that if a patient needs to gain 30 pounds, the process can take 10 weeks.

Hospitalizations of this length are almost invariably denied by insurance companies and managed-care case managers. This puts the clinician in a dilemma because the "experts" say that weight restoration is important, but if it cannot be accomplished outside of an inpatient setting, one frequently is asked to discharge the patient when they are medically and psychologically stable but have not yet reached ideal body weight. The use of alternatives to hospitalization, including intensive outpatient programs and day hospitals, has been initiated in order to deal with this problem.

If one has a treatment contract, hospitalization may not be the alternative to a violation of the treatment contract and other interventions such as those outlined above may be necessary.

Finally, managed care pushes one in the direction of shorter-term treatments which may or may not be adequate for some patients afflicted with chronic illness.

BIBLIOGRAPHY

1. Agras WS, Rossiter EM, Arnow B, et al: Pharmacologic and cognitive-behavioral treatment for bulimia nervosa: A controlled comparison. Am J Psychiatry 149:82–87, 1992.
2. Brotman AW, Rigotti NA, Herzog DB: Medical complications of eating disorders. Comp Psychiatry 26(3):258–272, 1985.
3. Fairburn CG, Jones R, Peveler RC, et al: Three psychological treatments for bulimia nervosa: A comparative trial. Arch Gen Psychiatry 48(5):463–469, 1991.
4. Garner DM, Garfinkel PE (eds): Handbook of Psychotherapy for Anorexia Nervosa and Bulimia. New York, Guilford Press, 1985.
5. Herzog DB, Keller MB, Lavori PW: Outcome in anorexia nervosa and bulimia nervosa: A review of the literature. J Nerv Ment Dis 176:131–143, 1988.
6. Jimmerson DC, Herzog DB, Brotman AW: Pharmacologic approaches in the treatment of eating disorders. Harvard Rev Psychiatry 1(2):82–93, 1993.
7. Mitchell JE: Subtyping of bulimia nervosa. Int J Eating Disorders 11(4):327–332, 1992.
8. Spitzer RL, Devlin M, Walsh TB, Hasin D, Wing R, et al: Binge eating disorder: A multi-site field trial of the diagnostic criteria. Int J Eating Disorders 11(3):191–203, 1992.
9. Steiner-Adair C: The body politic: Normal female adolescent development and the development of eating disorders. J Am Acad Psychoanalysis 14(1): 1986.
10. Walsh BT, Hadigan CM, Devlin MJ, Gladis M, Roose SP: Longterm outcome of antidepressant treatment for bulimia nervosa. Am J Psychiatry 148:1206–1212, 1991.
11. Walsh BT: Diagnostic criteria for eating disorders in DSM-IV: Work in progress. Int J Eating Disorders 11(4):301–304, 1992.

29. SLEEP DISORDERS IN PSYCHIATRIC PRACTICE

Martin Reite, M.D.

1. What are sleep disorders? How does the practitioner determine whether a sleep disorder is present?

Sleep disorders are initially indicated by the presence of sleep complaints, which generally are grouped into the following three categories:

1. "I can't sleep." This complaint most often indicates the presence of an insomnia disorder—insufficient sleep to permit the patient to feel refreshed and awake during the day. Insomnia, of course, is a complaint and not a disease; it has multiple causes. An accurate differential diagnosis is important to determine specific appropriate treatment.

2. "I'm too sleepy (or I fall asleep) during the day." This complaint usually indicates the presence of one of the disorders of excessive sleep. In about 80% of patients the cause is a sleep-related breathing disorder (such as sleep apnea) or narcolepsy. The symptom of excessive sleepiness demands careful work-up and often an all-night sleep study (polysomnogram) for accurate diagnosis. These disorders can be medically serious or result in serious accident or injury (for example, the patient may fall asleep while driving).

3. "Strange things happen while I'm asleep." This complaint often indicates a parasomnia disorder, which constitute a series of behaviors that would be normal while awake (e.g., walking, talking) but are not normal during sleep. Patients with parasomnia may arise from any sleep stage. Because the patient is asleep while they occur, they are usually not remembered but are complained about by bedpartners (or parents, in the case of children).

2. What is "normal sleep"?

Normal adults usually first enter slow-wave or non-REM sleep, which has four stages, depending on the nature of scalp-recorded EEG activity. Stage 1 is characterized by 5–6 Hz theta activity; stage 2, by 12–14 Hz sleep spindles and sharp, high-voltage K complexes; stage 3, by 20–50% high-voltage (over 75 μv amplitude) delta activity; and stage 4, by over 50% delta activity. After about 90 minutes, the EEG changes to a pattern of low-voltage, fast activity; the eyes move beneath the closed lids; and subjects report dreaming if awakened. This stage of sleep is termed rapid eye movement (REM) sleep, or dreaming sleep. This pattern of slow-wave stages followed by REM sleep is called a sleep cycle; a normal night's sleep is characterized by several such sleep cycles in sequence. Sleep cycles change as the night progresses. Stages 3 and 4 are usually confined to the first part of the night; REM periods become longer as the night progresses.

No hard and fast rule defines how much sleep is "enough"; individual variability is high. Most people need about $7\frac{1}{2}$ hours of sleep at night to feel rested and alert the following day. "Short sleepers" may get along with as little as 4 hours, whereas "long sleepers" may need up to 10 hours.

3. How does one approach the differential diagnosis of chronic insomnia?

Because insomnia is a complaint, not a disorder, accurate diagnosis requires the systematic evaluation and exclusion of the several etiologic factors that individually or together may result in chronic insomnia. Comorbidity is the rule in insomnia. The identification of one potential etiologic factor does not mean that the diagnostic work-up is complete. All possible contributing factors must be considered individually. The most frequent causes of insomnia are the following:

1. Many **medical disorders**, especially those associated with chronic pain, endocrine dysfunction, or chronic fatigue-like syndromes, may produce insomnia. In addition, many common

medications used in the treatment of medical disorder may result in side effects of insomnia. Such factors should be systematically excluded.

2. Many **psychiatric disorders**, especially anxiety and depression, are associated with insomnia. The complaint may include difficulty in getting to sleep (common in anxiety), difficulty in staying asleep, or early morning awakening (common in depression).

3. Chronic **sedative-hypnotic abuse**, especially involving older sedative-hypnotic agents or alcohol, may result in chronic insomnia in susceptible patients. Examples are medications started for transient (several days) or short-term (up to 3 weeks) insomnia but not stopped, and patients self-medicating with alcohol because of difficulty in getting to sleep.

4. **Nocturnal myoclonus** (periodic movements in sleep) may cause insomnia in some patients. Short (one-half to several second) bursts of muscle activity in the anterior tibialis muscles, accompanied by a leg jerk or kicking movement, occur about every 30 seconds in bouts during the night. Such movements are frequently seen in normal people with no sleep complaints, but if the leg jerks cause a transient EEG arousal several hundred times a night, the result is fragmented sleep and a complaint of insomnia (or excessive daytime sleepiness). Bedpartners usually complain that patients kick during sleep; if patients sleep alone, they may kick the bedclothes onto the floor during the night. A polysomnogram is usually necessary to establish the diagnosis. The important question is not only the number of leg jerks, but perhaps more important, how many are accompanied by transient arousals?

5. **Central sleep apnea** is a rare cause of chronic insomnia. Central apneas are usually short (about 20 seconds in duration) with little in the way of direct hemodynamic consequences, but they are frequently accompanied by arousals when breathing resumes. Several hundred short central apneas during the night, each accompanied by arousal, seriously fragment sleep and result in the complaint of insomnia. Patients usually are not aware of central apneas; bedpartners, however, frequently say that the patient frequently stops breathing for short periods during the night. Snoring may or may not be present, and the typical accompaniments of obstructive apnea (recent weight gain, mild hypertension, excessive daytime sleepiness) need not be present. A high index of suspicion is necessary, and a polysomnogram is required for accurate diagnosis. The condition, fortunately, is rare.

6. Circadian rhythm disorders, such as **delayed sleep phase syndrome**, may masquerade as an insomnia disorder. In delayed sleep phase syndrome the sleepy phase of the circadian sleep/wake rhythm is characteristically delayed about 6 hours, so that the patient is not ready to go to sleep until about 4 A.M. If allowed to sleep until 10 or 11 A.M., they have no sleep complaint and feel well rested; but if they have to get up early for work or school, they are fatigued and sleepy, perform poorly, and complain of insomnia. Such disorders are frequently familial, and many patients compensate by adopting a work schedule compatible with their phase delay. A careful history is most important in diagnosis; polysomnography is usually not necessary for diagnosis.

7. Finally, conditioned arousal, often termed **psychophysiologic insomnia,** is one of the most frequent causes of chronic insomnia and often complicates or is comorbid with other causes listed above. In such cases, a stress-related insomnia results, after several nights, in patients worrying about going to bed (and therefore becoming aroused) because they fear that once again they will not be able to sleep. In a short while, susceptible individuals are conditioned to arouse at the mere thought of going to bed or by going into the bedroom and getting ready for bed. This condition occurs most frequently in people with a history of fragile sleep (sleep easily disrupted by mild stress). Such cases of insomnias may become quite ingrained and persist for many years. When properly diagnosed (and other causes are excluded), patients frequently respond well to a combination of pharmacologic and behavioral therapies.

4. What is the difference between a nightmare and a night terror?

Nightmares are basically anxiety-filled dreams. They occur during REM sleep and may be quite frightening. Vivid dream content is the rule, but because REM sleep is associated with descending skeletal muscle inhibition, there is little motor activity during nightmares. Nightmares are most common in children but generally rare in adults except at times of stress. Most adults may expect to experience 1–2 nightmares per year. Nightmare content is usually remembered clearly on awakening.

Night terrors are parasomnias—that is, disturbances in arousal from slow-wave, usually stage 3 or 4 non-REM sleep. They may be accompanied by a feeling of terror or dread but as a rule are not associated with vivid dream activity. Autonomic arousal may accompany night terrors (rapid breathing, fast pulse), and some patients may exhibit considerable motor activity, such as sitting up in bed, striking out, or flailing about. Patients may injure themselves or others during parasomnia events. Patients usually do not remember parasomnia events clearly when they awaken. More complex parasomnias include somnambulism (sleep walking), a state that may include quite complex behaviors.

5. When is polysomnography necessary in the evaluation of a sleep disorder?
Polysomnography is rarely necessary for complaints of insomnia. Most causes can be identified by careful medical and sleep evaluation, and appropriate treatment may be instituted on the basis of the office evaluation. Two exceptions are insomnia related to central sleep apnea or nocturnal myoclonus, for which a sleep study is necessary to establish the diagnosis.

With excessive daytime sleepiness (EDS) complaints, polysomnography is usually necessary. Most EDS complaints are associated with sleep-related breathing disorders or narcolepsy; polysomnography and sometimes multiple sleep latency tests are necessary to establish the diagnosis.

Polysomnography is rarely necessary for parasomnia disorders. In most cases, a careful sleep evaluation strongly suggests a parasomnia disorder. In addition, it is often difficult to capture a parasomnia disorder during an all-night sleep study, because they rarely occur with sufficient frequency. However, if a parasomnia event occurs during a sleep study, the diagnosis is unequivocal.

6. Are all-night sleep studies useful in psychiatric disorders?
Probably not, at least on a routine basis. Certain changes in sleep are seen in affective disorders (depression and mania), including shorter than normal REM latency (minutes from sleep onset until the onset of the first REM period), increased REM density (number of REMS per minute of REM sleep), and decreases in slow-wave amplitude. Such changes, however, are not thought to be sufficiently specific to merit the cost of a sleep study. Sleep changes in other psychiatric disorders tend to be nonspecific and are unlikely to be of sufficient diagnostic utility to merit the cost and inconvenience.

7. Can patients commit violent or aggressive acts during parasomnia episodes?
Yes. Sleepwalkers often strike out if one attempts to awaken them forcibly, and patients may strike out and hit a bedpartner during other types of parasomnias. Patients also may injure themselves during parasomnia events. They may strike out at hard objects or walls and injure their hands, turn on the hot water and step into the bathtub, walk into traffic, or jump through a closed window. Violent acts such as killing other people have been reported during parasomnia events but are rare. Such cases have not been considered murder, because the intent to kill was not present.

8. Is it possible to screen for a sleep disorder during a routine medical evaluation without taking a detailed and time-consuming sleep history?
Yes. The following three questions may be incorporated into a routine medical history and will pick up the majority of significant sleep disorders:
1. Are you satisfied with your sleep? This question picks up most insomnia disorders.
2. Are you excessively sleepy during the day? This question picks up most of EDS disorders and severe insomnias that cause EDS.
3. Does your bedpartner (or parent, in the case of children) complain about your sleep? This question picks up most parasomnia disorders. Patients usually are not aware of parasomnia

events, nor do they remember them in the morning. Bedpartners (or parents), however, are aware of such unusual behaviors.

A positive answer to any of these three questions should be followed by a more detailed sleep history. If all three are answered negatively, a significant sleep disorder is unlikely.

9. If the three screening questions suggest the need for a more complete sleep evaluation, what does that consist of?

First and foremost is a careful sleep history. What is the nature of the complaint, how long has it been present, and how does it vary with time? Is it cyclic or periodic? Does it covary with stress or other symptoms or complaints? Is there a family history of similar sleep problems? A screen for medical, psychiatric, and other conditions known to be associated with sleep complaints or conditions is indicated. It may be helpful to have patients keep a sleep diary or detailed account of daily sleep patterns and symptoms to help determine periodicity, relationship to stressful events, and related issues. The important point is to keep in mind the differential diagnoses of the major sleep complaints (insomnia, excessive daytime sleepiness, parasomnias) and to include questions relevant to each.

10. What are the behavioral strategies for treating insomnia?
1. **Sleep hygiene education**
   - Provide time to relax and wind down before retiring.
   - Use the bed only for sleeping and sexual relations—not as a place to worry.
   - Do not vary the sleep schedule (especially time of arising) more than 1 hour from day to day.
   - Exercise regularly but not within 3 hours of bedtime.
   - A bedtime snack containing tryptophan (milk, cookies, banana) may be helpful.
2. **Biofeedback**
   - Both EMG and EEG (theta rhythm and sensorimotor rhythm) biofeedback may be useful to decrease arousal.
   - Perhaps best for patients with psychophysiological insomnia who have trouble turning off their thoughts at night.
3. **Stimulus control**
   - Go to bed only when sleepy.
   - If you cannot fall asleep within 20–30 minutes, get up and do something else and return to bed when sleepy.
   - Keep the bedroom dark and quiet.
4. **Sleep restriction**
   - Helpful for patients who spend considerable time laying awake in bed (e.g., 10 hours in bed with 6 hours sleep).
   - Have patients keep a 5-day sleep diary. Calculate time in bed (TIB), estimated total sleep time (TST), and sleep efficiency (SE) (SE = TST ÷ TIB × 100).
   - Restrict time in bed to patient's estimate of actual sleep time.
   - When SE reaches 90% for 5 days, increase TIB by 15 minutes.
   - Repeat until TST is adequate.
5. **Relaxation training**
   - Meditation training or Yoga.
   - Formal autogenic training or progressive muscle relaxation training.

Behavioral strategies work best when they are part of a treatment package that includes the appropriate use of hypnotic agents to assist with sleep onset until behavioral strategies become effective.

11. Episodic outbursts of violent behavior are noted during the night in an elderly man. What is the differential diagnosis?

One should rule out a parasomnia disorder (careful history, bedpartner interview, possibly a sleep study) or seizure disorder (EEG). Another problem not infrequently encountered in older men (rarely women) is REM behavior disorder, which is characterized by a failure of descending muscle inhibition normally seen during REM sleep; such patients act out their dream—not infrequently injuring themselves or others. Such violent behavioral outbursts are usually accompanied by vivid dream material, whereas parasomnia events usually are not accompanied by dreamlike mentation. A polysomnogram is usually required for accurate diagnosis, however.

12. Does melatonin have a role in the treatment of sleep disorders?
Melatonin is a natural hormone produced in the pineal gland. It has been shown to be important in the regulation of circadian rhythms. Melatonin levels are low during the day but increase during sleep. In preliminary studies low doses of melatonin have been found to improve sleep in neurologically disabled children, to facilitate phase advance in adolescents with delayed sleep phase syndrome, and to decrease sleep latency and increase total sleep time in normal adults. Definitive well-controlled studies have yet to be reported, and the FDA has not yet approved melatonin for medical use. Thus the answer to the question remains uncertain.

13. How does one use bright light in the treatment of sleep disorders?
Bright light acts on the superchiasmatic nucleus of the hypothalamus via the retinohypothalamic tract to alter the phase or timing of the circadian system. Bright light exposure in the evening at the beginning of the sleep cycle serves to advance the circadian system; light exposure in the early morning or at the end of the dark cycle serves to advance the circadian system. Thus exposure to a 10,000 lux bright light unit for 30–45 minutes in the early morning may be an effective treatment for delayed sleep phase syndrome. Similarly, bright light in the evening may help some patients with early morning awakening.

BIBLIOGRAPHY

1. Broughton R, Billings R, Cartwright R, et al: Homicidal somnambulism: A case report. Sleep 17:253–264, 1994.
2. Czeisler CA, Kronauer RE, Allan JS, et al: Bright light induction of strong (Type O) resetting of the human circadian pacemaker. Science 244:1328–1331, 1989.
3. Dollins AB, Zhdanova IV, Wurtman RJ, et al: Effect of inducing nocturnal serum melatonin concentrations in daytime on sleep, mood, body temperature, and performance. Proc Natl Acad Sci 91:1824–1828, 1994.
4. Jan JE, Espezel H, Appleton RE: The treatment of sleep disorders with melatonin. Dev Med Child Neurol 36:97–107, 1994.
5. Kryger MH, Roth T, Dement WC: Principles and Practice of Sleep Medicine, 2nd ed. Philadelphia, W.B. Saunders, 1994.
6. Morin CM, Culbert JP, Schwartz SM: Nonpharmacological interventions for insomnia: A meta-analysis of treatment efficacy. Am J Psychiatry 151:1172–1180, 1994.
7. Regestein QP, Monk TH: Delayed sleep phase syndrome: A review of its clinical aspects. Am J Psychiatry 152:602–608, 1995.
8. Reite M, Nagel K, Ruddy J: A Concise Guide to the Evaluation and Treatment of Sleep Disorders. Washington, DC, American Psychiatric Press, 1990.
9. Reite M, Buysse D, Reynolds C, Mendelson W: The use of polysomnography in the evaluation of insomnia. Sleep 18:58–70, 1995.
10. Van Cauter E, Sturis J, Byrne MM, et al: Demonstration of rapid light-induced advances and delays of the human circadian clock using hormonal phase markers. Am J Physiol 266(6 Pt 1):E953–E963, 1994.

30. IMPULSE-CONTROL DISORDERS

Michael H. Gendel, M.D.

1. What disorders are classified as impulse-control disorders (ICDs)?

Intermittent explosive disorder (IED), pyromania, kleptomania, trichotillomania (compulsive pulling of a patient's own hair), and compulsive gambling.

Disorders that involve the failure to resist impulses to use alcohol or drugs, to eat abnormally (including purging and food restriction), or to perform certain sexual behaviors are not classified in this group.

2. What fundamental features do these disorders have in common?

No one knows. Presumably they are grouped together because they are disorders of behavior resulting from the failure to resist a subjective impulse to perform that behavior. However, these irresistible impulses are very different in nature (e.g., violence and hair pulling), in frequency (rare violent outburst, hair pulling throughout the day), and resulting behavior (e.g., gambling and firesetting).

Many authors regard them as disorders of tension regulation. Feelings of excitement, tension, or arousal *before* acting; pleasure, euphoria, or relief *during* acting; and dysphoria or guilt *after* acting are more or less present in this cluster. Some empathic imagining of what this condition might be like should be attempted, if for no other reason than to help distinguish these illnesses from more ordinary experiences. For instance, in trichotillomania, one might become very agitated during any concerted attempt to stop hair pulling, such that focus on any other activity is impossible. Momentarily relieved by minutes to hours of hair removal, bitter depression and emptiness may envelop the sufferer as the day ends and the person imagines the next day as little more than the same struggle repeated.

A propensity of the person to act rather than express feelings is another common characteristic of this group. Many afflicted individuals are not aware of their feelings and cannot name or use them (alexithymia).

The biologic substrate of these disorders is not yet elucidated. Considerable evidence is mounting that abnormal serotonin metabolism is present, particularly low serotonin turnover with decreased CSF 5-HIAA, in some of these disorders. Intermittent explosive disorder is most clearly associated with these changes, though pyromania and trichotillomania are implicated in some studies. It is not yet clear whether all of these disorders share a common neurobiologic basis.

3. What is an impulse?

An impulse is a feeling to which an action is connected. It is an urge to act.

The issue of time course or urgency is very confusing. Commonly used expressions such as "impulsive decision" and "electrical impulse" suggest urgent action or immediate discharge. Some of these disorders conform clinically to these images, such as the sudden violence in IED. In pyromania, however, a fire might be intricately planned and executed, implying either that the concept of the firesetting impulse is not easily approached through common language paradigms or that tension relief begins with the **internal** act of planning the fire. Both these alternatives should be kept in the clinician's mind.

4. How does one resist or fail to resist an impulse?

In traditional psychiatry, impulses fail to result in actions because of adequate defenses. Defenses are ego functions, which themselves may be healthy (i.e., lead to better organismic adaptation) or less healthy (i.e., lead to problems of their own). Defenses also may be effective in preventing such expression of unwanted impulses. They are unconscious operations. They serve to reduce internal tension. One might imagine that those people with good defensive structures do not "leak" unwanted behaviors and those with poorer ones do. Unfortunately, such is not the case. Impulse control disorders involve, by definition, truly overwhelming internal states that sometimes coexist with sound psychological defensive structures which simply do not help with these behaviors. These problems occur in a variety of people. In fact, most of these diagnoses can only be made in the absence of a primary axis I or II illness, which suggests that there is no pervasive or typical deficiency in defenses. Treatments based on creating healthier defense structures have a poor track record in these disorders, as they do with substance abuse and sexual disorders.

Another framework from which to approach this question is that of the ability to defer an impulse-connected action. To what extent can a violent feeling be contained as just a feeling, and the urge to act on it be delayed, put off, or even permanently put aside. Here, we can examine the effect of conscious behavior-controlling schemes (such as using the knowledge that an act may be unlawful, dangerous, or unacceptable). Other such operations might include remembering a previous bad outcome, distracting oneself with other thoughts or actions, or calling a friend for support. The extent to which a patient has attempted to use such methods might also help a clinician understand the extent to which a person wanted to control an impulse.

It may ultimately prove more useful to examine the biology of the expression of specific behaviors when such information becomes available. This will allow understanding of the neurochemical regulation of impulses and actions in normal and pathologic states.

5. What does this have to do with Einstein?

General relativity teaches us to stop thinking about gravity as a force operating on an object. It suggests other metaphors. Gravity can be conceptualized as a property of mass that alters the shape of space in the vicinity of the mass, such that the motion of neighboring massful objects is changed. The earth thus alters nearby space such that the moon (which might otherwise travel in a different trajectory) orbits it; it does not "hold" the moon by force of gravity.

"Impulse," too, is an old concept which may profit from newer conceptualizations or metaphors. Perhaps acting on impulse is experiencing a particular internal mental state that is less separable from behavior: the "shape" of our being would be altered by a feeling of this type. An ICD might then be conceptualized as a condition of having more behavior-shaping feelings in which thoughts, fears, and concerns have less relevance. Although the underlying neurochemistry of such a condition is unclear, it is possible that the impulse-control-disordered phenomenon may be "wired" differently than ordinary feelings. If so, then gambling for the normal person may not be the same activity as gambling for the pathologic gambler.

One of the difficulties of working with patients with these sorts of problems is the negative feelings we have toward the behaviors themselves. Further, the problems tend to be repetitive and difficult to treat, leading to feelings of helplessness and powerlessness in the physician. Under these conditions we are likely to view such patients in moralistic and oversimplified ways. Anything we can do to generate intellectual interest, to conceptualize the issues differently, or otherwise tilt the problem on its end, will aid us in the effort to approach these disorders and the afflicted patients with scientific and humane interest.

6. What diagnostic problems are associated with impulse-control disorders?

As a group, these disorders are less well studied than most psychiatric conditions. When knowledge is sparse, diagnostic difficulty is inherent. Earlier versions of the DSM emphasized neurologic abnormalities in intermittent explosive disorder. In the current diagnostic schema, if a clearly diagnosable general medical condition is causing the explosive outbursts, one should diagnose "Personality Change Due to a General Medical Condition" rather than IED. However, soft neurologic signs and nonspecific EEG abnormalities do not constitute a diagnosable medical disorder and do not exclude the diagnosis of IED. Patients with IED demonstrate a greater frequency of EEG abnormalities when compared to various control samples.

Certain of these diagnoses cannot be made if the behavior is better accounted for by another condition, yet in reality it may rarely be seen in the absence of another serious disorder. For instance, IED should not be the diagnosis if antisocial or borderline disorders, in which explosiveness and poor temper regulation are common, better account for the behavior. However, many cases that conform well to the picture of the clinical entity of IED occur in the context of these serious character pathologies.

DSM-IV adds the "better accounted for" exception to the diagnostic criteria of all disorders in this group. For trichotillomania the accompanying condition is most likely dermatologic. For pathologic gambling, the other condition is specifically manic.

A patient's history is the most important diagnostic aid when two disorders may be present. If compulsive gambling clearly precedes the onset of identifiable manic symptoms, or is present in a euthymic period, both diagnoses may be appropriate. Many of those with any of these conditions suffer major depression. Such depression often results from the damage created by the disorder and historically will follow its onset. If the impulse disorder occurs only in the context of an affective episode, excluding or at least deferring the impulse disorder diagnosis is quite sensible.

In this chapter, characterizations of the diagnostic entities make use of and follow DSM-IV. DSM-IV is, however, not quoted exactly and is sometimes paraphrased.

7. What's the difference between intermittent explosive disorder and a bad temper?

A bad temper is not an illness; nor is explosive behavior. In IED, there are several episodes of aggression that result in serious destruction or assault and are not better accounted for by other psychiatric disorders including substance abuse or a medical condition. Some people known to have bad tempers may suffer from IED; most IED sufferers have bad tempers.

8. What is the difference between kleptomania and other forms of stealing?

The defining feature of kleptomania is that the sufferer steals in the absence of need for the stolen object or its monetary value. Kleptomaniacs tend to experience the impulse to steal as foreign and unwanted (ego-dystonic). They steal on the spur of the moment despite the more constant pressure of the urge to steal. Food, books, magazines, undergarments, or almost any item may be stolen. The article may be kept, hoarded, thrown away, or even returned. The individual may worry about getting caught but fail to plan the crime with such a consequence in mind. Kleptomaniacs are not more generally antisocial in their behavior. They steal alone, without accomplices. They are more often female than male.

Other stealing behavior has many forms. Shoplifters are often seeking the item stolen, even if it is small in value. Many individuals steal for profit, gain, or revenge. The stealing may be planned, and the thief may carefully consider the dangers and consequences of apprehension. These motives and thought patterns are not typical of kleptomania and if present should lead to doubt about such a diagnosis, as should a more general pattern of antisocial behavior. The cycle of tension building before the theft, pleasure or relief during its commission, and depression afterward is usually not present in criminal stealing, though sensation-seeking may be present. Accomplices are more common in other forms of stealing.

9. How does the clinician distinguish between trichotillomania and other causes of hair loss?

Trichotillomania consists of the pulling out of one's hair, resulting in noticeable hair loss, coupled with the cycle of tension preceding the act, gratification in doing so, and sometimes dysphoria afterward. Noticeable hair loss arises in other conditions, and because a patient with trichotillomania may be quite ashamed of the condition the patient may not report the true source of the hair loss. Hair may be pulled from any area of the body: most often from the head (eyelashes, eyebrows, scalp), and also from the axilla, pubic or perirectal areas. Other conditions with hair loss include alopecia areata, male-pattern baldness, chronic discoid lupus erythematosus, lichen planopilaris, folliculitis decalvans, pseudopelade, and alopecia mucinosa. Skin inflammation does not generally occur in trichotillomania, in contrast to alopecia areata. Biopsy shows short and broken hairs. Normal and damaged follicles will be seen in the same vicinity. Follicles often show trauma, or may be empty. More catagen hairs (those hairs in the short phase between growth and resting, or between anagen and telogen phases) are seen. Also look for evidence of nail biting and scratching behaviors. This condition may present with gastrointestinal symptoms caused by bezoars, generated by trichophagia (eating hairs).

10. What pharmacologic treatment(s) are useful in these disorders?

Medicines used to treat IED include anticonvulsants (especially carbamazepine, valproate, and phenytoin), beta blockers, lithium, neuroleptics, and calcium-channel blockers. Of these, anticonvulsants and beta blockers have recently shown promise.

Antidepressants, especially SSRIs, have been found useful in trichotillomania. Some suspect trichotillomania to be related to obsessive-compulsive disorder.

Anecdotally, kleptomania, pyromania, and pathologic gambling have responded to a variety of medicines, usually antidepressants or thymoleptics (mood stabilizers such as lithium, carbamazepine, or valproate).

11. If you suspect the diagnosis of pyromania, should steps be taken to ensure safety?

Anyone who sets fires may be dangerous, whether or not they meet the criteria for pyromania. Studies of mentally disordered arsonists generally reveal low rates of those who can be diagnosed as having pyromania, suggesting other firesetters may represent a more dangerous population. Potentially dangerous behavior should be evaluated systematically. Suicide and homicide risk assessments are models of this. Pyromaniacs should be queried about past fires, their scope, damage, and associated injuries or deaths. This is not for the purpose of reporting to authorities, but because it is one measure of the potential for danger. Similarly, current fantasies and plans for firesetting should be evaluated, including specific sites and individuals who may be involved. Even a general fantasy or plan, involving no definite place or person, particularly if the patient believes there is a likelihood of action, should be noted. These questions also address danger. Such patients may meet criteria for involuntary commitment. It is useful to be aware of the standards for civil commitment in each state.

Mental health professionals have been found liable for failure to warn possible victims of firesetting (*Peck v. Counseling Service of Addison County*, 146 Vt. 61, 499 A.2d 422 [1985]). The duties to warn and protect are clearly defined in some jurisdictions because of state law or case law, and each physician should be familiar with the applicable standards in the clinician's geographic area of practice. Depending on the jurisdiction, such duties may be carried out by warning the individual endangered, by calling the police or other authorities, by detaining the dangerous person, or other measures. Issues of confidentiality (and privilege, if court actions ultimately ensue) are raised if warnings are given without the patient's consent.

12. Is pathologic gambling an addiction?

This question is controversial in psychiatry and among addiction experts. It should not be construed to suggest that ICDs as a group are hard to distinguish from addictive disorders. Clinically, pathologic gambling has similarities to addictive behavior, and this resemblance is much closer than in the other ICDs (which are themselves so different from each other that it might be said that what they have most in common is being classified together). Below are arguments against and for this question.

Against:

1. Too many problems are already miscast as addictions. The word and concept are trivialized by such usage.

2. Such diagnosis lends an aura of respectability to behavior which is better thought of as simply impulse-ridden.

3. Addiction is a term that should be reserved for activities in which an exogenous chemical is introduced into the body, not for any other specific repetitive behavior.

4. Many conceptual models of pathologic gambling exist. No single model explains all such behavior. Any model may prove useful in a given case. Some cases might be best understood from a psychoanalytic or behaviorist perspective, as a habit disorder, or as a condition comorbid with other psychiatric illness or directly related to other psychiatric illness (especially manic state, depression, and obsessive-compulsive disorder).

5. Diagnosis implies treatment. One may too narrowly prescribe addiction-modelled treatment for a disorder with other available approaches.

For:

1. Loss of control over a compulsively repeated behavior (with resulting adverse consequences) is the hallmark of addiction. Pathologic gambling fits this model.

2. DSM-IV diagnostic criteria for pathologic gambling are strikingly similar to the criteria for addictive illness. This reflects the similarity in conditions.

SUBSTANCE DEPENDENCE	PATHOLOGIC GAMBLING
Tolerance: need for more substance to achieve desired effect or diminished effect with same amount of substance (1)	Needs to gamble with increasing amounts of money in order to achieve the desired excitement. (2)
Withdrawal: characteristic withdrawal syndrome or substance taken to relieve withdrawal symptoms. (2)	Is restless or irritable when attempting to cut down or stop gambling. (4)
Substance taken in larger amounts or longer than intended. (3)	After losing money gambling, often returns another day to get even ("chasing" losses). (6)
Persistent desire or unsuccessful attempts to cut down or control use. (4)	Has repeated unsuccessful efforts to control, cut back, or stop gambling. (3)
Much time spent in obtaining, using, or recovering from substance use. (5)	Is preoccupied with gambling (e.g., preoccupied with reliving past gambling experiences, handicapping or planning the next venture, or thinking of ways to get money with which to gamble). (1)
Important social, occupational, or recreational activities are given up or reduced because of substance use. (6)	Has jeopardized or lost a significant relationship, job, or educational or career opportunity because of gambling. (9) Lies to family members, therapist, or others to conceal the extent of involvement with gambling. (7)
Substance use continued despite knowledge of a physical or psychological problem likely caused or exacerbated by the substance. (7)	Gambles as a way of escaping from problems or relieving a dysphoric mood. (5) Has committed illegal acts such as forgery, fraud, theft, or embezzlement to finance gambling. (8) Relies on others to provide money to relieve a desperate financial situation caused by gambling. (10)

(The numbers in parentheses correspond to the numbered diagnostic criteria in the DSM-IV. The grouping of criteria is for the purpose of comparison and is *not* part of DSM-IV, and some material has been paraphrased or shortened.)

3. Some studies of compulsive gamblers document that upon cessation of gambling, physical withdrawal symptoms occur similar to those of opioid and central nervous system depressant withdrawal symptoms.

4. Gamblers Anonymous (GA), a 12-step program modelled on Alcoholics Anonymous (AA) has proved helpful to many pathologic gamblers, and may be as effective an intervention as is currently available. Gamblers have been successfully treated in programs with other addicts.

5. Addiction itself has many conceptual models. The notion of addiction should not impede thinking conceptually or diagnostically.

6. Medicine is eclectic and empiric. Any treatment that helps, does not pose excessive risk of harm, and is ethical, should be considered.

I side with the arguments for calling gambling an addiction. It may not be conceptually neat, but practically speaking, pathologic gambling behaves like an addiction, including its response to treatment and 12-step support programs. More knowledge or more effective treatment may lead to a reconsideration of this conclusion.

13. Isn't the expression of all impulse disorders more likely under the influence of substances of abuse?
Yes.

BIBLIOGRAPHY

1. American Psychiatric Association: Diagnostic and Statistical Manual of Mental Disorders, 4th ed. Washington, DC, American Psychiatric Association, 1994.
2. Drake ME, Hietter SA, Pakalnis A: EEG and evoked potentials in episodic-dyscontrol syndrome. Neuropsychobiology 26:125, 1992.
3. Gerner RH: Pharmacological treatment of violent behaviors. In Rosner R (ed): Principles and Practice of Forensic Psychiatry. NY, Chapman and Hall, 1994, pp 444–450.
4. Marohn RC, Custer R, Linden RD, et al: Impulse control disorders not elsewhere classified. In American Psychiatric Association: Treatments of Psychiatric Disorders: A Task Force Report of the American Psychiatric Association. Washington, DC, American Psychiatric Association, 1989, pp 2457–2496.
5. McElroy SL, Hudson JI, Pope HG, et al: The DSM-III-R impulse control disorders not elsewhere classified: Clinical characteristics and relationship to other psychiatric disorders. Am J Psychiatry 149:318, 1992.
6. Monopolis SJ, Lion JR: Disorders of impulse control: Explosive disorders, pathological gambling, pyromania, and kleptomania. In Curran WJ, McGarry AL, Shah SA (eds): Forensic Psychiatry and Psychology: Perspectives and Standards for Interdisciplinary Practice. Philadelphia, F.A. Davis, 1986, pp 409–424.
7. Murray JB: Review of research on pathological gambling. Psychol Rep 72:791, 1993.
8. Schalling D: Neurochemical correlates of personality, impulsivity, and disinhibitory suicidality. In Hodgins S (ed): Mental Disorder and Crime. Newbury Park, CA, Sage, 1993, pp 208–226.
9. Stein DJ, Hollander E, Liebowitz MR: Neurobiology of impulsivity and impulse control disorders. J Neuropsychiatry and Clin Neurosci 5:9, 1993.
10. Virkkunen M, Linnoila M: Serotonin in personality disorder with habitual violence and impulsivity. In Hodgins S (ed): Mental Disorder and Crime. Newbury Park, CA, Sage, 1993, pp 227–243.
11. Wolkowitz OM, Roy A, Doran AR: Pathologic gambling and other risk-taking pursuits. Psychiatr Clin North Am 8:311, 1985.

31. MEDICALLY UNEXPLAINED SYMPTOMS:

THE DIAGNOSIS AND THERAPEUTIC APPROACH TO SOMATOFORM AND FACTITIOUS DISORDERS AND MALINGERING

Alan M. Jacobson, M.D.

1. To what does the term "medically unexplained symptoms" refer?

Patients commonly present to their primary physicians with medical symptoms that cannot be fully explained by specific somatic illnesses. Such unexplained symptoms may vary considerably in duration and severity; often they are transient and mild and resolve without specific apparent intervention. Simple explanation and reassurance, supported by physician assessment (history, physical exam, and basic office-based laboratory tests) may significantly reduce others. The severity, intensity, or persistence of the symptom dictates consideration of in-depth diagnostic evaluation that may include more extensive medical and psychiatric work-ups. Even with more detailed assessment, a clear somatic explanation may not become apparent, yet the symptom persists. The more severe and/or persistent presentations of medically unexplained symptoms may be the manifestation of four groups of psychiatric disorders and conditions: somatoform disorders; factitious disorders; other psychiatric disorders (e.g., anxiety and depression); and/or malingering. The assessment of patients with medically unexplained symptoms that are more than mild or transient should consider etiologies in all four spheres.

Even after careful medical assessment, some unexplained symptoms are due to organic syndromes that are not yet diagnosable. Thus persistent and disruptive symptoms always involve a certain tension. The clinician must balance between helping the patient with underlying psychiatric problems and remaining attuned to unfolding medical conditions. Indeed, in the course of ongoing somatoform and other psychiatric disorders, patients may develop medical problems that require treatment. This can be especially demanding when somatization occurs in the context of chronic medical illness. Careful psychiatric assessment helps to identify classic patterns of psychopathology, which in turn may guide the evaluator to consider the possibility of unrecognized medical conditions.

2. What are the common characteristics of somatoform disorders?

Somatoform disorders present with physical symptoms that are not fully explained by clear medical disorder, the effects of substance abuse, or other psychiatric syndromes. The physical symptoms are *not intentional.* In other words, in somatoform disorders, the symptoms are not simply under voluntary control. Five general categories of somatoform disorders have been described:

Somatoform Disorders

CATEGORY	KEY CHARACTERISTICS
Somatization disorder	Multiple symptoms—pain, gastrointestinal, sexual dysfunction Symptoms vary over time Chronic condition—often with extensive treatment history Not intentional
Conversion disorder	Symptoms affect voluntary motor or sensory system Symptoms do not conform to neuroanatomic structures May reflect, symbolically, past or current stressor

Table continued on following page.

Somatoform Disorders (Cont.)

CATEGORY	KEY CHARACTERISTICS
Conversion disorder *(cont.)*	Patient may not be upset by the symptoms Not intentional
Hypochondriasis	Chronic preoccupation with having a serious disease Patient misattributes symptom or test results Preoccupation not solely due to affective status
Body dysmorphic disorder	Preoccupation with an imagined defect in physical appearance May exaggerate mild anomaly
Chronic pain syndrome	Pain is the central feature May begin after specific injury Can lead to serious functional impairment and medication overuse

3. Describe somatization disorder.

Previously, somatization disorder was referred to as hysteria or Briquet's syndrome. It is a chronic fluctuating condition that usually begins before the age of 30 and extends over many years. The patient presents with multiple symptoms that may vary considerably over time, including pain, gastrointestinal symptomatology, neurologic symptoms, and sexual dysfunction. When the patient presents, he or she may have a long history of past extensive treatment, including surgery. In practice the patient may seek out multiple providers because of dissatisfaction with prior treatment and may end up on complex combinations of medications because of frustration on the part of both patient and physician. It is common for patients to have significant impairments in work and social functioning.

As described in the *Diagnostic and Statistical Manual–IV,* patients should have a history of pain in at least four different sites, two different gastrointestinal symptoms other than pain, at least one sexual symptom, and one neurologic symptom. The work-up of the patient with somatization disorder usually reveals a positive history of multiple medical and surgical treatments, current symptoms without abnormal laboratory test results, and a physical exam that fails to identify objective findings that explain subjective complaints. As with other patients with unexplained medical symptoms, past treatment may lead to clear physical findings that explain some persisting symptoms that overlie the original complaints. For example, the patient may have had an exploratory laporatomy that now leads to persistent symptomatic cramping pain due to adhesions.

The presentation of symptoms may vary across cultures and countries and varies in frequency among men and women of different cultures. In North America somatization disorder is more commonly found in women than men; up to 2% of women and less than 0.2% of men have a lifetime prevalence of this disorder.

4. Describe conversion disorder.

Conversion disorder presents with symptoms or deficits that affect the voluntary motor or sensory neurologic system. The presentation often mimics or appears similar to recognized neurologic or other medical conditions. As with somatization disorder, the symptoms are not intentionally produced or faked; rather, underlying psychological factors are expressed in physical symptoms. Common presentations include loss of sensation in a single limb or part of a limb, double vision, blindness, deafness, difficulty with swallowing, and paralysis. On careful exam, the symptoms typically do not conform to recognized anatomic pathways. For example, a classic sensory loss due to conversion disorder may conform to a glove or stocking distribution. It is important to recognize that unusual distributions of sensory and motor loss may occur in some neurologic disorders, such as multiple sclerosis. Historically, conversion reactions have been thought to symbolize unresolved conflict. For example, the patient who feels guilt-ridden because he or she stole something loses all ability to move the hand that grabbed the object. Such conversion symptoms also may occur in patients with a history of physical and emotional abuse as well as borderline personality disorder. Conversion disorders are likely to be associated closely in time with an acute stressor. However, the stressor itself may be mild and important only as a symbolic representation of past psychological trauma or conflict. For example, the patient may develop trouble with swallowing (sometimes called globus hystericus) on viewing a movie that depicts sexual violence and thus symbolizes earlier oral rape that the patient experienced. In such instances, most patients (but not all) do not concurrently remember the earlier events; the symptoms of gagging are felt without accompanying memories of trauma or conflict.

Whereas the symptoms of conversion disorder may generate social responses that are reinforcing, conversion symptoms typically are thought to derive primarily from inner psychic gain rather than so-called secondary social gains. In the previous example, the muffled inability to speak may represent the individual's earlier sense of suffocation and gagging as an abused child. The inner conflict also may have been caused by the authority figure's threat to kill the patient if he or she talked about the event and/or by the patient's inner shame or guilt about speaking of the event, now brought near the psychological surface by exposure to the movie. Because the early event is commonly forgotten or very poorly remembered and only the symbolic physical symptom is experienced, the patient with a conversion disorder may present with minimal upset associated with the physical symptom. This reaction has been termed "la belle indifference." However, in other instances, the patient may be confused and even terrified by the new symptom.

5. Describe hypochondriasis.

Hypochondriasis refers to a chronic preoccupation and fear of having a serious disease. It is typically based on the individual's continual misperception of bodily symptoms and/or test results, which may occur in the context of a well-recognized and diagnosed illness, such as diabetes, or in the absence of known illness. The preoccupation in hypochondriasis persists despite all reasonable medical testing and reassurance; it may cover a wide range of body functions and systems and vary over time as evaluation demonstrates healthy functioning in a particular body system. Although the preoccupation cannot be attributed simply to the presence of comorbid anxiety, depression, obsessive-compulsive disorder, or psychotic disorder, hypochondriasis may be associated with such comorbid conditions. It is differentiated from body dysmorphic disorder (see below) because it is not focused on a specific, circumscribed concern about appearance.

Hypochondriasis may occur at any age. The course is usually chronic with waxing and waning symptoms and presentations. It appears to be equally common in men and women and may be made worse by the diagnosis of new medical problems. Hypochondriacal patients frequently "doctor shop" when dissatisfied by the responsivity of their current physician. "Doctor shopping" may occur in response to failure to diagnose a condition but more commonly occurs when a physician unwittingly becomes irritated by the patient's persistent complaints. Such irritation may manifest as avoidant behavior, such as failure to return phone calls, abrupt referral to a psychiatrist without careful preparation, or unwillingness to reassure the patient for the "umpteenth" time that the dark urine does not represent kidney failure.

Treatment of the hypochondriacal patient should include careful assessment and reassessment for comorbid psychiatric disorders. Particularly important is aggressive treatment of symptomatic anxiety and depression, which may worsen hypochondriacal complaints and/or occur in response to the chronic fear of disease. Although hypochondriasis and chronic somatization disorder should be considered as separate entities and are differentiated by the hypochondriacal patients' intense preoccupation, in practice somatization disorder and hypochondriasis exist on a continuum.

6. Describe body dysmorphic disorder.

Body dysmorphic disorder refers to preoccupation with an imagined defect in physical appearance. The sense of defect may occur in response to a mild physical anomaly or with no identifiable trace of abnormality. A common example is the person obsessed with the ugliness of his or her nose because of a small bump. Distress over such abnormalities frequently leads to a search for cures through techniques such as plastic surgery or dental treatment. The patient is frequently tormented with these feelings and may go to extreme lengths to resolve them; make-up, exercise, and diet may be part of important rituals. Clearly the intense focus of western culture on physical beauty provides a setting for a continuum of concern about bodily perfection. Body dysmorphic disorder represents the extreme of this continuum. In anorexia nervosa the focus is on being too fat; thus the patient uses diet-related methods rather than surgery to cure the problem.

7. Describe pain disorders.

Pain disorders are characterized by specific predominant focus on pain as the presenting symptom. The pain usually does not follow established anatomic patterns. However, it may be impossible to differentiate from established medical conditions such as lumbar disc disease. Although work-ups are usually negative, prior invasive treatment may lead to physical findings that completely muddy the diagnosis. Indeed, pain disorders may develop after prior injury or treatment, which provides some pathophysiologic explanations for the symptoms. Pain disorders may occur throughout the lifespan. The course may be persistent and lead to severe functional impairment and extensive use of pain medication. It is more common in women than men.

The assessment should include careful attention to the presence of comorbid depression, which may present with pain symptoms. Psychotic and anxiety disorders also may involve pain as one symptom. The management of chronic pain syndromes is described at length in chapter 68. Rehabilitation programs combining behavioral and physical therapies may be helpful in some patients. External gains may affect the success of treatment, but as with somatization disorder, the primary cause is not social and financial gain.

8. How are malingering and factitious disorder distinguished from somatoform disorders?

Malingering	Factitious Disorder
Intentionally causes or feigns symptoms	Motivated by assumption of the sick role
Poor cooperation in evaluation and treatment	Involves fabrication of symptoms and/or self-inflicted injury
Motivated by external gain (e.g., winning a lawsuit	History vague and confusing
	Often chronic
May be accompanied by antisocial personality disorder	Patients may go from hospital to hospital seeking care

The essential feature of malingering is an *intentional* causing or faking of physical or psychological symptoms motivated by external incentives. Such incentives may be monetary or related to avoidance of work, prosecution, or military service; they also may involve the goal of obtaining drugs.

Several factors can be used as suggestive indicators of underlying malingering, such as association of a medical-legal issue with the presenting problem. Most commonly, the symptom is complex and/or vague, and the patient is involved in a law suit because of an injury or accident. The discrepancy between the symptomatic presentation and the apparent physical findings may be marked. Lack of cooperation in the evaluation process and poor compliance with recommended treatment are also common. Finally, the presence of an antisocial personality disorder may suggest malingering in a patient presenting with unexplained symptoms associated with possible external rewards or motivations. Thus malingering, unlike somatoform disorder, is motivated primarily by external gain.

In factitious disorder external factors, such as financial gain, may be present but play a minor role in providing support or reinforcement for symptoms. The motivation for a factitious disorder appears to derive from assuming the role of a sick person. Factitious disorders may involve fabrication of subjective complaints, such as headache; self-inflicted injury; and/or exaggeration of preexisting medical conditions.

Patients with factitious disorder usually engage in some form of lying. They may present with vague, inconsistent histories, often with a dramatic flair. Patients often have prior experience with medical routines and are also usually knowledgeable about medical terminology. Their complaints may change as the work-up returns with normal or negative findings. To the nurses and physicians caring for them, patients may seem to await eagerly and even to ask for multiple invasive procedures. They usually deny any suggestion that symptoms are self-induced or exaggerated and with confrontation usually discharge themselves, only to appear in another emergency department or clinic. In some instances the hospitalizations may involve traveling to multiple cities and even countries. The onset of factitious disorder is usually in adolescence or early adulthood. Although it may involve only a few episodes, chronic patterns often develop, leading to successive experiences with hospitals, emergency departments, and other treatment facilities.

In its most extreme form factitious disorder has often been termed **Münchausen's syndrome,** which refers to a chronic recurrent factitious disorder that typically involves wandering from place to place and taking on a lifestyle that centers on repeated evaluation, treatment, and hospitalization. Some have suggested that the extensive wandering and recurrent search for different treatments are reflections of patterns of treatment; i.e., the typical confrontation of an angry staff is said to be one reason that patients scurry from hospital to hospital. However, it is not entirely clear whether the wandering and the accompanying chronic factitious disorder can be prevented by alternative treatment approaches.

Severe, factitious disorders also have been described in children. The parent reports symptoms in the child in the manner described in adults. Termed **Münchausen's by proxy** (see chapter 80), this syndrome should be considered as a possible instance of child abuse and reported to appropriate authorities under the guidance of state and local laws.

9. Describe a general approach to the patient with unexplained medical symptoms.

The management of unexplained medical symptoms may be considered as a series of recurring steps. In the acute or first presentation, careful diagnosis and assessment of the medical symptoms and physical findings, together with the associated psychological responses, may be followed by thoughtful, nonjudgmental reassurance when the symptoms are relatively mild, circumscribed, and of recent origin. The psychoeducational approach of information combined with reassurance and careful explanation of probable causation is often sufficient, and the symptoms remit. For example, a child may present with headaches before school is to begin. Exploration of possible particular aspects of the stress may help the parents and child to find methods of reassurance that alleviate the source of the anxiety-related symptoms.

Such an approach can be used in combination with more in-depth medical assessment. For example, a patient on an orthopedic floor at a general hospital for treatment of a compound fracture of the left leg spontaneously developed paresis in the good leg. The paresis had no anatomic basis. Careful assessment by a consulting neurologist confirmed the initial evaluation by the primary physician. The consultant's suggestion that the symptoms would improve gradually over time was sufficient; over the following several days of recuperation the symptoms completely remitted.

When symptoms are persistent and/or severe, further steps are warranted, including more careful medical evaluation and detailed psychosocial assessment to identify psychological factors and social triggers. As information is gathered and a diagnosis formulated, the laboratory and physical findings should be presented unambiguously and in a nonjudgmental manner. The treatment plan may require negotiation with the patient to set limits on the nature of investigations, specialty referrals, and unwarranted treatment. It is important with chronic somatisizers to avoid simplistic dual models in which the diagnosis is either physical or mental. Indeed, it is often helpful to present, as part of the medical evaluation, a psychological explanatory model of the symptom process using words that are both understandable and safe. The model may include the understanding that the symptoms may be stress-related. It is important to underline that stress-related symptoms are just as real as symptoms produced by a clear medical illness. For example, the patient fearing cancer needs to understand that the presenting symptom, if it is said to be stress-related, is just as real to the doctor as if it were caused by cancer. Furthermore, it is important to emphasize that the suggested treatments for somatoform disorders are just as real, even though they differ from treatments for feared medical conditions.

Careful assessment also should include evaluation for comorbid psychiatric conditions such as depression, anxiety, personality disorders, and psychosis, which may provide direction for future treatment. It is helpful to have a single medical doctor or team approach in treating the chronic somatizing patient. The team may include a physician and psychiatrist or other mental health professional who work either in the same institution or in close collaboration. It is important to be open and honest at all steps of the treatment. Sneaking in a psychiatric referral will lead only to greater mistrust and resistance to treatment recommendations.

Consistency and flexibility may seem to represent opposite poles, but both are important. Consistency involves avoidance of unnecessary, new medical assessments and a clear, sensible, recurrent pronouncement of the physician's findings and recommendations. Patients often need to hear repeatedly what the doctor thinks, why he or she thinks it, and why a specific treatment is or is not recommended or pursued. On the other hand, at times of increased anxiety, flexibility may be required. For example, the patient who is chronically worried about developing renal failure may require periodic (and superficially unnecessary) simple kidney function tests to demonstrate that there is no sign of kidney failure. Letting the patient's concerns help to dictate evaluation and treatment decisions provides a sense of control. Continual renegotiation with the patient is essential. Flexibility is also warranted because in the course of chronic somatizing problems other psychiatric disorders commonly develop. The patient who is chronically hypochondrically worried may become depressed and require antidepressant treatment. Likewise, inflexibility may lead to missing the diagnosis of newly emerging medical illness.

Finally, by maintaining a consistent, stable, nonjudgmental attitude the physician helps the patients to feel understood and therefore to continue in treatment, thereby avoiding "doctor shopping."

10. Are specific treatment approaches applied differentially to the different forms of somatoform disorders?

There are more similarities than differences in the approach to treating patients with medically unexplained symptoms. As noted, the severity and chronicity of the complaint are important determinants of the initial therapeutic approach. Nonetheless, certain therapeutic variations may derive from differentiating among types of somatoform disorders. For example, patients with body dysmorphic disorder have a more narrowly defined concern involving perception of the body. The focused concern about bodily shape or deformity may benefit from a supportive therapeutic approach that helps the patient to understand possible sources of the distorted beliefs. Cognitive-behavior therapy, described in chapter 41 for treating depression, may be useful. Beliefs about body shape and deformity, however, are so powerful that short-term cognitive approaches are unlikely to lead to radical changes in imagery. Thus, such approaches need to be considered in the context of chronic management that helps the patient to avoid recurrent invasive treatment. The distorted perception of body dysmorphic disorder may be so severe as to become delusional; such patients may respond to judicious use of low doses of antipsychotic medications.

A focused approach is less likely to be effective in the patient with somatization disorder because of the broad range of symptoms and complaints. Hypochondriacal patients similarly may vary their bodily concern, thereby making a specific therapeutic focus more difficult. In all instances the therapy for chronic conditions needs to be considered as long-term and supportive; the therapist and physician must recognize that such patients often produce intense emotional reactions in the caretaker. They may arouse anger for repeated complaints and disturbance as well as for potential embarrassment when they make multiple visits to the emergency department, seeming to represent treatment failures in the eyes of the clinician and possibly his or her colleagues. Furthermore, chronic demands for pain medications and letters to housing boards and employers may lead the clinician to feel used by the patient. While external gain may be a secondary motivation for some symptoms in some patients, it is usually not the primary causal factor. Recognition of serious underlying psychological problems may not only guide therapy but also serve to allay the sense of being used and abused by the patients, thereby helping to maintain a positive therapeutic alliance.

Especially in patients with conversion disorder, hypnotherapy and/or other methods for exploring sources of particular stress may bring out unresolved conflicts and concerns that were not previously identified. Uncovering such issues can be useful in treating conversion symptoms. Simple suggestion combined with reassurance also may be beneficial for mild conversion disorders as well as other mild somatoform conditions. As noted before, conversion symptoms that appear in the context of a chronic pattern of somatization require supportive, nonjudgmental approaches by the health care team.

11. How do approaches to treatment differ for patients with factitious disorder or malingering?
In many ways the approaches to treatment are similar. The critical differential with the malingering patient is recognizing that the patient always has another, external goal; consistency and clarity are required so that the patient understands what the physician is recommending. Many such patients leave treatment because they do not obtain an external reward. The patient with factitious illness also may leave treatment if the drive for the sick role comes in conflict with the physician's unwillingness to perform more invasive tests.

12. How are medical symptoms associated with other psychiatric conditions differentiated from those associated with somatoform, factitious disorders, and malingering?
Three psychiatric syndromes most commonly present with subtle and sometimes vague physical symptoms: (1) depression, (2) anxiety, and (3) psychosis. Diagnosis depends on a careful history that explores for the symptoms of each psychiatric disorder. Headaches and other bodily pains commonly present in the context of depression and anxiety disorders. When the patient presents with other symptoms suggestive of either condition, a trial of appropriate medication may be useful. Such therapeutic trials are also valuable because anxiety and depressive disorders may well coexist with somatoform conditions. It is not unusual for the hypochondriacal patient also to have intense anxiety or depression. Treatment of the comorbid psychiatric condition may lead to considerable improvement in the somatoform disorder. In addition, symptomatic treatment of depression, anxiety, and psychosis is often more effective than treatment of chronic somatisizing conditions.

BIBLIOGRAPHY

1. Bass C, Benjamin S: The management of chronic somatisation. Br J Psychiatry 162:472–480, 1993.
2. Folks DG, Freeman AM: Münchausen's syndrome and other factitious illness. Psychiatr Clin North Am 8:263–278, 1985.
3. Kellner R: Psychosomatic syndromes, somatization and somatoform disorders. Psychother Psychosom 61:4–24, 1994.
4. Kellner R: Somatization: Theories and research. J Nerv Mental Dis 178:150–160, 1990.
5. Lipowski ZJ: Somatization: The concept and its clinical application. Am J Psychiatry 145:1358–1368, 1988.
6. Margo KL, Margo GM: The problem of somatization in family practice. Am Fam Physician 1873–1879, 1994.
7. Mayou R: Somatization. Psychother Psychosom 59:69–83, 1993.
8. Somatoform disorders. Diagnostic and Statistical Manual–IV. Washington, DC, American Psychiatric Association, 1994.

32. GRIEF AND MOURNING

Stephen R. Shuchter, M.D., and Sidney Zisook, M.D.

All psychiatrists will encounter patients whose loved one has died either just recently or in the near or distant past. Such losses often are quite traumatic and painful and can precipitate both psychological and medical sequelae which may require intervention. Appreciating the consequences of death on its survivors can be a crucial element in assessing the patient.

1. What is grief?

Grief is a term that is applied to the myriad psychological, physiologic, and behavioral responses which accompany the human awareness of an irrevocable loss, such as a pending or actual loss of a close friend or relative.

Manifestations of Normal Grief

Psychological
  Numbness or dissociation
  Sense of loss
  Anguish
  Yearning
  Anger
  Guilt
  Apathy
  Anxiety and fear
  Intrusive images
  Cognitive disorganization
  Distractibility
  Hallucinatory experiences
  Regression

Physiologic
  Autonomic discharge: gastrointestinal, cardiovascular,
      respiratory, neuromuscular
  Insomnia
  Agitation
  Anorexia

2. What are the psychological aftereffects?

The psychological sequelae may include experiences of intense anguish and emotional pain accompanied by crying, feelings of loss, and yearning for the one who has died; feelings of anger or guilt; transient periods of numbness, shock or disbelief when the loss does not register emotionally; a sense of apathy or directionlessness in the face of a profound loss; the appearance of anxiety and fearfulness; the intrusion of painful images and memories, especially if the nature or course of death was traumatic to the survivor; and cognitive disorganization. Behaviorally, survivors frequently search for evidence that their loved one is still alive. They may experience multiple sensory hallucinations of the deceased, most often in the form of sensing their presence but also including auditory, visual, haptic and olfactory hallucinations.

Many grieving persons attempt to isolate themselves from social contacts which are made too painful because of the memories they evoke. They may avoid discussing their loss or even confronting those mundane experiences of life or possessions of the deceased which can trigger their anguish. The aggregation of all of these powerful emotional and cognitive forces often leads to a regression: an emotional state in which the grieving person feels overwhelmed, out of control, helpless, and child-like in heightened dependency.

3. What forms of physiologic responses are common?

Physiologic responses occur frequently, often in reaction to reminders of the loss. These occur in the form of sudden autonomic discharge with acute symptoms reflecting the *pangs* of grief: chest pain ("heartache"), gastrointestinal distress ("a knife in the belly"), dyspnea, paresthesias, palpitations, dizziness, nausea, tremulousness, and others. Acutely grieving survivors may demonstrate hypercortisolism, sleep and appetite disturbances, and continuous heightened autonomic arousal.

4. Are all losses the same?

Although the word "grief" is often reserved for the feelings and behavior associated with death (e.g., bereavement), the same sort of reaction is seen after any loss considered important by the individual. Examples are stillbirth and miscarriage, loss of a job, failing health, disability, amputation, loss of home, or divorce. Indeed, divorce, especially when dependent children are involved, can lead to some of the most tumultuous and persistent grief reactions. Sometimes a loss which to the outside observer may seem quite trivial, such as the death of a pet or a favorite celebrity, or losing an object of sentimental value, will be followed by a severe grief reaction because the loss has a disproportionate significance. The grief reaction can also occur even when the loss is intangible, such as after a stroke or cataract, when the loss involved is a *function* of a part of the body. In each of these examples, the individual loses someone or something that is emotionally or physically "part of themselves." The meaning of such losses, the intensity of the grief, and the way people ultimately cope with the changes in their lives vary from person to person.

5. What is mourning?

An important aspect of the total grief reaction, mourning refers to the culturally prescribed set of experiences which may include a time-frame and a series of behaviors, rituals, and observances which reflect a given culture's or religion's views about the meanings of life and death and the role of the individual survivor within this context. Mourning customs may be strictly defined: the widow should wear black and avoid pleasantries for a year; the funeral and memorial services should contain certain elements; prayers for the dead are said on particular occasions. Some grief experiences, such as hallucinations, may be more acceptable or even desirable in certain cultures. In the United States, no standard traditions dictate the decisions and behavior of survivors. There are few tight-knit communities where widowed men and women are scrutinized or monitored. Individuals' religious beliefs may dictate some traditions, but for the most part, mourning has also evolved toward a more individualized and relatively unstructured experience.

6. What is pathologic grief?

Pathologic grief is a commonly used term whose definition has remained elusive. It originally referred to those patients whose grief was absent or excessively intense or prolonged. It also referred to situations where grieving patients developed medical or psychiatric illnesses. Although clinicians will likely continue to encounter references to pathologic grief, we do not believe it is a useful concept. First, we have come to appreciate that the spectrum of normative responses to loss is enormous. There are people whose grief is brief and limited in terms of their emotional responses and sequelae. On the other hand, a substantial number of people grieve profoundly for a long time. Furthermore, particularly following the death of a spouse or a child, survivors are likely to continue to manifest elements of grief intermittently throughout their lives. Responses at both ends of this continuum are normal and not pathologic.

At the same time, other individuals are vulnerable to the development of medical and psychiatric illnesses in the context of grief. Here again, such illnesses do not constitute pathologic grief but idiosyncratic vulnerability (genetic and developmental), as expressed at a point of an enormous stressor.

7. How long does grief last?

There is great variability in the course of grief. The most important determinant of the length and intensity of grief is the closeness of the relationship between the deceased and survivor: how central was that person to the survivor's emotional life. For the closest of relationships, there will be an acute period of grief that may last from a few weeks to several months, but protracted grief may last for years. If the clinician encounters such extended grief or such a persistent intense level of grief that extends for a year or more, a possibility that the person has developed a major depression must be considered.

The most common and clinically normal forms of protracted grief occur on an intermittent basis for several years, or forever. A person who has lost a child may experience elements of acute grief every time she hears the name of the child, on special occasions (birthdays, holidays, anniversaries) or whenever the survivor sees the child's picture on the nightstand. Such grief, often referred to as anniversary reactions, will usually be short-lived and dissipate in minutes. Similarly, when a clinician makes an inquiry into the emotions of any patient's loss, it should be recognized that in such a regressively oriented exploration, elements of grief are likely to appear and are normal. It is a mistake to think that grief "resolves" in the sense that it disappears or goes away. In most people, grief becomes circumscribed and suppressed only to reemerge in response to familiar triggers.

8. What is the relationship between grief and depression?

Acute grief represents one of the most powerful paradigms for the stress-diathesis model of medical illness, including psychiatric illness, as depicted in the figure below. The death of a loved one is likely to be the most profound and intense stressor that most people will encounter. Studies have repeatedly demonstrated the association between grief and the development of numerous stress-related medical disorders, including heart disease, cancer, and the common cold. The bereaved are vulnerable, as well, to psychiatric syndromes, especially depression.

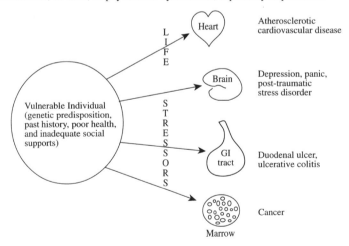

Stress-diathesis model of medical illness.

Historically, bereaved individuals, their families, and physicians have taken the position that grief is "depressing" and that "mourning" and "melancholia" are inseparable phenomena. No one is ever surprised when a widow is depressed. This fact seems normal and natural, giving rise to less zeal from the physician to treat a disorder that otherwise would be the object of aggressive therapy. At some time during the first year after the death of a spouse, 30 to 50% of widows and widowers meet the criteria for a major depressive episode. Recognizing the ubiquity of depressive symptoms in grief, the DSM–III and DSM–III–R introduced the term *Uncomplicated Bereavement* to demarcate depressive syndromes occurring shortly after the death of a close friend or relative from a major depressive disorder. Because uncomplicated bereavement is not considered an illness, the clinical rule-of-thumb has been benign neglect rather than active treatment of the depressive episode. Such depressions often are persistent, however, and may be associated with substantial morbidity. Therefore, the DSM–IV changed the term uncomplicated bereavement to *Bereavement*, suggesting that only mild depressive syndromes beginning and ending within 2 months of the death should be considered "normal."

9. Can they be distinguished?

Although manifestations of acute grief frequently mimic or overlap with those of depression, they can be differentiated by the intermittent and trigger-related quality of grief symptoms and the *autonomous* quality of depressive symptoms. Once depression has a "life of its own," the clinician is much less likely to see the intermittent periods of good functioning and relatively normal affects that punctuate the lives of the nondepressed grieving individual. Other differential points are: (1) the constellation of *several* symptoms of depression occurring simultaneously most of the time, for at least 2 weeks; and (2) the presence of relentless anhedonia so often seen in depression but less frequently in grief uncomplicated by major depression.

The DSM–IV lists several additional factors that should alert the clinician that a major depression may be present. These include (1) guilt unassociated with the death; (2) preoccupation with death independent of the specific death of the loved one; (3) morbid preoccupation with worthlessness; (4) marked psychomotor retardation; (5) prolonged and marked functional impairment; and (6) hallucinations not involving the deceased.

Differentiation of Mourning and Melancholy

	NORMAL DEPRESSION OF BEREAVEMENT (DSM–IV)	MAJOR DEPRESSIVE EPISODE (MDE)
Onset	Within 2 months of death	Any time after death (or before death in response to prolonged "dying")
Duration	Less than 2 months	Weeks to years; typically at least 6–9 months
Course	Circumscribed episode: symptoms associated with "triggers" then resolve	Often chronic, intermittent, or recurrent symptoms, autonomous, usually present
Symptoms	Rarely include severe guilt, suicidal ideation, morbid worthlessness, psychomotor retardation or psychosis	Any and all symptoms of MDE positive/negative melancholia
Impairment	Brief and mild to moderate	May be prolonged and marked
Self-perception	Normal	Ill

10. Are grief and depression intrinsically connected?

Yes. Another complicating element in the relationship between grief and depression is that depression recruits grief; that is, depressive states have a tendency to exacerbate prior experiences of grief. It is not uncommon that one encounters patients with a major depression whose focus is on some relationship that ended, or on the death of someone important in their lives. Such losses may have been years before. This presentation often leads a clinician to believe that this depressive episode is a manifestation of "unresolved grief" and to begin to focus treatment on the grief. Remembering that grief does not resolve but only subsides, the correct assessment will reveal that the grief displayed is simply a manifestation of depression which will subside once the depression is treated. In this scenario, depression "begets" grief, rather than the converse.

11. Should grieving patients be treated with psychopharmacologic agents?

It depends. Grief itself is a normal response to loss. At times, people feel overwhelmed by the power of their emotions: the anguish, sadness, sense of loss, and other forms of emotional pain. They will frequently try to "dose" themselves by allowing exposure to stimuli which will evoke such anguish and then avoiding such when it becomes too much. People learn what is painful and what is not, which activities they can do safely and which are "dangerous" as triggers for their grief. For those who are experiencing this type of distress, there is no indication to medicate despite what may be a perceived need by the patient for relief. However, there are exceptions.

12. When should grieving patients be treated by psychopharmacologic agents?

When grief-related symptoms of anxiety are expressed so continuously that they are interfering with cognitive and other functions of living in a substantial way, the use of a benzodiazepine should be considered. This may also be considered in those patients who have a higher risk of developing or exacerbating a major depression or anxiety disorder. Usually, benzodiazepines are used as needed for relatively brief periods.

For individuals who develop substantial sleep disorders, short-term intervention with pharmacology can be both humane and helpful, using agents from any of the three classes of (1) hypnotics (e.g., chloral hydrate, 500 mg), (2) short-acting anxiolytics, or (3) low-doses of sedating antidepressants (e.g., trazodone, 50 mg). A persistent and continuous sleep disorder with features of early, middle, or late insomnia may indicate the onset of major depression, requiring closer monitoring and possible use of an antidepressant in standard doses.

Depression is very under-diagnosed and is often under-treated even when diagnosed. Historically, physicians have been reluctant to treat the depression of bereavement aggressively, feeling that treating such depression interferes with normal grief and with nature's restorative properties. However, depression is depression, regardless of the context in which it appears or even the existential reasonableness of its presentation. Depression carries with it substantial morbidity, both medical and psychological. We strongly encourage physicians to treat major depression aggressively, even if it appears in the context of bereavement.

13. How can I help to counsel the bereaved to get past their loss or to put it behind them?

You cannot and you ought not try. The death of one's spouse or child or sibling is forever, and elements of the survivor's grief will also last forever. Healthy people find many ways to cope with their losses and their grief. One of the most "human" capacities to deal with such loss has been to mitigate against it by keeping the loved one alive. In other words, it is normal and healthy for survivors to maintain a relationship with the deceased.

Survivors frequently have a sense that their loved one is with them, watching over them, protecting them. It is not uncommon for a widow to carry on conversations with her dead husband or to ask for his advice. These and similar phenomena occur in healthy people with intact reality-testing whose sensory perceptions are highly directed toward keeping their loved ones alive. As time goes by, the actual sense of their loved one's presence evolves into an emotional feeling of the person's place in their heart. Qualities of the deceased may become incorporated into the identity of the survivor. Cherished possessions and memories keep the deceased alive for those who have physically lost them. Important emotional ties do not disappear when our loved ones die, and clinicians must learn to appreciate these connections, respect them, and even foster communication about them. For survivors, life will go on, and more comfortably once they have established an emotionally viable way of sustaining their relationship with the deceased.

Therefore, it is not helpful to convince a bereaved individual to "let go" or get on with life in a way that disregards the loved one. What is helpful is to let such patients know you care, to listen when they feel like talking, to offer the perspective of someone who identifies with the painful and often protracted course of grief, and to be ready to step in when, and if, a major depression or other medical or psychiatric complications develop.

14. What are the other common problems of the bereaved?

Grief is an extraordinarily powerful emotion. We have examined some of the problems such feelings create for the bereaved: their suffering, their vulnerability to illness, and their needs to re-order their relationships. Frequently, problems develop because of the reactions of others to grief.

Friends and family may be unable to tolerate grief and may avoid the bereaved or, when with them, discourage them from expressing what they feel. A grieving person may feel more isolated from others, at times because of their reluctance to inflict their own suffering on others. With time, they will find closeness and comfort from others who have felt such pain and with whom they feel a common bond. For this reason, involvement in a bereavement support group is usually very helpful.

Of particular concern is the difficulty physicians and therapists may find in dealing with the bereaved, particularly those in the most acute throes of grief. Empathetic clinicians may find themselves experiencing much anguish and helplessness in the face of their patients' suffering. At times, this may feel intolerable, and clinicians may become inclined to push their patients away or to divert them from their grief. Other therapists may fear being "swallowed up" by the intense need of the grieving person. The intense regression of grief is, however, a time-limited phenomenon, and the clinician's emotional availability is central to their ability to help the bereaved. The healthy clinician will emerge from this suffering and will often feel stronger for the experience.

BIBLIOGRAPHY

1. Burnell GM, Burnell AL (eds): Clinical Management of Bereavement: A Handbook for Healthcare Professionals. New York, Human Sciences Press, 1989.
2. Clayton PJ: Mortality and morbidity in the first year of bereavement. Arch Gen Psychiatry 30:747–750, 1974.
3. Jacobs S (ed): Pathologic Grief: Maladaptation to Loss. Washington, DC, American Psychiatric Association, 1993.
4. Osterweis M, Solomon F, Green M (eds): Bereavement: Reactions, Consequences, and Care. Washington, DC, National Academy Press, 1984.
5. Parkes CM (ed): Bereavement: Studies of Grief in Adult Life, 2nd ed. New York, International Universities Press, 1972.
6. Raphael B: Preventive intervention with the recently bereaved. Arch Gen Psychiatry 34:1450–1454, 1977.
7. Raphael B (ed): The Anatomy of Bereavement. New York, Basic Books, 1983.
8. Rynearson EK (ed): Bereavement. Psychiatric Annals (Special Issue) 16:268–318, 1986.
9. Rynearson EK (ed): Pathologic Bereavement. Psychiatric Annals (Special Issue) 20:294–348, 1990.
10. Shuchter SR (ed): Dimensions of Grief: Adjusting to the Death of a Spouse. San Francisco, Jossey-Bass, 1986.
11. Silverman PR: Widowhood and preventive intervention. Family Coordinator 21:95–102, 1972.
12. Stroebe MS, Stroebe W, Hansson RO (eds): Handbook of Bereavement: Theory, Research and Intervention. Cambridge, Cambridge University Press, 1993.
13. Worden JW (ed): Grief Counseling and Grief Therapy: A Handbook for the Mental Health Practitioner, 2nd ed. New York, Springer, 1991.
14. Wortman CB, Silver RC: The myths of coping with loss. J Consult Clin Psychol 57:349–357, 1989.
15. Zisook S, Shuchter SR: Major depression associated wit widowhood. Am Assoc Geriatr Psychiatry 1:316–326, 1993.
16. Zisook S (ed): Grief and Bereavement. Psychiatr Clin North Am 10:329–510, 1987.

IV. Organic Mental Syndromes

33. BEHAVIORAL PRESENTATIONS OF MEDICAL AND NEUROLOGIC DISORDERS

C. Alan Anderson, M.D., and Christopher M. Filley, M.D.

1. Why is the identification of an underlying medical or neurologic disorder important?
What initially seems to be a standard psychiatric illness on closer examination may prove to be a medical or neurologic disease. Patients who present with behavioral or psychiatric symptoms as the major manifestation of such a condition have been shown to have significant morbidity and mortality that worsens with delay in diagnosis and treatment. Illnesses as diverse as brain tumors and renal failure may present with behavioral syndromes, and for many of the conditions there are specific and effective therapies. Treatment is unlikely to be effective and the condition may worsen unless the primary problem is addressed. Hence the timely and expeditious identification of patients with secondary or induced behavior syndromes is crucial.

2. What are the typical behavioral presentations of medical and neurologic diseases?
Whereas nearly every symptom, syndrome, and psychiatric diagnostic category has been described, several presentations are particularly common. Confusional states, psychosis, depression, and personality changes are the most frequent, with anxiety, mania, and conversion disorder occurring less often. All varieties of presentation are seen. Affected patients may present with isolated symptoms or with multiple symptoms of sufficient duration and severity to meet DSM–IV criteria. The problem may be acute and progressive, or it may present as a chronic condition with little or no change over months to years. The bad news, therefore, is that we need to consider an underlying medical or neurologic problem in nearly every patient that we see. The good news, however, is that clinical clues help to identify patients at higher risk and assist in focusing the evaluation.

In general, the absence of prior psychiatric problems, lack of family history of psychiatric illness, and onset of symptoms after age 40 should raise the suspicion of medical or neurologic illness. A thorough review of systems may uncover other problems that otherwise would be overlooked in the face of major behavioral disturbances. A history of headaches, syncope, seizures, head trauma, focal neurologic problems (i.e., visual disturbance, weakness, incoordination), cardiopulmonary complaints, incontinence, weight change, or fevers should prompt further investigation. Finally, presenting complaints that have a higher likelihood of representing medical illness include progressive intellectual deterioration, apathy or indifference, and visual hallucinations.

3. Which disorders may present with confusion?
Because of its everyday use, confusion as a medical concept has confused many. In clinical terms, confusion means the inability to maintain a coherent line of thought. Confusional states are exceedingly common, and most arise acutely because of a reversible toxic or metabolic disorder with prominent effects on the brain. The patient with an acute confusional state typically presents with impaired attention, disorientation, incoherent thinking, hallucinations, delusions, illusions, disturbed sleep-wake cycles, and variable alterations in level of consciousness. The cardinal feature

is the disturbance of attention; other symptoms present in varying combinations and degrees. Synonymous terms include delirium and metabolic or toxic encephalopathy, and each may be used to emphasize certain aspects of the syndrome. The term acute organic brain syndrome, however, is inadequate, both because it lacks specificity and because it promulgates the unlikely belief that some behavioral disorders do not result from brain dysfunction. This terminology has been deleted from the DSM–IV, and we suggest that it be dropped from common medical usage as well.

All clinicians encounter the acute confusional state, but patients at higher risk include the elderly, patients with prior brain disease or injury, postoperative or burn patients, and patients with acquired immunodeficiency syndrome (AIDS). The list of causes for the acute confusional state is long but the more common disorders associated with confusion are listed below:

Common Causes of the Acute Confusional State

Intoxications—alcohol; prescription, over-the-counter (OTC), and street drugs; solvents; heavy metals; pesticides; carbon monoxide.

Withdrawal states—alcohol, sedative-hypnotic drugs.

Nutritional deficiencies—thiamine (Wernicke's encephalopathy), vitamin B_{12}, folate, niacin.

Metabolic disorders—electrolyte and acid-base disturbances; hepatic, renal, pancreatic disease.

Infections—pneumonia, urinary tract infection, sepsis, AIDS.

Endocrinopathies—hypo- and hyperthyroidism, hypo- and hyperglycemia, hypo- and hyperadrenocorticism.

Structural brain disease—traumatic brain injury, seizure disorders, stroke, subarachnoid or parenchymal hemorrhage, epidural or subdural hematoma, encephalitis, brain abscess.

Postoperative state—anesthesia, electrolyte disturbances, fever, hypoxia, analgesics.

4. Which disorders may present with psychosis?

The essence of psychosis is loss of contact with reality. This breakdown in perception, thought content, and communications takes various forms, including hallucinations, delusions, motor disturbances, paranoia, and changes in affect. Although the typical constellation of symptoms and signs of schizophrenia has been described in medical and neurologic illness, usually other clues suggest an underlying pathologic process. Secondary or induced psychosis often has a more abrupt onset, more prominent alterations in level of consciousness, and more evidence of intellectual deterioration. The character of symptoms may also be different, with induced psychosis more likely to cause visual hallucinations and poorly defined delusions. Functional psychosis more often manifests auditory hallucinations, preserved level of alertness and orientation, and more complex and stable delusions. The following table lists some of the medical and neurologic disorders presenting with psychotic features.

Disorders Associated with Secondary Psychosis

Complex partial seizures	Traumatic brain injury
Alcohol withdrawal	Stroke
Drugs (prescription, over-the-counter, street; for example amphetamines, diet pills, levodopa, bromocriptine)	Brain infections
	Brain neoplasms
Metabolic disorders (hepatic, renal, thyroid disease; vitamin deficiencies)	Dementia (Alzheimer's disease, Pick's disease, Huntington's disease, Wilson's disease)
	Multiple sclerosis

5. Which disorders may present with depression?

The depressed patient presents with low mood, psychomotor retardation, apathy, and anhedonia plus the vegetative signs of decreased appetite, diminished libido, and sleep disturbance. The more common concern is overlooking functional depression while searching for medical and neurologic illness, but the reverse situation also occurs. Systemic illnesses can present with a clinical picture typical of major depression in every respect. Clues to distinguishing these patients include the absence of previous psychiatric problems or family history, no precipitating event, older age at onset, and associated medical and neurological signs and symptoms. The following table lists frequent causes of secondary depression.

Frequent Medical and Neurologic Causes of Depression

Drugs (oral contraceptives, diltiazem, isoniazid, benzodiazepines, barbiturates, methyldopa)	Metabolic disorders (thyroid disorders, adrenal disorders, hepatic disease, hypoglycemia, pancreatic and gastrointestinal cancer)
Stroke, especially left frontal	
Brain neoplasms	Dementia (Alzheimer's disease, Parkinson's disease, Huntington's disease)
Traumatic brain injury	Neurosyphilis
Multiple sclerosis	Systemic lupus erythematosus

6. Which disorders may present with mania?

Manic patients present with increased energy, flight of ideas, grandiosity, and impaired judgment against a background of an abnormally elevated or irritable mood. There may be delusions and hallucinations as well. Mania has been described as the presenting symptom of many medical disorders and also as a consequence of head trauma and seizure disorder. The diagnosis of secondary or induced mania is suggested by associated neurologic signs and symptoms and initial presentation after the age of 40. The following table lists frequent causes of secondary mania.

Common Medical and Neurologic Causes of Mania

Drugs (e.g., excessive thyroid hormone, amphetamines, cocaine, monoamine oxidase inhibitors)	Multiple sclerosis
	Dementia (Huntington's disease, Wilson's disease, Pick's disease)
Hyperthyroidism	
Seizure disorders, especially complex partial	Herpes simplex encephalitis
Traumatic brain injury	Neurosyphilis
Stroke	Brain neoplasms

7. Which disorders may result in personality change?

Personality changes are like good art: they are hard to describe and categorize, but we know them when we see them. Subtle alterations in basic character and temperament often herald the onset of neurologic illness. Comportment, motivation, affect, judgment, and impulse control may change dramatically in the face of disease or injury of the brain. Pathologic processes affecting the frontal lobes have been frequently described in this regard. Personality change also may result from involvement of the temporal lobes, including the controversial entity of behavioral changes that develop over many years in patients with complex partial seizures of temporal lobe origin. Whereas nearly any illness or injury may alter personality, the following list provides a clinical guide.

Medical and Neurologic Causes of Personality Change

Traumatic brain injury	Complex partial seizure disorder
Dementia (Pick's disease, Alzheimer's disease, Huntington's disease, Wilson's disease, normal pressure hydrocephalus)	Drug and alcohol abuse
	Neurosyphilis
	Infection with human immunodeficiency virus (HIV)
Brain neoplasms	
Stroke	Hypothyroidism
Multiple sclerosis	

8. Which disorders may present with anxiety?

Patients with anxiety typically display apprehension, fear, hyperattentiveness, trembling, restlessness, dizziness, dry mouth, and palpitations. These are common autonomic responses to psychological stress but also may represent an undiagnosed medical or neurologic illness. As in the examples above, absence of related history, lack of precipitating event, and older age at onset suggest an underlying disorder. In large series of patients, endocrine diseases and cardiopulmonary conditions were most likely to present with anxiety. Likely disorders include:

Hyperthyroidism	Pulmonary disease
Hypoglycemia	Drugs
Pheochromocytoma	Alcohol or sedative-hypnotic withdrawal
Hypoparathyroidism	Systemic lupus erythematosus
Cardiovascular disease	Wilson's disease

9. Why is it important to recognize conversion disorder?

Many patients present with symptoms and signs that suggest medical or neurologic illness but are due to unconscious manifestations of emotional conflict. The clinician needs to be able to recognize this pattern, both for accurate diagnosis of psychiatric illness and for isolation of hysterical clinical features from those that may be due to medical or neurologic illness. An important point to remember is signs and symptoms of conversion disorder are common in patients with known neurologic illness. For example, nonepileptic seizures may be encountered in patients with established seizure disorders. Such traditional signs of conversion disorder as give-way weakness, nonanatomic sensory changes, and la belle indifference may be seen in patients with multiple sclerosis and other neurologic disorders (see chapter 31 for further discussion of conversion disorder). Disorders that frequently accompany hysteria include:

Multiple sclerosis	Complicated migraine
Systemic lupus erythematosus	Neurosyphilis
Seizure disorders	Endocrine disorders

10. What is an appropriate evaluation of patients presenting with behavioral syndromes?

As with all medical disciplines, it is wise to start with a detailed history, paying close attention to onset and course of symptoms, past and present medical and surgical history, and complete review of medications and drugs (prescription, over-the-counter, borrowed, stolen, or obtained on the street). The family history should be reviewed for both medical and psychiatric illness. A complete review of systems is also necessary. At this point, we suggest "going where the money is" and reviewing medications and drugs again. A detailed general physical examination, including neurologic and mental status testing is next. Laboratory evaluations should include a complete blood count, urinalysis, thyroid function studies, and toxicology screen. For example, one may encounter delirium due to hypoglycemia or psychosis related to hyperthyroidism. Pulse oximetry or arterial blood gas studies, lumbar puncture, syphilis serology, HIV testing, B_{12} and folate levels, vasculitis screening, and measurements of heavy metals, copper, ceruloplasmin, and porphyrins may be indicated. These tests should be considered when signs and symptoms suggest particular organ system involvement or the presence of reversible disorders.

Additional tests include electroencephalography (EEG) and neuroimaging studies. EEG provides information about the physiology of the brain and is safe and readily available at modest cost. Another advantage is that it can be performed at the bedside if necessary. The utility of EEG is best documented in seizure disorders, but it is often useful in the diagnosis of acute confusional states, dementia, and focal brain lesions. Both computerized tomography (CT) and magnetic resonance imaging (MRI) generate detailed anatomic information, and MRI in particular shows elegant views of brain regions that may be implicated in the pathogenesis of behavioral and psychiatric disorders. Because of high cost, however, the indications for obtaining such scans have been controversial. Several behavioral presentations should generally prompt a neuroimaging scan, including acute confusional state or dementia of unknown cause, the initial episode of undiagnosed psychosis, and the first presentation of personality change after age 40. Other indications include focal neurologic findings, movement disorders, incontinence, or evidence of increased intracranial pressure such as headache, nausea, vomiting, and papilledema on funduscopic examination.

BIBLIOGRAPHY

1. Cummings JL: Organic delusions: Phenomenology, anatomical considerations, and review. Br J Psychiatry 146:184–197, 1985.
2. Cummings JL: Psychosis in neurologic disease: Neurobiology and pathogenesis. Neuropsychiatry Neuropsychol Behav Neurol 5:144–150, 1992.
3. Cummings JL, Miller BL: Visual hallucinations: Clinical occurrence and use in differential diagnosis. West J Med 146:46–51, 1987.
4. Gorman DG, Cummings JL: Organic delusional syndrome. Semin Neurol 10:229–238, 1990.
5. Gould R, Miller BL, Goldberg MA, Benson DF: The validity of hysterical signs and symptoms, J Nerv Ment Dis 174:593–597, 1986.
6. Larson EW: Organic causes of mania. Mayo Clin Proc 63:906–912, 1988.
7. Mackenzie TB, Popkin MK: Organic anxiety syndrome. Am J Psychiatry 140:342–344, 1983.
8. Skuster DZ, Digre KB, Corbett JJ: Neurologic conditions presenting as psychiatric disorders. Psychiatr Clin North Am 15:311–333, 1992.
9. Strub RL: Mental disorders in brain disease. In Frederiks JA (ed): Handbook of Clinical Neurology, vol 2. Amsterdam, Elsevier, 1985, pp 413–441.
10. Taylor D, Lewis S: Delirium. J Neurol Neurosurg Psychiatry 56:742–751, 1993.
11. Weinberger DR: Brain disease and psychiatric illness: When should a psychiatrist order a CAT scan? Am J Psychiatry 141:1521–1527, 1984.
12. Winokur G, Clayton P (eds): The Medical Basis of Psychiatry, 2nd ed. Philadelphia, W.B. Saunders, 1994.
13. Yudofsky SC, Hales RE (eds): Neuropsychiatry, 2nd ed. Washington, DC, American Psychiatric Press, 1992.

34. DEMENTIA

Roberta M. Richardson, M.D.

1. Define dementia.

Dementia is an impairment in intellectual functioning in at least two spheres. One of the spheres is memory; the second may be any other area of cognition.

Cognitive Functions that May Be Impaired in Dementia

Language	Ability to dress and do other
Visuospatial ability	semiautomatic tasks
Personality	Abstraction
Judgment	Calculation
Object recognition	Information synthesis
	Problem solving

In contrast to delirium, the deficits of dementia are relatively stable over at least a few months. In contrast to mental retardation, the deficits are acquired. Memory disturbance is an early feature. It may be evidenced by inability to learn new material or loss of ability to recall previously learned material.

The degree of interference in the patient's life should be taken into account, as should education and intelligence. For example, a highly educated man may "pass" a screening test but still have significant impairment in his usual complex occupation. Alternatively, a retired manual laborer may show some deficits on exam but have no problems in his daily life. Third-party informants are helpful. People who know the patient best can report changes in functioning from a previous level as well as notice signs or symptoms of which the patient is unaware. More extensive, formal neuropsychological testing may be helpful if the diagnosis is in doubt.

2. Why is dementia an increasingly important problem?

The population of the U.S. is aging. It is estimated that by the year 2010 about 15% of Americans will be 65 or older, and 25% will be 55 or older. Currently the fastest growing segment of the population is people over the age of 85. The incidence of dementia rises steadily with age. About 5% of people over 65 have severe dementia, and another 10–15% show mild-to-moderate symptoms. Of people over 80, one-fourth have severe dementia. Dementia is presently the fourth leading cause of death in the U.S. Death occurs because so much of the nervous system has failed that the entire body is profoundly affected. Such patients are mute, unable to eat, incontinent, and immobile. The immediate cause of death may be pneumonia, dehydration, malnutrition, or sepsis.

3. What are the causes of dementia?

Alzheimer's disease is the most common cause of dementia, accounting for about 50% of cases. Multiinfarct dementia accounts for about 25%, and the remaining 25% are caused by a wide variety of other conditions or agents.

Causes of Dementia

Cortical dementias	Normal pressure hydrocephalus
Alzheimer's disease	Dementia syndrome of depression
Pick's disease (frontal lobe degeneration)	
Vascular dementias	Chronic confusional states
Multiinfarct dementia	Infections
Lacunar state	Toxic-metabolic encephalopathies
Binswanger's disease	Trauma
	Neoplasms
Movement disorders	Demyelinating diseases
Parkinson's disease	
Huntington's disease	
Wilson's disease	
Progressive supranuclear palsy	
Spinocerebellar degeneration	

4. What are the differences between cortical and subcortical dementias?

Subcortical dementias are caused by disorders that affect mainly the basal ganglia, thalamus, and brainstem. Clinical characteristics contrast with those of the cortical dementias, which, as the name implies, affect mainly the cerebral cortex. Recognizing this distinction assists in differential diagnosis. Movement disorders exemplify the subcortical dementias. In addition to effects on the motor system, cognition and comprehension are slowed. The ability to synthesize and manipulate information for problem solving and decision making is impaired. Memory deficits are characterized by retrieval deficits. Clinically, patients with subcortical dementias may be helped by clues, structure, and prompting. Information registers, but it is difficult to retrieve from storage. Such strategies do not help patients with Alzheimer's disease, because the information was not learned.

Cortical dementias are characterized by language disturbances, agnosia and apraxia, visuospatial deficits, and impairment of judgment, abstraction, and calculation. Memory deficits are characterized by problems with registering new information and, as the dementia progresses, with remote recall. For example, the patient with Alzheimer's disease has great difficulty recalling the three objects commonly requested during mental status screening. Clues do not help. The patient may not even remember that three objects were mentioned, because the information was not registered in the memory. In the later stages, things that were previously learned are forgotten. The neurologic exam shows no abnormalities in motor function, gait, reflexes, or posture. Alzheimer's disease is the prototypic cortical dementia.

Many dementias have features of both cortical and subcortical type. Multiinfarct dementia is the most common example.

5. What conditions are commonly mistaken for dementia?

Normal aging is associated with some alterations in mental functioning. Benign senescent forgetfulness refers to alterations in memory function with age; it is characterized by decreased retrieval of learned information rather than inability to learn. Word-finding difficulties, especially proper names, are common in the elderly. If cognitive decline does not interfere with social or occupational functioning, it is not considered to indicate dementia.

Delirium is an acute or subacute decline in mental functioning associated with a specific organic cause. Because patients with dementia are predisposed to delirium, the two conditions may be superimposed. Delirium is temporary and should remit when the underlying organic cause is treated.

Focal brain syndromes, such as isolated amnesias or aphasias, may be mistakenly diagnosed as dementia. Dementia, however, involves disturbances of memory and at least one other area of cognition. The careful clinician is not fooled by the aphasic patient who at first glance seems to have memory deficits. Nor does the careful clinician assume that an amnestic patient has dementia. All areas of cognition must be considered and tested.

Major depression may cause reversible dementia, especially in the elderly. It may also cause symptoms that may be misdiagnosed as dementia: apathy, withdrawal, decrease in attention to personal grooming, personality changes, and loss of interest in activities. Such symptoms are prominent features of major depression as well as common symptoms of senile dementia. Because major depression may cause memory loss and actual decrease in cognitive abilities, it is considered a reversible cause of dementia. Careful attention to full mental status testing, including subtleties of mood and thought, is essential for proper diagnosis and treatment. Like delirium, depression also may coexist with dementia.

6. How is delirium distinguished from dementia?

It is important to distinguish delirium from dementia, but the distinction is especially difficult when delirium overlies preexisting dementia. The main distinguishing feature is **level of attention**, which is impaired in patients with delirium. When interviewed patients answer a question asked of the person in the next bed rather than the question just posed to them, impairment of attention is suggested.

An easy and accurate bedside test of attention is the so-called A test. The examiner recites a series of random letters at a steady rate of about one per second and asks the patient to indicate by a gesture every time he or she hears the letter A. The examiner should sometimes say the letter A two or three times in a row and also allow a long list of letters to pass by without an A. The patient should be able to perform this task for about a minute without error. Errors indicating impairment of attention include omissions, gesturing for the wrong letter, and perseverating after a series of As.

Other features that suggest delirium rather than dementia include:

- **Acute or subacute onset**. Family and friends of the demented patient will have noticed problems for at least a few months.
- **Fluctuating course**. The delirious patient may be confused one hour, clear the next, and confused again a few hours later.
- **Clouding of consciousness**. The delirious patient may not be fully alert or aware of surroundings.
- **Florid hallucinations**, most often visual or tactile.
- **Illusions**, or misrepresentations of sensory stimuli, such as believing that the coat rack is a person or the stethoscope a snake.

7. How are depression and dementia related?

Both depression and dementia are common in the elderly. They may coexist, either in a causative manner or coincidentally, and at times they are difficult to distinguish.

Depressive pseudodementia describes what once were thought to be apparent but not real cognitive deficits associated with severe major depression. More recent research indicates that major depression is a cause of reversible dementia; that is, major depression may cause true cognitive deficits that resolve with successful treatment of depression. The term **depressive pseudodementia** should be replaced by the more precise term, **dementia syndrome of depression**.

If the clinician is uncertain whether major depression is a part of a presentation that includes dementia, it is best to treat depression empirically, not only for the emotional well-being of the patient, but also because cognition may improve. The classic clue to the diagnosis of dementia syndrome of depression is the occurrence of many "I don't know" answers. Patients with pure dementia are likely to try their best or even to invent answers when memory is poor. But severely depressed patients have a motivational deficit and negative attitude. They may even emphasize and complain about thinking problems in a catastrophic way, whereas patients with Alzheimer's disease are often poorly aware or in denial of cognitive difficulties. Rapid decline in functioning, inconsistency in the mental status exam, pervasively dysphoric mood, and suicidal ideation or expressions of a wish to die are other important clues to major depression.

8. Describe the elements of the work-up for dementia.

There is no definitive work-up for dementia. The astute clinician takes a careful history, completes a careful examination, and orders further tests as indicated in each case. However, certain chronic confusional states are difficult or impossible to rule out by history and physical exam but common enough to warrant routine laboratory investigation. Others should be considered if the history, physical exam, or preliminary blood tests are suggestive.

Laboratory Tests for Work-up of Dementia

Routine	Supplementary
Complete blood count	Serum antibody for human immunodeficiency virus (HIV)
Syphilis serology	Electroencephalogram
Chemistry panel	Computed tomography scan of head
Thyroid functions tests	Magnetic resonance imaging of head
Vitamin B_{12} and folate	Heavy metals screen
Sedimentation rate	Lumbar puncture
Urinalysis	Antinuclear antibody test
	Pulse oximetry
	Serum amylase

9. Describe the most common cause of nontraumatic dementia in young people.

HIV encephalopathy, also known as AIDS dementia complex (ADC), was first described in detail in 1986. Nearly all patients with AIDS develop HIV encephalopathy at some time during the course of the disease. In 20% of HIV-infected people, changes in mental status precede immunologic abnormalities, and in another 10% changes in mental status and immunologic abnormalities are recognized simultaneously. All persons with changes in mental status should be questioned about risk factors for HIV exposure; if any are present, serum testing should be performed.

HIV encephalopathy is the most common but by no means the only neurologic manifestation of HIV infection. Although a wide variety of infectious and neoplastic brain diseases may occur, the dementia syndrome progresses in a fairly predictable fashion. Forgetfulness, poor concentration, and slowing of thought are early symptoms. Apathy and social withdrawal often appear early and become progressively severe. Psychomotor retardation occurs. Memory impairment and disturbances of higher cortical functioning become apparent as the disease progresses. Delusions, hallucinations, and agitation may occur. The terminal state is usually characterized by "quiet confusion."

10. Name the two behaviors of patients with dementia that most commonly lead to nursing home placement.

The two behaviors of demented individuals most commonly leading to nursing home placement are insomnia and aggression. Caregivers often feel helpless to deal with these problems, which are distressingly frequent and extremely difficult to tolerate.

11. Discuss the management of insomnia in patients with dementia.

Normal sleep patterns are disrupted in many patients with dementia. In addition to actual brain changes that can be demonstrated in sleep EEGs, changes in behavior and lifestyle may cause the demented patient to be awake and active at night. For example, disinterest and inability to participate in usual activities may lead to excessive napping during the day. Decreased sensory stimulation at night may foster hallucinations or confusion. Inability to recall structure and social norms may encourage arousal and activity at night.

Increasing structure and activity during the day should be the first approach to insomnia. Senior centers and day programs for patients with dementia are excellent resources. Exercise, especially in the late afternoon, encourages appropriate desire for rest at night. Routine bedtime and rising, with structure and ritual as cues, also may be helpful. The caretaker should react calmly if the person arises at night. Often guiding to the bathroom or giving a drink of water or milk, then leading back to bed allow a return to sleep.

If such approaches are not enough, medication may be considered. Sedatives-hypnotics should be used sparingly in patients with dementia, because they may further impair memory, cause paradoxical excitement, and interfere with balance, leading to falls. Anticholinergic medications, such as Benadryl, also may increase confusion. The sedating tricyclic antidepressants and antipsychotics are also highly anticholinergic and may cause significant orthostatic hypotension, increasing the risk of falls as well as cardiovascular complications. Sometimes a low dose of trazodone is effective. Trazodone is not sedating for all individuals but may be effective without the hazards of more traditional sleeping medications. A dose as low as 25 mg may be sufficient.

12. How should aggression be approached in patients with dementia?
Aggression is a disturbing problem for caregivers and frequently brings the patient to the attention of a physician. The first response that comes to mind for many doctors and caregivers is sedating medication. However, medications involve significant risks and are usually only partially effective. It is best to attempt behavioral approaches first.

Caregivers should be instructed to note the circumstances that commonly precede outbursts of aggression. Usually, there is a period of increasing agitation in response to something that the patient has difficulty in understanding or handling. Often the responses of caregivers increase rather than resolve the agitation. For example, caregivers may argue, raise their voice, or use physical force to make patients do something that they are resisting. It is much more effective to stop immediately whatever is happening when the patient begins to show warning signs of aggression and to initiate more soothing and relaxing activity. If possible, the patient's underlying concern should be addressed. For example, if the patient is accusing someone of stealing, help the patient to find what has been lost. The Alzheimer's Association, a national organization with chapters in many cities, is an invaluable asset for educating caregivers in how to deal with these and other difficult behaviors associated with dementia. *The 36-hour Day*, by Nancy Mace and Peter Rabins, is an excellent reference to recommend to caregivers.

13. If pharmacologic treatment of aggression becomes necessary, how should it be managed?
The first step is to consider carefully the cause. If delusions or hallucinations are present, the **antipsychotics** are the treatment of choice. High-potency agents, such as haloperidol and thiothixene, are preferred, because the anticholinergic and orthostatic properties of low-potency agents such as chlorpromazine and thioridazine outweigh any advantage in sedation. Very low doses may be effective. It is important to watch for significant extrapyramidal side effects, particularly parkinsonism, over time. Such symptoms may emerge after weeks of continuous use. If Parkinson's disease is present, the antipsychotics must be avoided.

Propranolol may be useful in the management of chronic organic aggression. Careful consideration must be given to the patient's medical condition. This approach is contraindicated in patients with asthma, insulin-dependent diabetes mellitus, congestive heart failure, angina, hyperthyroidism, and clinically significant peripheral vascular disease. Latency of onset of action is 4–8 weeks. Yudofsky et al.[10] published specific guidelines for exact dosing. Dosages in the range of 400–800 mg/day may be required and must be titrated upward gradually, with careful monitoring of the patient.

Buspirone and trazodone have been reported to be helpful in managing chronic organic aggression. Their benefits may derive from effects on serotinergic brain systems. Latency of onset of action of buspirone is usually 4–8 weeks. Dosages should be increased to 30–60 mg as tolerated. Trazodone may be effective at the higher dosage range of 150–300 mg/day. The patient must be monitored for orthostatic hypotension.

Benzodiazepines may be used carefully, in small doses, to treat aggression. Lorazepam or oxazepam is preferred; both are metabolized at the same rate in the old as in the young and therefore do not accumulate in the aging body. Caution is necessary because more than the smallest doses often cause postural instability and falls. If aggression is chronic, one of the medications discussed above should be instituted and an attempt made to taper the benzodiazepine after the latency period passes.

BIBLIOGRAPHY

1. Cummings JL, Benson DF: Dementia: A Clinical Approach, 2nd ed. Boston, Butterworth-Heinemann, 1992.
2. Eberling JL, Jagust WJ: Neuroimaging and the diagnosis of dementia. Psychiatr Ann 24:178–185, 1994.
3. Horowitz GR: What is a complete work-up for dementia? Clin Geriatr Med 4:163–180, 1988.
4. Kim E, Rovner BW: Depression in dementia. Psychiatr Ann 24:173–177, 1994.
5. Mace NL, Rabins PV: The 36-Hour Day, rev. ed. Baltimore, Johns Hopkins University Press, 1991.
6. Mortimer JA: The dementia of Parkinson's disease. Clin Geriatr Med 4:785–797, 1988.
7. Moss RJ, Miles SH: AIDS dementia. Clin Geriatr Med 4:889–895, 1988.
8. Strub RL, Black FW: Neurobehavioral Disorders: A Clinical Approach. Philadelphia, F.A. Davis, 1988, p 58.
9. Warheit GJ, Longino CF, Bradsher JE: Sociocultural aspects. In Sadavoy J, Lazarus LW, Jarvik LF (eds): Comprehensive Review of Geriatric Psychiatry. Washington, DC, American Psychiatric Press, 1991, pp 100–116.
10. Yudofsky SC, Silver JM, Hales RE: Pharmacologic management of aggression in the elderly. J Clin Psychiatry 51(Suppl 10):22–28, 1990.

35. DELIRIUM

Joyce S. Kobayashi, M.D.

1. Why should the psychiatrist be concerned about the recognition of delirium or delirious states?

Delirious patients may present with various psychiatric symptoms and are often referred to a psychiatrist for evaluation. Misdiagnosis results in delay of appropriate medical intervention. Delirium may be the initial presentation of a number of medical conditions; it is common among medically ill populations that psychiatrists are asked to assess, and the cause of delirium is often iatrogenic.

Delirium, therefore, should be considered in the differential diagnosis of any change of mental status and should be ruled out in any initial assessment, particularly in the emergency room. Psychiatrists who readily diagnose intoxication and withdrawal states from alcohol and other substances or confusional states from the side effects of psychotropic medications such as anticholinergics may not be as familiar with the specific manifestations of toxicity from other medications or are not likely to monitor routinely for other common causes of delirium, such as fluid and electrolyte imbalance. They should be able to diagnose delirium solely on the basis of the acute presentation and to refer appropriately or to initiate a diagnostic work-up. Among medically ill, geriatric or substance-abusing patients, the possibility of a delirium acutely superimposed upon a more chronic psychiatric disorder, should be carefully considered.

2. What are the common clinical symptoms and findings in the initial presentation of delirious patients?

1. Intermittent disorientation to time or place (fluctuating course)
2. Easy distraction by irrelevant stimuli during interview (reduced ability to focus or shift attention)
3. Mumbling or muttering (dysarthric speech)
4. Hyper- or hypoactivity (agitation or hypersomnolence)
5. Worsening over the course of the day (i.e., "sundowning," in which the patient is consistently more confused in the early evening than morning hours)
6. Mistaken perceptions (illusions) such as thinking that a loud sound is gunfire or believing a spot on the wall is a spider
7. Inability to remember activities of the previous day (memory deficit)
8. Transient difficulties in word-finding, or disorganized speech (language disturbance)

Careful clinical observation assists in the differentiation of these common symptoms from psychiatric symptoms of other disorders. For example, illusions are generally a misperception or misinterpretation of some real object of sensation, whereas hallucinations are devoid of reality or without a reality-based stimulus. In a manic flight of ideas, it is often possible to find a cognitive (or affective) thread connecting the sequence of topics spewed out by the acutely manic patient, whereas in the delirious patient's meanderings a change of topic may be secondary only to a sudden change in the direction of gaze and new focus of attention or be altogether unrelated to the previous thought. This is often accompanied by the clinical feeling that the patient no longer has a sense of connection to, or even memory of, the previous topic. Dysarthric speech, which is mispronounced or poorly articulated, may be differentiated from the neologisms (newly created words) or idiosyncratic speech (new meanings or usage) of the schizophrenic patient, who rarely has trouble with actual pronunciation. Intermittent word-finding difficulties may be easily differentiated from the profound and consistent inability to express oneself verbally that is observed in a patient with expressive aphasia. Mood disorders are similarly profound and consistent over time; they do not fluctuate acutely and intermittently or manifest the emotional lability of the delirious patient, who may cry and laugh and cry again in short sequences unrelated to external stimuli.

When symptoms such as paranoid delusions are manifested in delirium, they are indistinguishable from other major psychiatric disorders, making the identification of associated characteristic symptoms (see list) critical in the differential diagnosis. Serial mental status exams also may be useful in such cases, particularly in identifying the cardinal difference between symptoms that fluctuate and symptoms that remain stable over time. Finally, as discussed in question 8, systematic consideration of risk factors, history, acuity of onset, course, and probable causes readily assists the psychiatrist in differentiating delirium from other psychiatric disorders.

In addition to toxicologic or other laboratory findings related to the specific cause of delirium, patients frequently have an abnormal electroencephalogram, with either diffuse slowing (which also may be present at therapeutic levels of benzodiazepines, narcotics, or neuroleptics) or low-voltage fast activity (delirium tremens).

3. What are the formal criteria for diagnosing delirium?

There are four primary elements in the diagnosis of a delirium: time course, disturbance of consciousness, change of cognition, and evidence of medical cause. Change in mental status usually occurs over a period of hours to days, and tends to fluctuate during the day. Disturbance in consciousness (i.e., reduced clarity of awareness of the environment) is probably the core dysfunction and results in reduced ability to focus, sustain, or shift attention. Changes in cognition (e.g., memory deficit, disorientation, language disturbance) or perceptual disturbance should not be attributable solely to dementia, and the history, physical examination, or laboratory findings should provide evidence that symptoms are caused by the direct physiologic consequences of a general medical condition.

Presumptive causes are among the changes in the DSM-IV categorization of delirium. Substance-induced delirium, for example, includes intoxication and withdrawal syndromes from substances of abuse as well as medication toxicity.

4. What premorbid clinical and historical factors should be considered in a patient with delirium?

Dementia, head injury, mental retardation, or other neurologic disorders may predispose a patient to delirium of any etiology. Other risk factors include:

1. Age over 65 years, with or without prior psychiatric history
2. History of significant substance abuse
3. Advanced medical illness or organ failure
4. Easy susceptibility to infection
5. Transient vulnerability due to other specific medical circumstances (e.g., postsurgical patients, patients with major changes in fluid or electrolytes)

A good history is necessary to determine exposure to medications, substances, or toxins, and both intoxication and withdrawal syndromes should always be considered. It is also important to determine the premorbid level of function, psychiatric history, and timing of onset in relation to the presumed cause. The history usually must be obtained from knowledgeable family members, close friends, nursing home staff, or housekeepers in addition to medical records of prior functioning, and possible precipitants.

5. What medications may cause delirium?

Although any centrally active medication has the potential for toxicity in high-risk patients, or at high levels in most patients, a number of the most common offenders should be kept in mind. Such agents may cause delirium in either therapeutic or toxic levels, depending on the premorbid susceptibility of the patient, and also may be associated with withdrawal syndromes. Medications that are not toxic in oral forms may cause a delirium when administered intravenously.

Common Pharmacologic Causes of Delirium

Narcotics	Beta blockers
Barbiturates	Cimetidine
Benzodiazepines	Clonidine
Anticholinergics	Digitalis
Medications with anticholinergic side effects	Pressors (lidocaine)
(e.g., amitriptyline, thioridazine, some anti-	Theophylline derivatives
histamines)	Bromides
Steroids	Antibiotics (cephalosporins, aminoglycosides)
Sympathomimetics	(less common)
Anticonvulsants	Antifungals (amphotericin B) (less common)
Antihypertensives	Over-the-counter agents (e.g., antitussives and
Antiarrhythmics	sedatives)
Antidepressants	
Antineoplastics (e.g., 5-fluorouracil)	

6. What common medical disorders may be associated with delirium?

In addition to medications, substances, and toxins (e.g., heavy metals), delirium may be caused by infection, hypoxia or hypoglycemia, metabolic or fluid and electrolyte disturbance, trauma, vitamin deficiencies, endocrinopathies, cerebrovascular events (strokes, hemorrhage), seizures, and other CNS pathology (e.g., tumors, infections or abscesses, cerebritis, acute hypertensive crisis, hydrocephalus). Finally, a summation effect may occur in which subclinical factors may combine to cause delirium, particularly in predisposed patients. For example, such factors as sleep deprivation, dehydration, anemia, or stress may precipitate delirium in conjunction with a clinical condition such as a low-grade infection in an elderly patient.

7. What is the differential diagnosis of delirium in psychiatric patients?

Substance intoxication or substance withdrawal are differentiated from substance intoxication delirium and substance withdrawal delirium "if the symptoms of the delirium are in excess of those usually associated with the intoxication or withdrawal syndrome and are sufficiently severe to warrant independent clinical attention" (DSM-IV). If hallucinations and/or delusions are present, all psychotic disorders should be considered: brief psychotic disorder, schizophrenia, schizophreniform disorder, and mood disorders with psychotic features. In older or predisposed individuals an important differential is whether dementia is either underlying or confounding the diagnosis.

8. How can the psychiatrist readily differentiate delirium from psychotic disorders?

In general, systematic consideration of risk factors, history, acuity of onset, course, associated symptoms, and probable causes helps the psychiatrist to differentiate delirium from other major psychiatric disorders. Serial mental status exams may be extremely useful, particularly in identifying a fluctuating course. As mentioned in question 2, careful clinical observation assists in the differentiation of illusions from hallucinations, cognitive distractibility from manic flight of ideas, dysarthric from idiosyncratic speech, word-finding difficulties from expressive aphasias, and emotional lability from mood disorder.

In **schizophrenia**, age of onset is rarely after the fifth decade, speech usually is not dysarthric or muttering, auditory hallucinations are more common than visual hallucinations, disorientation is uncommon, and memory may be fairly normal. Symptoms generally do not worsen at the end of the day as they often do with the delirious patient. It has also been observed that schizophrenic individuals misinterpret the familiar as unfamiliar (for example, believing that someone else has inhabited the body of a family member, as in Capgras syndrome), whereas the delirious patient more commonly misinterprets the unfamiliar as familiar (mistaking an unknown nurse for a relative). The positive psychotic symptoms observed in schizophrenia usually occur in the context of a more gradually deteriorating ability to function and are frequently associated with a more extensive course of deficit symptoms, such as marked social isolation or withdrawal, peculiar or bizarre behavior, marked impairment in personal hygiene, blunted or inappropriate affect, poverty of speech or speech content, or marked lack of initiative. The onset of delirium usually is rapid, over the course of hours or days.

Mood disorders with psychotic symptoms may be differentiated from delirium because emotional lability is more common in delirium than a persistently disordered mood (see question 10). The depression of hypothyroidism, for example, is diagnosed in DSM–IV as a mood disorder due to a general medical condition rather than as chronic delirium or reversible dementia. A manic flight of ideas is often distinguishable from simple cognitive distractibility, and, except in the most acute states, disorientation in mood disorders is unusual. Cognitive performance in specific areas, such as serial calculation, timed tasks, abstraction, and memory, may be improved in manic states. Mood congruent psychotic features are relatively rare in delirium.

A **brief reactive psychosis** should be differentiated from delirium by the relationship in time to an acute major emotional precipitant and lack of disorientation and memory disturbance. Symptoms may or may not fluctuate over time, particularly if complicated by acute grief.

Although many patients with **dementia** experience paranoid delusions or hallucinations, they usually demonstrate some decline over time in higher cortical functions, such as abstract reasoning, judgment, language, or personality, before manifesting frank psychotic symptoms. Such patients rarely have muttering, mumbling, or dysarthric speech until late in the course of illness and generally do not fluctuate as significantly or frequently in level of function or as suddenly in level of activity as delirious patients. Overlapping symptoms may include distractibility, memory disturbance and disorientation, confabulation, word-finding difficulties, and emotional lability. The possibility of superimposed delirium in demented patients should be reviewed routinely and considered specifically with acute change in presentation, given the predisposition of demented patients to delirium. "Secondary dementias" also should be considered, because they may present with mild cognitive dysfunction and prominent psychotic symptoms. Examples include porphyria, Huntington's chorea, endocrinopathies, nutritional deficiencies, temporal lobe epilepsy, and heavy metal toxicity (see questions 5 and 6).

9. In which medical conditions may mood disturbance—instead of or in conjunction with cognitive dysfunction—be a prominent manifestation of delirium?
Steroid toxicity, hypocalcemia and hypercalcemia, exacerbations of thyroid disease and tertiary syphilis may result in prominent disturbance of mood.

10. How do the terms toxic psychosis, ICU psychosis, acute confusional state, organic psychosis, and organic mental syndrome relate to the formal diagnosis of delirium?
Delirium should replace all of these historic terms, which reflect the presumed causes of the delirium. As mentioned, numerous medications, substances, and other toxins may cause delirium. Theories about the causes of delirium in the intensive care unit (ICU) include sensory deprivation, sensory overload, and sleep deprivation as well as all of the medical causes of delirium to which ill patients may be susceptible. Psychoses caused by identifiable biologic factors were historically termed "organic" to differentiate them from the "functional" psychoses such as schizophrenia, but this distinction is no longer useful and no longer used in DSM-IV. Although the term "organic" may be useful as a descriptive term referring to the spectrum of possible causes (physiologic, metabolic, and structural), the general terms organic mental syndrome and organic brain syndrome should be discarded for a specific diagnosis of delirium or dementia.

11. What are useful behavioral, environmental, and pharmacologic approaches to treatment of delirious patients?
The first step in taking care of delirious patients is to address the underlying disorder. This may not be so obvious, however, when there is more than one cause, when a number of additional factors complicate delirium, or when delirium persists for a period of time or becomes a more chronic state. In such cases, additional interventions to make the patient more comfortable should be initiated whenever it is clear that delirium will not be rapidly reversed. Such interventions

orient the patient, structure activities, and make the environment feel more familiar. Examples include (1) introducing anyone who enters the patient's room and reminding the patient of the date and purpose of the visit; (2) maintaining a regular daily schedule without abrupt changes in location; (3) keeping a diary, appointment book, or calendar visible in the room; (4) having a nightlight, clock, and familiar objects nearby; (5) asking friends or relatives to accompany or visit the patient frequently; (6) keeping information and discussions simple and brief; and (7) writing down specific instructions about medications or activities.

The most useful pharmacologic agents for delirious patients, besides those that may reverse the underlying disorder, are low-dose neuroleptic medications. High-potency antipsychotic medication in divided doses, such as haloperidol (0.5–2.0 mg/day) or trifluoperazine (1.0–4.0 mg/day), may have a remarkable effect on agitation, behavioral dyscontrol, and confusion without significant orthostatic hypotension, whereas medications of lower potency, such as perphenazine (2.0–8.0 mg/day), thiothixene (2.0–10.0 mg/day), or loxapine (5.0–10.0 mg/day), may be substituted in patients with extrapyramidal side effects, rather than treating the side effects with anticholinergics or using thioridazine. Risperidone (0.5–1.5 mg/day) may also be tried Benzodiazepines such as lorazepam (1.0–6.0 mg/day), alone or in combination with antipsychotic medication, may be useful acutely in managing significant physical agitation but risk further confusion. Anticonvulsants at low doses and methylphenidate at titrated doses may be useful in chronic or intermittent delirious states such as in medically ill patients with dementia.

12. What psychotherapeutic issues should be considered in delirious patients?
As with any patient, the clinician must be aware of specific countertransference to delirious patients, who may range from passive and unresponsive to agitated and alarming. It is also helpful (but often not done) for a clinician to process the experience of the delirious episode with the patient for four reasons:

1. Delirious states, known to the Greeks as the "waking dream," often produce material that may be helpful for a patient to understand with a clearer consciousness at a later time.

2. It helps to allay patients' fears, which otherwise may remain unaddressed, that they are going crazy or will lose their minds.

3. The experience may be followed by posttraumatic sequelae, and patient education as well as support and monitoring may be useful, particularly if the causes is iatrogenic.

4. If factors predispose to another episode of delirium, intervention or patient education may be appropriate as soon as the initial episode has resolved.

BIBLIOGRAPHY

1. Lipowski ZJ: Delirium. Springfield, IL, Charles C Thomas, 1980.
2. Lipowski ZJ: Update on delirium. Psychiatr Clin North Am 15:335–346, 1992.
3. Wise MJ: Delirium. In Hales RE, Yudofsky SC (eds): Textbook of Neuropsychiatry, 2nd ed. Washington, DC, American Psychiatric Press, 1992.
4. Westreich L, Bialer PA: Delirium and acute psychosis. Mental states calling for clear diagnostic thinking and careful management. Postgrad Med 92:319–320, 326–328, 332, 1993.
5. Popkin MK, Tucker GJ: Secondary and drug-induced mood, anxiety, psychotic, catatonic, and personality disorders: A review of the literature. J Neuropsychiatry Clin Neurosci 4:369–385, 1992.
6. Pompei P, Foreman M, Rudberg MA, et al: Delirium in hospitalized older persons: Outcomes and predictors. J Am Geriatr Soc 42:809–815, 1994.
7. Marcantonio ER, Juarez G, Goldman L, et al: The relationship of postoperative delirium with psychoactive medications. JAMA 272:1518–1522, 1994.
8. Mcartney JR, Boland RJ: Anxiety and delirium in the intensive care unit. Crit Care Clin 10:673–680, 1994.
9. Crippen DW: Pharmacologic treatment of brain failure and delirium. Crit Care Clin 10:733–766, 1994.
10. Inouye SK, Viscoli CM, Horwitz RI, et al; A predictive model for delirium in hospitalized elderly medical patients based on admission characteristics. Ann Intern Med 119:474–481, 1993.
11. Inouye SK: The dilemma of delirium: Clinical and research controversies regarding diagnosis and evaluation of delirium in hospitalized elderly medical patients. Am J Med 97:278–288, 1994.
12. Stoudemire A, Fogel BS (eds): Principles of Medical Psychiatry. New York, Grune & Stratton, 1987.
13. Diagnostic and Statistical Manual of Mental Disorders, 4th ed. Washington, DC, American Psychiatric Association, 1994.

36. ORGANIC PSYCHOSIS

C. Munro Cullum, Ph.D.

1. What are "organic" psychoses?

Psychosis is an impairment of reality testing as evidenced by any of a number of abnormal symptoms outlined in DSM–IV. Organic psychosis refers to the development of psychotic symptoms secondary to neurologic disease or dysfunction. Whereas the organic vs. nonorganic distinction serves a useful purpose in some situations, it often becomes blurred, particularly as researchers discover the organic or neurobiologic underpinnings for more psychiatric syndromes. For example, it may not be appropriate to classify the spectrum of schizophrenic disorders as "functional" or "nonorganic" in view of the plethora of data indicating various functional and structural CNS abnormalities in such patients. In the acute phase, schizophrenia may be indistinguishable from psychosis secondary to neurologic disease (see question 3).

2. What are some of the more common symptoms of psychosis?

- Hallucinations (most commonly visual or auditory)
- Delusions (e.g., paranoid, bizarre, grandiose, somatic)
- Aberrant or bizarre, disorganized thinking
- Bizarre, disorganized behavior
- Loosening of associations
- Incoherent and/or neologistic speech
- Inappropriate or flat affect

As is the case with most other aspects of medical diagnosis, such symptoms are not diagnostic of a particular condition but rather indicative of an underlying abnormal process. The development of psychotic behavior de novo in a previously normal patient clearly requires prompt attention, because it may be related to any of numerous neuromedical factors. Metabolic, medication, and illicit drug effects must be considered early in the diagnostic process so that appropriate (and possibly life-saving) interventions can be instituted.

3. Give the differential diagnosis of organic and nonorganic psychosis.

Despite many similarities, some psychotic symptoms associated with neurologic disease tend to show qualitative differences compared with symptoms of primary psychiatric disorders. The examples in the table below serve as general observations and guidelines; many exceptions exist.

Common Qualitative Features of Selected Psychotic Symptoms in Psychiatric and Neurologic Disease

SYMPTOM	PSYCHIATRIC DISORDER	NEUROLOGIC DISORDER
Delusions	Typically fixed, with more stable themes and elaborate contents	Tend to be more transient and less systematized
Hallucinations		
Auditory	Prominent in psychiatric disorders, especially schizophrenia	Less common in neurologic disorders
	Often developed and related to themes and other symptoms	Often ill-developed
Visual	Somewhat less common; typically consistent and related to delusional themes	Common in delirium; often less defined and variable

Table continued on following page.

Common Qualitative Features of Selected Psychotic Symptoms in Psychiatric and Neurologic Disease (Cont.)

SYMPTOM	PSYCHIATRIC DISORDER	NEUROLOGIC DISORDER
Hallucinations *(cont.)*		
Tactile	Uncommon	More common, especially in delirium
Olfactory	Uncommon	More common in delirium or temporal lobe disorders
Incoherent or neologistic speech	Meanings of neologisms tend to be consistent and context-specific	"Word salad" more generalized and inconsistent; characteristic aphasic symptoms per syndrome
Bizarre behavior	May be related to delusional themes and may tend to be stereotyped	Often less organized or purposeful

As with any symptom or set of symptoms, a critical diagnostic point is to examine the history: initial onset, frequency, changes over time, and context in which they occur. Psychotic symptoms in a person with a history of psychiatric hospitalizations and diagnosis of schizophrenia present a different clinical picture from the case of the business executive with an unremarkable neuromedical/psychiatric history who suddenly begins to believe that he or she is being followed by the FBI and plotted against by family members. Information about premorbid personality and behavioral characteristics can be quite useful in the differential diagnosis. Nonorganic psychotic symptoms are more common in people with poorer social and vocational adjustment.

Regardless of previous history, a thorough medical work-up is indicated in any patient with new psychotic symptoms. Patients with schizophrenia may develop neurologic disease and should not be subjected to clinical bias. The qualitative nature of psychotic symptoms can be useful in differentiating primary psychiatric from neurologic disorders, as outlined below.

4. What is the frequency of psychotic symptoms in neurologic disorders?
Psychotic symptoms may arise in association with a host of disorders affecting the CNS. Acute metabolic disturbances or drug effects are common causes, although given the overlap between some psychiatric and neurological symptoms, it is not surprising that many neurologic conditions result in at least transient psychotic symptoms.

Neurologic Conditions Sometimes Associated with Psychotic Symptoms

Epilepsy	Delirium
Head injury	Confusional state
Dementia	Systemic lupus erythematosus
Alzheimer's disease	Metabolic disturbances
Parkinson's disease	Hydrocephalus
Huntington's disease	Korsakoff's syndrome
Alcoholic dementia	Intracranial hematoma
Pick's disease	Encephalitis and meningitis
Other dementias (e.g., AIDS)	Alcohol intoxication
Stroke	Acute or chronic substance abuse
Brain tumor, abscess	Acute fever or infection

The above categories obviously represent only a subset of neuromedical illnesses in which psychotic symptoms have been reported. Specific estimates of the frequency of psychotic symptoms or full-blown psychosis in any of these diagnostic categories are not easily derived from the existing literature. Some reliable data exist for Alzheimer's disease: 5–20% of patients have been reported to demonstrate hallucinations, and 10–50% experience delusions at some point during their illness. Similar estimates of psychotic symptoms in general have ranged from 4–50% among patients with various types of epilepsy. Estimating the frequency of psychotic symptoms in neurologic disorders involves inherently complex methodologic issues that have been the subject of much interest and investigation in some cases (e.g., epilepsy), yet little attention has been given to many of the other areas.

5. How can organic and nonorganic psychotic symptoms be distinguished?
One of the best means is to obtain a good history. A good history requires interview material as well as neuromedical records, including notes and evaluation results (when available) from medicine, psychiatry, neurology, psychology, and neuropsychology. Depending on the patient and symptoms, many of the following studies may be useful in the differential diagnosis.

Diagnostic Procedures to Be Considered in the Evaluation of the Patient with Psychosis

---

* Routine laboratory studies (e.g., B_{12}, Sequential Multiple Analysis, VDRL test for syphilis, HIV)
* Physical examination
* Psychiatric interview and history
* Mental status examination
* Neurologic examination
* Neuropsychological evaluation
* Neuroimaging (MRI, CT, functional imaging)
* Electrophysiological studies (e.g., EEG, evoked potentials)

Good premorbid adjustment is more often seen in patients with organic psychosis, whereas poorer adjustment is more common in patients with major psychiatric disorders. Baseline behavior is also a useful discriminator. Patients with schizophrenia, for example, often demonstrate evidence of disturbed thinking between psychotic episodes. Likewise, interpersonal relationship and work histories tend to be more disrupted in patients with primary psychiatric disease. Thus, a variety of background information and historical data can be useful in helping to delineate the nature of psychotic symptoms.

Various neurodiagnostic procedures (see above) are useful in estimating the likelihood of neurologic disease in patients with major psychiatric illnesses, although this task is challenging and sometimes impossible. Neurobehavioral examination, including formal neuropsychological studies, may be helpful, particularly when emphasis is placed on qualitative as well as quantitative aspects of test performance. Establishment of a patient's intellectual status and assessment of relative strengths and weaknesses across cognitive domains (e.g., memory, attention/concentration, language, visuospatial function) are also useful in evaluating medication effects and planning for general treatment and discharge.

6. Discuss the treatment of psychotic symptoms.
Treatment of psychotic symptoms varies, depending on the underlying causative factors. Resolution of acute neuromedical conditions (e.g., delirium) often results in the amelioration of psychotic symptoms without additional interventions. In more chronic neurologic disorders, traditional antipsychotic medications may be indicated to control more severe symptoms. In general, lower doses of antipsychotic medications are used in psychoses due to medical conditions than in primary psychiatric disorders. Psychological interventions also may be effective in managing psychotic symptoms, however, and should not be overlooked. In some cases, even simple behavioral and/or environmental manipulations are surprisingly efficacious. For example, extinction, positive and negative reinforcement, and/or successive approximation techniques to shape various behaviors often maintain their utility. The simple rewarding of desirable behaviors and

lack of reinforcement for undesirable behaviors are basic tenets of behavior modification. Such interventions, furthermore, may enhance the effects of medication or decrease the need for heavier-dose medications in some patients. Multidisciplinary treatment approaches are often indicated.

BIBLIOGRAPHY

1. Cullum CM, Heaton RK, Nemiroff B: Neuropsychology of late-life psychoses. Psychiatr Clin North Am 11:47–59, 1988.
2. Cummings JL: Organic delusions: Phenomenology, anatomical correlations, and review. Br J Psychiatry 146:184–197, 1985.
3. Cummings JL: Clinical Neuropsychiatry. San Diego, Grune & Stratton, 1985.
4. Gorman DG, Cummings JL: Organic delusional syndrome. Semin Neurol 10:229–238, 1990.
5. Grant I, Adams KM: Neuropsychological Assessment of Neuropsychiatric Disorders. New York, Oxford, 1986.
6. Lishman WA: Organic Psychiatry, 2nd ed. Boston, Blackwell, 1987.
7. Rubin EH: Psychosis in neurologic diseases: Delusions as part of Alzheimer's disease. Neuropsychiatry Neuropsychol Behav Neurol 5:108–113, 1992.
8. Strub RL, Black FW: Neurobehavioral Disorders. Philadelphia, F.A. Davis, 1988.
9. Yudofsky SC, Hales EE (eds): The American Psychiatric Press Textbook of Neuropsychiatry. Washington, DC, American Psychiatric Press, 1992.

V. Personality Disorders

37. PERSONALITY AND PERSONALITY DISORDERS

Alexis A. Giese, M.D.

1. What is the difference between a personality and a personality disorder?

Everyone has a distinct personality style, which includes typical ways of perceiving the self and the world, preferred coping mechanisms in response to stress, and values derived from cultural, familial, and individual experiences. Although personality development continues throughout life, most characteristic traits are formed by early adulthood, including the tendency to be passive or active, the intensity with which one expresses emotion, and the degree of social extroversion. Adverse events may exacerbate negative aspects of personality; however, positive or adaptive traits also surface, and baseline personality remains generally intact after a crisis has passed.

Personality disorders, on the other hand, are distinguished by chronically inadequate adaptive capacities affecting several realms of functioning, such as social relationships or occupational performance. The DSM–IV also includes in its general definition of personality disorders the criteria of pervasiveness across a broad range of situations and long duration with onset by early adulthood. People with personality disorders have chronic problems dealing with responsibilities, roles, and stressors; they also have difficulty understanding the causes of their problems or changing their behavior patterns.

For example, a person with dependent personality traits may be somewhat overreliant on others but generally functions fairly well. During a crisis (such as an acute medical illness) the person may exhibit exaggerated neediness in the health care setting or increase demands on family and friends to make decisions and provide care. When the illness is over, the person returns to the previous pattern of relating and functioning. By contrast, someone with dependent personality disorder has trouble making even routine decisions without extensive support and advice, is underfunctioning socially and occupationally because of the inability to initiate things independently, and is submissive, clinging, and fearful of loss of nurturance, even in everyday situations.

2. What is the natural history of personality disorders?

In most cases, early manifestations of personality disorders are evident in adolescence or even childhood. By young adulthood, maladaptive traits, causing major problems in social or occupational functioning or significant distress to the individual, are more clearly evident. Developmental tasks common to late adolescence or early adulthood, such as completing an education, emancipation from the family of origin, obtaining employment, and pursuit of romantic relationships, are often mishandled or delayed. Impairment from a personality disorder (especially antisocial and borderline personality disorders) is usually most pronounced during the third and fourth decades and decreases thereafter. However, some personality disorders, such as obsessive-compulsive and schizotypal, are less likely to remit with age.

For example, a typical chronology of borderline personality disorder may present first in the middle or late teens with onset of self-mutilatory behaviors, eating disorder symptoms, depression, or suicide attempts. Sometimes such behaviors present after leaving home for the first time or after the breakup of an early marriage. The twenties and thirties can be tumultuous, with frequent crises and hospitalizations. By 40 years of age, however, the features of borderline personality disorder have typically attenuated, with decreased impulsive behaviors, but possibly with residual emptiness and identity disturbance. Crises that occur in mid-life (e.g., loss of employment) may precipitate a recurrence of some borderline symptoms such as self-mutilatory or suicidal behavior, but such symptoms tend to be more limited than earlier in the illness because of some degree of social stability and coping skills.

3. Describe the clinical features that help to distinguish an axis I disorder from an axis II disorder.

Axis I disorders (clinical syndromes) are conceptualized as primarily focal disturbances affecting one particular dimension, such as thought (as in psychotic disorders) or mood (as in mania). Axis I disorders may be episodic, chronic, or progressive, but in general they represent a distinct departure from premorbid functioning. Many axis I disorders are highly amenable to specific pharmacotherapeutic and psychotherapeutic interventions.

Axis II (personality) disorders, on the other hand, represent an impairment in baseline functioning, in which the person generally functions below the level that would be expected for his or her intelligence, education, and resources; the impairment is most evident in self-perceptions and interpersonal and social functioning. By definition the personality impairment has an early onset and pervades a wide variety of situations. Stressors may exacerbate axis II symptoms, but dysfunction is not limited to certain contexts or crises.

Clinical tip-offs to the presence of an axis II problem include atypical presentations that do not fit readily into the usual axis I categories. For example, a patient who complains of mood swings and depression that are of insufficient severity and duration to meet criteria for bipolar disorder or cyclothymia may have histrionic or borderline personality disorder. Another clue is the presence of multiple conflicting previous psychiatric diagnoses. For example, a patient seen in several clinics and diagnosed variably with schizophrenia, chronic depression, and social phobia may have schizotypal personality disorder. A high degree of chaos and emotional response is sometimes a tip-off to personality disorder, especially the cluster B group (e.g., some relatives are furious at the patient, other family members are highly sympathetic and make unreasonably demands of the health care system, and members of the treatment team see the patient in widely disparate ways). In addition, failure to respond to appropriately aggressive treatment of an axis I disorder may suggest an underlying axis II problem.

The distinction between axis I and axis II symptoms is often quite difficult and sometimes can be made only after extensive longitudinal data are obtained. The clinician must conduct a thorough diagnostic evaluation for axis I disorders before attributing symptoms to a personality disorder or risk failing to make an accurate diagnosis and provide appropriate care for what may be a highly treatable problem.

4. Name the three clusters of personality disorders in DSM–IV, and describe the general characteristics of each.

Cluster A is the odd or eccentric group, which includes paranoid, schizoid, and schizotypal personality disorders. This group is characterized by a general distrust of others, misinterpretation of others' actions, odd or idiosyncratic beliefs, and a tendency toward social isolation. The assessment that beliefs and behaviors are abnormal must take into account the patient's cultural and religious background and whether the findings occur commonly in his or her cultural group. Some religious and ethnic traditions may appear bizarre on the surface (e.g., voodoo, dietary restrictions) but are pervasive in certain cultures. The distinction that the finding is pathologic is strengthened by evidence that the belief or behavior puts the patient at odds with his or her society and interferes with social or occupational functioning.

The initial presentation of cluster A personality disorders is often hostility or conflict with others; the underlying mistrust and unusual ideas usually become apparent over time. Only rarely do people with cluster A disorders self-present for treatment. Referral for psychiatric evaluation may be prompted by primary medical providers when depression or frank psychotic symptoms develop or when the patient's odd beliefs interfere with treatment of a general medical condition. Occasionally, such persons come to psychiatric attention through the legal system when idiosyncratic behaviors conflict with social convention or laws. For example, a person with schizotypal personality disorder may live an isolated lifestyle with dozens of cats, ignoring hygiene and health codes; he or she may refuse to leave the home when it is condemned by health or housing authorities and ultimately be brought to mental health care by the police.

Cluster B is the dramatic, overly emotional, or erratic group, including antisocial, borderline, histrionic, and narcissistic personality disorders. Such people are often characterized as labile, unpredictable, unlikable, or impulsive. The initial clinical presentation of the cluster B patient is typically crisis-related and chaotic, often involving severe symptoms (that may decrease after the crisis has passed), substance abuse, and conflicts with family members, employers, or the health care system. Such people have difficulty establishing and maintaining interpersonal relationships (e.g., with medical providers) and often have a history of discharge against medical advice, doctor shopping, or failure to follow recommended treatment. Awareness of a cluster B personality disorder may help the practitioner to anticipate such problems and to undertake treatment in a more sophisticated way.

Cluster C is the anxious or fearful group, including avoidant, dependent, and obsessive-compulsive personality disorders. Patients are often anxious, timid, perfectionistic, and conflict-avoidant; presentation is frequently triggered by depression or somatic complaints. Although sometimes initially reluctant to engage in general medical or psychiatric treatment, they may become highly attached because they have few other important relationships and have difficulty disengaging at the appropriate time.

DSM-IV Personality Disorder Clusters

CLUSTER	DESCRIPTION	PERSONALITY DISORDERS
A	Odd/eccentric	Paranoid Schizoid Schizotypal
B	Dramatic/erratic	Antisocial Borderline Histrionic Narcissistic
C	Anxious/fearful	Avoidant Dependent Obsessive-compulsive

Reprinted with permission from the Diagnostic and Statistical Manual of Mental Disorders, 4th ed. Copyright 1994 American Psychiatric Association.

5. How frequently do personality disorders occur in the general and psychiatric populations?
Standardized, structured diagnostic interviews estimate the lifetime prevalence of personality disorders in the general population at 10–13%. Schizotypal personality disorder is the most common cluster A disorder in the general population, borderline personality disorder the most common in cluster B, and dependent personality disorder the most common in cluster C.

The overall prevalence of personality disorders in clinical psychiatric populations is, of course, much higher than in the general population. Psychiatric inpatients have prevalence rates of personality disorders ranging from 30–60%. Factors that affect the frequency and distribution of personality disorders in an inpatient setting include the method of determining the axis II diagnosis (e.g., structured interview vs. chart review) and the types of patients at the institution (e.g., chronically vs. acutely mentally ill, employed vs. unemployed). In most studies, borderline personality disorder is the most frequently found axis II condition in hospitalized psychiatric patients, 20–30% of whom meet the diagnostic criteria. In outpatient psychiatric clinics prevalence rates of personality disorder fall between those for the general population and inpatients, ranging from 20–40% in some estimates. Avoidant, dependent, and borderline personality disorders have been reported most frequently in psychiatric outpatient clinics.

Many persons meet criteria for more than one personality disorder. Multiple diagnoses of axis II disorders are allowed in DSM-IV, and the clinician should list all disorders in order of clinical importance.

6. Describe comorbid psychiatric conditions that often lead persons with personality disorders into treatment.

Mood disturbances, such as depression, intense anger, and anxiety, are frequent complaints of people with personality disorders. Major depressive episodes and suicide attempts are more common in persons with a personality disorder than in those without. Anxiety disorders such as social phobia are sometimes comorbid diagnoses in the cluster C group, particularly avoidant personality disorder. Posttraumatic symptoms (e.g., intrusive memories and flashbacks of traumatic events) are common in borderline personality disorder, although only a minority of cases meet full criteria for posttraumatic stress disorder.

Substance abuse is a frequent comorbid diagnosis with personality disorders, especially in cluster B. Substance intoxication or withdrawal may contribute to some of the presenting symptoms, including depression, anxiety, irritability, and impulsivity, and also may explain why some of the symptoms are severe at presentation yet remit fairly quickly.

Transient psychotic symptoms may lead to treatment, especially in the cluster A group and borderline personality disorder.

Many people with personality disorders initially present to primary medical providers with physical complaints rather than seek psychiatric help; in addition to medical problems, some patients also may have a somatization disorder. A personality disorder may complicate or prolong medical treatment and result in higher service utilization and costs if unidentified.

7. What types of psychiatric treatment approaches are useful for treating personality disorders?

By definition, personality disorders are chronic and relatively fixed and thus are not easily "cured." In short-term treatments, adaptational approaches that help the patient to cope with the current crisis and solve problems more effectively are most helpful. Commonly used treatment modalities include crisis intervention, supportive psychotherapy, environmental manipulation (such as change in living situation), and treatment for substance abuse. Behavioral therapies (such as assertiveness training or systematic desensitization) may be helpful for avoidant and obsessive-compulsive personality disorders. Careful consideration of comorbid axis I disorders may lead to a diagnosis with specific treatment implications, including pharmacotherapy.

Certain patients with personality disorders may require long-term psychotherapy that attempts to restructure the faulty coping mechanisms. Because of the intensity and complexity of the therapeutic relationship, such treatment is best undertaken by professionals with specific expertise (such as a psychiatrist, psychologist, or psychiatric social worker with psychodynamic training). This type of treatment is not without its risks and should be recommended only to patients who are not in crisis, who have some degree of stability in their lives (e.g., are productively employed), and who have addressed substance abuse problems.

8. What personality changes are commonly seen when underlying organic brain disease is present?

Personality changes are a feature of many organic brain diseases, sometimes presenting as the earliest signs of illness or even its major manifestation. Dementias due to Alzheimer's disease and other neurodegenerative disorders often begin with subtle personality changes that are typically recognized in retrospect after other findings, such as memory deficits, are also noted. Structural damage to the brain may result from tumors, trauma, or infarcts and may cause significant permanent personality changes, especially if the frontal and/or temporal lobes are involved. The abrupt or late onset of personality changes should not be attributed to a personality disorder until a thorough diagnostic investigation (e.g., premorbid functioning, neurologic history, review of systems, physical exam) has been conducted. Examples of personality changes in common neurologic disorders are listed below:

Disorder	Common personality changes
Dementias (e.g., Alzheimer's)	Early: apathy, narrowing of interests, loss of sense of humor, lack of social judgment, impulsivity, immaturity
	Late: irritability, oppositionality, aggressive outbursts, suspiciousness
Frontal lobe damage	Apathy, indifference
	Depression
	Disinhibition, excitement
Temporal lobe epilepsy	Heightened emotional tone
	Rigidity, hypermoralism
	Circumstantiality, loquaciousness
	Dissociative symptoms
	Temper outbursts
Acquired immunodeficiency syndrome (HIV)	Early: social withdrawal, apathy, agitation
	Late: progressive dementia, paranoia, manic symptoms

9. Are personality disorders caused by environmental or constitutional factors?

The DSM–IV avoids the question by taking an empirical, atheoretical approach; the disorders are defined by descriptive criteria emphasizing observable behaviors. In the past, personality was traditionally viewed as a product of upbringing, whereas the major mental illnesses were thought to be related to biologic vulnerabilities. However, such issues are now understood to be much more complex, and a substantial body of evidence suggests that both biologic and environmental variables play important and interacting roles in personality development and disorders.

A familial relationship may exist between schizophrenia and cluster A personality disorders, as evidenced by elevated rates of schizophrenia in relatives of patients with cluster A disorders. This relationship is especially strong for schizotypal personality disorder and less conclusive for paranoid and schizoid personality disorders. Family studies have also suggested a hereditary component to antisocial personality disorder. Borderline personality disorder clusters in families, although this trend is not clearly genetically determined. Some axis I illnesses such as depression are present at elevated rates in families of personality disordered probands, giving rise to the hypothesis that in some cases personality disorder symptoms may be inherited subsyndromal forms of axis I problems.

Data supporting the role of environmental factors are strongest in the cluster B group, including high rates of childhood sexual and physical abuse as well as higher rates of childhood stressors such as divorce, loss of a parent, inconsistent or inadequate parenting, frequent moves, and institutional placements. Although the association between borderline personality disorder and childhood abuse is the most strongly established (70–80% prevalence in most studies), other personality disorders have been estimated to have childhood trauma prevalence rates of approximately 50% compared with estimates of 20–40% in mixed psychiatric populations and 10–15% in the general population. Narcissistic personality disorder has been postulated to develop in the context of impaired parent-child relationships, particularly failure of parents to meet the child's need for attention and admiration at critical stages of development; little empirical evidence, however, supports this formulation.

10. Are psychotropic drugs useful in treating personality disorders?

Most clinicians agree that psychotropic drugs have at least limited usefulness. In patients with an axis I disorder that usually responds to pharmacologic intervention, such as a major depressive episode, treatment should not be withheld because a personality disorder is suspected. Some of the apparent character symptoms may remit with adequate treatment of depression and anxiety.

Even in the absence of a formal axis I diagnosis, medications are sometimes moderately effective for certain target symptoms in personality disorders. For example, the perceptual distortions and brief psychotic symptoms in paranoid or schizotypal personality disorders may respond to low doses of antipsychotics (e.g., trifluoperazine 5 mg/day or thioridazine 100 mg/day). Severe behavioral dyscontrol (as sometimes seen in antisocial and borderline personality disorders) may respond to carbamazepine (with blood levels at the low end of the anticonvulsant range) or beta blockers at high doses (e.g., propranolol 250–400 mg/day or more).

On the other hand, a treatment plan that focuses largely or exclusively on medications may ill serve the needs of patients with a personality disorder. Many such patients desperately want amelioration of their distress and seek pharmacologic intervention as a panacea. Multidrug regimens carry the risk of combined toxicity and provide a ready means of suicide and drug dependence, particularly if substance abuse is a comorbid diagnosis. The definitive resolution of many problems faced by personality disordered patients requires the development of new coping mechanisms and better social skills; even with aggressive pharmacotherapy, such goals are usually best reached through psychotherapeutic processes.

BIBLIOGRAPHY

1. American Psychiatric Association: Diagnostic and Statistical Manual of Mental Disorders, 4th ed. Washington, DC, American Psychiatric Association, 1994.
2. Andreasen NC, Black DW (eds): Introductory Textbook of Psychiatry. Washington, DC, American Psychiatric Press, 1991.
3. Gorton G, Akhtar S: The literature on personality disorders, 1985–88: Trends, issues, and controversies. Hosp Community Psychiatry 41:39–51, 1990.
4. Oldham JM: Personality disorders: Current perspectives. JAMA 272:1770–1776, 1994.
5. Oldham JM, Skodol AE: Personality disorders and mood disorders. In Tasman A, Riba MB (eds): Review of Psychiatry, vol 11. Washington, American Psychiatric Press, 1992, pp 418–435.
6. Shea MT, Pilkonis PA, Beckham E, et al: Personality disorders and treatment outcome in the NIMH treatment of depression collaborative research program. Am J Psychiatry 147:711–718, 1990.
7. Siever LJ, Davis KL: A psychobiological perspective on the personality disorders. Am J Psychiatry 148:1657–1658, 1991.
8. Turkat ID: The Personality Disorders: A Psychological Approach to Clinical Management. Elmsford, NY, Pergamon Press, 1990.
9. Tyrer P: Personality Disorders: Diagnosis, Management and Course. London, Butterworth, 1988.

38. BORDERLINE PERSONALITY DISORDER

Elissa M. Ball, M.D., and Robin McCann, Ph.D.

1. What is borderline personality disorder?

The key to recognizing borderline personality disorder (BPD) is instability—instability in affect, interpersonal relationships, and self-identity. The emotional instability of patients with BPD is characterized by vulnerability, intensity, and poor regulation. Emotions are quickly and easily aroused and more intense than those of others; patients often experience difficulty soothing themselves and returning to a stable emotional baseline. People with BPD are particularly vulnerable to perceived or actual abandonment and often react with rage, panic, and despair. As they have difficulty in soothing themselves, they may attempt to block the experience of pain by experiencing, if not inducing, changes in consciousness, including feelings of derealization, depersonalization, and brief psychotic reactions with delusions and hallucinations. Substance use, gambling, overspending, eating binges, and/or self-mutilation, including suicidal threats, gestures, and attempts, are often used to escape intensely painful affect. People with BPD frequently engage in self-injurious acts, ranging from minor scratches or self-inflicted cigarette burns to overdoses or other acts requiring ICU admissions; such nonfatal, intentionally self-harmful acts are referred to as parasuicidal behaviors. The criteria for BPD were developed by consensus rather than empirical study and were first published in 1980 in DSM III. Specific DSM IV diagnostic criteria[1] for BPD are as follows:

A pervasive pattern of instability of interpersonal relationships, self-image, and affects, and marked impulsivity beginning by early adulthood and present in a variety of contexts, as indicated by five (or more) of the following:

1. Frantic efforts to avoid real or imagined abandonment. Note: Do not include suicidal or self-mutilating behavior covered in Criterion 5.

2. A pattern of unstable and intense interpersonal relationships characterized by alternating between extremes of idealization and devaluation.

3. Identity disturbance: markedly and persistently unstable self image or sense of self.

4. Impulsivity in at least two areas that are potentially self-damaging (e.g., spending, sex, substance abuse, reckless driving, binge eating). Note: Do not include suicidal or self-mutilating behavior covered in Criterion 5.

5. Recurrent suicidal behavior, gestures, or threats, or self-mutilating behavior.

6. Affective instability due to a marked reactivity of mood (e.g., intense episodic dysphoria, irritability or anxiety usually lasting a few hours and only rarely more than a few days).

7. Chronic feelings of emptiness.

8. Inappropriate, intense anger or difficulty controlling anger (e.g., frequent displays of temper, constant anger, recurrent physical fights).

9. Transient, stress-related paranoid ideation or severe dissociative symptoms.

Reprinted with permission from the Diagnostic and Statistical Manual of Mental Disorders, 4th ed. Copyright 1994 American Psychiatric Association.

Emotional lability is often associated with a cognitive style characterized by all-or-nothing, either-or thinking. Patients vacillate suddenly between rigidly held, yet contradictory points of view and find it extremely difficult to formulate compromise positions. This cognitive style contributes to an unstable self-concept and unstable interpersonal relationships. For example, the belief that Dr. X is totally trustworthy leads to worship or idealization of Dr. X. When Dr. X inevitably disappoints the patient, perhaps by saying no to a particular request, the patient predictably decides that Dr. X is a totally untrustworthy individual who deserves punishment and denigration; Dr. X's reasons for denying the request are not considered. Thus, relationships between patients with BPD and their significant others, including spouses, children, and treatment providers, often begin on a highly positive note (idealization), but deteriorate quickly into a chronically irritating and often emotionally and physically abusive interchange (devaluation).

Unstable self-concept and emotional lability predict difficulty in maintaining commitment to long-term goals. Commitment to school, occupation, friends, mores, and treatment plans is erratic. Behavior is impulsive and unpredictable and further contributes to unstable relationships. People with BPD often frantically seek the company and attention of others to avoid feeling lonely, empty, and worthless. Examples of such characters in literature and film include Alex in *Fatal Attraction* and Natalya Fillipovna in Dostoyevsky's *The Idiot*.

2. How common is BPD?

BPD is commonly diagnosed, particularly among women. Approximately 10% of psychiatric outpatients and 20% of psychiatric inpatients meet criteria for BPD. Approximately 75% of patients diagnosed with BPD are women.

3. Explain the origin of the term *borderline*.

The term *borderline* has both historical and colloquial uses extending beyond the DSM IV criteria. Historically, the term described individuals with both neurotic and psychotic symptoms who were believed to be on the borderline or continuum between psychosis and neurosis. Some patients diagnosed with schizophrenia before 1980 (when DSM III criteria for schizophrenia were constricted and refined) probably would be diagnosed with BPD today. Historically, the term also described a pathologic level of personality organization, subsuming some but not all of the characteristics of the current DSM IV criteria, including instability of self-concept and poor differentiation between self and others. Colloquially, the term sometimes has been used pejoratively to describe patients who evoke anger or hate in treatment providers.

4. What causes BPD?

The many proposed etiologies reflect a variety of theoretical paradigms. From a **psychodynamic paradigm**, BPD is the result of poor mothering. Because the mother-child relationship serves as a template for later relationships, it is important that it is "good enough." A "good-enough" mother adequately responds to her child's needs and fosters an adequate balance between dependence and independence. Without a mother who is adequately reflective and responding, the child who later develops BPD is unable to develop a sense of self that is strong, cohesive, and good. Without a strong sense of self, the child is unable to separate and differentiate self from mother. Thus, without a sufficiently cohesive sense of self, the child is unable to differentiate self from others. To an excessive degree, the child seeks self-definition and safety through others.

A **biologic paradigm** suggests that BPD is the result of an innate inability to modulate or tolerate emotion. Regulation of emotion is complex and involves multiple areas of the brain. Research to date does not suggest any single neurologic or genetic factor common to all borderline patients. Abnormalities in limbic system reactivity have been suggested as causal factors of emotion dysregulation. Limbic abnormalities may result from genetic influences, intrauterine events, or negative effects on brain development of early childhood environments. Some researchers have suggested that chronic sexual abuse and other severe, recurrent traumas (more common in patients with BPD than in those without BPD or normative samples) may physiologically alter the limbic system and thereby cause permanent adverse effects on emotional arousal, sensitivity, and modulation. Some studies have suggested additional biologic vulnerability; first-degree relatives of borderline patients were found to have a higher prevalence of mood disorders than relatives of control groups.

Biologic and psychodynamic paradigms have been incorporated into a variety of **interactional or diathesis-stress models**. An example of an interactional or diathesis-stress model is the biosocial model described by Linehan,[6] who attributed BPD to an interaction between biologic vulnerability to intense and unmodulated emotionality (the diathesis) and an invalidating, unpredictably punishing environment (the stress). Invalidating environments are environments in which a child's perception of personal experience is trivialized, punished, disregarded, or dismissed. A mother may insist that a child feels what the child says that he or she does not feel. A sexually abusive father states that his sexual molestation is an expression of his love, then states that it is all the child's fault and the the child must tell no one. An invalidating environment teaches children to mistrust their own observations, emotions, and reactions and to search the immediate environment for social cues about how to feel, think, and behave. According to Linehan, the borderline patient's innately intense, emotional nature collides with this invalidating environment again and again and predictably produces the instability of affect, interpersonal relationships, and identity characteristic of BPD. Some believe that such interactions lead to biologic changes in the brain, e.g., reinforced learned emotional pathways. Thus, in contrast to nature vs. nurture, nature and nurture may interact.

5. Why is BPD more frequently diagnosed among women?

Some theorists argue that at best the paradigms described above miss the point and at worst (particularly the psychodynamic paradigm) are "women-blaming." Such theorists argue that the cause of BPD—a disorder so overwhelmingly diagnosed among women—is a society that disempowers and victimizes women.

Extensive research has confirmed differences in the interpersonal relationship styles of men and women. Such studies suggest that socialization, beginning in infancy, may render women generally more affectively connected and interpersonally perceptive than men. By age 6, girls and boys already communicate and socialize in significantly different ways. Girls are more likely to play in intimate, confiding dyads; boys are more likely to play in rough-and-tumble, competitive groups. Studies have shown that rough-and-tumble play is aversive to some girls. Thus, when girls play with boys, they become relatively passive, allowing the boys to monopolize or control the game. This pattern may be reinforced by adults, who consciously or unconsciously encourage aggression in boys yet discourage identical behavior in girls.

Perhaps as a result of such socialization, emotional health and sense of well-being among women is highly correlated with the degree of social support and intimacy. This socialization leaves women especially vulnerable to the needs, whims, and vicissitudes of others. Given a pathologic, invalidating environment, this vulnerability may lead to the instability of self, affect, and relationships of BPD. Such gender role socialization also may be related to the increased sexual victimization experienced by girls compared with boys. Although most theorists focus on the effects of early invalidating experiences, similar effects may result from later spouse abuse, especially if such experiences are cumulative.

In addition, the high frequency of diagnosis among women may reflect clinician bias. It has been suggested that clinicians attribute specific symptoms in women to BPD yet attribute the same symptoms in men to antisocial or narcissistic personality disorder.

6. Is BPD caused by sexual and/or physical abuse?

Data suggest that the risk of sexual abuse is 2–3 times greater for girls than boys. Physical abuse rates are not significantly different for boys and girls, yet rates of physical abuse for patients with BPD are reported to be as high as 76% vs. 38% for patients without BPD. Eighty-six percent of inpatients with BPD report a history of sexual abuse compared with 34% of inpatients without BPD; 70% of outpatients with BPD compared with 26% of outpatients without BPD report such a history. Studies also have suggested a predictive relationship between both sexual and physical abuse in childhood and adult suicidal behavior. Although childhood victimization appears to be tragically common, data suggest a unique relationship among female gender, sexual abuse, perhaps physical abuse, and BPD.

7. List and discuss the differential diagnosis of BPD. What particular disorders are associated with BPD?

1. Major depression
2. Bipolar disorder
3. Substance abuse or dependence
4. Posttraumatic stress disorder

Major depression and bipolar disorder are commonly considered in the differential diagnosis. Up to 50% of individuals diagnosed with BPD also may have concomitant diagnoses of either major depression or bipolar disorder. BPD can be described as marked *instability* of self, mood, interpersonal relationships, and symptoms. In contrast, a diagnosis of major depression requires *stability* of affective symptoms, notably a period of at least 2 weeks in which the patient experiences depression or anhedonia every day. The marked changes in mood in BPD generally occur within hours or days rather than within weeks or months as in bipolar disorder.

Substance abuse frequently results in impulsive, emotionally labile behavior and unstable interpersonal relationships. The impulsivity associated with BPD often results in substance abuse or dependence. Studies suggest that 10–50% of hospitalized chemical abusers meet criteria for BPD.

The high prevalence of physical and sexual trauma among patients with BPD suggests a differential diagnosis of posttraumatic stress disorder (PTSD). However, whereas rates of abuse and BPD in the general population are high, baseline rates for PTSD in the general population are low (1%). Whereas patients with either PTSD or BPD may have histories of abuse and experience intense emotional arousal, patients with PTSD avoid the feared stimuli and yet reexperience the trauma through dreams, flashbacks, or intrusive thoughts. For example, a rape victim with PTSD may avoid all men and experience nightmares of the rape. If a patient with BPD has a recent history of trauma but does not actively avoid similar stimuli or reexperience the trauma, a concomitant diagnosis of adjustment disorder may be more appropriate.

8. Describe the main risks involved in the treatment of BPD. How significant is the risk of suicide in such patients? How are the risks assessed?

Symptoms of BPD such as impulsivity, anxiety, anger, and concomitant affective and substance abuse disorders result in a high risk of suicide. Between 70–75% of patients with BPD have histories of at least one self-injurious act. Rates of completed suicides are about 9% for patients with BPD vs. 1% in the general population. In one longitudinal study in which psychiatric inpatients were followed for 10–23 years after discharge, patients who met all 8 of the DSM III criteria for BPD had a suicide rate of 36% vs. 7% for patients who met 5–7 of the criteria. Suicidal threats should be taken seriously and warrant psychiatric consultation. Suicidal threats are particularly worrisome if the patient:

- Is a white male over age 45
- Is recently separated, divorced, or widowed
- Is unemployed or retired
- Is in poor physical health
- Has previously attempted suicide with a highly lethal method (e.g., firearms, hanging)
- Currently threatens to complete suicide with a highly lethal method
- Experiences intense anxiety
- Expresses hopelessness

9. What feelings are commonly generated in professionals by patients with BPD? What do such feelings mean? Can they be useful?

Patients with BPD often live in a state of chaos. Their moods shift rapidly and without apparent cause. They often appear to have normal cognitive abilities and yet demonstrate extremely poor judgment. They repeatedly present to emergency departments for treatment of self-inflicted injuries or overdoses. They overdramatize or give inconsistent reports of symptom history. One minute they appear to have a good relationship with their doctor and the next minute they are angry, hostile, and critical. They report an understanding of the risks and benefits of recommended treatment but then are noncompliant. They miss scheduled follow-up appointments yet demand immediate attention or call at all hours to discuss new symptoms.

Such behaviors not surprisingly engender feelings of anger, irritation, confusion, helplessness, and hopelessness in providers. Professionals respond in different ways to such feelings. Anger engenders feelings of guilt in some. For example, one doctor may feel hopeless or think,

"It might be better if this patient *did* kill herself." Feeling guilty, the physician then may become overly solicitous of the patient, agreeing to unreasonable demands and reinforcing negative behavior. Physicians may find themselves wanting to exert control or to reject the patient and refuse provision of further needed treatment. Others find themselves mirroring the patient's attitudes and extreme reactions and worry that they themselves are borderline. For example, they find themselves siding with the patient and devaluing clinic staff or other doctors. When the patient's criticism is directed at them, they are filled with self-doubt and question their own professional competence or find themselves becoming argumentative and unreasonable with the patient, staff, or another doctor.

Borderline patients also may induce intensely positive feelings in treatment providers. Their propensity to idealize may cause some physicians to become quite protective and nurturing. Some providers suddenly may want to rescue patients from various crises. Physicians may find themselves feeling unusually powerful and competent. Another doctor may unconsciously blur professional-patient boundaries in response to the positive feelings elicited by idealization; this may take the form of romantic or sexual fantasies. Physicians sometimes find themselves agreeing to keep certain information secret and then feel trapped or paralyzed.

All of these reactions are especially likely to arise when care providers are particularly stressed (e.g., sleep deprivation during internship or in marital discord). It is often helpful to recognize that many such feelings are engendered simply by contact with the borderline patient. Borderline patients experience a broad range of emotions; all-or-none, black-and-white thinking; idealization-devaluation of relationships; self-esteem vulnerability; and difficulties with loss of significant relationships. All humans are familiar with such experiences to some degree. Borderline patients simply experience emotions and defenses with less ability to modulate reactions and to maintain or regain a balanced perspective. When care providers become involved, they also may experience some loss of their normal ability to maintain balance. This emotional experience can be a highly useful tool to help professionals recognize that a patient suffers from BPD. The cognitive and behavioral techniques that the professional uses to reestablish balance also provide useful clues to treatment and management of the patient. Thus, a physician's acknowledgment of his or her own feelings, obtaining consultation or peer supervision, and possibly limiting clinical contact may be useful strategies.

10. What are some clues that the doctor-patient relationship is in trouble?

1. Rescue fantasies ("Only I can treat this patient")

2. Defensive posture with colleagues, family, or other staff; concern expressed by clinic or hospital staff about the physician's involvement with the patient.

3. "Special" behaviors or deviation from routine behaviors or procedures, including keeping secrets from supervisors, staff, or consultants; making house calls; giving out personal information; talking to the patient about personal stress in an intimate way; agreeing "just to have coffee"; feeling sexual tension when the patient is present; or feeling guilty about time spent with the patient, or thoughts or feelings about the patient.

Most of these clues were previously listed as clues that the patient suffers from BPD. They become clues to problems within the doctor-patient relationship when they become reciprocal or when they become the pattern rather than the unusual event. The common denominator for each of these clues is loss of equilibrium and objectivity in the professional's thinking, feelings, or behavior in regard to the specific patient. The key to reestablishing the necessary objectivity is recognition that something within the relationship is out of balance and must be rectified to provide competent treatment. Formal or informal consultation with a colleague is often helpful.

11. Are there guidelines for successful management of the behavior of patients with BPD when the physician's primary goal is medical stability and compliance with treatment?

Management of emotional dyscontrol

1. Provide structure. Patients with BPD experience intense, poorly understood emotions, and their thinking becomes diffuse and disorganized. They have difficulty consistently providing

order to internal experience. At times, self-destructive behaviors are their best, although primitive, attempt at "grounding" their emotional state. Borderline patients experience significantly less turmoil and engage in fewer negative behaviors if the environment around them is clearly structured. They need clear expectations and clear role definition.

2. Be matter-of-fact. Patients with BPD become overwhelmed by emotions and are reassured by a professional who calmly addresses affect-laden issues. Avoid expression of extreme emotions.

3. Help patients to validate their own experience by acknowledging their feelings while also clearly stating the expectation of behavior control. Many (perhaps most) patients with BPD were raised in traumatic and abusive environments. The child's feelings and needs were ignored. Such children grow into adults who, on the one hand, overvalue the importance of their emotions and, on the other hand, are profoundly confused and distrustful of their emotional experience.

4. Consider frequent, brief, scheduled contacts for needy, demanding, or somaticizing patients with BPD. Gently encourage patient the patient to consider the relationship between psychological stressors and emotional stress and somatic symptoms.

5. Be alert to the risk of suicide. Discuss this risk openly with the patient. Weigh potential overdose potential when deciding to prescribe medication, amount to be dispensed, and number of refills.

6. Have a low threshold for seeking psychiatric or psychological consultation. Consider a referral for psychotherapy. Take care to make this referral in a nonrejecting manner, clearly defining the roles of medical and psychotherapy professionals.

Management of interpersonal boundaries

1. Interact in a genuine manner, balancing appropriate warmth and concern with appropriate professional boundaries. Avoid interactions conveying either unresponsiveness or overinvolvement.

2. Convey a demeanor of professional competence, yet also openly and matter-of-factly acknowledge minor errors. Presentation of oneself as infallible or omnipotent plays into the borderline patient's idealization. Idealization invariably leads to devaluation and rage; no one can live up to the fantasy of perfection. Model comfort with nonperfection to decrease the intensity of expressed anger in response to expected disappointments.

3. Perform physical examinations with a chaperone present, regardless of gender of doctor or patient. Patients with BPD have significant boundary problems and may misinterpret the meaning of physical exams or other procedures. When angry, patients also may consciously or unconsciously distort their recall of physical contact.

Additional general guidelines

1. Be aware of the high risk of comorbid substance abuse and major depression. Avoid prescription of addictive medications. Consider providing treatment or referring the patient for treatment of these conditions.

2. Confront noncompliance in a direct, calm, nonjudgmental manner; consider use of written contracts.

3. Avoid global, black-white, all-or-none statements and thinking. Present the patient with choices. Think compromise.

4. Set limits in a calm, nonhostile, nonjudgmental manner.

5. Think balance. Continually ask, "Am I over- or underreacting to the patient's complaints?" Aim for the middle ground.

12. Are patients with BPD competent to make medical decisions?

Generally, yes. Patients with BPD are prone to brief psychotic episodes and to distortions in thinking, especially under stress; this at times may interfere with competency. Providing information about risks and benefits in a calm, structured manner often is sufficient to reestablish their capacity to participate in medical decisions. When in doubt, consult a mental health professional.

CONTROVERSY

13. Patients with BPD just need to try harder and be more motivated to act in a mature, adult manner; thus psychotropic medications have no place in treatment.

For:

1. Although studies support biologic, genetic, and environmental contributions to the development of BPD, studies support no pharmacologic "treatment of choice." Effects of all classes of medication studied are modest at best.

2. Patients with BPD have inadequate coping skills; medication does not replace the need to learn new coping skills.

3. Evidence suggests that the behavioral dyscontrol exhibited by patients with BPD is within their control. For example, when limits are set firmly, behavior improves. All medications have associated risks, which are not justified if control can be attained through behavioral interventions.

4. Patients with BPD cannot be trusted. They will use the medications in an attempt to kill themselves, will self-medicate their unstable moods and become addicted psychologically or physiologically, or will simply comply with prescribed medication in such an erratic manner that treatment trials are inadequate and inconclusive.

Against:

1. Having BPD does not provide protection from the typical medication-responsive axis I disorders. In fact, mood disorders, substance use disorders, anxiety disorders, gender identity disorders, eating disorders, and other personality disorders often coexist with BPD. BPD has the greatest overlap with other personality disorders; comorbidity with mood disorders (particularly dysthymia and major depression) and substance use disorders is extensive. At times, comorbidity may be due to overlap in diagnostic criteria, but studies suggest that, at least for some patients, borderline symptoms represent a characterologic variant within the affective spectrum. Clinicians must consider additional syndromes that may warrant separate treatment approaches. Withholding effective medications for coexisting psychiatric conditions cannot be justified.

2. Psychopharmacologic interventions reduce specific target symptoms (anxiety, behavioral dyscontrol, acute or chronic perceptual disturbances, and emotional lability). Symptom reduction may increase the patient's ability to benefit from other psychosocial interventions.

3. Low-dose neuroleptics have been shown to decrease cognitive symptoms such as magical thinking, illusions, ideas of reference, tangentiality, and circumstantiality. Studies have shown superiority over placebo in measures of global functioning, hostility, anger, impulsivity, and subjective feelings of depression. Most patients, however, show only modest improvement and continue to meet criteria for BPD. Other patients show no improvement and/or cannot tolerate side effects. Because of the risk of tardive dyskinesia, antipsychotics are used more frequently during periods of acute stress or decompensation rather than for long-term maintenance.

4. Controlled pharmacologic trials and clinical experience suggest that some patients with BPD symptoms experience a decrease in emotional lability and impulsivity with use of carbamazepine, lithium, and monoamine oxidase inhibitors.

5. The minor tranquilizers generally should be avoided in patients with BPD because of their potential for abuse and disinhibition of impulses. Despite this relative contraindication, some patients benefit from cautious, controlled use.

6. Although the risk of suicide must be weighed in the decision to use any medication, overdose is commonly an interpersonal event and patients provide extensive opportunity for "rescue." Many physicians find that when this issue is addressed in a serious, matter-of-fact manner, patients with BPD consciously and consistently avoid overdose of physician-prescribed psychotropic medications.

14. Is BPD treatable? How is it treated?

By definition, a personality disorder is a disorder with an enduring pattern. Hence, some theorists suggest that BPD is not treatable and that therapy, particularly analytic therapy, may have a worsening effect. More recent theorists (particularly brief dynamic and cognitive-behavioral theorists) have suggested that the symptoms of BPD can be significantly ameliorated and perhaps resolved. For example, Linehan[6] successfully taught patients with BPD to monitor, recognize, and regulate painful affect; to inhibit inappropriate behaviors associated with affect; and to refocus attention on nondistressing stimuli. This technique ameliorates the negative effects of intense affect on interpersonal relationships. In clinical practice, when feeling angry, patients may be taught first to recognize the anger, to analyze its causes, to soothe themselves and then consciously to initiate a behavior that is the opposite of anger. For example, after recognizing anger related to her husband's interest in a friend's art work, the patient may gently avoid discussion of the work and instead ask about her husband's work day, thereby resisting the impulse to attack. The success of this approach has been validated with controlled empirical data. Compared with controls, patients with BPD who were treated with Linehan's approach were less likely to engage in parasuicidal acts and to receive inpatient hospitalizations and more likely to remain in treatment and to rate themselves higher on measures of occupational and other role performance.

BIBLIOGRAPHY

1. American Psychiatric Association: Diagnostic and Statistical Manual of Mental Disorders, 4th ed. Washington, DC, American Psychiatric Association, 1994.
2. Beck AT, Freeman A: Cognitive Therapy of Personality Disorders. New York, Guilford Press, 1990.
3. Bernstein AE, Warner GM: An Introduction to Contemporary Psychoanalysis. New York, Jason Aronson, 1981.
4. Cowdry RW: Psychopharmacology of borderline personality disorder: A review. J Clin Psychiatry 48:15–22, 1987.
5. Kreisman JJ, Straus H: I Hate You—Don't Leave Me: Understanding the Borderline Personality. New York, Avon, 1989.
6. Linehan M: Cognitive-behavioral Treatment of Borderline Personality Disorder. New York, Guilford Press, 1993.
7. Paris J: The treatment of borderline personality disorder in light of the research on its long term outcome. Can J Psychiatry 38:S28–S34, 1993.
8. Sansone RA, Sansone LA: Borderline personality disorder: Office diagnosis and management. Am Fam Physician 44:194–198, 1991.
9. Sedright HR: Borderline personality disorder: Diagnosis and management in primary care. J Fam Pract 34:605–612, 1992.
10. Tasman A, Hales RE, Frances AJ (eds): American Psychiatric Press Review of Psychiatry, vol. 8. Washington, DC, American Psychiatric Press, 1989.

39. ANTISOCIAL PERSONALITY DISORDER

Robin A. McCann, Ph.D., and Elissa M. Ball, M.D.

1. What is antisocial personality disorder?

Clues to a diagnosis of antisocial personality disorder include (1) a high frequency of behaviors that violate rules or the rights of others and (2) a cognitive style characterized by lack of motivation to understand the world from any point of view except one's own. To meet criteria for the diagnosis of antisocial personality disorder, such behaviors must begin in childhood (before age 15 years) and persist through adulthood. Childhood behaviors that violate rules or the rights of others include frequent lying, stealing, and physical fights; fire setting and other destruction of property; and cruelty to people or animals. For adults such behaviors include impulsivity, consistent failure to follow through with occupational and family commitments, frequent lying, and lack of remorse. Examples of such characters in literature and film include Fagin in Dickens' *Oliver Twist*, the Benefactor in Dickens' *David Copperfield,* and the title characters in *Bonnie and Clyde.* The specific criteria for the DSM IV[1] diagnosis are presented below:

A. There is a pervasive pattern of disregard for and violation of the rights of others occurring since age 15, as indicated by 3 or more of the following:
   1. failure to conform to social norms with respect to lawful behaviors as indicated by repeatedly performing acts that are grounds for arrest.
   2. deceitfulness, as indicated by repeated lying, use of aliases, or conning others for personal profit or pleasure.
   3. impulsivity or failure to plan ahead.
   4. irritability and aggressiveness, as indicated by repeated physical fights or assaults.
   5. reckless disregard for safety of self or others.
   6. consistent irresponsibility, as indicated by repeated failure to sustain consistent work behavior or honor financial obligations.
   7. lack of remorse, as indicated by being indifferent to or rationalizing having hurt, mistreated, or stolen from another.

B. The individual is at least 18 years.

C. There is evidence of conduct disorder with onset before age 15 years.

D. Occurrence of antisocial behavior is not exclusively during the course of schizophrenia or a manic episode.

From American Psychiatric Association: Diagnostic and Statistical Manual of Mental Disorders, Fourth Edition. Washington, DC, American Psychiatric Association, 1994, with permission.

Antisocial personality disorder, as currently conceptualized in DSM IV, is a quantitative (behaviorally anchored) rather than qualitative (trait- or predisposition-based) diagnosis. However, it is important to recognize the difference between specific antisocial acts and the chronic maladaptive pattern of antisocial behavior that characterizes the patient with antisocial personality disorder. For example, most adolescents have committed the following illegal activities at least once: driving a car without a license, skipping school, fist fighting, stealing, drinking alcohol, or using marijuana. Similarly, many adults have committed some of the following illegal or hurtful behaviors: lying, use of marijuana and other illegal drugs, extramarital affairs, failure to provide child support, and spouse and child abuse. In a randomly sampled survey, 25% of married individuals reported that their spouse had physically abused them in the past year. Despite a few behaviors that particularly distinguish the antisocial individual (vagrancy, the use of aliases, impulsivity, and a poor marital history), the differentiation between antisocial personality disorder and normative legal and social violations is largely quantitative. Individuals with antisocial personality disorder, beginning in childhood, consistently and inflexibly commit a higher frequency of antisocial behaviors resulting in maladaptive social or occupational functioning.

The credo of the individual with antisocial personality disorder can be summarized as "I believe; therefore, it is so." Such individuals are 100% certain of the veracity of their viewpoint, 100% certain that because they want something, they should receive it. They are 100% certain that because they believe that a particular rule is silly, they need not follow it. Because they believe that they can avoid negative consequences, they are 100% certain that they will not happen. Because they believe that another is not worthy of respect, they feel 100% justified in denigrating the person. The high frequency of antisocial behaviors may be maintained by this egocentric cognitive style, notable for a lack of motivation to understand events from any other point of view. Such individuals do not think about how others perceive them and are not concerned about the effect of their behavior on others. Qualities such as empathy, remorse, reliability, and sincerity depend on understanding events from the vantage of others. Low motivation to do so may account for the limited ability to demonstrate empathy, remorse, sincerity, or reliability.

2. List clues for the general practitioner that he or she is treating a patient with antisocial personality disorder.
Such clues include physical, historical, and interpersonal characteristics of the patient and the practitioner's response to the patient. **Physical characteristics** of the patient include (1) multiple tattoos, especially "jail-house" tattoos, which generally are of poor quality and completed by nonprofessional tattoo artists or the patient; and (2) "biker" or otherwise nonconformist appearance modeled after groups known to approve or sanction violence or disregard for the rights of others. **Historical characteristics** include (1) multiple injuries or scars not explained by occupation or involvement in sports and (2) unstable lifestyle. **Interpersonal characteristics** include an ingratiating interaction style, (2) entitled attitude with frequent demands, (3) superficial charm with overall functioning and level of success well below the level anticipated on the basis of perceived level of intelligence, (4) references in the interview to prison time or use of prison slang (e.g., "the man," "snitches," "hooch," "the joint,"), (5) unsolicited statements that "I'm telling you the truth, doc!" and (6) statements suggesting a pattern of projecting blame onto others. Examples of such statements include, "Yeah, doc, those doctors in the pen, they're not like you, they don't know what they're doing. They never told me I shouldn't drink . . . smoke . . ." or "yeah, they really screwed up" or "yeah, those fast food restaurants, they really ought to be sued by somebody . . . it is their *fault* we all got this cholesterol problem."
The **practitioner's responses** often include:
1. A perception that the patient's complaints or requests are manipulative, including an uncomfortable feeling that the patient is seeking drugs. Suggestive evidence includes an unusual degree of knowledge about pain medication, a request for *specific* addictive medication, vague responses to questions about prior treatment providers, or subjective complaints justifying addictive medication without supportive physical findings.
2. Suspicion that the patient is not being truthful about the medical history. This suspicion may be based on inconsistencies in the patient's report, vague answers to many questions, or an irritable, defensive response to detailed questioning.
None of these clues are pathognomonic for the diagnosis of antisocial personality disorder. They are sufficiently suggestive to warrant particular notice and consideration of more detailed questioning, special precautions, or external validation of history before implementing treatment.

3. How common is antisocial personality disorder?
It is estimated that 4% of men and 1% of women meet criteria for a diagnosis of antisocial personality disorder.

4. What is a psychopath? What is a sociopath? Are these terms synonymous with antisocial personality disorder? What is the diagnostic reliability of antisocial personality disorder?
Currently the terms psychopath, sociopath, and antisocial personality disorder are loosely used synonymously. This usage is unfortunate because it fosters poor communication and poor diagnostic

reliability. Historically, the term psychopath referred to people with a wide range of problems, including not only antisocial behaviors but also depressed mood and histrionic behaviors. The term sociopath, as delineated by Cleckley,[3] includes the following traits: superficial charm, low anxiety, irresponsibility, insincerity, lack of remorse, impulsiveness, egocentricity, and a failure to learn from experience. Cleckley's trait-based description of sociopathy was incorporated into the DSM II criteria in 1968. However, because the criteria were based on traits rather than behaviors, they were not diagnostically reliable. A trait approach requires the diagnostician to determine absolutely the presence or absence of qualities such as irresponsibility and insincerity in an either/or and all/nothing fashion. However, in actuality, traits such as irresponsibility and insincerity reflect a continuum of behaviors rather than a dichotomy. In contrast to DSM II, the DSM IV criteria are behaviorally anchored, resulting in considerably increased diagnostic reliability. For example, it is difficult for a clinician to determine whether one is or is not "irresponsible" but relatively easy to determine whether one has or has not failed to honor financial obligations or provide regular child support. Although clinicians can diagnose reliably the presence or absence of a personality disorder, they are not able to distinguish reliably between the different personality disorders. Because of its behavioral anchors, however, the diagnosis of antisocial personality disorder has the highest diagnostic reliability of all personality disorders.

5. Discuss the differential diagnosis of antisocial personality disorder.

Antisocial personality disorder must be differentiated from antisocial behavior. Antisocial behavior may be committed intermittently by many people without mental disorders or may be a symptom of another disorder. To differentiate between antisocial behavior and antisocial personality disorder it is necessary to consider whether the patient meets criteria for a personality disorder. Patients must demonstrate a pervasive, enduring, and inflexible antisocial pattern of perceiving, relating to, and thinking about themselves, others, and their environment.

Although antisocial personality disorder, not unexpectedly, is represented disproportionately in prison populations, a pattern of criminal behavior (beginning before or after age 15) is insufficient to make the diagnosis. Studies of prison populations have reported prevalence rates of antisocial personality disorder as low as 40% and as high as 75%. Prisoners without antisocial personality disorder may include "professional criminals," those involved in organized crime, and one-time offenders. Many such persons clearly disregard the rights of others and may have no remorse for their harmful effects. However, if they are neither aggressive nor impulsive, they probably do not meet criteria for antisocial personality disorder.

Criminal or antisocial behavior is commonly associated with substance use disorders. Correlations between the diagnoses of antisocial personality disorder and alcohol or other substance abuse or dependence are statistically significant. The presence of one of the three diagnoses increases the probability of the presence of the others. Despite this association, the diagnosis of antisocial personality disorder should not be given if criminal behavior and other antisocial behavior occur only in the context of addiction.

Specific symptoms of antisocial personality disorder are associated with many psychiatric disorders. Patients with schizophrenia, mania, sexual perversions, mental retardation, organic brain syndromes, and other personality disorders (including narcissistic personality disorder) may demonstrate some but not all features of antisocial personality disorder. For example, patients with schizophrenia, mental retardation, and organic brain syndromes are likely to demonstrate impaired occupational and parental functioning. All of these disorders are sometimes associated with impulsive acts, including repeated unlawful behavior. Sometimes such impulsive acts may be associated with lack of remorse. For example, sex offenders may not experience remorse with regard to their sexual victims because of false beliefs that their behavior is not harmful or in fact is desired by the victim. At times, only the absence of symptoms of a conduct disorder as a child clarifies that the patient does not have antisocial personality disorder.

6. What is the cause of antisocial personality disorder?

Antisocial personality disorder is likely the result of the interaction among multiple factors, including individual vulnerabilities and environmental stressors. Individual vulnerabilities include characteristics that have been correlated with antisocial personality disorder such as low intelligence and impulsivity. Impulsivity may be the result of a biologic predisposition, learning, or both. Environmental stressors include low socioeconomic status, antisocial and other poor parenting, academic failure, delinquent siblings or peers, and substance abuse.

The many proposed etiologies of antisocial personality disorder reflect a variety of theoretical paradigms. A biologic model suggests a genetic vulnerability. Adoptee studies have found higher rates of criminality and sociopathy in biologic opposed to adopted relatives of criminal or sociopathic individuals. EEG studies have found a high frequency of abnormalities in sociopaths.

Despite the various theories, a behaviorally based developmental theory of antisocial behavior is presented here. This theory is empirically anchored and has generated interventions, primarily prevention, with demonstrated success. Patterson et al.[6] hypothesized the following sequence in the etiology of antisocial behaviors. First, parents teach their children antisocial behavior through inappropriate and inconsistent parenting. Inappropriate parenting may occur when the parent positively reinforces the child for antisocial acts. For example, the parent may laugh or praise the child when the child hits another. Inconsistent parenting may occur when the parent negatively reinforces the child. For example, a mother asks her son to clean his room (an example of responsible goal-directed behavior). Like most children, he does not comply immediately, so the mother asks again. The child throws a tantrum. The mother experiences his tantrum as aversive and stops asking him to clean his room. Thus the child is negatively reinforced for his tantrum; in other words, when he throws a tantrum, the mother stops asking him to be responsible. The mother also learns that if she does not ask her child to be responsible, he will not throw a tantrum. Thus the child learns to use aversive behavior to avoid responsibility.

The second step in the development of antisocial behavior occurs when the child begins school. Aversive behavior leads to a predictable social outcome: the child is rejected. He or she does not following instructions, is unable to complete a task on time, and does not cooperate with others. The child lacks the skills to do well academically and thus may fail to learn to read or compute math. Such failures have dire consequences for occupational and social future. Step three of the inexorable sequence occurs when after being rejected, the child gravitates towards deviant peer groups. Such peers are likely to provide positive feedback for antisocial behaviors and punishment for prosocial behaviors. Studies suggest that about 50% of children who have demonstrated antisocial behavior maintain antisocial behavior through adolescence and that 50–75% of adolescents who have demonstrated antisocial behavior maintain antisocial behavior through adulthood.

7. What is the prognosis for the patient with antisocial personality disorder?

Impairment is the rule, although it may range from mild to severe. Not uncommonly, professionals or laypersons refer to various prominent persons, such as politicians, as "sociopaths." Sociopathic qualities such as disregard for the truth and lack of remorse are perhaps present in many individuals drawn to positions of national recognition or power. However, economic or political success is unlikely if a person truly meets criteria for antisocial personality disorder. Characteristics of antisocial personality disorder such as early onset, related impairment in educational achievement, impulsivity, and aggression generally preclude success.

Impairment due to the disorder is frequently severe. Typically, such individuals fail to become independent, experiencing years of institutionalization, usually penal rather than medical. Although estimates vary, such individuals appear significantly more likely to die prematurely as a result of suicide, homicide, or complications of drug or alcohol abuse.

Although people who meet criteria for antisocial personality disorder are at risk of early death, the prognosis for those who live to middle-age is somewhat encouraging. Spontaneous improvement with age appears to be the rule rather than the exception. In one large study, 50% of adults who met criteria for antisocial personality disorder at some point in their lives had experienced the first symptom by age 9; 80% experienced a symptom by age 11. One-half of adults no longer met criteria for the disorder by age 29; 80% recovered by age 45. The median duration of symptoms was 20 years.

8. What kind of difficulties do professionals have with patients diagnosed with antisocial personality disorder?

Health care professionals frequently experience the following problems with patients diagnosed with antisocial personality disorder: (1) difficulty in collecting reliable history, (2) difficulty in managing the patient, (3) conflict between responsibility to the patient and responsibility to society, and (4) because of the conflict, negative feelings such as anger, boredom, and hopelessness.

The dishonesty of patients with antisocial personality disorder makes it difficult to collect reliable history. Inconsistency or vagueness is a clue that the patient may be lying. Nonverbal cues include stammering, short answers, hesitations, excessive blinking, dilated pupils, and excessive touching of clothing. The patient is likely to blame the clinician who questions inconsistencies (e.g., "aren't you listening?" "you heard that wrong," "I didn't say that," or "use your head, doc"). In such situations, straightforward delineation of the costs and benefits of presenting an accurate history is useful. Patients with antisocial personality disorder respond best to an approach based on self-interest. Fortunately, they typically have the capacity and motivation to discuss honestly their physical history (in contrast to social or occupational history).

Keys to the second difficulty, difficulty in management, include the following:

1. It is the patient's responsibility to deal with the consequences of antisocial behavior.
2. The clinician must set clear expectations regarding acceptable behavior.
3. The clinician must take a nonjudgmental stance and objectively help the patient to consider the costs and benefits of his or her behavior to self.

For example, the patient may wish to consider whether the benefits of denigrating nursing staff (reduction in tension) outweigh the costs (probable reduction in care). Given the patient's difficulty appreciating any point of view other than his or her own, it is more effective to emphasize the effects on self than on others.

The health care provider also may experience conflict between responsibility to the patient and responsibility to the patient's dependents or society. Informing the patient of the limits of confidentiality at the onset of treatment helps to ameliorate such problems. For example, the patient should be informed that the clinician will be unable to maintain confidentiality if the patient threatens to harm self or others, or reveals plans to commit a crime. Similarly, the patient should be informed that the clinician is unable to maintain confidentiality if the patient reports physical abuse or neglect of a child or, in some states, an elderly person. Before breaking confidentiality, the clinician is well advised to consult. Consultation not only provides information but also enables the clinician to wear one rather than multiple hats. For example, in the case of mandated reporting of child abuse, by consulting with specialists in psychiatry and social work the clinician avoids the potentially conflicting roles of investigator, therapist, and physician. Data indicating that hospital personnel report less than 50% of child abuse cases suggest a conflict between medical and social responsibilities.

The above difficulties may result in the fourth difficulty: the health professional may experience negative feelings such as anger, boredom, hopelessness, and hatred toward the patient. Whereas it is the patient's responsibility to deal with the consequences of his or her behavior, the provider must deal appropriately with her or his own feelings. The clinician's perusal of police reports may result in anger, fear, or horror. Some clinicians avoid reading police reports for fear that such feelings may prevent them from providing adequate care. As a result of the marked tendency of patients with antisocial personality disorder to project blame and responsibility, the clinician may experience guilt, impotence, and hopelessness. It is important, particularly for the introspective health care provider, to study the patient's behavior, not his or her own. Finally, it is important to recognize that feelings of apathy or boredom may shield more intense feelings. Signs that clinicians may be acting out their feelings inappropriately include forgetting appointments and other commitments, colluding with staff in denigrating the patient, colluding with the patient in denigrating staff, giving the patient special consideration, or giving the patient less than appropriate consideration.

9. What are the guidelines for management of medical conditions in patients with antisocial personality disorder?

1. Err on the side of caution. If anyone (clinician, spouse, colleague, or support personnel) expresses concern about personal safety, whether based on clearcut logic or "gut" feeling, evaluate the patient with a chaperone present.

2. The clinician at times will be required to evaluate patients in restraints or chains. The patient should be evaluated as thoroughly as possible with restraints in place. If adequate assessment is not possible, adequate security personnel should be obtained before removal of restraints and completion of physical examination. The clinician should defer security assessment decisions to security personnel. The clinician must not try to be a hero.

3. The clinician should consider a diagnosis of malingering (exaggeration or complete fabrication of symptoms for secondary gain). For example, the patient may wish to avoid work, military conscription, or prison time or to obtain financial gain, disability payments, or drugs. Clinicians should ask themselves, "Why is this patient in my office right now?" "What does this patient really want?"

4. The clinician should be cautious in prescribing medication and avoid prescription of addictive medications when possible. When such medications are prescribed, the clinician must be explicit and write out exactly how much is to be dispensed—e.g., "dispense 4 (four)." The clinician must think, "Is this written in such a way that the patient could alter what the pharmacy dispenses?" "No refills" should be specified. If the clinician follows a patient with antisocial personality disorder or antisocial symptoms, precise amounts should be prescribed from visit to visit. The patient should be notified that the clinician will not provide extra prescriptions if they are "lost," "stolen," or "accidentally flushed down the toilet."

CONTROVERSY

10. Is antisocial personality disorder a treatable condition?

Against:

1. Prior comprehensive, costly programs in which offenders were diverted to secure treatment facilities rather than prison demonstrated no sufficient improvement or decrease in recidivism to warrant the cost to society.

2. Psychiatric or psychological treatment of individuals with antisocial personality disorder is a poor allocation of financial and social resources.

3. Psychiatric or psychological treatment of incarcerated individuals is coercive, unethical, and unconstitutional.

For:

1. Previous treatment outcome studies of patients with antisocial personality disorder involve significant methodologic problems: (1) Few outcome studies identified subjects by DSM-III or DSM-III-R criteria; (2) no studies in which diagnostic criteria were well-defined employed nontreated control group; and (3) although expert opinion supporting the lack of benefit of individual psychodynamic treatment is pervasive, no information in the literature addresses outcome for patients with antisocial personality disorder treated with other modalities for an extended time in a forensic setting. Schizophrenia does not respond to psychodynamic psychotherapy but is generally agreed to be a treatable condition. Depression does not generally improve with psychoanalysis but often responds to cognitive therapy, antidepressant medication, or a combination of the two.

Studies of treatment outcome with conduct-disordered children, who may potentially become adults with antisocial personality disorder, suggest that antisocial personality disorder can be prevented. Parent-management training, cognitive therapy, and court-diversion appear to be promising approaches. In summary, conclusions about the treatability of antisocial personality disorder are premature; it is as scientifically valid to say that such patients are treatable as it is to say that they are not.

2. Patients with antisocial personality disorder have a significant risk of early death but also a good chance of spontaneous remission (or at least substantial improvement) if they live till age 30 or 35. At a minimum, this observation supports crisis intervention strategies aimed at decreasing the risk of early death and minimizing negative effects of antisocial behaviors on both the patient and others.

3. For unclear reasons, the standard for psychiatric medical conditions appears to equate "treatment" with "cure." Diabetes mellitus, coronary artery disease, and chronic obstructive pulmonary disease are only three of the many medical diseases that are "treatable" (i.e., morbidity and mortality can be reduced by medical interventions) but not currently "curable." Accurate assessment of treatability of antisocial personality disorder requires clear definition of the target symptoms to be reduced or relieved. Target symptoms may include prevention or treatment of violent death, aggression, substance abuse, impulsivity, or concomitant major mental disorders. Individuals with antisocial personality disorder have a 5–20-fold increased risk of experiencing concurrent mania, schizophrenia, and alcohol or drug abuse. Prognosis is improved by treatment of concurrent anxiety and depression. Treatment of such disorders may prolong life and decrease personal and societal damage while awaiting possible spontaneous remission.

BIBLIOGRAPHY

1. American Psychiatric Association: Diagnostic and Statistical Manual of Mental Disorders, 4th ed. Washington, DC, American Psychiatric Association, 1994.
2. Beck AT, Freeman A: Cognitive Therapy of Personality Disorders. New York, Guilford Press, 1990.
3. Cleckley H: The Mask of Sanity, 5th ed. St. Louis, Mosby, 1976.
4. Frances AJ, Hales RE (eds): American Psychiatric Association Annual Review, vol 5. Washington, DC, American Psychiatric Press, 1986.
5. Oltmanns TF, Neale JM, Davison GC: Case Studies in Abnormal Psychology. New York, John Wiley & Sones, 1991.
6. Patterson GR, DeBaryshe BD, Ramsey E: A developmental perspective on antisocial behavior. Am Psychol 44:329–335, 1989.
7. Reid WH: The antisocial personality: A review. Hosp Community Psychiatry 36:831–837, 1985.
8. Schubert DS, Wolf AW, Patterson MB, et al: A statistical evaluation of the literature regarding the associations among alcoholism, drug abuse, and antisocial personality disorder. Int J Addict 23:797–808, 1988.
9. Treatment outlines for antisocial personality disorder. The Quality Assurance Project. Aust N Z J Psychiatry 25:541–547, 1991.
10. Widiger TA, Corbitt EM, Millon TM: Antisocial personality disorder. APA Rev Psychiatry 11:63–79, 1992.

VI. *Therapeutic Approaches in Psychiatry*

40. PSYCHOANALYTICALLY ORIENTED PSYCHOTHERAPIES

James L. Jacobson, M.D., and Alan M. Jacobson, M.D.

1. Describe psychoanalytically oriented psychotherapy.

Psychoanalytically oriented psychotherapy (sometimes called psychodynamic psychotherapy) encompasses a group of psychotherapeutic approaches founded on the discoveries of Sigmund Freud and later refined and expanded by a number of other researchers, clinicians, and theoreticians. This group of approaches is based on the belief that current behavior, emotions, capacities for functioning, and patterns of relationship are deeply influenced by one's experiences throughout life. Initially attention was focused more on specific early developmental periods, although current analytic beliefs look at all developmental stages and processes.

Psychoanalytically oriented therapists believe that early developmental experiences continue to exert influence over later behavior and that such influences are often outside of normal awareness; that is, earlier life experiences continue to be retained in the unconscious mind as memories, expectations about relationships, beliefs about ourselves and the world around us, and mechanisms to control uncomfortable feelings, thoughts, and experiences from coming into the conscious mind. Such unconscious processes continue to be active in determining present feelings and actions. Simply put, the past shapes the present through forces that are sometimes known and sometimes not known. For example, one person may maintain a haughty, aloof attitude toward others that results in a painful lack of emotional closeness. In the course of therapy, it may be discovered that this way of relating was developed to protect the person earlier in life against a hostile relationship with a caregiver who may have been demeaning, imparting an inferior self-image. Hence, the person develops false superiority to protect from internal feelings of inferiority and aloofness to maintain distance from relationships that may be perceived as threatening to self-esteem.

Psychoanalytically oriented psychotherapy is a method of treatment that takes place through verbal interaction between patient and therapist in an effort to elucidate unconscious past forces that affect current emotions and actions. Intensive therapy often is paced at 1–2 sessions per week over several weeks to years. In psychoanalysis, the most involving approach based on psychodynamic principles, the course of treatment is often longer, with more frequent meetings (up to 4–5 times per week). This process allows the patient to reexperience with the analyst, in a deeply felt way, earlier emotional involvements. The bringing forward of past experiences and reexperiencing them in the present is called **transference**. Generally speaking most people are unaware of transference, although it frequently shapes the way in which they relate to other people.

Such unawareness is maintained by unconscious mental processes known as **defense mechanisms**. Although defense mechanisms are widely varied (e.g., repression of memory, denial, disconnection of emotion from event known as isolation, externalization of blame, internalization, and sublimation), their common purpose is to keep out of awareness potentially anxiety-provoking events and feelings. In psychoanalysis and in some forms of psychodynamic therapy the therapist or analyst interprets (i.e., comments on) defensive maneuvers in a spirit of gradually

uncovering their origins by expanding the patient's awareness of current (defensive maneuvers) and historical (origins) events. Through this process, the patient is helped to achieve a
broader range of options in behavior, emotions, and relationships. Because this process may
bring forth uncomfortable feelings and seemingly unacceptable thoughts, defense mechanisms
may be activated in the relationship with the therapist. Such mechanisms may present as apparent resistances, such as reactions to the therapist that lead to breaks in the free flow of discussion. In such cases, the therapist offers further commentary on the nature of the resistance,
which may lead to further understanding or insight into the difficulties in the interpersonal
relationship.

Through repeated, successive interpretation and intense experience of the connection between current personal involvement, with both the therapist and other people, and past events,
the patient learns about the forces at work in his or her own behavior. Such understanding
then may lead to a broader choice of behavior and relief of emotional suffering. Hence, as unconscious sources of difficulties gradually emerge in the way the patient relates to the therapist or analyst, the therapist or analyst explains them to the patient over and over again in an
effort to expand understanding of unconscious forces. Such forces are demonstrated in daily
life, in work, in dreams, and in every human endeavor. The patient, in an intimate evolving relationship with the therapist or analyst, experiences increasingly deep emotional and intellectual understanding of such unconscious forces. As the patient becomes more aware of the
forces at work in shaping attitudes and relationships, he or she can compare previously unconscious perceptions with current experiences with the therapist. This comparison provides
an opportunity to gain control over the previously unknown impulses and defensive reactions,
leading to changes in the nature of feelings about oneself and in the quality of relationships
with others. The result is greater freedom to make choices in work and in establishing loving
relationships. Often, new developmental processes or the reestablishment of normal development ensues.

In practice, the original psychoanalytic understandings have been modified significantly.
Clinicians have come to recognize limitations and risks in pursuing psychoanalytic therapy, such
as overdependence on the clinician and increased anxiety and depression when previously unconscious information is brought to the surface. Analysis, in particular, is time-consuming and
usually costly. As a result, various alternatives have been derived from psychoanalysis. Some derivatives (e.g., supportive therapies) seek to strengthen existing defense mechanisms and to
expand the repertoire of defense to assist the patient in maintaining basic day-to-day functioning
instead of attempting to uncover unconscious origins. The decisions made in the therapeutic
process may be based on a similar understanding of unconscious process, although the goals and
intent are quite different in supportive psychotherapy.

2. Define transference and countertransference.
In its broadest form transference is bringing into a current life experience, such as an interpersonal relationship, the beliefs, expectations, and perceptions from previous relationships. In analytic therapy transference often refers to relationships from particular stages of development. For
example, a patient may see his wife in a similar way to the way he experienced one of his parents
during a particular time in childhood. Although there may be some similarity to the way his wife
behaves, the total perception is colored by the early experience; hence, this is termed a transference relationship.

Countertransference is a specific reaction of the therapist to the same types of phenomena.
Examples include feelings, thoughts, and attitudes that are reactions to specific events in therapy.
The therapist may experience such a reaction or feeling as being unlike him- or herself; this is
often a hint to the presence of a countertransference reaction. Both transference and countertransference can be elucidated to increase understanding of behavior and to assist in the progress of
therapy. If not addressed and commented on, such reactions may stall the therapeutic endeavor or
lead to negative reactions (e.g., the therapist gets angry at the patient or the patient prematurely
ends treatment because of strong emotional reactions).

3. How are dreams used in psychodynamic psychotherapy and analysis?

Dreams were initially seen by Freud as "the royal road to the unconscious." Dreams were thought to contain a direct view into the unconscious life of the individual. Thus dream interpretation was once considered the central method for understanding unconscious phenomena. Dream elements represent current life events as well as earlier life experiences and conflicts. Images in dreams are thought to be symbolic representations of such events and conflicts. Although dreams still play an important role in psychodynamic psychotherapy, they are now seen as one of many sources of information about hidden wishes and fears that are relevant to both current and past functioning. The therapist or analyst may focus on current concerns manifested by the content of the dream or on representations of the past. The therapist may ask a patient to associate (i.e., let the mind wander and freely react to different thoughts or feelings) to the dream as a whole or the different elements of the dream to unmask and elaborate what the symbols in the dream represent. Such thoughts or associations are termed the latent content.

Current analytic thought places as much or perhaps more emphasis on transference than on dreams as the royal road to the unconscious. Other phenomena that help to elucidate unconscious processes include slips of the tongue (known as parapraxis), fantasies, daydreams, resistance, and virtually any recurrent way of relating in life.

4. What are defense mechanisms?

Freud's initial theory of personality placed importance on conflict between the desire for gratification of basic instincts and the need to control unwanted or dangerous pressure for gratification of instincts. Instincts may be thought of primarily as aggressive and sexual. The methods of control, termed defense mechanisms, regulate such inner urges. Defense mechanisms are conceptualized as part of a process called the ego or the "I." Originally Freud conceptualized repression as the ego's central mechanism of defense, although various defense mechanisms are now recognized. Repression refers to the mechanism by which internal urges, thoughts, and feelings and memory of events are "forgotten." They are contained in unconscious (or repressed) memory. The repressed is not recognized, but the effects of what has been repressed may remain. For example, a person may "forget" or repress a traumatic event yet retain an emotion that he or she cannot connect to a particular event. Inexplicable sadness unattached to a particular memory is one example. Other mechanisms of defense include denial, altruism, intellectualization, projection, internalization, and sublimation. Each mechanism represents a somewhat different method of dealing with unacceptable thoughts, feelings, wishes, or events. Although such defensive operations occur largely outside the individual's awareness, they become manifest as types of behavior in all relationships, including the therapeutic relationship. The therapist helps the patient to understand such defensive maneuvers as ways of dealing with unacceptable memories, thoughts, and feelings; therefore, the individual becomes more aware of the influence of unconscious defenses on everyday functioning and, with the therapist's help, may change behavioral patterns.

5. Who is treatable with psychoanalysis or psychoanalytic psychotherapy?

In assessing who will benefit from psychoanalysis or psychoanalytic therapy, the clinician must assess the patient's relative strengths and capabilities as well as relative weaknesses and difficulties. Psychoanalysis or psychoanalytic psychotherapy are not specifically indicated or contraindicated by particular psychiatric disorders. Psychoanalytic psychotherapy is not a specific treatment for depressive illness, bipolar illness, schizophrenia, or personality disorder. Rather, the individual who may benefit from psychoanalytic psychotherapy may suffer long-standing symptoms such as depressed mood, anxiety, and repetitive patterns of behavior that result in a sense of limited choices and enjoyment. The person's capacities may be thwarted by his or her own actions, or the person may sense that he or she is falling short or be disappointed with the outcome of behavior and ways of relating. The person may sense difficulty in being spontaneous or feeling close to others. There may also be a sense of inordinate suffering. Concurrently there must be adequate psychological and emotional strength to endure the explorations of psychoanalytically oriented therapy. For example, the person must have demonstrated some capacity to achieve, such as history of satisfaction in relationships with friends or work. The capacities to form relationships, to self-observe, and to contain strong feelings adequately are also strengths that may aid in the psychotherapeutic process. The psychoanalyst or therapist assesses specific patterns of defensive functioning and the nature of relationships to evaluate the required sturdiness and the degree of symptoms that would motivate someone to pursue and succeed in therapy oriented toward exploring unconscious forces behind current problems. Exploratory and exposing approaches demand considerable resilience as well as support from the clinician.

6. Are risks associated with exploratory psychoanalytic psychotherapy or analysis?

Yes. As with any treatment, risks are involved. Dynamic analytic therapy is often anxiety-provoking because of its attempt to take away the comforting defensive operations used by the patient to cope with unwanted feelings. Therefore, such unwanted feelings may gradually emerge into awareness. The therapist must first determine whether the patient is prone to impulsive actions that may be quite dangerous if anxiety-provoking feelings and instincts become more accessible. Likewise, the therapist must assist in managing the expression of such impulses. The therapist balances with the patient the goal of uncovering unconscious elements against the need to maintain current emotional stability. Along similar lines, psychoanalytically oriented psychotherapy is designed to promote a transitory regression in which the patient experiences earlier ways of relating to people. Regression by definition means returning to a former state. Earlier states of development may be painful to experience and lead to behavior that is no longer appropriate. The result may be transient functioning that is less adaptive. For example, a patient may reexperience the full force of a humiliating experience with his or her father and hence be left more vulnerable. A criticism from a supervisor may be felt as humiliating and responded to angrily or by quitting work. Furthermore, such regression may persist and lead to chronic over dependence on the therapist.

7. Differentiate exploratory (or uncovering) versus ego supportive approaches.

The psychodynamic framework includes therapies that are deemed more or less uncovering of unconscious motives and experiences. The use of psychoanalytic understanding to strengthen rather than diminish defenses is called ego supportive psychotherapy. Some of the techniques of supportive psychotherapy are similar to those used in cognitive and behavioral therapies (see chapters 41 and 42). One particularly well-defined method of therapy, which is based in part on psychodynamic principles, was developed by Klerman and Weissman and has been termed interpersonal psychotherapy. This approach is one commonly used and well-described method of short-term dynamic psychotherapy that contains supportive therapy principles.

8. Describe interpersonal psychotherapy.

Interpersonal psychotherapy was designed as a short-term treatment model for patients with depression and has been empirically evaluated in a series of studies. A manual provides therapists with a basis of understanding the methods and techniques of this model of therapeutic intervention in a consistent, reproducible fashion. Interpersonal therapy focuses primarily on the social roles and interpersonal interactions in the patient's past and current life experiences. Although it focuses on the entire life span, including early life experience and personality patterns, the interpersonal therapist places a clear emphasis on current factors. Particular emphasis is placed on a patient's disappointment in personal role expectations as well as disputes and problems in relationships. The interpersonal therapist helps to direct the patient to one or two problem areas in current functioning. Such problem areas become the primary focus of the therapy. Examples include grief over a loss; disputes in marriage, family, and work; role transitions such as retirement or job demotion; and loss through divorce. In other words, the focus is a current developmental process. Although the interpersonal therapist recognizes the importance of defense mechanisms, he or she does not attempt to address internal conflict as a source of current problems. Instead, behaviors and emotions are examined as they relate to current interpersonal problems.

Thus, the focus of interpersonal therapy, as a supportive approach, helps to build on current capacities to function rather than uncovers inner conflict. The primary focus is not enduring personality and character problems or earlier life experiences, although they may play a role in the development of a current bout of depression. The primary focus attempts to relieve the symptoms through reduction of grief and helping the patient to develop better strategies for dealing with current problems associated with the onset of depressive symptoms.

Comparison of Interpersonal Psychotherapy with Uncovering Analytic Psychotherapies

INTERPERSONAL PSYCHOTHERAPY	UNCOVERING ANALYTIC PSYCHOTHERAPIES
What has contributed to the patient's current depression?	Why did the patient become what he or she is and/or where is the patient going?
What are the current stresses?	What was the patient's childhood like?
Who are the key persons involved in the current stress? What are the current disputes and disappointments?	What is the patient's character?
Is the patient learning how to cope with the problem?	Is the patient cured?
What are the patient's assets?	What are the patient's defenses?
How can I help the patient to ventilate painful emotions and talk about situations that evoke guilt, shame, resentment?	How can I find out why this patient feels guilty, ashamed, or resentful?
How can I help the patient clarify his or her wishes and have more satisfying relationships with others?	How can I understand the patient's fantasy life and help him/or her to gain insight into the origins of present behavior?
How can I correct misinformation and suggest alternatives?	How can I help the patient discover false or incorrect ideas?

Adapted from Klerman G, Weissman M, Rovsanville B, Cherron E: Interpersonal Psychotherapy of Depression. New York, Basic Books, 1984.

9. How long do psychoanalytically oriented therapies take?

Therapeutic approaches range from short-term, well-defined therapies with specific focus, which may take as little as 2–8 sessions, to psychoanalysis, which may require 4 or 5 sessions per week for many years. Brief forms of treatment attempt to focus on specific current problems that result in an outbreak of particular symptoms, such as anxiety or depressed mood. The longer-term forms of psychoanalytic psychotherapy and psychoanalysis do not address only the source of current difficulty but attempt to understand and change basic long-held patterns of relating to others and feelings about oneself that have developed over the patient's lifetime. Hence, the goals of each particular form of therapy are related directly to the length of treatment. In addition, the longer forms of treatment involve the development of an intense interpersonal relationship, the elucidation of multiple aspects of that relationship, and the development of the personal strength and ability to move beyond that relationship. Hence, it may be viewed similarly to other important interpersonal relationships which enhance development, such as a parent, sibling, friend, grandparent, or mentor. The length of treatment is influenced, therefore, by the goals of therapy and the degree to which the primary focus is on the relationship between patient and therapist. Supportive psychotherapies also vary greatly in duration. Support through a specific life event (job change, divorce, grief over the death of a parent) may be approached in brief supportive therapy. On the other end of the continuum, long-standing therapeutic relationships may help to support *fragile* patients sufficiently to allow them to function at work and to avoid suicide attempts or costly hospitalizations.

10. Differentiate dynamic analytic therapies from behavior therapy.

In simple terms, behavior therapies attempt to modify observable behavior through various reinforcement strategies. For example, if an individual is afraid of snakes, behavioral therapy may define a gradual approach to desensitize the patient to his or her fear. This goal may be accomplished by having the patient learn a specific method of attaining a relaxed state, free of fear, and then introducing the idea of a common earthworm. Subsequently, a picture of an earthworm is followed by the idea of a common, nonthreatening snake, then by a picture, with gradual steps that may lead to viewing a snake in a contained environment such as the zoo. There is no focus on the origin or symbolic representation of the fear. In psychodynamic psychotherapy the therapist would focus on both. Thus, behavior therapy focuses on a strategy of managing a symptom without the necessity of understanding their meaning or origin. Psychodynamic psychotherapy places emphasis on understanding the meaning and origin of the symptom; management strategies are developed secondarily.

11. Are there uses of psychoanalytic principles other than for psychotherapy?
The psychoanalytic method in which the patient says everything that comes to mind in the context of an interpersonal relationship is both a method of psychotherapy and a tool for learning about human mental functioning. Based on such information, various theories of human mental functioning and normal development from infancy to old age have evolved. Hence, the school of psychotherapies also provide a tool for investigating inner life, a theoretical framework for human development, and a mechanism of viewing the functioning of the human mind.

From the more practical viewpoint, the principles of understanding derived from psychoanalysis can be used to understand patients' reactions to medical illness, compliance and adherence problems in outpatient medical and psychiatric practice, and also to gain a view of the complexities of human behavior as manifest in any form of clinical practice. It may well be that the psychodynamic perspective has its broadest application in understanding doctor-patient interchange rather than as a specific method for therapy. Indeed, clinicians using psychopharmacologic, behavioral, and other techniques can use this approach to enrich their understanding of the patient.

BIBLIOGRAPHY

1. Balint M, Balint E: Psychotherapeutic Techniques in Medicine. London, J.B. Lippincott, 1961.
2. Greenson RR: The Technique and Practice of Psychoanalysis, vol. 1. New York, International University Press, 1967.
3. Haley J: Strategies of Psychotherapy. New York, Grune & Stratton, 1963.
4. Jacobson AM, Parmelee DX: Psychoanalysis: Critical Explorations in Contemporary Theory and Practice. New York, Brunner/Mazel, 1982.
5. Klerman G, Weissman M, Rovsanville B, Chevron E: Interpersonal Psychotherapy of Depression. New York, Basic Books, 1984.
6. Mann J: Time-Limited Psychotherapy. Cambridge, MA, Harvard University Press, 1973.
7. Menninger K: Theory of Psychoanalytic Technique. New York, Harper & Row, 1958.
8. Sloane RB, Staples FR, Cristol AH, et al: Psychotherapy Versus Behavior Therapy. Cambridge, MA, Harvard University Press, 1975.
9. Wachtel PL: Psychoanalysis and Behavior Therapy. New York, Basic Books, 1977.
10. Stern DN: The Interpersonal World of the Infant. New York, Basic Books, 1985.
11. Rothstein A: Models of the Mind. New York, International Universities Press, 1985.
12. Vaillant GE (ed): Ego Mechanisms of Defense: A Guide for Clinicians and Researchers. Washington, DC, American Psychiatric Press, 1992.

41. COGNITIVE THERAPY

Jacqueline A. Samson, Ph.D.

1. What is cognitive-behavioral therapy?

The techniques of cognitive-behavioral therapies are based on the premise that dysphoric emotions arise from faulty cognitive processing that selectively filters incoming information. One identifies faulty processing by examining "automatic thoughts"—spontaneous thoughts that occur throughout the day or following specific events. Treatment takes the form of helping the patient to become aware of his or her automatic thoughts and the underlying assumptions. The patient is then encouraged to seek evidence by which to support or refute the assumptions and to modify assumptions based on a more balanced view of all available information.

For example, one depressed patient reported to her cognitive therapist that she felt sad over the weekend. In reconstructing the events of the weekend, she noted that the sadness began during a telephone call on Saturday morning from an old friend. The therapist then encouraged her to remember the conversation and the point at which she first felt sadness. She remembered that her friend Sarah was discussing her plans to take a vacation but did not invite the patient to come along. The patient then remembered her first "automatic" thought: "Sarah doesn't want me along because I'm no fun." Her next thought was, "Nobody wants to be with me. I have no friends." She then thought, "I will be alone for the rest of my life." Gloomy thoughts indeed! The patient's thoughts began with her first reaction to the news of Sarah's vacation. When the therapist asked the patient to examine the evidence for her assumption that Sarah did not want to be in her company, she had to say that there was no evidence; the fact that Sarah called indicated that Sarah enjoyed her company. Once the distortion in the automatic thought was worked through, the patient felt more hopeful about the future and was able to say that she might ask Sarah if they could plan to do something together soon.

2. What is the cognitive triad?

The cognitive triad refers to negative biases that are characteristic of depressed patients. The first component consists of the patient's tendency to view him- or herself in a negative light and to assume excessive responsibility for failures or negative experiences. The second component consists of the patient's tendency to view his or her world in a negative light and as presenting obstacles that cannot be overcome. The third component consists of the tendency to view the future negatively, consisting only of more failures and insurmountable obstacles.

3. What are the main types of cognitive processing errors that contribute to maintaining negative biases?

In general cognitive errors involve (1) making predictions about the future or how others will behave without sufficient evidence; (2) selectively focusing only on information that is consistent with one's expectations and ignoring information that runs counter to expectations; (3) assuming too much responsibility for negative events without acknowledging the contributions made by others or the situation; and (4) seeing situations as all or none and failing to acknowledge partial successes or progress.

Cognitive Processing Errors

1. **Emotional reasoning:** A conclusion or inference based on an emotional state; i.e., "I feel this way; therefore, I *am* this way."
2. **Overgeneralization:** Evidence drawn from one experience or a small set of experiences to reach an unwarranted conclusion with far-reaching implications.

Table continued on the following page.

Cognitive Processing Errors (Cont.)

3. **Catastrophic thinking:** An extreme example of overgeneralization, in which the impact of a clearly negative event or experience is amplified to extreme proportions; e.g., "If I have a panic attack I will lose *all* control and go crazy (or die)."

4. **All-or-none (black-or-white; absolutistic) thinking:** An unnecessary division of complex or continuous outcomes into polarized extremes; e.g., "Either I am a success at this, or I'm a total failure."

5. **Shoulds and musts:** Imperative statements about self that dictate rigid standards or reflect an unrealistic degree of presumed control over external events.

6. **Negative predictions:** Use of pessimism or earlier experiences of failure to prematurely or inappropriately predict failure in a new situation; also known as "fortune telling."

7. **Mind reading:** Negatively toned inferences about the thoughts, intentions, or motives of another person.

8. **Labeling:** An undesirable characteristic of a person or event is made definitive of that person or event; e.g., "Because I *failed* to be selected for ballet, I am a *failure.*"

9. **Personalization:** Interpretation of an event, situation, or behavior as salient or personally indicative of a negative aspect of self.

10. **Selective negative focus (selective abstraction):** Focusing on undesirable or negative events, memories, or implications at the expense of recalling or identifying other, more neutral or positive information. In fact, positive information may be ignored or disqualified as irrelevant, atypical, or trivial.

11. **Cognitive avoidance:** Unpleasant thoughts, feelings, or events are misperceived as overwhelming and/or insurmountable and are actively suppressed or avoided.

12. **Somatic (mis) focus:** The predisposition to interpret internal stimuli (e.g., heart rate, palpitations, shortness of breath, dizziness, or tingling) as *definite* indications of impending catastrophic events (i.e., heart attack, suffocation, collapse, etc.).

Adapted from Thase ME, Beck AT: Overview of cognition therapy. In Wright JG, Thase ME, Beck AT, Ludgate JW (eds): Cognitive Therapy with Inpatients. New York, Guilford, 1993, pp 3–34.

4. How do patients learn to correct cognitive processing errors?

Patients learn to correct cognitive errors by working with a therapist who questions their logic. The therapist may use the socratic method and encourage the patient to identify errors in rational thinking by asking questions such as: "What is the evidence that this is true? What is the evidence that this is not true? Is there another way of looking at this?" Once alternative explanations have been generated, the therapist may collaborate with the patient to design a miniexperiment through which the patient may gather information by which to confirm, refute, or modify the assumption.

5. How does correction of cognitive errors result in mood change?

Although the exact mechanisms involved in clinical change are not known, it is hypothesized that the tendency to filter incoming information through a negative lens systematically excludes the positive information needed to maintain a balanced perspective. The process of change involves completing homework assignments. This is a critical step because it requires that the patient take concrete action to gather data (i.e., fill out daily activity monitoring forms). It is more likely that patients will follow through on such assignments if they understand the rationale of the treatment and if evidence of its usefulness is demonstrated in the initial therapy sessions (see question 1). This behavioral component to cognitive-behavioral therapy not only results in an increased activity level but also is likely to increase the patient's sense of self-efficacy. Once the patient becomes more active and is feeling somewhat empowered, opportunities for positive feedback from others increase. Mood improves as the negative cognitive biases are refuted by experience or evidence and the patient begins to see more options.

6. How is the role of the cognitive-behavioral therapist different from other more psycho-dynamically oriented therapists?

The cognitive-behavioral therapist takes an active, problem-oriented, and directive stance in the therapy relationship. Early in the relationship, the therapist assumes a direct teaching role and conveys the basic principles of cognitive therapy to the patient. In later sessions, the therapist assumes the role of coach, as the patient takes on more responsibility. Sessions are structured: the therapist and patient (1) jointly set an agenda, (2) briefly review the previous session, (3) review homework completed since the last session, (4) work on additional topics spurred by the homework or events of the week, (5) set up homework for the following week, and (6) end with a summary of the key points from the session. Throughout the session the therapist actively summarizes and highlights points as they occur and selectively pursues issues for further work.

Structure of a Typical Cognitive Therapy Session

1. Mood check
   Examine symptom severity scores from a questionnaire such as the
      Beck Depression Inventory.
2. Set the agenda
3. Weekly items
   • Review of events since last session
   • Feedback on reactions to previous session and review of key points
   • Homework review
4. Today's major topic
5. Set homework for next week
6. Summarize key points of today's session
7. Feedback on reactions to today's session

7. How many sessions are typically involved?

Protocols for cognitive therapy of depression and anxiety disorders are relatively brief (typically 12–20 sessions). It is expected that the patient will gradually master the skills of the method so that he or she may continue to monitor automatic thoughts and test assumptions independently after therapy termination. For patients with multiple diagnoses or comorbid personality disorders, more sessions may be needed to address target problems.

8. To what degree is early developmental experience examined in cognitive-behavioral therapy?

In general, cognitive-behavioral therapists are oriented toward the present and encourage patients to examine how present thoughts affect specific behaviors. Examination of a number of automatic thoughts may reveal recurring themes. Such themes may then be examined in more detail to understand core beliefs or "schemas" about oneself or the world that may be driving the thoughts. Although it is acknowledged that core beliefs are likely to have developed as a result of early experiences, it is not necessary to spend a great deal of therapy time exploring such experiences. Rather, the patient may be encouraged to write a brief autobiography outside the session from which likely links between schemas and early experiences may be drawn with the therapist in the next session. The therapist can help the patient to trace how the core beliefs may have evolved from painful early experiences and to see how they are understandable in that light. However, the emphasis is primarily on examining the ways in which old beliefs distort present thinking and behaviors and on developing an action plan for change.

9. Is there research evidence that cognitive therapy works?

Yes. A growing number of well-designed therapy studies have demonstrated that cognitive therapy is effective for patients with depression or anxiety disorders. Studies also show cognitive therapy to be as effective as antidepressant medication in mildly to moderately depressed patients. In patients with severe depressions, the evidence is mixed. Some studies show cognitive therapy to be equally effective as medication, whereas others show medication to be more effective. No clear evidence suggests that a combination of the two approaches is superior to either alone or that the combination is less effective than either alone.

Studies comparing cognitive therapy to psychodynamically oriented therapies have not been conclusive, partly because of differences in the length of the treatments and difficulties in establishing standardized treatment protocols.

10. How do relapse rates compare?
Follow-up studies find that 70–80% of patients treated with cognitive therapy alone continue to be well 2 years later. These rates are significantly higher than the maintenance rates in patients who are withdrawn from antidepressant medication after a comparable initial trial and equal to the rates in patients who continue on antidepressant medication.

11. Are there patients for whom cognitive therapy does not work?
Studies predicting outcome based on patient characteristics are only now being completed. Preliminary work suggests that patients who have borderline personality disorder or a great deal of difficulty forming a working alliance with the therapist may show poor response to a brief trial of cognitive therapy. However, such patients are also likely to show poor response to other forms of brief therapy. By and large, patients who have been diagnosed with bipolar depression or who show psychotic features have been excluded from research trials and are assumed to be less responsive to intervention with cognitive therapy alone.

BIBLIOGRAPHY

1. Beck AT: Depression, Causes and Treatment. Philadelphia, University of Pennsylvania Press, 1967.
2. Beck AT, Emery G: Anxiety Disorders and Phobias: A Cognitive Perspective. New York, Basic Books, 1985.
3. Beck AT, Rush AJ, Shaw BF, Emery G: Cognitive Therapy of Depression. New York, Guilford Press, 1979.
4. Beutler LE, Engle D, Mohr D, et al: Predictors of differential response to cognitive, experiential and self-directed psychotherapeutic procedures. J Consult Clin Psychol 59:333–340, 1991.
5. Dobson K: A meta-analysis of the efficacy of cognitive therapy for depression. J Consult Clin Psychol 57:414–419, 1989.
6. Elkins I, Shea T, Watkins J, et al: National Institute of Mental Health Treatment of Depression Collaborative Research Program. Arch Gen Psychiatry 46:971–982, 1989.
7. Evans M, Hollon SD, DeRubeis RJ, et al: Differential relapse following cognitive therapy and pharmacotherapy for depression. Arch Gen Psychiatry 49:802–808, 1992.
8. Fennell MJ: Depression. In Hawton K, Salkovskis PM, Kirk J, Clark DM (eds): Cognitive Behavior Therapy for Psychiatric Problems. A Practical Guide. New York, Oxford University Press, 1989, pp 169–234.
9. Hollon SD, DeRubeis RJ, Evans MD, et al: Cognitive therapy and pharmacotherapy for depression: Singly and in combination. Arch Gen Psychiatry 49:774–781, 1992.
10. Hollon SD, Shelton RC, Loosen PT: Cognitive therapy and pharmacotherapy for depression. J Consult Clin Psychol 59:88–99, 1991.
11. Thase ME, Beck AT: Overview of cognitive therapy. In Wright JG, Thase ME, Beck AT, Ludgate JW (eds): Cognitive Therapy with Inpatients. New York, Guilford, 1993, pp 3–34.

42. BEHAVIOR THERAPY

Garry Welch, Ph.D., and Alan Jacobson, M.D.

1. What is behavior therapy?

Behavior therapy is a scientifically based approach to the understanding and treatment of human problems. It arose from laboratory experiments of animal behavior conducted in the early 1900s and has developed since from a large body of clinical research and experience. The goals of behavior therapy are to improve daily functioning, to reduce emotional distress, to enhance relationships, and to maximize human potential. It first came into common use in the 1960s and is now applied to a wide range of human problems. Originally, the emphasis in behavior therapy was on overt, measurable behavior and the application of classical and operant conditioning principles. However, since the 1980s it has been expanded to include cognitive aspects that emphasize the role of inner mental processes and emotional states. In addition, a new consideration of the broader social context of behavior has developed. The focus of behavior therapy is therefore not only what we overtly do but also what we think and feel; all of these elements are influenced by the fundamental principles of learning.

2. To what problems is behavior therapy applied?

Behavior therapy has been used successfully in the treatment of a wide range of psychiatric disorders, notably anxiety disorders, eating disorders, addictions, conduct disorders, and sexual deviations. It also has been used to modify problematic behaviors in classrooms, psychiatric wards, and adult workshops; to assist with lifestyle change (e.g., weight control, smoking cessation); to improve interpersonal relationships (e.g., marital counseling); and to enhance self-growth. Poor compliance, severe comorbid conditions, and drugs that depress the central nervous system may interfere with behavior therapy.

3. How do operant and classical conditioning differ?

Behavior therapy draws heavily on principles derived from **classical (or pavlovian)** and **operant (or instrumental)** conditioning. Both forms of conditioning are important influences in daily life because they permit a rapid behavioral response and adaptation to inner changes and external events. Learning may occur through personal experience or the experience of others (i.e., through vicarious learning and modeling). Classically conditioned reflexes generally function to maintain internal bodily processes, and the conditioned responses that arise from this conditioning are stereotypic. Operant behaviors, on the other hand, are typically instrumental in managing the external environment. They involve skeletal muscles under voluntary control and the ongoing learning of a changing repertoire of new and varied behaviors.

4. Describe classical conditioning.

Classical conditioning involves the acquisition of new cues (or triggers) to "wired-in" physiologic reflexes. These reflexes, which function naturally to protect us and to maintain our inner physiologic state, are principally linked to the autonomic nervous system. They are found in many internal bodily systems and are triggered by specific, unconditioned stimuli. For example, a nausea-vomiting reflex typically occurs in response to the eating of overly rich, diseased, or poisonous food (this reflex helps to protect us from sickness). Classical conditioning occurs when a neutral stimulus that normally does not evoke a given reflex is paired repeatedly with the unconditioned stimulus that naturally provokes the reflex. Under such conditions, the neutral stimulus will take on the ability to evoke the reflex. For example, the nausea reflex in response to eating rich or poisonous food can become linked to the sight or smell of the food (or even just the thought of it). As another example, because nausea and sickness are side effects of chemotherapy treatment, cancer patients may develop anticipatory nausea on entering the hospital for treatment. This reflex results from prior classical conditioning of the nausea side-effect of chemotherapy treatment in the hospital.

5. Give examples of classically conditionable reflexes.

Many potential reflexes in the reproductive, muscular, respiratory, and circulatory systems can be classically conditioned. Of importance, the emotional components of reflexes (e.g., fear, pleasure, anxiety) can be conditioned as well as the physical components. In daily life, classical conditioning can be **adaptive** (e.g., it helps us learn quickly to avoid danger or unpleasantness) or **maladaptive**. For example, the normal adult response of sexual arousal and pleasant feelings with genital stimulation can become classically conditioned to inappropriate cues such as children (as in pedophilia) or nonanimate objects (as in fetishism).

Examples of Internal Reflexes and Conditioned Stimuli

Digestive system
  Vomiting and nausea in response to food poisoning (e.g., nausea on sight or smell of target food
Reproductive system
  Sexual arousal and pleasurable feelings in response to genital stimulation (e.g., arousal on viewing erotic books or videos)
Respiratory system
  Asthma attack in response to allergens (e.g., an asthma patient feels the beginning of an attack on seeing an allergy-producing cat enter the room)
Circulatory system
  Pounding heartbeat and anxiety produced by involvement in an auto accident on the freeway (subsequent fear and anxiety when driving in similar circumstances)
Muscular system
  Relaxation response to ingestion of alcohol (relaxation felt on pouring the first drink at home at the end of a tense day)

6. Describe important principles of classical conditioning that are used in behavior therapy.

Classically conditioned responses will be weakened and become less frequent (be **extinguished**) if the conditioned stimulus is not subsequently paired with the original unconditioned stimulus. **Generalization** occurs when similar stimuli evoke a similar conditioned response. For example, a child frightened by the barking of a large dog may develop an anxious, fearful response to all dogs. **Discrimination** occurs when the individual learns to respond differently to two similar or related stimuli. For example, the child frightened of dogs may subsequently learn that large dogs that bark aggressively are more dangerous than small, quiet dogs.

    Counter-conditioning occurs when a conditioned stimulus is paired with a new stimulus that produces an incompatible or opposite response. The original, problematic conditioned response is extinguished by this technique, and new, healthy conditioning is introduced simultaneously. For example, a patient with a spider phobia can be taught relaxation techniques and then in therapy be asked to recreate the relaxed feeling during simultaneous exposure to the anxiety-provoking spider stimulus. Under such conditions, the old conditioned anxiety response to spiders will weaken (extinguish). **Aversive counter-conditioning** is used to reduce problematic behaviors that are pleasurable. For example, an alcoholic patient may be given disulfiram (Antabuse) so that drinking alcohol becomes associated with nausea and unpleasantness, thereby helping to reduce the frequency of later drinking. **Covert conditioning** is classical conditioning that occurs through imagery techniques rather than actual (in vivo) experience.

7. Describe operant conditioning and its important principles.

In operant conditioning (also known as trial-and-error learning) behavior is shaped and modified by its **consequences**. Behavior that produces good effects becomes more frequent (positive reinforcement occurs), whereas behavior that produces bad effects becomes less frequent (negative reinforcement occurs). Learning occurs when the consequences are **contingent** (interpreted to be causally linked) on the operant behavior.

Of importance, behavior in operant conditioning is influenced by the **situational or antecedent cues** that precede it; any given operant behavior may produce good effects in one situation but bad effects in another. Thus we learn to discriminate between situations in which behavior may be rewarded or punished. For example, stepping on the gas pedal when driving a car produces good effects when traffic lights are green (the driver can proceed quickly with the intended journey) but bad effects when they are red (the driver may receive a speeding ticket or have a serious accident).

Shaping occurs when new, complex behaviors are learned through reinforcement of successive approximations of the desired goal behavior. **Discrimination** occurs when an individual learns to respond differently to two similar predictive cues through differential reinforcement (i.e., one predicts reinforcement and the other does not, or one predicts more reinforcement than the other). For example, a shopper may drive to store A rather than store B because he or she has learned that store A has better bargains. **Generalization** occurs when stimuli that resemble a predictive cue become cues to the operant behavior. For example, a child who learns to bang in a nail with a hammer may then enjoy hammering many objects that look like a nail. Understanding important situational cues and the negative or positive consequences of behavior are the two keys to understanding how operant behavior arises and is subsequently maintained, shaped, or extinguished.

8. Describe systematic desensitization.

Systematic desensitization, which is used principally in the treatment of phobias and obsessive-compulsive disorders, combines counter-conditioning with extinction. It can be carried out through patient imagination or (more effectively) in vivo. This approach reduces the conditioned anxiety response by pairing incompatible, positive feelings (e.g., relaxation, calm) with the original anxiety-provoking, conditioned stimulus. In systematic desensitization, the patient first learns relaxation techniques. Then a hierarchy of anxiety-provoking situations is identified by the therapist and patient to guide treatment planning. The patient is taught to rate the conditioned anxiety and fear he or she feels on a scale from 0 (e.g., no fear or anxiety) to 10 (e.g., extreme fear, panic) to provide immediate feedback during each treatment exercise. Then, in therapy and in homework, the patient is systematically exposed to graded levels of conditioned anxiety through imagination or in vivo. At each anxiety-provoking level, the patient pairs relaxed feelings and thoughts with the conditioned stimulus and endures the conditioned stimulus until the anxiety subsides to a low level. For example, a patient with a fear of flying may work through a hierarchy of fears by going through airport procedures before a flight, sitting in a plane, taking off, and then finally flying and landing. This process is often preceded by practice sessions in the office in which each phase is imagined along with a paired relaxation exercise. The aim of treatment is for the patient to feel little anxiety in the most difficult flying-related situations. Research has shown that the relaxation component of systematic desensitization is not always necessary for successful treatment.

9. Describe the use of exposure with response prevention in the treatment of simple phobias.

Exposure with response prevention for a simple phobia involves extinction of the conditioned anxiety reaction through enduring exposure to the feared phobic object. This strategy is combined with prevention of usual escape (avoidance) behaviors that provided reinforcement in the past through negative reward (i.e., relief from phobic anxiety). For example, if a patient with a spider phobia is exposed to pictures or thoughts of spiders without escape or avoidance, he or she will experience a gradual reduction of anxiety and fear as the presence of the unconditioned stimulus (the spider) persists. In therapy, patients are initially taught the rationale behind the treatment, receive specific exposure with response prevention treatments, practice homework assignments at fixed times, discuss homework with the therapist, receive new assignments, and carry out maintenance exercises in follow-ups if needed. For simple phobias, exposure in vivo is generally preferred to exposure through imagination of the phobic object. Exposure and cognitive restructuring approaches (used to overcome irrational fears and negative thoughts) have become the psychosocial treatments of choice for panic, agoraphobia, and social phobia (see chapters 14 and 15).

10. Name the essential elements of behavior therapy for obsessive compulsive disorder.

1. Behavioral assessment is carried out to identify the nature of obsessional thoughts and compulsive rituals and related fear and anxiety responses.

2. Gradual exposure in vivo to the problematic, conditioned stimuli (e.g., exposure to dirty objects for patients with fears of dirt and contamination) is based on a hierarchy drawn up by the patient and therapist. This exposure allows extinction of the conditioned anxiety response.

3. Response prevention is applied to obsessive rituals (e.g., compulsive hand-washing behaviors) used by the patient to alleviate anxiety after exposure to feared situation.

4. Faulty patient cognitions (self-talk) are modified.

5. Ongoing structured homework includes further exposure and response prevention assignments and correction of maladaptive self-talk.

11. Describe flooding.

In flooding patients are exposed in vivo or through imagination to their conditioned object of fear at the most anxiety-provoking level possible until the fear and anxiety responses have been extinguished. Flooding differs from systematic desensitization, in which graded levels of exposure are introduced. Furthermore, in flooding the therapist controls the exposure, whereas in systematic desensitization the patient determines progression through the hierarchy of conditioned fears. Flooding may be poorly tolerated by some patients because of the high level of unpleasant feelings. In vivo flooding is generally considered more effective than flooding through imagination.

12. What is the Premack principle?

If, as a precondition made in therapy, the patient must complete desired low-frequency behavior before high-frequency behavior can be carried out, the desired behavior will increase in frequency. For example, if an obese patient in behavior therapy for weight control contracts to complete a 20-minute walk each evening before sitting down to watch a favorite television show (something the patient does often), regular walking will increase in frequency and weight loss and health gains will be more likely to occur. The high-frequency behavior typically is pleasurable and provides positive reinforcement for the low-frequency behaviors. This principle is applied in many forms of behavior therapy.

13. What is the role of cognitive factors in behavior therapy?

An understanding of the role of cognitive factors in the development and maintenance of problem behaviors enables the therapist to identify cognitive distortions (negative self-talk and beliefs) arising from false assumptions or interpretations of life experiences and fear-inducing self-instructions. Cognitive interventions aim to teach the patient to recognize distortions of thinking and to replace them with more realistic, positive thoughts. They are particularly helpful in the treatment of anticipatory anxiety, demoralization, avoidance behaviors, and low self-esteem (see chapter 41).

14. What is assertiveness training?

Assertiveness training uses principles of operant reinforcement to improve social skills through shaping, modeling of appropriate social behaviors by the therapist, role rehearsal of new skills in therapy sessions, and patient homework assignments. Typical problems include poor refusal skills; difficulties with self-disclosure, expression of negative emotions, and giving or receiving criticism; and opening, maintaining, and closing conversations. Such deficits can be incorporated into a broader treatment plan for the presenting clinical problem. Treatment begins with a careful recording of the problematic social situations and the circumstances under which problem behaviors and thoughts arise. Patients are taught new social responses for each specific problematic social situation. Problem solving is used in reviews of patient homework exercises, and new goals are set as the patient progresses to more challenging social situations based on a previously agreed hierarchy of social difficulty. Reinforcement of the new social behaviors after mastery of problem situations may combine with newfound enjoyment of social activities to strengthen the frequency of new behaviors through positive reward.

15. Describe token economies and their use.

Token economies are based on the operant conditioning principles that positive reward of a desired behavior increases its frequency. Token economies often involve the use of behavior shaping (i.e., the selective reinforcement of successive approximations to the target behavior). All token economies have in common a clear definition of the appropriate behavior that the therapist wishes to promote and a contract with the patient that details the explicit rewards for carrying out desirable behaviors. Target behaviors may range from simple tasks related to feeding, personal hygiene, or politeness to complex social interaction behaviors that are the end result of a systematic behavior-shaping schedule. Token economies may be based on the use of primary reinforcers (e.g., food, drink) or secondary (or acquired) reinforcers (e.g., tokens, points, praise, smiles). Tokens or points are accumulated by the patient and exchanged for tangibles such as television time, toys, or privileges. Points or tokens also may be taken away for inappropriate behavior (negative punishment). Use or primary reinforcers such as food (e.g., candy) may be problematic as they can reach levels of satiation, whereas secondary rewards (e.g., tokens) cannot. Token economies have been used to promote adaptive, normal, or healthy behaviors in classrooms, adult day hospitals, sheltered workshops, and patient psychiatric settings; to help family functioning; and to promote individual self-development.

16. What is stimulus control?

Large numbers of stimuli from the environment and from within our bodies influence behavioral responses in any given situation and at a given point in time. Depending on past learning, significant stimuli may be (1) unconditioned or conditioned stimuli that produce classical responses, (2) discriminant stimuli that predict operant responses, or (3) stimuli that operate in both capacities. Treatment approaches based on stimulus control involve the identification of this array of antecedent stimuli through a careful behavioral assessment and implementation of strategies to limit their influence. Stimulus control approaches have been used notably in the management of obesity and smoking cessation. For example, obese patients are taught to recognize conditioned stimuli (from previous classical learning) and predictive stimuli (from previous operant learning) that may promote eating when the patient is not hungry. A patient who eats when depressed, bored, or angry is taught to recognize these cues and instructed to carry out healthier, incompatible behavior instead (e.g., go for a walk, phone a friend). Food also may be hidden from view outside of mealtimes and eating restricted to the dining table only (instead of while watching television or reading). The patient may be given specific exercises to slow down the rate of eating and to increase awareness of consumption. A slower eating speed with improved awareness of the pleasurable, hedonic value of food may reduce overall calorie intake. In addition, slower eating is thought to give the brain sufficient time to respond appropriately to rising blood glucose levels that provide feedback signals of satiety.

17. How does biofeedback work?

Biofeedback involves the use of specific machines that provide information (feedback) about variations in one or more of the patient's physiologic processes that are not ordinarily perceived (i.e., brain wave activity, muscle tension, blood pressure). Feedback over a period of time may help the patient to learn to control certain target physiologic processes (i.e., anxiety, muscle tension responses) through operant conditioning. For example, awareness of alpha wave patterns through a graphic representation of wave activity on a biofeedback monitor may help the patient to elicit a relaxation response (see chapter 46).

18. How is behavior therapy structured?

The foundation of behavior therapy is the initial behavior analysis, a process of careful documentation and recording of the specific conditions under which presenting problem behaviors arose and are maintained. Based on the behavioral analysis, a specific series of treatment tasks devised by the therapist and patient are implemented in therapy sessions and in regular patient homework. Because behavior therapy is highly goal-oriented, treatment goals are clearly spelled out for the patient, progress is assessed and discussed, and new goals are set for the next stage of treatment. Treatment gains are maintained with follow-up sessions and ongoing homework assignments. Through this process, behavior therapy reshapes the problem behavior in a more desirable direction. The treatment plan may include a microanalysis that focuses on the conditions surrounding th presenting clinical problem and a macroanalysis that relates the presenting problem to other broader problem areas (e.g., social skill deficits, marital problems).

19. What differentiates behavior therapy from psychodynamic therapy?

Although both approaches are based on careful and detailed collection of information about patient's problems, the psychodynamic therapist principally focuses on historical and early life experiences, parenting dynamics, enduring personality traits, and links between these and current life experiences and problematic emotions and behaviors. The behavior therapist focuses on the conditions surrounding current problematic behavior and past circumstances that may highlight maladaptive learning relevant to the current problems. In psychodynamic therapy the fundamental goal is to reshape the intrapsychic structure of the patient to produce favorable symptom change based on specific theories about the nature of early childhood nurturance experiences and parenting dynamics. In behavior therapy the goal is to improve problematic behaviors, cognitions, and emotions directly, through application of principles of classical and operant learning theory and cognitive therapy.

As in behavior therapy, information gathering is important in psychodynamic treatment as part of the continual exploration for new ideas and connections. Behavior therapy is highly structured and goal- and outcome-oriented, whereas the psychoanalytic therapist deliberately uses an unstructured approach to facilitate unexpected associations and to derive new information and insights into the causes of current problems. Techniques such as free association and dream analysis are similarly unstructured to produce new clinical insights into current problems.

Although behavioral and psychodynamic therapies differ markedly in theoretical basis and treatment approach, elements of each may be found in the other. For example, repeated discussion of anxiety-producing concerns in the comfortable environment of psychodynamic therapy sessions may lead to extinction of a conditioned anxiety response (as in systematic desensitization). In behavior therapy open-ended questions and chance discussions in unstructured parts of a treatment session may lead to important insights into the broader psychosocial context of specific problematic behaviors (e.g., the presence or marital or work difficulties that exacerbate problem behaviors).

BIBLIOGRAPHY

1. Baldwin JD, Baldwin J: Behavior Principles in Everyday Life. Englewood Cliffs, NJ, Prentice-Hall, 1981.
2. Emmelkamp PMG, Bouman TK, Scholing A: Anxiety Disorders. A Practitioner's Guide. Chichester, John Wiley & Sons, 1992.
3. Griest JH: Behavior therapy for obsessive compulsive disorders. J Clin Psychol 55:60–68, 1994.
4. Noyes R: Treatments of choice for anxiety disorders. In Coryell W, Winokur G (eds): The Clinical Management of Anxiety Disorders. New York, Oxford University Press, 1991.
5. Sloane R, Staples F, Cristol A, et al: Psychotherapy Versus Behavior Therapy. Cambridge, MA, Harvard University Press, 1975.
6. Wachtel P: Psychoanalysis and Behavior Therapy. New York, Basic Books, 1977.

43. PLANNED BRIEF PSYCHOTHERAPY

Mark A. Blais, Psy.D.

1. How did brief psychotherapy develop?

Freud was one of the first practitioners of brief psychotherapy. A review of his early cases reveals that he treated many patients in a span of weeks to months rather than years. Over time, as psychoanalytic theory became more complex, the goals of psychoanalysis became more ambitious, and the length of treatment increased greatly. As early as 1925 this trend had become a concern to some.

Alexander and French can be considered the true fathers of brief psychotherapy. Their book *Psychoanalytic Psychotherapy* outlined the first systematic attempt to develop a shorter and more efficient form of psychotherapy. Although not generally accepted in its time, this work laid the foundation for both psychoanalytic psychotherapy and modern brief psychotherapy.

The modern era of brief treatment began with the work of Malan and Sifneos, who, working independently, developed detailed brief psychoanalytic psychotherapies. At present, brief psychoanalytic psychotherapies are supplemented by several other effective time-limited treatments, such as Beck's cognitive therapy, Mann's "existential" psychotherapy, and Klerman's interpersonal treatment of depression.

2. How does brief psychotherapy differ from long-term psychotherapy?

Four dimensions are generally considered to be common to all brief therapies and are also seen as differentiating short-term or brief psychotherapies from the more traditional long-term therapies. These common dimensions include (1) the setting of a fixed time limit for the treatment, (2) holding to specific patient selection criteria, (3) using a treatment focus to limit the scope of the therapy, and (4) requiring increased activity by the therapist.

Summary of Selected Planned Brief Psychotherapies with Their Common Aspects

THERAPY SCHOOL	NUMBER OF SESSIONS	TYPE OF FOCUS	PATIENT SELECTION
Analytic			
Sifneos Anxiety suppressing	4–10	Crisis and coping	Fairly open, less healthy
Sifneos Anxiety provoking	12–20	Very narrow, Oedipal conflict and grief	Very selective, top 2–10% outpatients
Malan	20–30	Very narrow, similar to Sifneos	Responds to trial interpretation
Davanloo	1–40	Resistance and suppressed anger	Less healthy, top 30% outpatients
Existential			
Mann	12 exactly	Central issue and termination	Broad patient selection (passive-dependent)
Cognitive			
Beck	1–14	Automatic thoughts	Very broad, not psychotic
Interpersonal			
Klerman	12–16	Patient's interpersonal experience	Depressed patient, any level of health
Eclectic			
Budman	20–40	Interpersonal, developmental, and existential	
Leibovich	36–52	One borderline trait	Borderline outpatients

Adapted from Groves J: The short-term dynamic psychotherapies: an overview. In Ritan S (ed): Psychotherapy for the 90's. New York, Guilford Press, 1992.

Comparison of Brief and Long-term Therapy

BRIEF	LONG-TERM
Specific focused goals	Broad goals: "insight and character change"
Specific time frame	Time unlimited
Emphasizes patient selection	Down-plays patient selection
Here and now focus	Inner life, historical focus
Attempts to restore psychologic functioning quickly	Employs techniques which can cause increased psychological distress and temporary dysfunction
The therapist is active and directive	The therapist is nondirective; therapy unfolds
Uses between-session homework	Is mostly limited to the treatment hour

3. What is the best attitude for learning brief therapy?

1. From the start there must be a willing suspension of disbelief and cynicism about brief treatment. Trainees are frequently taught that quick improvement is suspect and likely represents a transient "flight into health." This can be a hard lesson to unlearn. Remember, brief therapy is not a fad, but rather a form of treatment developed and refined over many years, based upon clinical experience and treatment outcome studies.

2. Psychotherapy must be conceived of as time-limited. It must be recognized from the outset that therapy will end after a set number of sessions (or in some cases on a planned date). This can be difficult, particularly for therapists trained in long-term therapy, because this mindset has ramifications for all treatment decisions and requires a clinician to reconsider every intervention during the treatment.

3. The brief therapist should accept (and expect) that patients will return to therapy periodically across their life span. This perspective allows a brief therapist to focus on the patient's current difficulties rather then attempting a "total" lifelong cure.

4. For which patients is brief therapy appropriate?

Patient selection is an important (and distinguishing) part of brief therapy. Basically, patient selection is the art of finding the right patient with the right problem for brief psychotherapy. A two-session format is recommended for evaluating potential brief therapy patients. This format allows the clinician to conduct a complete psychiatric evaluation while also assessing the appropriateness of the patient for brief psychotherapy without feeling excessive time pressure.

5. Name some useful criteria for excluding or including a patient for brief psychotherapy.

Exclusion criteria are best seen as categories (either the condition is present or absent); if any is present, the patient should be considered a poor candidate for brief treatment. The brief therapy patient should *not be* (a) actively psychotic, including odd idiosyncratic thinking which is not severe enough to require antipsychotic medication; (b) currently abusing substances (if there is a history of substance abuse, a detailed evaluation of recovery, and current support systems, should be undertaken because brief therapy can be stressful and may put recovery at risk); and (c) at significant risk for self harm with either current active suicidal ideation or a past history of suicide attempt.

Inclusion criteria are best viewed as dimensions, and as such they are likely present to a varying degree in every patient. The more of these qualities a patient has, the better the candidate for brief psychotherapy. The potential candidate for brief therapy should (a) be in moderate emotional distress; (b) want relief from pain; (c) be able to articulate a fairly specific formulation of their problem; (d) have a history of at least one positive mutual interpersonal relationship; (e) still be functioning in at least one area of life (work or love); and (f) have the ability to commit to a treatment contract.

Patient Selection Criteria for Brief Therapy

Exclusion criteria
The candidate should **not** be:
(these are categories)
    Actively psychotic
    Abusing substances
    At significant risk for self harm

Inclusion criteria
The candidate should:
(not all required, but the more the better)
    Be in moderate emotional distress
    Want relief from pain
    Be able to articulate or accept a specific cause or circumscribed problem as a focus of treatment
    Have a history of at least one positive mutual interpersonal relationship
    Be functioning in at least one area of life, and
    Have the ability to commit to a treatment contract

6. How does the brief therapist focus the treatment?

Developing a treatment focus is probably the most misunderstood aspect of brief therapy. Many writers talk about "the focus" in a mysterious and circular manner. It often appears as if the whole success of the treatment rests on finding the *one* correct focus. Rather, what is needed for a successful brief treatment is the establishment of a "functional focus;" that is, a focus on which both the therapist and patient can agree to work.

7. How is this established?

One powerful technique for finding a functional focus is the "Why now?" question used by Budman and Gurman (1988). This technique is straightforward. It is applied by repeatedly asking the patient ("Why did you come for treatment now?" "Why are you here now?") rather than last week or tomorrow (you really need to try this simple technique a few times to see how effective it can be).

For example, a male patient **(Pt)** presents to a therapist **(Th)** in a walk-in clinic with significant depressive symptoms.

Th   "I hear from what you say that you are depressed and are feeling terrible, but I wonder what made you come in today?"

Pt   "I can't take it any more. I know I need help."

Th   "You can't take it. What makes it impossible to take it now?"

Pt   "It's getting too bad. I just can't take it any more."

Th   "It sounds like something happened recently that made you realize how bad things were. What made you realize that you had to get help now?"

Pt   "I just felt so bad I couldn't go to work yesterday. I stayed home in bed all day. I never miss work. I must be falling apart."

This line of questioning led to establishing the patient's physical inactivity as a functional focus for treatment. As a result, his depression was successfully treated by getting him physically active.

In addition to the "Why now?" question, Budman and Gurman describe five common treatment foci:

    1. Losses past, present, or pending.
    2. Developmental dyssynchronies (being out of step with expected developmental stages). (Therapists should be able to identify with this because years of extended schooling and training usually keep life events such as marriage and children on hold.)
    3. Interpersonal conflicts (usually repeated disappointments in important relationships).
    4. Symptomatic presentations and desire for symptom reduction.

5. Severe personality impairment (it is possible in brief therapy to select one aspect of personality impairment as the focus of therapy).

Beginning brief therapists should use these five common foci to help organize their patient's complaints and problems. The most important thing to remember is that you are not finding **the** focus, only **a** focus for the therapy.

8. How does the therapist complete the evaluation?

Right from the start, brief therapy is demanding for the therapist and patient. In addition to doing a full psychiatric interview, by the completion of the second evaluation session you need to have (1) determined whether the patient is suitable for brief treatment; (2) developed a functional focus; and (3) articulated a clear treatment contract.

The patient and the therapist must agree on a treatment contract. In addition to identifying the focus of the treatment, this contract will spell out details, such as the number of sessions, how missed appointments will be dealt with, and how post-termination contact will be handled. Brief therapy typically lasts from 10 to 24 sessions; however, some are as long as 50 sessions. A 15-session treatment, not including the evaluation sessions, is a good length for a beginning brief therapist to start with. Both patient and therapist must initially clarify how missed appointments are to be handled. A flexible approach is recommended, and if the patient has a valid reason for missing a session, the therapist should try to reschedule. If a session is missed without a valid reason, the missed session should be counted and the patient's motivation for missing the session should be explored, because this is a resistance to treatment.

Another advantage to the two-session evaluation is that it allows an evaluation of how the patient responds to the therapy (and therapist). The patient's response can provide important additional information about the patient's appropriateness for brief treatment. Some form of intervention at the end of the first evaluation session is helpful in this regard. This initial intervention can be as simple as summarizing the patient's problem and offering a tentative treatment focus or as complex as requiring filling out a psychological questionnaire. At the start of the second session, inquire about the intervention. If the patient reports positively (e.g., found it helpful to think of her problem in this new light or is interested in what the psychological test showed), it is a sign that brief therapy may work. If the patient has not followed up on the intervention (e.g., did not think about the potential focus) or reacted angrily to it, it is a negative sign. Also an initial positive response, such as feeling a little better by the second session, can be taken as a positive sign (whereas a strong negative reaction would be considered a negative sign).

9. Is there one general approach that should be used in brief therapy?

Once a functional focus has been established, the therapist must maintain it. One way is by working consistently from within one style or orientation, of which there are basically three: (1) psychodynamic, (2) interpersonal, or (3) cognitive/behavioral. The one you use will depend upon your preference and, to some extent, your patient's problem.

More psychodynamic treatments are limited in their range of application and are appropriate for only a small percentage of the typical clinic patients. The psychoanalytic techniques tend to be limited to patients suffering from reactive or neurotic forms of depression (such as a failure to grieve, fear of success and competition, and triangular, conflicted love relationships). These are demanding treatments for the therapist to undertake and require that the patient be able to tolerate considerable affective arousal.

The cognitive-behavioral brief therapies, like Beck's, are more broadly applicable, both in percentage of patients who can benefit from them and the range of problems that can be treated by them. These therapies aim at bringing the patient's "automatic" (pre-conscious) thoughts into awareness and demonstrating how these thoughts maintain negative behaviors and feelings.

Brief interpersonal psychotherapy (IPT) was developed by Klerman and colleagues specifically to treat depression. It is a highly formalized (manualized) treatment often used in research studies. IPT focuses on the patient's depressive symptoms from within an interpersonal context. This type of treatment can be considered a mix of psychoeducation and supportive therapy. In

IPT, the patient's symptoms are explained (psychoeducation) and their interpersonal interactions, interpersonal expectations, and experiences are all explored. IPT seeks to clarify what the patient wants to receive from relationships and helps patients develop necessary social-interpersonal skills. In IPT no effort is made to understand the deeper unconscious meanings of the patients' social interactions or desires.

Regardless of the adopted orientation it is important to conceptualize and work predominantly from within one orientation or approach to keep treatment focused and clear. However, in brief treatment, therapeutic flexibility is necessary, and a moderate amount of thoughtful mixing of techniques from different therapy styles is acceptable. Avoid uncritical wholesale mixing of styles and orientations, because such "wild" treatment confuses and disappoints both the therapist and patient.

10. What does it mean to be an active therapist?

Completing a psychotherapy in 12 to 15 sessions requires the therapist to be very active. The activities of the brief therapist aim at maintaining treatment focus and keeping the process of therapy moving forward.

The brief therapist works to structure and make productive every session. One way is starting each session with a summary of important material from the last session and restating the treatment focus. This activity organizes therapy and keeps the treatment on tract. Homework is often given to the patient to be completed between sessions to help increase the impact of therapy on the patient's current life situation and to monitor the patient's motivation for change. If the patient does not complete the homework, the motivation for change must be explored.

The "working alliance" between therapist and patient must be developed quickly. It will be frequently invoked to return the patient to the treatment focus. Patients may attempt to escape the anxiety inherent in brief therapy by bringing up interesting but diverting material. The therapist should meet such tactics by gently reminding the patient of the agreed-upon focus (thus invoking the working alliance) and by asking how new material relates to it. Prolonged silences (by either the therapist or patient) are considered unproductive in brief therapy and are also quickly confronted as resistance.

To whatever extent possible, deep or prolonged regressions in the patient's functioning are best avoided, and the brief therapist must know how to cut short potentially regressive interventions. Two useful techniques are (1) organizing interpretations around events in the "here and now," using either the therapy relationship or the patient's current life situation, rather than around early developmental traumas; and (2) moving a patient away from feelings and into thoughts, "What are you thinking?" rather than asking "What are you feeling?" Regressions within sessions are permitted and even encouraged in some short-term work. For example, it is quite common, when employing a treatment modeled after that of Sifneos, to keep a patient focused upon an anxiety-provoking conflict even if this results in mild confusion or panic for the patient.

The brief therapist makes heavy use of *confrontation* and *clarification*. Confrontation helps the patient recognize when he or she is avoiding or resisting the treatment focus, usually resulting from anxiety provoked in the patient by the treatment focus itself. Clarification techniques are used whenever the patient is communicating in a vague or incomplete manner. It usually entails the therapist asking for specific examples of vaguely described situations or feelings. Finally, the brief therapist must always be ready to deal quickly with manifestations of transference. Regardless of the style of therapy you employ (psychodynamic, cognitive, or interpersonal) patients will inevitably react to some of your interventions based upon past experiences (transference). When such reactions are negative ("You always criticize me") or excessively positive ("You know me better than anyone on earth"), they must quickly be explored and interpreted. Rapid attention to both negative and overly positive feelings can help keep the patient's transference under control and reduce the likelihood that it may become a major resistance to treatment.

Brief therapist activity includes the use of supervision. As in all psychotherapy, supervision is important in both learning and practicing brief psychotherapy. For beginning therapists supervision with an experienced colleague provides an excellent learning vehicle for mastering brief therapy. Whereas for the more advanced practitioner some form of ongoing supervision, either formal or informal, helps maintain the treatment focus and aids the therapist in identifying subtle, but often important, changes in the patient's manner. Such subtle changes can represent the first signs of transference.

Being an Active Therapist

The short-term therapist is an active therapist
  Structure each session
  Give homework assignments
  Develop and use the working alliance
  Limit silences and vagueness
  Use confrontation and clarification
  Quickly deal with both negative and overly positive transference distortions
  Limit regressions
  Use supervision

---

11. What are the phases of brief therapy?

The **initial phase** includes evaluating and assessing patient appropriateness for brief therapy, selecting a treatment focus, and establishing the main treatment orientation. For the patient this phase is usually accompanied by mild symptom reduction and development of a mildly positive transference. Both of these factors should help with the quick development of the working alliance.

At the **middle phase,** the work gets more difficult. Typically the patient becomes concerned about the time limit and, in addition to the treatment focus, issues of dependency become important. The patient often feels worse and the therapist's faith in the treatment process is tested. The **early middle phase** of brief therapy can be particularly hard for the therapist, who during this period must be active in keeping the treatment focused, keeping the patient working, and countering patient skepticism while keeping her or his own optimism visible. Because this phase of the treatment can be difficult for the beginning brief therapist, good supervision is invaluable.

In the **termination phase,** therapy tends to settle down. The patient accepts that treatment will end as planned and that symptoms will decrease. Now, in addition to the treatment focus, post-therapy plans and the patient's feelings about termination should also be explored.

Among the most common **termination problems** is the introduction of new material or information by the patient. As treatment ends, the patient will often bring up some new and psychologically rich information or symptom. The therapist will be tempted to explore this and extend the therapy but this is usually a mistake, because introduction of new material at termination should be treated like all previous attempts to avoid the treatment focus, and in most cases the treatment should end as planned.

12. How do I handle post-treatment contact with the patient?

This difficult question must be answered individually by each therapist. During training, the beginning therapist should experience the intense feelings (for both patient and therapist) that accompany the termination of a treatment in which there will be no post-therapy contact. This teaches the therapist how to deal openly with these powerful and important feelings. In ongoing practice, however, it is important to encourage patients to return for treatment when new difficulties develop, and to foster the understanding that help is available if needed. Patient care should be guided by the understanding that, "Therapy is for living and not vice versa." From this perspective the brief psychotherapist practices as a primary care physician, available to help patients with (psychological) troubles or crises that develop throughout patients' lives.

13. How does brief psychotherapy relate to managed care?

In managed care, payers are encouraging the use of shorter treatments such as planned brief psychotherapy. However, one should not mistakenly think of managed mental health care and brief psychotherapy as being identical. Managed health care is primarily concerned with controlling cost. Planned brief psychotherapy represents a clinically proven procedure for helping some patients who present in need of psychiatric services. To be administered properly, brief psychotherapy must be based on clinical, not financial, considerations. Although many patients covered by managed care contracts will benefit from brief psychotherapy, not all patients are appropriate. Selecting patients for brief psychotherapy includes many variables; mental health insurance coverage is not one of them. Finally, therapy which is considered brief for clinical work (i.e., 15 to 20 sessions) may be considered too long by managed care companies who often suggest that six to eight sessions are sufficient.

BIBLIOGRAPHY

1. Alexander F, French T: Psychoanalytic Psychotherapy. New York, The Ronald Press, 1946.
2. Beck S, Greenberg R: Brief cognitive therapies. Psychiat Clin North Am 2:11–22, 1979.
3. Budman S, Gurman A: Theory and Practice of Brief Therapy. New York, The Guilford Press, 1988.
4. Burk J, White H, Havens L: Which short-term therapy? Arch Gen Psychiatry 36:177–186, 1989.
5. Davanloo H: Short-Term Dynamic Psychotherapy. New York, Jason Aronson, 1980.
6. Ferenczi S, Rank O: The Development of Psychoanalysis. New York, Nervous and Mental Disease Publishing Company, 1925.
7. Flegenheimer W: History of brief psychotherapy. In Horner A (ed): Treating the Neurotic Patient in Brief Psychotherapy. New Jersey, Jason Aronson, 1985, pp 7–24.
8. Goldin V: Problems of technique. In Horner A (ed): Treating the Neurotic Patient in Brief Psychotherapy. New Jersey, Jason Aronson, 1985, 56–74.
9. Groves J: The short-term dynamic psychotherapies: An overview. In Rutan S (ed): Psychotherapy for the 90's. New York, Guilford Press, 1992.
10. Hall M, Arnold W, Crosby R: Back to basics: The importance of focus selection. Psychotherapy 4:578–584, 1990.
11. Horner A. Principles for the therapist. In Horner A (ed): Treating the Neurotic Patient in Brief Psychotherapy. New Jersey, Jason Aronson, 1985, 76–85.
12. Horath A, Luborsky L: The role of the therapeutic alliance in psychotherapy. J Consult Clin Psychol 61:561–573, 1993.
13. Klerman G, Weissman M, Rounsaville B, Chevron E: Interpersonal Psychotherapy of Depression. New York, Basic Books, 1984.
14. Leibovich M: Short-term psychotherapy for the borderline personality disorder. Psychother Psychosom 35:257–264, 1981.
15. Malan D: The Frontier of Brief Psychotherapy. New York, Plenum Medical Book Company, 1976.
16. Mann J: Time-Limited Psychotherapy. Cambridge, Harvard University Press, 1973.
17. Marmor J: Short-term dynamic psychotherapy. Am J Psychiatry 136:149–155, 1979.
18. Sifneos P: Short-Term Anxiety Provoking Psychotherapy: A Treatment Manual. New York, Basic Books, 1992.

44. MARITAL AND FAMILY THERAPY

Margaret Roath, MSW, LCSW

1. What are marital and family therapy?

Marital and family therapy are therapeutic modalities whose focus of assessment and treatment is on the relationship, not on the individual. Assessment includes gathering data related to the following areas:

- History of the relationship
- Goals of the individuals in the relationship
- Coping mechanisms which have been unsuccessful
- Precipitant for seeking therapy—"why now?" or what changed?

- Communication patterns, both constructive and destructive
- Description of the strengths of the relationship
- Unmet needs of the individuals in the relationship

Assessment of the precipitant for seeking marital and family therapy is especially important in determining the relationship equilibrium which may have previously worked for all members of the relationship but is now out of balance. The precipitant might be a change in external circumstances or a change within an individual that is affecting the relationship.

Marital and family therapy identify these changes and then examine patterns of communication, behavior, and coping mechanisms which may have been destructive, not constructive, in responding to the identified changes. The goal of therapy is to provide the marriage and the family with new ways of responding that are helpful and constructive to the relationships. Sometimes, there is no acute precipitant to the request for marital and family therapy, but instead there are long-standing destructive patterns of communication that have been identified and the married couple or the family are interested in changing those patterns.

2. What are the indicators for marital and family therapy?

Statements or complaints expressed by individuals that reflect concerns about the relationship and also show the inability to resolve those concerns. Indications might include internal and external changes within individuals in the relationship or changes within the relationship itself.

Internal and External Indicators for Marital and Family Therapy

INTERNAL CHANGES	EXTERNAL CHANGES
A person, through individual therapy or through life experience, is making a decision about whether to remain in the relationship	Recently diagnosed illness of one of the marital or family members—the illness may mean death or adjustment to changing abilities
A person, through experience or therapy, realizes that he or she is of a different sexual orientation than originally believed	Change in financial status through loss of a job or a decrease in pay
A person may be experiencing an internal crisis, such as a mid-life crisis, and desires to change or maybe end the relationship	Addition of members to the marriage or family: the birth of a child, an in-law or children of a previous marriage joining the family
Normal developmental changes of children, such as adolescence	Children leaving home, which may exacerbate unresolved relationship issues for the marriage
Developmental changes of adults, such as the wife desiring to return to a career after being a homemaker	A decision to divorce which causes all relationships to be renegotiated

3. What treatment models are used for marital and family therapy?

The most common model for marital therapy is one in which both partners of the marriage are seen together by one therapist. Sometimes one or both partners will also be in individual therapy. In preparation for the marital sessions, the individuals may be working on issues pertinent only to themselves or developing a better understanding of their needs as partners in a marriage. It is usually optimal for the individual's therapist not to be the couple's therapist because the therapist may learn secrets which would compromise the marital therapy. However, when it is not possible or deemed optimal for separate therapists for each treatment modality, (e.g., in rural areas), the therapist and the patients must establish clear boundaries regarding the content discussed in each treatment modality. When several therapists are involved, communication among them can be helpful to clarify that they are working together and not at cross-purposes. Confidentiality needs to be addressed by each therapist with their respective patient or patients.

The most common treatment model for family therapy is one in which all members of the immediate family are seen together. Issues involving individual therapy should be handled much as those noted for marital therapy.

Marital group therapy and family group therapy are other possible modalities. They afford the possibility of learning from others in similar situations and also the benefit of feeling less alone with the issues being addressed. Couples and families can often listen and integrate advice from others in similar situations better than they can integrate advice from therapists. A disadvantage is that each couple's or family's specific issues may take longer to address because time is spent on developing relationships among couples or families. In marital and family group therapy, the therapist's role is one of facilitating interaction among participants.

4. What is the role of the therapist in marital and family therapy?

Typically quite active. The therapist assists marriage and family members in defining the problem and determining goals to address it. The therapist may need to stop certain behaviors and encourage others within therapy—for example, stopping one person from doing all of the talking and encouraging another to talk more. The therapist may also have to direct marriage and family members to stop certain behaviors outside of the treatment session, such as marathon discussions which might escalate into arguments or physical actions. The therapist might suggest a time limit for all discussions which have not resolved an issue, and also set very specific rules prohibiting physical violence, both in and out of therapy. When individuals in a marriage or family cannot stop physical violence, a separation with strict guidelines for being together may be suggested.

The therapist also reframes problems or feelings among marriage and family members by removing labels of good and bad and making statements about differences among the members. The therapist may suggest problem-solving with the directive that, if the solution is not effective, it only means that the participants, including the therapist, did not have all of the information necessary to develop a better solution. The therapist may give homework to the marriage and family members so that the therapy does not just take place in the office, but also becomes a part of daily home life. The therapist may serve as coach, educator, or mentor to the marriage and the family when destructive communication is observed, by giving specific examples of what to say or by participating in role-playing. Overall, the therapist is active and joins with the marriage and the family to develop new coping mechanisms, communication skills, and negotiation skills to address the identified problems in the marriage and the family.

5. What assessment and treatment techniques are used by the therapist?

The techniques of marital and family therapy focus on the relationships and relationship issues.

Assessment Techniques

- Ask each individual to describe their sense of the problem and its history
- Ask each individual the same question that has been asked of another
- Identify nonverbal communication
- Ask each individual's reaction to what another has said
- Identify themes common to the relationship and individuals within that relationship

Treatment Techniques
- Ask individuals to speak with "I" phrases, not "you" phrases, which sound accusatory
- Ask that each expressed need be accompanied by a proposed solution
- Assign homework or tasks that respond to the assessed problem
- Clarify—repeat what the other said and ask if the repeated statement was heard as intended

Many other techniques exist; they have a common goal of strengthening the marriage or the family's bond even when the individuals feel polarized, disappointed, and angered at the time of therapy.

6. How long does marital or family therapy take?

It is not possible to say specifically. However, it is possible to establish specific goals and assess at the end of each session or after an agreed-upon number of sessions whether the goals have been met and what will need to happen for any remaining goals to be met. The length of time needed for marital and family therapy depends on how much blame is present, how much desire or ability there is for the participants to move from blame to identification and problem solving, and how much empathy all members have for other marriage and family members. The more blaming, the less problem-solving behavior, and the less empathy, the longer the therapy will take. The more willingness for each individual within the relationship to examine his or her behavior and develop solutions for changing it, the less time therapy is likely to take.

7. Are there any patients with specific psychiatric diagnoses who should not be referred to marital and family therapy?

Yes. If one member of a marriage or family is psychotic or so severely depressed that he or she is unable to focus cognitively on marriage and family issues, then such therapy would not be recommended. Once treatment for psychosis or depression has occurred, however, there can be a referral for marriage and family therapy if the issues identified indicate the need for it. Otherwise, because marriage and family therapy focus on changes in behavior, coping mechanisms, and problem-solving, they have the potential to be successful if the members are motivated to pursue those changes, irrespective of the members' DSM-IV diagnoses. Some research shows that marital and family problems may increase vulnerability to mood disorders, and those same problems may slow recovery or cause exacerbations of additional episodes of severe illness. Treatment to promote marital and family harmony may prevent recurrences of the illness.

Family therapy may be very helpful in reducing severity or relapses for persons with schizophrenia. Family members often respond very positively to information about mental illness and coping strategies and feel less alone when professionals are interested in working with them in management and caretaking. Partners and families of schizophrenics usually identify relapses earlier than the patient does; if they are working collaboratively with professionals, they can provide data which increase services being provided. Also, partners and families who have a positive relationship with professionals and are able to express their feelings and worries in marital and family therapy sessions are less likely to be intrusive or hovering with the patient to express hostility and anger, which could precipitate a relapse. The intrusive or hovering behavior is referred to as expressed-emotion behavior. The greater the level of this behavior, the more likely a relapse by the patient; the lower the level, the less likely.

8. Can marital and family therapy be effective if one of the members is resistant?

If one of the members displays resistance by not attending meetings, the issues in the marriage and the family may still be addressable, but with the understanding that the only ones who can change behavior are those willing to attend meetings. The focus cannot be on the person not present. If the resistant person attends the meetings, it may be possible to lessen the resistance by having everyone listen to and understand the reasons for the resistance. If an individual maintains resistance, a decision can be made for that person not to attend, and therapy can proceed for those members who are motivated.

9. Are marital and family therapy different for different cultures, races, ages, and sexual orientation?

No. The assessment process remains the same, as does the treatment process. In other words, assessment and treatment will always focus on needs, expectations, complementarity of roles, communication, and behavior patterns. However, cultural differences between individuals in a marriage or a family may lead to different goals or expectations, and those differences need to be elucidated and clarified by the therapist.

10. Does there have to be a match with the therapist in the areas of culture, race, age, and sexual orientation?

No, although couples and families will request it. Accommodating that request may facilitate the beginning process of therapy. However, it is not necessary because a competent therapist will address the lack of complementarity in the beginning, which creates alliance-building. It encourages the members of a marriage or family to express feelings, either negative or positive, about the lack of complementarity and allows the therapist to empathize with those feelings. The therapist may also encourage the couple or family to share information about culture, history, traditions, or life-style as a way to bridge the gap between those differences.

11. Are marriages and family therapy always successful in keeping marriage and family together and improving the relationships?

No. Approximately 50% of the marriages which enter marital therapy end in separation or divorce. Some couples come to marital therapy when anger has created too great a distance and one, if not both, partners have already decided on separation or divorce. At those times the therapy can be a forum through which to accomplish this goal. One partner is sometimes hoping the other will be able to connect with the therapist as a source of support in order to feel less guilty or fearful about abandoning the partner.

Marital and family therapy are sometimes unable to promote change because the desire to change and enter into the unknown is weaker than the comfort of the known. The therapist shares that observation with a marriage and family in a nonjudgmental way, encouraging them to return should the situation change. Some marriages and families will experience several attempts at therapy before they decide to make changes and risk the unknown. Part of the process in marital and family therapy is learning whether the members of a marriage or family can meet the needs expressed. If, through therapy, it is learned that needs cannot be met, decisions may be required to meet those needs other than through the marriage or family.

12. What are some of the controversial issues?

1. The issue today is "Who is the Family?" when the therapist is making decisions such as who to invite to family therapy sessions. The divorce rate has altered the composition of family systems and relationships. There are often parents, step-parents, children, step-children, half-siblings, grandparents, and step-grandparents who are now forming this new family. There are also gay and lesbian couples who may have ex-spouses by previous marriages. Children of those marriages will most likely be sharing time with both their homosexual and heterosexual parents. Another recent social phenomenon is the choice being made by both men and women to have children outside of marriage. Children of such relationships may be living with both biologic parents, a single parent, or one biologic parent and a significant other of that biologic parent.

2. Another controversial issue is whether or not couples and families in which domestic violence has taken place should be treated with marital or family therapy. Some professionals say "never," because marital and family therapy support blaming the victim. Those professionals will say that only the perpetrator needs to be in therapy whereas the basic tenet of couples' therapy is that both people contribute to destructive behavior. Other professionals argue that the domestic violence occurred in the context of a relationship and that the most helpful treatment program is individual help for the perpetrator in addition to therapy which addresses marital or family relationships. It may be that the therapy program should not be viewed as "either-or" but

that the decision of when to add marital or family therapy to individual therapy needs to be viewed as a clinical decision and depends on whether or not the goal is to reunite the couple or family.

BIBLIOGRAPHY

1. Balcom D, Lee R, Tager J: The systemic treatment of shame in couples. J Marital Family Ther 21:55–65, 1995.
2. Beck RL: Redirecting the blaming in marital psychotherapy. Clin Soc Work J 15:148–158, 1987.
3. Berg KI, Jaya A: Different and same: Family therapy with Asian-American families. J Marital Family Ther 19:31–38, 1993.
4. Carter B, McGoldrick M: The Changing Family Life Cycle, A Framework for Family Therapy. New York, Gardner Press, 1988.
5. Dattilio F, Padesky C: Cognitive Therapy with Couples. Sarasota, FL, Professional Resource Exchange, 1990.
6. Glick ID, Clarkin JF, Spencer JH, et al: A controlled evaluation of inpatient family intervention: Preliminary results of the six-month follow-up. Arch Gen Psychiatry 42:882–886, 1985.
7. Gottman J, Notarius C, Gonso J, Markman H: A Couple's Guide to Communication. Champaign, IL, Research Press, 1976.
8. Greenspan R: Marital therapy with couples whose lack of self-sustaining function threatens the marriage. Clin Soc Work J 21:395–404, 1993.
9. Guerin PP, Fayu L, Burden S, Kautto G: The Evaluation and Treatment of Marital Conflict. New York, Basic Books, 1987.
10. Gurman A, Kniskern D: Handbook of Family Therapy. New York, Brunner/Mazel, 1981.
11. Hugen B: The effectiveness of a psychoeducational support service to families of persons with a chronic mental illness. Res Soc Work Pract 3:137–154, 1993.
12. Marley J: Content and context: Working with mentally ill people in family therapy. Soc Work 37:412–417, 1992.
13. Moltz D: Bipolar disorder and the family: An integrative model. Family Process 32:409–423, 1993.

45. GROUP THERAPY

John F. Zrebiec, M.S.W.

1. What is group psychotherapy?
It has often been defined in the broadest terms, encompassing many kinds of groups with goals that range from behavioral change to educational exchange. It will be considered here as a field of clinical practice and as a specific approach within the realm of psychotherapy. All group therapy is aimed at alleviating illness or distress with the help of a trained leader. What distinguishes group treatment from other methods is the use of group interaction as the agent for change.

2. How did group therapy begin?
In 1905, Dr. Joseph Pratt, a Boston physician, brought his tuberculosis patients together for weekly discussion groups and found that these meetings seemed to provide mutual support, alleviate depression, and decrease isolation. Moreno, who is best known for developing psychodrama, first used the term "group therapy" in the 1920s. Group treatment was largely considered ineffective until World War II. The large number of neuropsychiatric casualties returning from the war compelled the governments of the United States and England to find ways to treat these veterans more efficiently and economically. Since then, the group therapy field has mushroomed in many directions and is now applied in many different clinical settings for many different types of problems.

3. What are the advantages of group therapy?
1. The patient recreates characteristic difficulties in the group. Interactions in the group quickly expose patterns of behavior.
2. The "hall of mirrors" concept refers to the group's ability to confront an individual with behavior he or she had been unable to recognize. Individual members will more likely accept feedback about their behavior if it comes from multiple observers.
3. Multiple supporters who empathize with the patient's struggle can make confrontation more tolerable and dealing with intense affect more possible.
4. The revelation of shameful secrets can lead to immense relief.
5. Group interactions pull for socially appropriate responses and interchanges.
6. The group offers alternative models for behavior.
7. Group therapy is often experienced as less regressive than individual therapy.

4. What are the disadvantages?
1. Patients get less exclusive time and attention than in individual therapy.
2. Groups can create a feeling of being lost in the crowd, and of not being appreciated for one's uniqueness.
3. Confidentiality has limitations. The group leader cannot guarantee that members will maintain confidences.
4. Termination is more complicated (less flexible, more final) than in individual therapy.

5. Are there different theoretical viewpoints?
Originally, most group therapy was established on psychodynamic principles; now most group therapists use a combination of theories. For example, a common blend of models is psychodynamic (focused on individual group members), interpersonal (focused on interactions between members), and group as a whole (focused on the group processes). This chapter blends those models into some general principles that are broadly applicable to a wide variety of groups, of any length and type, in any clinical setting.

6. What do I need to do first?

A successful group requires thoughtful planning:

1. Clarify your own values about why group treatment is valuable.

2. Assess the institution in which you work and whether it values group treatment. Will the institution and your colleagues be friend or foe in your attempts to start a group? Who values or devalues groups? Who has the authority to help you start a group? What kinds of groups are already in existence? What kinds of patients need a group? How will you get your group members? How much competition is there between professionals for these patients?

3. You need to be clear about the type of group you are offering. Groups range from discussion and theme-centered or supportive/educational to process-oriented therapy. It is essential to be clear about the type of group because that will help in explaining the purpose of the group to potential patients and referral sources, and it will define your role as leader. For example, in a social skills training group, the leader's primary role would be as a teacher, whereas in a psychodynamic group, the leader's role would be as an interpreter of unconscious phenomena.

7. Who is appropriate to select for groups?

There are many different criteria that have been proposed for selecting patients. In general, most patients can work effectively in some type of group therapy. If patients are willing to listen to others and talk about themselves, then they are group therapy candidates. Exclusionary criteria are (1) patients who refuse to enter a group or who refuse to abide by group agreements, and (2) patients who have serious problems with interpersonal relatedness. Contrary to popular opinion, people who do not do well in groups are not the prime candidates for groups. Caution also needs to be exercised in including patients who are highly impulsive, acutely suicidal, homicidal, or psychotic.

8. Which group for which patient?

Groups are not random collections of strangers thrown together because a clinic has too few therapists and too many patients. It is important not only to select patients who will benefit from a group but to place them in a group from which they will benefit. Patients have traditionally been placed in beginning groups along the guideline of being similar in terms of ego development but different in terms of interpersonal style. For example, the ability to establish trust or capacity for concern is similar, but degrees of shyness or submissiveness are different. Most important is that no one in a group sees themselves as one of a kind in the group because they will be at high risk to drop out. To use a broad example, the only elderly, widowed man in a group with young, new mothers is going to find little common ground with other members and is likely to quickly leave the group.

There are three reasons why patients drop out of groups:

1. The right group at the wrong time (the patient is not ready for group).

2. The wrong group at the right time (for example, the elder widower with the young mothers).

3. The patient is not suited for group treatment.

9. Should I have a screening interview?

Ideally, there should be at least one individual interview before a patient is accepted into a group. Some patients may require more if they are unfamiliar with therapy or very ambivalent about joining the group. In order to assess whether a patient is suitable for group therapy in general and for your group, in particular, some face-to-face contact is necessary. This interview also helps form an alliance between leader and member, establish goals, provide education about the role of the leader and the members, review the group agreements, and answer questions and address potential problems. It gives the patient an opportunity to make an informed decision about joining the group, and the leader an opportunity to assess whether the patient is appropriate for this particular group.

Common Questions or Issues Raised During the Screening Interview

1. What do you want to get out of this group?
2. Why do you want to join this group at this time?
3. What is your experience in groups (prior treatment, but also including family, school, job, social groups)?
4. What do you imagine this group will be like?
5. What do you think you will contribute to this group?
6. What will be the most difficult aspect of this group for you?
7. May we review group agreements?

10. Should I have a group agreement?

All groups need some operational guidelines which provide structure and a baseline for addressing any future behavior that jeopardizes the group. The following guidelines have been traditionally used by psychodynamic group therapists. They can be modified for time-limited groups, and for groups with a variety of patients in different settings:

- To attend each meeting, to be on time, and to remain for the entire meeting.
- To work on the problems which brought them to the group.
- To realize that communication is verbal and not physical.
- To protect the names and identities of other group members.
- To use relationships therapeutically and not socially.
- To remain in the group until the problems which brought them to the group are resolved.
- To understand that when they decide to leave the group they will give appropriate time to themselves and to the group to understand the reasons for leaving and to say good-bye.
- To give the leader permission to speak with their individual therapist (if they have one) at any time that the leader feels it is in their best interests.
- To be responsible about payment.

11. What are the basics in terms of place, time, size?

Most groups meet weekly, although there are some groups which meet twice weekly, and others which meet twice monthly. The important point for therapeutic benefit is that patients do not lose contact with the affect and process of the previous meeting.

Most groups meet for 90 minutes, with the range from 75 to 120 minutes. Less than 75 minutes is not enough time for members to get their fair share, and meetings longer than 120 minutes can be exhausting for members and leaders.

The range for a group is four to ten members. Fewer than four members provides a temptation to focus on individuals, not group processes, more than ten seems to become unmanageable and less productive. Most group experts recommend seven as the ideal number with higher-functioning patients, and starting with at least that many patients in order to compensate for some potential early drop-outs.

It is the group leader's responsibility to arrange for a comfortable, private room with enough chairs for everyone. Most group leaders prefer chairs in a circle where members are not physically hidden from one another by tables or other furniture.

12. What is the role of the leader?

To help the group members understand themselves by understanding their behavior in the group. The leader, then, has the challenge of deciding how the group can best be helped. There are several decisions that the leader will need to make:

- What to say, how much to say, and when to say it.
- How much to pursue the present experience while welcoming reports of past events or future hopes.
- How much attention to give to individuals while still observing interactions between members or the entire group.

- How much value to give to feelings and emotional experience without ignoring reason and intellectual understanding.
- How to integrate dialogue about group members with discussions about people outside the group.
- How to blend understanding of the content (obvious meaning) with the process (symbolic meaning).
- How much to respond to group demands or wishes.
- How much personal information to share.

All these leadership decisions are influenced by theoretical orientation, personality, and context of the group. Moreover, all these decisions are a matter of degree, not all or nothing, and each will have consequences for the group.

All these variables may seem overwhelming, so here are ten useful rules to live by so that you will not feel lost in a sea of group words:

- Each meeting is in a context (time, place, purpose).
- Each group member has a context. Try to keep in mind their history and presenting problems.
- Pay attention to what is happening in the group at that very moment . . . the "here and now" focus. Ask yourself: What is happening? Why is it happening now?
- Remember everything that happens in the group has something to do with the group.
- Each group meeting has a theme or connecting thread.
- Pay special attention to the beginning words and behaviors which might predict the theme.
- Think in terms of metaphors or analogies as a clue to the theme of the group.
- Pay attention to your own emotional response to the group as a barometer of what is happening in the meeting.
- Do not panic if you do not always know what is happening in the group. This is a common experience. Remember the above points and try to formulate hypotheses which should help in making an educated guess about the theme.
- Prepare a summary statement, whether you actually state it or not, as a way of organizing the group theme.

13. Are there advantages to co-leadership?

Co-therapy is a frequently used model, primarily for training. The most important and time-consuming aspect is the need for the co-therapists to maintain their communication and attend to their relationship.

Co-leadership has certain advantages for the patients because it (1) enhances continuity in the case of leader absence, (2) may provide a constructive relationship model for imitation, (3) replicates a two-parent family, and (4) provides more limit-setting capability.

Co-leadership has certain advantages for the leaders because it (1) provides mutual support and co-supervision, (2) offers two vantage points on the group, (3) allows leaders to share or change roles from verbal to observational and focus from whole group to individual, and (4) helps in dealing with crises and concrete tasks.

Co-leadership also has certain disadvantages, which include the potential for (1) increased cost; (2) destructive competition; (3) lack of communication; (4) serious disagreement based on each leader's different professional, clinical or administrative role; (5) distancing oneself from the emotional impact of the experience; and (6) operating by one leader in the shadow of the more experienced group leader.

14. Are there stages in group development?

It is valuable for the group leader to have a developmental framework for understanding group themes and the myriad interactions of group process. Yalom has a useful framework for thinking about these four developmental stages.

The initial stage is concerned with "in or out": searching for purpose, getting to know other members, finding similarities, and learning the ground rules. Members are primarily concerned with acceptance and nonacceptance. Do the others like me? Are there others like me? Communication in this stage is often superficial, polite, focused on giving or seeking advice, and gaining approval from the leader. The leader's primary role is to promote trust and safety, and to help members find common ground.

The second stage is concerned with "top or bottom": jockeying for positions of control, dominance, and power among members, but above all, between members and the leader. The honeymoon comes to an end as safety and trust are established. Now, members want to know how they are different, how much autonomy the group leader will permit, and how much they can challenge one another and the leader? How can they batter, bend, and break group guidelines? Who are the strong ones? Whereas in the first stage members were primarily concerned with being seen as the same, now they are primarily concerned with being accepted as different. Criticism of one another, hostility toward the leader, and disenchantment with the group are more often heard. The group has great expectations from the leader so it should come as no surprise that they are disappointed in the leader's failure to fulfill their dreams. What is essential is that the group leader tolerate their disappointment, encourage their confrontation, and not respond punitively. It can help to remember that this rebellious, emotionally stormy phase is a sign that the group is moving ahead.

The third stage is concerned with "near or far": the chief concern of the group is with intimacy and closeness. How close to get to others? How many secrets to share? Following the previous stage of conflict there is more trust, cooperation, openness in communication, and group spirit among the members. The leader sets the stage for progress by making sure that the group does not suppress all negative affect for the sake of group cohesiveness. The group is now ready to become a mature working group where there is focus, flexibility, compassion, a greater tolerance for affect, a realistic appraisal of the leader, and a recognition of the value of other members.

The fourth and last stage is termination. It is the leader's job to draw the attention of the group members to the loss. Ordinarily, termination resurrects feelings around three themes: mortality and death, separation, and hope.

These stages are present in all groups but the depth and breadth of expression will differ depending upon goals, time, and leadership style. These stages will also overlap with no clear boundary among them or consistency between groups. Groups never ultimately resolve these developmental issues, but periodically cycle through them at progressively deeper levels as stresses and conflicts emerge during the group.

15. How do you handle difficult patients?
The difficult patient, often self-centered or demanding, can create a difficult group and a scapegoated group member. Volumes have already been written about managing difficult patients, but it is worth mentioning one particularly constructive approach in groups. This is based on the premise that the difficult patient plays an important role for the group and represents aspects of everyone else in the group. Then, the most therapeutic response is to focus on the reaction of other group members rather than on the pathology of the individual patient. This avoids further attack on the individual patient and encourages others to take responsibility for their share of the interaction.

16. What about combining group therapy with pharmacotherapy or individual therapy?
It is very common for group members to receive psychotropic medications and it is essential in groups for psychotic patients. Attitudes about and reasons for medication will likely become a topic for group discussion.

Many patients are also seen in concurrent individual and group therapy, which can be a powerful therapeutic combination. There are two variations: (1) combined therapy—the same therapist sees the patient in both individual and group therapy, (2) conjoint therapy—the patient is seen in individual and group therapy by two different therapists. Group therapy is often added to individual treatment, but patients can be referred for individual treatment from group. It is very important that neither mode of treatment be viewed as better than the other. It is also crucial to consider the repercussions for communication, confidentiality, and countertransference.

17. How do you decide when to terminate?

Time-limited groups come to a preordained ending. Other groups end because of the leader's decision to terminate. Patients leave groups because they have successfully completed treatment or leave prematurely for a variety of personal, group, and circumstantial reasons. This whole process is more complicated than individual therapy because it affects a number of people, not just the therapist. The leader should attempt to prevent premature termination and should draw attention to the feelings surrounding termination. There are two helpful questions to ask: (1) Has the patient leaving gained the most possible from the group? (2) Why is the patient leaving at this particular time? The decision can also be examined on the basis of the original goal for joining the group and whether that goal has been accomplished. It is not uncommon for a group to assess the constructive changes and continuing conflicts exhibited by the terminating member.

18. Is there a place for brief group therapy?

Time-limited treatment is becoming more common because of cost-limited care. Time-limited groups are often formed around specific symptoms, crises, or common issues (for example, medical illness, divorce, or adolescence) with limited goals of symptom relief, crisis management, or support and psychoeducation. There are also brief-treatment groups designed for more aggressive interpersonal intervention and more ambitious therapeutic change. They have in common a careful selection of patients, explicit goals, a well-defined working focus, rapid application of learning, active leaders, the use of interpersonal resources, and the use of time limits to accelerate behavior change. Unlike longer-term groups, patients often can return for several courses of treatment, but as in longer-term groups, success is predicated upon careful pregroup preparation. Time-limited groups can also be conceptualized as having developmental stages, as already described. Progression through stages may be intensified because of the time limit.

19. Can the leader guarantee confidentiality?

There is a legal and ethical responsibility to protect the patients' privacy and confidentiality which is uncompromised and uncomplicated for the therapist doing individual treatment. Although the same standard applies for the group therapist, group therapy poses special problems because patients are generally expected to respect the identities and protect the information shared by other group members. In actuality, group therapy places limits on confidentiality (where one group member violates the confidentiality of another) because neither the leader nor the other group members have any legal means of enforcement.

BIBLIOGRAPHY

1. Alonso A, Swiller HI (eds): Group Therapy in Clinical Practice. Washington, DC, American Psychiatric Association Press, 1993.
2. Brabender V, Fallon A: Models of Inpatient Group Psychotherapy. Washington, DC, American Psychological Association, 1993.
3. Budman SH, Gurman AS: Theory and Practice of Brief Therapy. New York, Guilford Press, 1988.
4. Dies RR: Models of group psychotherapy: Sifting through confusion. Int J Grp Psychol 42:1–17, 1992.
5. Gans JS: The leader's use of metaphor in group psychotherapy. Int J Grp Psychol 41:127–143, 1991.
6. Grunebaum H, Kates W: Whom to refer for group psychotherapy. Am J Psychol 134:130–133, 1977.
7. Guttmacher JA, Birk L: Group therapy: What specific advantages? Comp Psychol 12:546–556, 1971.
8. Horowitz L: Projective identification in dyads and groups. Int J Grp Psychol 33:259–279, 1983.
9. MacKenzie KR (ed): Classics in Group Psychotherapy. New York, Guilford Press, 1992.
10. Ormont L: Group resistance and the therapeutic contract. Int J Grp Psychol 18:147–154, 1968.
11. Roth BE, Stone WN, Kibel HD (eds): The Difficult Patient in Group. Madison, CT, International Universities Press, 1990.
12. Rutan JS, Stone WN: Psychodynamic Group Psychotherapy. New York, Guilford Press, 1993.
13. Scheidlinger S: Focus on Group Psychotherapy. New York, International Universities Press, 1982.
14. Stone WN: The curative fantasy in group psychotherapy. Group 9:3–14, 1985.
15. Yalom ID: The Theory and Practice of Group Psychotherapy. New York, Basic Books, 1985.

46. RELAXATION TRAINING

William H. Polonsky, Ph.D.

1. What are the major forms of relaxation training?

Interventions to promote relaxation include meditation, progressive muscle relaxation, hypnosis, autogenic training, and biofeedback.

Major Forms of Relaxation Training

TYPE	DESCRIPTION
Meditation	Self-guided, passive attention to a single object of focus
Progressive muscle relaxation	Systematic contraction and relaxation of the major muscle groups
Hypnosis	Verbal and repetitive suggestions, often involving mental imagery, to relax the mind and body
Autogenic training	Structured series of formalized suggestions directed toward promoting body sensations associated with relaxation
Biofeedback	Machine-based detection and amplification of tension-related physiologic signals which are fed back to the patient, who then learns to sense and modify the signal

Meditation, usually of the concentrative form, have become increasingly popular in the West. In concentrative meditation, the patient is taught to attend passively to a single object of focus that is unchanging or repetitive (e.g., a visual image, a repeated word or mantra, or a body sensation such as breathing). The emphasis is on present-centered, effortless attention, often without any directive guidance that relaxation or any other psychophysiologic change should occur. Nonconcentrative forms are similar, though usually more difficult, with the attention directed in a more expansive or "mindful" manner towards the ever-changing flow of mental activity.

In **progressive muscle relaxation,** the patient is guided in the tensing and relaxing of 16 major muscle groups, one at a time. Of the major relaxation forms, progressive muscle relaxation may be the simplest, most straightforward, and most teachable. Through voluntary muscle contraction, the patient is thought to be better able to sense the difference between tension and relaxation in each of the muscle groups and thus is able to promote the subsequent muscle relaxation more easily. Recent research, however, suggests that the tensing component may not be necessary; techniques involving awareness of each muscle group followed by suggestions for relaxation may be just as effective. As the progressive muscle relaxation skill is developed, patients are encouraged to combine muscle groups, until relaxation is achievable through simple recall.

Hypnosis and self-hypnosis focus on the use of formalized suggestion, often involving the use of mental imagery. Hypnotic suggestion may be applied to a variety of different ends, of which the most well-known is relaxation. With a rhythmic and calming voice, repetitive suggestions are used to guide the patient toward somatic relaxation (e.g., "the muscles of your body are relaxing more and more") and cognitive relaxation (e.g., "slowly letting go of the day's worries"). Of all hypnotic suggestions, relaxation is one of the easiest to attain, although considerable evidence exists that individuals differ greatly in their abilities to respond to hypnotic suggestion.

Autogenic training may be conceptualized as a standardized form of hypnosis, involving a series of six self-suggestions referring to specific body sensations. In the course of treatment, patients are slowly guided in the promotion of each group of sensations (e.g., "the heart is beating quietly and strongly," "the forehead is cool") in a step-by-step manner, which is believed to promote relaxation. There is a strong emphasis on "passive concentration," whereby the patient is encouraged to allow, rather than force, changes in body sensations to occur. As in progressive muscle relaxation, after autogenic skills are acquired, abbreviated forms are introduced so that the patient can more reliably and rapidly achieve states of deep relaxation.

Biofeedback systems are used to detect small changes in relevant physiologic systems (including autonomic systems as well as striated muscle) and then immediately to transform and relay this information, by means of visual and/or auditory signals, back to the patient. With such feedback, the patient may learn to modify the signals (and, thus, the associated physiologic system) in the desired direction. Thus, biofeedback interventions may be used to promote states of deep relaxation through directed reductions in electrodermal activity, heart rate, muscle tension, and other physiologic systems. With further training, the patient may learn to sense and modify the subtle internal sensations which correspond with the desired physiologic change, and may thus be slowly weaned from the biofeedback system.

2. How is biofeedback training different from other forms of relaxation training?
Biofeedback may be viewed as a more multidimensional tool than relaxation training; specifically, it may promote potentially valuable physiologic changes not necessarily associated with relaxation. For example, electromyographic biofeedback training is used in neuromuscular rehabilitation to help patients in relearn to perceive, activate, and/or relax specific muscles, followed by the regaining of patterned muscle movement. The complexity and specificity of such training is clearly distinct from relaxation training. Biofeedback training has proved useful with other syndromes, including Raynaud's disease and encopresis.

3. What is the "relaxation response"?
Benson suggested that all types of relaxation training are remarkably similar. They involve verbal repetition and a passive attitude toward external stimuli and all lead to the same, generic result, the "relaxation response," which is characterized by muscle relaxation, diminished heart rate, reduced blood pressure, and other psychophysiologic changes indicative of a broad reduction in sympathetic arousal.

4. Do all types of relaxation training actually produce this result?
This is a point of considerable controversy. In contrast with the relaxation response model, some researchers have argued for a "specific effects" model, suggesting that somatic versus cognitive forms of relaxation may be more effective when matched with the appropriate form of anxiety (e.g., complaints of chronic muscle tension versus "racing thoughts"). Evidence to date suggests that compromise is warranted. Each form of relaxation training has been shown to promote general, stress-reducing effects. Specific effects apparent for each of the techniques exist, however. For example, progressive muscle relaxation and biofeedback (relaxation forms with a more somatic focus) have more powerful effects on somatically based anxiety (where the experience of anxiety is primarily body-oriented, such as a rapid heart rate) than meditation (a more cognitive form of relaxation). In turn, meditation appears to have more impact on cognitively based anxiety (where the experience of anxiety is primarily psychological, such as excessive worrying). In summary, unique effects of the various relaxation techniques are apparent and may be overlaid on a more general relaxation response. For a more comprehensive discussion, see Lehrer and Woolfolk, 1993.

5. For which psychiatric problems has relaxation training been shown to be of value?
Although relaxation training is widely viewed as a panacea across a wide range of conditions, evidence to date suggests that relaxation training, at least as a stand-alone treatment, is rarely the most effective intervention. Especially for anxiety-related diagnoses, powerful and effective stress management treatment packages have been developed, many of which include relaxation training, but as a solitary intervention, relaxation training is unlikely to be sufficient for most

conditions. In treating agoraphobia and panic disorder, for example, cognitive intervention and therapist-directed exposure have been shown to be remarkably effective in promoting long-term reductions in symptoms. As part of a comprehensive treatment program, relaxation training may also be included and, indeed, may add to treatment efficacy (especially when focused on breathing retraining, a relaxation technique involving slow, paced diaphragmatic breathing) but it is clearly a second-tier therapy. Relaxation training may be valuable in the treatment of generalized anxiety disorder, social phobia, and depression, but it is commonly included as only one component of a larger treatment plan, where cognitive therapy interventions are central and relaxation techniques are directed toward situation-specific practice (e.g., learning to relax before and during difficult social situations).

In other conditions, relaxation training may be of special value to specific subsets of patients; for example, chronic substance abusers for whom anxiety is a central factor in their abusive behaviors. In sum, simple relaxation practice is far from being a cure-all for any of the psychiatric diagnoses. Relaxation training may be valuable when included as a component in broader stress management programs, when intervention is directed toward situation-specific practice of relaxation skills (especially for anxiety-related diagnoses), and when appropriate subpopulations of patients are targeted.

6. How are stress management programs different from relaxation training programs?

Stress management programs commonly involve a broad range of techniques, usually including relaxation training, directed toward the amelioration of stress-mediated conditions. In contrast to relaxation training, stress management programs tend to be multi-component in nature. One well-known program is "anxiety management training," which packages a number of cognitive therapy techniques along with progressive muscle relaxation. In this program, the goal is applied relaxation, in which patients are trained to repeatedly imagine anxiety-provoking scenes and to use their relaxation skills to reduce anxiety, to recognize and treat early signs of stress, and to practice relaxation skills during anxious moments. Other programs focus more directly on specific psychiatric conditions. For example, Barlow and colleagues have developed a multicomponent treatment program for panic disorder which uses relaxation techniques, cognitive restructuring (to identify the common cognitive errors that contribute to panic), and graded exposure to fearful body sensations (to promote desensitization to those sensations).

7. Given these data, should patients be discouraged from the broad usage of relaxation techniques?

Not at all! In addition to its role as a potentially valuable component in the treatment of anxiety and other psychiatric disorders, relaxation training can be potent for relieving daily stress and attenuating psychophysiologic stress responses (i.e., chronically exaggerated reactions to stressful stimuli in any of a variety of organ systems, including blood pressure, heart rate, muscle tension, and peripheral vasoconstriction). For alleviation of subclinical anxiety disorders, as an alternative coping response to self-destructive behaviors, as an adjunct to psychotherapy, and as a preventive to the accumulation of daily stress, it can be a rewarding and effective practice. In addition, accumulating data suggest that relaxation training may be useful in the treatment of certain physical illnesses.

8. For what medical conditions has relaxation training been shown to be of value?

As reviewed in the table, the strongest and most positive effects of relaxation training are apparent in headache disorders. Both progressive muscle relaxation and electromyographic biofeedback are effective in promoting a clinically significant reduction in tension headache symptoms (50% reduction in self-reported symptoms) in approximately 40 to 50% of sufferers, although cognitive therapy (focusing on such tasks as identifying situations where headaches occur, improving recognition of the early warning signs of headache, and learning to practice relaxation skills immediately before headache onset) appears to be even more effective. Recent evidence suggests that cognitive therapy in combination with relaxation training may be more effective in reducing symptoms than amitriptyline. Relaxation training, especially autonomic-directed approaches (temperature biofeedback and autogenic training) is also of value in the treatment of migraine, although the effects are generally not as large as those seen for tension headaches. Temperature biofeedback in combination with autogenic training, however, has been found to be as effective in promoting long-term reductions in migraine frequency as ergotamine tartrate and propranolol.

For the management of low back pain and other chronic conditions involving pain, relaxation training may be of some benefit (in particular, hypnotic interventions have been popular), although more comprehensive, cognitive-behavioral treatment programs are clearly the treatment of choice. Similarly, relaxation strategies are commonly effective in reducing chronic insomnia complaints, though other cognitive-behavioral interventions (e.g., stimulus control) are likely to be even more effective. Thus, for both conditions, relaxation training may be best regarded as merely one component of effective treatment programs.

For irritable bowel syndrome, stress management programs promote significant and long-term clinical improvement in reported symptoms. The degree to which the relaxation component contributes to these effects, however, is not clear. Relaxation training has also been considered as a treatment for hypertension. Research findings, however, have been generally disappointing. Significant decrements in blood pressure have been apparent, through quite small, and antihypertensive medications have consistently been found to produce much more powerful results. Similarly, in bronchial asthma, relaxation training leads to significant improvement in pulmonary function, although the effects are consistently modest. Discouraging results have also been found with diabetes. Relaxation training does not promote consistent, direct effects on blood glucose in insulin-dependent diabetes mellitus, though the effects in non-insulin-dependent diabetes mellitus are more equivocal. Although evidence for broad relaxation effects in hypertension, bronchial asthma, and diabetes is disappointing, suggestive data point to small subgroups of patients (e.g., the highly anxious) where relaxation training may lead to significant clinical improvement.

The Efficacy of Relaxation Training for Medical Conditions

MEDICAL CONDITION	DEGREE OF BENEFIT	PREFERRED METHOD
Tension headache	**	Progressive muscle relaxation EMG biofeedback
Migraine headache	*	Autogenic training Temperature biofeedback
Chronic pain	*	Hypnosis Meditation EMG biofeedback
Chronic insomnia	*	Progressive muscle relaxation Meditation
Irritable bowel syndrome	*	Progressive muscle relaxation Temperature biofeedback
Hypertension	—	
Bronchial asthma	—	
Diabetes	—	

— Small, often transitory improvements are apparent, but not clinically significant.
* Clinically significant effects of minor degree.
** Clinically significant effects of moderate degree.

9. Which is the most effective type of relaxation training?

Meditation is increasingly popular in hospital-based programs around the country and, indeed, for the management of cognitive anxiety, it is often an excellent choice. It must be remembered, however, that there are many cases where somatic anxiety is paramount (e.g., chronic muscle tension), where symptom-specific training is necessary (e.g., breath retraining), or where patients do not respond well to the relatively unstructured directions for meditation. As an introduction to relaxation training, progressive muscle relaxation—an easy and nonthreatening technique with very concrete directions—is often chosen. It is especially useful in cases where somatic anxiety is central, thus helping to sensitize patients to their own patterns of muscle tension. Biofeedback may be of great value to patients in whom concrete feedback is essential for further training. When immediate progress can be observed (e.g., an on-screen display of a slowly increasing finger temperature), the skeptical patient may be more likely to appreciate relaxation. Growing evidence suggests that the various forms of relaxation can promote uniquely different effects. Thus, there cannot be a relaxation type that is most effective for all cases.

10. Under what conditions are antianxiety medications a better choice?

In the treatment of anxiety, drug treatments and stress management approaches which include relaxation training appear to have similarly potent, short-term effects. In long-term studies, stress management training appears to be somewhat more effective than antianxiety medication. In certain circumstances, however, antianxiety medication are often a better choice for *initial* treatment than relaxation training. When anxiety is overwhelming, for example, patients are unable to concentrate on the tasks of relaxation training (or other stress management instructions). Psychopharmacologic agents may facilitate later introduction and use of relaxation training. In addition, when time and/or finances are limited, referral for relaxation training may not be practical. Given the high relapse rates for anxiety conditions following the discontinuation of drug therapy, however, practitioners should be wary of limiting their intervention to antianxiety medication, especially when the presenting problem does not appear to be transient. At the very least, inclusion of stress management interventions, which work toward expanding the patient's range of coping strategies, significantly lowers the rate of long-term relapse. For treatment of anxiety conditions, therefore, stress management approaches should be included in treatment as often as possible.

11. Is providing patients with relaxation tapes as clinically effective as live training?

No. Live training has been consistently shown to be more effective than taped instruction in providing patients with the skills to lower physiologic arousal. In live training, the patient has the opportunity to benefit from an individualization of training and ongoing feedback. Interpersonal factors, especially the therapist's involvement and warmth, may also be important contributors.

12. How important is home practice?

For clinical success, home practice of relaxation techniques appears to be essential. However, few differences are observed between those who practice daily and those who practice only occasionally, and frequency of home practice is commonly found to be uncorrelated with degree of clinical improvement. Thus, although home practice may be necessary, extensive and regular practice is not necessarily more advantageous than occasional practice.

13. What are the best methods for encouraging home practice?

Greater levels of self-efficacy (high expectations of personal success) and higher expectations of benefits are both associated with more regular practice, suggesting that the therapist may be most successful in promoting home practice by encouraging the patient to believe that relaxation training is a worthwhile endeavor and that he or she can be successful at relaxation practice. In addition, written prescriptions for home practice (detailing the specifics of practice duration, frequency and timing) may be effective in promoting greater practice.

14. What is relaxation-induced anxiety?

Although adverse effects are not common, a subset of patients experience paradoxic sensations of transient anxiety when beginning relaxation training. On rare occasions, severe anxiety may develop (referred to as "relaxation-induced panic"). Anxiety responses appear to be more common with cognitive forms of relaxation (e.g., meditation) than with somatic forms (e.g., progressive muscle relaxation). The causes of relaxation-induced anxiety are not clear, but cognitive factors (e.g., fear of losing control) as well as somatic factors (e.g., subtle hyperventilation) are suspected. In autogenic training, such responses (termed autogenic discharges) are not considered abnormal, and are thought to reflect the unloading of pent-up thoughts or muscular activity. A similar perspective is seen in many forms of meditation, where such anxiety is viewed as a too-rapid release, an "unstressing," of emotional tension. Given the aversive nature of such responses, relaxation-induced anxiety could be a major contributor to the high dropout rate often seen in relaxation training. In the hands of a skilled therapist, however, it may become a valuable part of ongoing training (as well as potentially useful in associated psychotherapeutic interventions) as the patient learns to relax and accept such experiences. Alternatively, when anxiety responses occur (especially during meditation), it is often recommended that therapist switch, at least initially, to a more structured form of relaxation (e.g., progressive muscle relaxation or biofeedback).

BIBLIOGRAPHY

1. Barlow DH, Craske M, Cerny J, Klosko J: Behavioral treatment of panic disorder. Behavior Therapy 20:261–282, 1989.
2. Benson H: The Relaxation Response. New York, Morrow, 1975.
3. Borkovec TD, Mathews AM, Chambers A, et al: The effects of relaxation training with cognitive or nondirective therapy and the role of relaxation-induced anxiety in the treatment of generalized anxiety. J Consult Clin Psychol 55:883–888, 1987.
4. Craske MG, Barlow DH: Panic disorder and agoraphobia. In Barlow DH (ed): Clinical Handbook of Psychological Disorders, 2nd ed. New York, Guilford Press, 1993.
5. Gatchel RJ, Blanchard EB (eds): Psychophysiological Disorders: Research and Clinical Applications. Washington, American Psychological Association, 1993.
6. Lehrer PM, Woolfolk RL (eds): Principles and Practice of Stress Management, 2nd ed. New York, Guilford Press, 1993.
7. Russell ML (ed): Stress Management for Chronic Disease. New York, Pergamon Press, 1988.
8. Suinn RM: Anxiety Management Training: A Behavior Therapy. New York, Plenum Press, 1990.

47. MEDICAL TREATMENT OF DEPRESSION

Russell G. Vasile, M.D.

1. What factors in clinical presentation would lead one to prescribe an antidepressant medication?

Antidepressant medications exert their effects on the psychological symptoms and neurovegetative physical symptoms of depressive illness, including lack of energy, trouble with concentrating, insomnia or hypersomnia, appetite disturbance (with weight loss or, less commonly, weight gain), diminished interest and/or pleasure in daily activities, and symptoms of psychomotor agitation or retardation. Additional physical or so-called neurovegetative symptoms of depression include diminished libido, increased anxiety and/or agitation, and impaired cognitive function. The psychological symptoms of depression include feelings of sadness, hopelessness, helplessness, worthlessness, guilt, and suicidal ideation.

The persistent presence of five or more physical features, together with psychological symptoms, for a period of 2 weeks is a strong indication for antidepressant medications. Additionally, evidence suggests that the persisting presence of psychological symptoms (sad mood and feelings of depression), even in the absence of marked neurovegetative depressive features, may be sufficient indication to prescribe antidepressant medications.

2. What do antidepressants accomplish? How do they work?

Antidepressant medications reverse the neurovegetative and psychological symptoms of depression, restoring the patient's sense of well-being and function to the levels before onset of the depressive episode. Antidepressant medications typically take at least 2 weeks to exert their therapeutic effects, and up to 6 weeks at adequate dosage may be required before full therapeutic effect occurs. They are not euphoriants and do not induce elevation of mood in the absence of a depressive disorder. Before prescribing antidepressant medication, the clinician should establish that no organic factor (such as anemia, frontal lobe tumor, or hypothyroidism) has initiated and maintains the depressive symptoms.

Current understanding of the mechanism of action of antidepressant medications suggests that they work by blocking the reuptake and degradation of important neurotransmitters (such as serotonin, norepinephrine, and epinephrine), enhancing their availability at the synaptic level, and facilitating the transmission of neurochemical impulses in brain regions rich in noradrenergic and serotonergic neurons that contribute to the regulation of neurovegetative and psychological function.

3. Can antidepressants be used in conjunction with psychotherapy?

Antidepressants are commonly used in conjunction with psychotherapy. Psychotherapy exerts its primary effect on the psychosocial and interpersonal adaptation of the patient but has little impact on the neurovegetative symptoms of depression and is not effective for the treatment of severe depressive symptoms. Most clinicians recommend that once a diagnosis of major depression is established, antidepressant medications should be initiated to afford relief of major depressive symptoms and that psychotherapy should be supportive in nature, emphasizing psychoeducational approaches that enable the patient to maintain hope and realistic perspective and marshaling social supports from family and others in the environment. Once the major symptoms of depression are resolved, many patients find insight-oriented psychotherapy helpful in reducing stress by altering patterns of behavior that have become maladaptive. Several studies have suggested that the combination of antidepressant medication and psychotherapy is the most comprehensive and effective approach for resolving an acute depressive episode.

4. What are the common antidepressant treatments?

The most commonly used antidepressants are the selective serotonin reuptake inhibitors (SSRIs), fluoxetine (Prozac), sertraline (Zoloft), and paroxetine (Paxil); cyclic antidepressants, including tricyclic antidepressants, such as imipramine (Tofranil) and amitriptyline (Elavil); and heterocyclic or atypical antidepressants, such as amoxapine (Asendin), maprotiline (Ludiomil), bupropion (Wellbutrin), trazodone (Desyrel), and venlafaxine (Effexor). Monoamine oxidase (MAO) inhibitors, another distinct class of antidepressants, include phenelzine (Nardil), tranylcypromine (Parnate), and isocarboxazid (Marplan). Venlafaxine, a novel antidepressant with a unique chemical structure, has been introduced within the past year. In addition to effects on the neurotransmitter systems noted above, venlafaxine has dopamine-blocking properties.

The tricyclic antidepressants were first used in the early 1960s and long remained the standard treatment. The MAO inhibitors were also discovered over 20 years ago but fell out of popularity for a time because of adverse reactions, often severe and rarely fatal, with ingestion of foods containing tyramine. Prevention of such adverse side effects requires a special tyramine-free diet. The heterocyclic antidepressants vary from the classic tricyclic molecular structure and have found a specific role in selected circumstances. Commonly prescribed heterocyclic antidepressants include amoxapine, bupropion, and trazodone. Each has specific clinical features that may be advantageous in specific circumstances. Amoxapine has significant dopamine-blocking properties and may play a particular role in the treatment of psychotic depression. Trazadone has highly sedating properties and is often useful in the treatment of depressed patients with insomnia; it is also commonly used in low dosage (25–50 mg in the evening) in conjunction with SSRIs, which are usually activating and may induce insomnia. Bupropion is a highly stimulating antidepressant that may be of particular value in bipolar patients in the depressed phase of illness. Some clinical studies have suggested that it induces mania or hypomania less frequently than other antidepressants. The heterocyclic antidepressants were introduced in the 1970s and 1980s.

SSRIs, developed in the mid 1980s, have become the most popular antidepressants in the world because of their relatively benign side effect profile and their relative safety in overdose.

Similar rates of response to all antidepressant drugs have been documented (see question 2). The choice of antidepressant is predicated on factors specific to the particular patient, such as tolerance to specific side effects and previous history of response to a given antidepressant.

5. What are the common side effects of antidepressant treatment?

Pharmacology of Antidepressant Medications

DRUG	MOST COMMON SIDE EFFECTS
Tricyclics Amitriptyline Clomipramine Desipramine Doxepin Imipramine Nortriptyline	Anticholinergic side effects predominate, including dry mouth, constipation, drowsiness, orthostatic hypotension, and urinary hesitancy. Weight gain, excessive sweating, and increased intraocular pressure may occur. Side effects vary within the group; amitriptyline and clomipramine are the most anticholinergic, whereas desipramine and nortriptyline are the least.
Heterocyclics Amoxapine Bupropion Maprotiline Trazodone	Amoxapine may induce mild parkinsonian symptoms. Bupropion may be associated with agitation and insomnia. Trazodone is highly sedating and has been associated with priapism in men. Maprotiline is sedating.

Table continued on following page.

Pharmacology of Antidepressant Medications (Cont.)

DRUG	MOST COMMON SIDE EFFECTS
Selective serotonin reuptake inhibitors Fluoxetine Paroxetine Sertraline	The most common side effects in the SSRI group are erectile dysfunction in men, anorgasmia in women, insomnia, agitation, headache, and gastrointestinal upset, typically nausea and cramping. Fluoxetine is generally more activating than the other SSRIs. Sertraline may have more pronounced gastrointestinal side effects. Paroxetine has mild anticholinergic properties and may cause mild dry mouth.
Mixed reuptake blockers Venlafaxine (Effexor)	SSRI-like side effects include agitation, nausea, headache, and gastrointestinal distress. Because hypertension may also occur over time, ongoing blood pressure monitoring is required.
Monoamine oxidase inhibitors Isocarboxazid Phenelzine Tranylcypromine	Orthostatic hypotension, weight gain, and adverse interactions with tyramine-containing foods may occur. The adverse food interaction is characterized by throbbing headache and blood pressure elevation with marked pressor response. Tranylcypromine is the most activating MAO inhibitor and causes the least hypotension. Tranylcypromine may induce insomnia, whereas phenelzine can be sedating, and has a greater effect on lowering of blood pressure.

Cyclic antidepressants, SSRIs and MAO inhibitors are not uncommonly associated with sexual dysfunction, including diminished libido, delayed ejaculation, and anorgasmia. Such side effects are less likely to occur with bupropion.

Weight gain is a side effect that may be encountered with cyclic antidepressants and MAO inhibitors but is less likely with SSRIs. Weight loss has been reported in conjunction with the use of SSRIs. The SSRI antidepressants are therefore contraindicated in the treatment of anorectic or underweight patients.

Neurologic side effects include an approximate 1% risk of induction of seizures. This risk is associated with elevated antidepressant blood levels and is more commonly associated with tricyclic antidepressants than with SSRIs and MAO inhibitors. Mild myoclonus and toxic confusional states may also be encountered, particularly in the elderly, and in association with elevated blood levels of tricyclic antidepressants.

Cardiovascular side effects of antidepressant medications include orthostatic hypotension, commonly seen with tricyclic antidepressants, MAO inhibitors and trazodone. Among the tricyclic antidepressants, nortriptyline (Pamelor, Aventyl) and desipramine (Norpramin) induce less orthostatic hypotension. In patients with sinus node dysfunction, treatment with tricyclics may on occasion induce bradyarrhythmias. Therapeutic concentrations of tricyclic antidepressants may lengthen the QT interval, which predisposes to the development of ventricular tachycardia. Cardiovascular side effects are less commonly observed with the SSRI antidepressants.

The cyclic antidepressants have a range of side effects that vary from medication to medication. Certain antidepressants have side effect profiles worth noting. Bupropion is quite activating and is associated with less sexual dysfunction than other antidepressants, but it has a tendency to induce insomnia and in high doses has caused a significant incidence of seizure in underweight patients. Trazodone has been associated with priapism in men, yet in low doses is often used adjunctively with SSRI antidepressants to facilitate sleep.

6. What factors influence the choice of antidepressant medications?
Because all antidepressants are equally effective in clinical trials, factors specific to a given patient influence choice of antidepressant. Depressive illness is heterogeneous in symptom expression.

Individual patients differ in their profile of acute depressive symptoms and exhibit different patterns of side effects and response to antidepressants. If a patient has had an excellent response to a specific antidepressant in the past, that antidepressant is likely to be the best choice for future administration. Similarly, if a first-degree relative has had an excellent response to an antidepressant, the likelihood of a good response to that antidepressant is enhanced. In addition to patient and family history of response, the profile of antidepressant side effects becomes an important consideration. If a patient has insomnia, an antidepressant with sedative properties is advantageous. Conversely, if a patient experiences lethargy and hypersomnia as symptoms of depression, a more activating antidepressant is advantageous. Antidepressants that induce orthostatic hypotension should be avoided in the management of patients at risk for falls, such as the elderly.

Another factor related to choice of antidepressant may be safety in overdose. The SSRI antidepressants, trazodone, and bupropion are substantially safer than other antidepressants, especially tricyclic antidepressants. Ingestion of 2,000 mg of a tricyclic antidepressant, a 10-day supply of 200 mg/day, may be fatal.

Antidepressant medications may be combined with adjunctive medications that may enhance antidepressant efficacy, such as lithium carbonate (600–1200 mg/day) or triiodothyronine (25–50 µg/day). In some treatment-resistant patients combinations of antidepressant medications, such as low-dose Prozac (10–20 mg/day) and low-dose desipramine (25–50 mg/day), may be considered, provided that antidepressant blood levels are carefully monitored; toxic levels of desipramine may result from medication interactions.

7. Do specific types of depression respond more consistently to specific antidepressant treatments?

Major Depressive Disorder Subgroups and Selection of Treatment

SUBGROUP	ESSENTIAL FEATURES	DIAGNOSTIC ISSUES	TREATMENT ISSUES	PROGNOSTIC FEATURES
Psychotic	Delusions Hallucinations	More likely to be bipolar than nonpsychotic types; may be misdiagnosed as schizo-phrenia	Antipsychotic med plus antidepressant is more effective treatment than antidepressant alone; ECT is highly effective	Usually a recurrent illness Subsequent episodes are usually psychotic Psychosis is affect consonant in depressed patients Patients with mood incongruent features have a poorer prognosis
Melancholic	Anhedonia Unreactive mood Severe vegetative depressive symptoms	May be misdiagnosed as dementia; more common in elderly patients	Antidepressant medication is essential ECT is highly effective if medications fail to produce remission of depression	Maintenance treatment should be considered if recurrent episodes occur
Atypical	Reactive mood Overeating and oversleeping Rejection sensitivity Waves of fatigue Prominent anxiety Irritability	Patients tend to be younger May be misdiagnosed as a personality disorder	TCAs are less effective than MAO inhibitors SSRI show promise as therapeutic agents	Unclear

Table continued on following page.

Major Depressive Disorder Subgroups and Selection of Treatment (Cont.)

SUBGROUP	ESSENTIAL FEATURES	DIAGNOSTIC ISSUES	TREATMENT ISSUES	PROGNOSTIC FEATURES
Seasonal	Onset in low light months	More frequent in nonequatorial latitudes	May respond to antidepressant medication Phototherapy is an effective option	Recurs seasonally
Postpartum depression	Acute onset (< 30 days) in postpartum period Severe, labile mood symptoms	Often heralds bipolar disorder	Hospital treatment required Medical treatment necessary	50% chance of recurrence in next postpartum period

ECT = electroconvulsive therapy, TCA = tricyclic antidepressants, MAO = monoamine oxidase, SSRI = selective serotonin reuptake inhibitors.

Although all antidepressants are equally effective in general, evidence indicates that specific subtypes of depressive disorder appear to respond preferentially to different antidepressant treatments.

MAO inhibitors (especially phenelzine) are more efficacious for the treatment of atypical depression than classic tricyclic antidepressants. A dramatic, histrionic yet dysthymic interpersonal style (sometimes termed hysteroid dysphoria) also may characterize patients with atypical depression, as may the sensation of episodic waves of leaden fatigue. SSRIs are currently under investigation for the treatment of atypical depression and have shown promise in early clinical trials. MAO inhibitors also may have a preferential role in the treatment of patients with panic and/or phobic symptoms with concurrent depressive features.

Some clinicians believe that amoxapine may have superior efficacy to other antidepressants in the treatment of psychotic depression.

Many clinicians believe that the antidepressant bupropion is a superior choice for the treatment of manic-depressive patients in the depressed phase of their illness, because it may result in less of a tendency towards inducing mania than other antidepressants.

Clinical trials currently under way suggest that SSRI antidepressants may have specific benefits in depressed patients with a proclivity towards inappropriate anger and impulsivity.

The antidepressant clomipramine (Anafranil) has specific beneficial effects on obsessive-compulsive symptoms and may be a preferential choice for patients with depression and associated obsessive-compulsive disorder or obsessive compulsive symptoms.

Imipramine has distinct antipanic properties and may be a preferential choice for patients with comorbid panic and depressive illness.

In some patients who characteristically experience depression during low-light months, bright white artificial light in the morning and/or evening hours for 30 minutes or more may be effective in reducing symptoms. Phototherapy responsive patients may also respond to antidepressant medication; phototherapy and antidepressant medication may be used in combination. Phototherapy is not generally associated with side effects, but some patients may report irritability or increased anxiety during the course of treatment, particularly if phototherapy is combined with antidepressant medication.

8. When should electroconvulsive therapy be considered?
Electroconvulsive therapy (ECT) is a treatment to consider in the following circumstances:
1. When the patient has failed to respond to several antidepressant medication trials.
2. When the patient is experiencing threatening acute symptoms, such as intense suicidal pressure, food refusal, or catatonic stupor, that require a rapid antidepressant response; ECT

often exerts a therapeutic effect within days, whereas antidepressant medications commonly take 2–3 weeks to exert a therapeutic effect.

3. When the patient has prominent features of agitation and/or psychotic symptoms, characterized by delusions or hallucination.

4. When antidepressant medications are associated with unacceptable side effects.

5. When the patient has a history of a positive response to previous ECT treatments.

6. When the patient has a medical condition that precludes the use of antidepressants.

During the course of ECT, antidepressant medication is suspended, although low-dose antianxiety medication may be used. High-dose antianxiety medications may interfere with the efficacy of ECT and should be discouraged during ECT treatments.

ECT has shown a high rate of success in patients exhibiting marked neurovegetative symptoms, including marked agitation or psychomotor retardation, and in patients with psychotic depression. ECT has a demonstrated excellent safety profile and rapid onset of action. Although there are no absolute contraindications, ECT causes a transient elevation in blood pressure, heart rate, cardiac workload, and blood-brain barrier permeability. Therefore, ECT should be considered with caution in patients with recent myocardial infarction, cardiac arrhythmias, and intracranial space-occupying lesions. In such circumstances consultation is advised.

The most common side effects of ECT include a transient postictal confusional state and anterograde and retrograde periods of memory disturbance that may take 2–3 weeks to resolve after completion of the course of ECT. ECT treatments usually consist of 3 treatments per week for up to 4 weeks. Recent advances in ECT instrumentation have resulted in a reduction in cognitive side effects and permitted some patients to be treated as outpatients with careful day program and/or family monitoring. The two standard electrode placement positions are unilateral nondominant hemisphere placement and bilateral electrode placement, which utilizes a bitemporal positioning of electrodes. Generally, bilateral electrode placement is reserved for patients who fail to respond optimally to unilateral treatment. Bilateral treatments generally cause somewhat more confusion and transient memory impairment than unilateral treatments.

9. What approaches are useful in patients who fail to respond to initial pharmacologic interventions to treat depression?

In 20–30% of patients with a major depressive disorder, initial pharmacologic interventions are not effective. The most common factors in failure to respond to initial antidepressant treatment include inadequacy of dosage and duration of treatment and failure to detect and treat a coexisting medical or psychiatric disorder. The duration of treatment required before a medication trial should be ruled a failure can be as long as 6 weeks. Antidepressant medication blood levels are also available to assess adequacy of dosage, although they are not precisely established for every antidepressant medication.

If a patient fails to respond to an antidepressant medication, given adequate dosage and sufficient duration, other interventions are likely to be required. Possible medical factors contributing to treatment resistance should be reassessed. Comorbid psychiatric conditions, including anxiety disorders, alcohol or substance abuse, neuropsychiatric disorders, and personality disorders, should be ruled out. Chronic psychosocial stressors should be identified as potential complicating factors.

Assuming that none of the above issues is operative, modification of antidepressant treatment may include the following interventions: (1) changing to an alternate class of antidepressant medication; (2) using adjunctive medications to boost antidepressant response; (3) using combinations of antidepressant medications; and (4) considering the use of ECT as a treatment alternative.

In shifting to an alternative antidepressant, using an SSRI if a tricyclic antidepressant has failed and considering an MAO inhibitor are possible strategies. Serious adverse reactions may occur if SSRIs and MAO inhibitors are combined; therefore, a waiting period of up to 6 weeks is required before beginning an MAO inhibitor after a trial of an SSRI agent.

Adjunctive medications commonly used with antidepressants include lithium carbonate in a standard dosage of 300 mg 3 times/day. The addition of lithium carbonate frequently boosts antidepressant response and may restore a patient to a response if it has begun to fail. Other adjunctive medication strategies include the addition of Cytomel (T3) (25–50 µg). Finally, some clinicians use low doses of stimulants such as methylphenidate (Ritalin), 5–10 mg/day to enhance antidepressant efficacy. Hormonal treatments, such as the use of estrogen in women, are less well established as adjunctive agents.

Combinations of antidepressants may be tried in treatment-resistant patients failing to respond to the above measures. A commonly used combination is low-dose SSRI with low-dose tricyclic, typically fluoxetine (10–20 mg/day) and desipramine (10–20 mg/day). It is not advisable to combine any antidepressant with an MAO inhibitor; a 2-week washout period is advisable before beginning an alternative antidepressant trial after a failed MAO inhibitor trial. In addition, when switching from an SSRI to a MAO inhibitor, a longer waiting period of 4–6 weeks is advisable.

In treatment-resistant cases failing to respond to any of the interventions above, ECT may be a reasonable alternative. Approximately 50% of medication-resistant patients exhibit a positive response to ECT. The novel antidepressant, venlafaxine, which acts on both noradrenergic and serotonergic neuronal systems, has shown promise in a subgroup of patients who fail to respond to trials of antidepressants. Venlafaxine, which is generally well tolerated, has a spectrum of side effects similar to the SSRIs, including nausea, insomnia, and induction of anxiety.

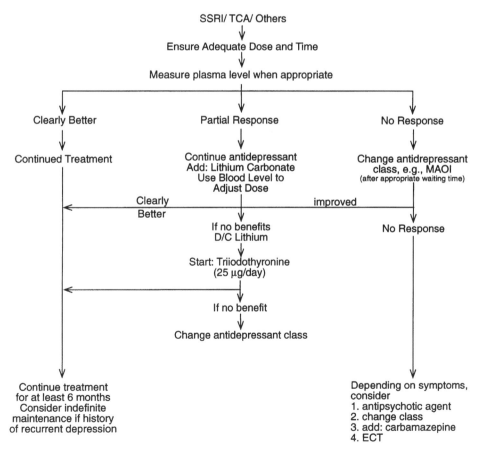

Flow chart for approaching treatment-resistant depressions.

10. How long and at what dosage should medical treatment for depression be continued?
Antidepressant medication treatment may be conceptualized as divided into three phases: acute treatment, continuation treatment, and maintenance treatment. Acute treatment refers to the initial stages of a depressive episode; continuation treatment, to the 6 months after the acute phase; and maintenance treatment, to chronic prevention.

Increasing evidence suggests that patients who have had 3 or more major depressive episodes or histories of chronic low-grade depressive symptomatology are candidates for maintenance antidepressant medication. Recent studies also have suggested that adequacy of dosage is an important factor in effective prophylaxis of depression and that full dosage of medications should be administered for maintenance treatment. If a patient has had one initial depressive episode and exhibits none of the risk factors noted above, treatment should be continued for a full 6 months to 1 year before attempting gradual tapering on an individual basis. Decisions about precisely when to taper medication are best evaluated collaboratively between patient and doctor with full consideration of the patient's life circumstances, including the likelihood of a recurrent episode of depression.

Withdrawal symptoms may occur with the abrupt discontinuation of antidepressant medications, including feelings of malaise, agitation, confusion, and increased feelings of dysphoria.

No well-established long-term risks are associated with chronic administration of antidepressant medications. Monitoring of cardiac status in the elderly by obtaining serial electrocardiograms and episodic assessment of liver function tests are recommended. Chronic administration of lithium carbonate requires periodic assessment (every 6–12 months unless symptomatic) of complete blood count with differential, thyroid tests, and measures of renal function, including urine-concentrating capacity after water restriction. Because an increasing number of patients require maintenance antidepressant treatment, problems that occur after years of treatment may necessitate changes in antidepressant medications. For example, the development of coronary vascular disease may lead to the risk of arrhythmia and therefore to an alternative antidepressant with less cardiac toxicity, such as an SSRI.

11. What other psychiatric conditions commonly influence the medical treatment of depression?
It is crucial to have a high index of awareness of other psychiatric conditions that influence and adversely affect the treatment of depressive disorder. Common conditions include (1) substance abuse, in particular alcoholism; (2) anxiety disorders, including panic disorder, and (3) personality disorders, most commonly borderline personality disorder. It has been repeatedly demonstrated that these common comorbid conditions enhance morbidity and exert an adverse impact on the treatment outcome of depressive disorders. In elderly patients, dementia is commonly superimposed on depression. Increased sensitivity to the adverse cognitive side effects of antidepressant medication is particularly important to note in this population.

12. What common medication interactions may influence antidepressant treatment?
Antidepressants may potentiate the sedative and central nervous system effects of various medications, including antihistamines, barbiturates, and anticonvulsants. Particular attention needs to be placed on avoiding the use of barbiturates and MAO inhibitors—a potentially fatal combination. Blood levels of tricyclic antidepressants may be sharply increased by concomitant use of SSRIs. MAO inhibitors and SSRIs should not be combined, because a potentially fatal "serotonergic syndrome" may occur.

13. What are the treatment implications of concurrent general medical disorders?
- Patients requiring sympathomimetic bronchodilators for the treatment of asthma should be cautioned about the use of MAO inhibitors.
- Patients with cardiac disease, including subclinical sinus node conduction disease or a history of ventricular arrhythmia, are best treated with bupropion, fluoxetine, sertraline, or ECT as opposed to tricyclic antidepressants.

- Patients with dementia do well with low doses of antidepressants, given their vulnerability to adverse cognitive side effects of anticholinergic antidepressants. If tricyclic antidepressants are to be used, low-dose desipramine or nortriptyline, which have low anticholinergic properties compared with other tricyclics, are advised. Bupropion, fluoxetine, or trazodone, which have even lower anticholinergic effects, may be preferable.
- Narrow-angle glaucoma is a relative contraindication to anticholinergic antidepressants.
- Obstructive uropathy, usually secondary to prostatism, mitigates against the use of highly antimuscarinic antidepressants. SSRIs, desipramine, or bupropion is advised in this circumstance.
- Severe depression in pregnancy can be treated safely with ECT. The relative risk (particularly in the first trimester of pregnancy) of inducing birth defects, versus the benefits of antidepressant medication, need to be reviewed on a case-by-case basis.

BIBLIOGRAPHY

1. Depression Guideline Panel: Depression in Primary Care. Vol. 2: Treatment of Major Depression. Clinical Practice Guideline, Number 5. Rockville, MD. U.S. Department of Health and Human Services, Public Health Service, Agency for Health Care Policy and Research. AHCPR Publication No. 93-05551, 1993.
2. De Vane CL: Pharmacokinetics of the selective serotonin reuptake inhibitors. J Clin Psychiatry 53(Suppl):13–20, 1992.
3. Gelenberg AJ: New horizons in the management of complicated anxiety and depressive disorders. J Clin Psychiatry 55(Suppl): 1994.
4. Guscott R, Grof P: The clinical meaning of refractory depression: A review for the clinician. Am J Psychiatry 148:695–704, 1991.
5. Kupfer DJ, et al: Three year outcomes for maintenance therapies in recurrent depression. Arch Gen Psychiatry 47:1093–1099, 1990.
6. Manning DW, Frances AJ (eds): Combined Pharmacotherapy and Psychotherapy for Depression. APA Press, 1990.
7. Maxmen JS: Psychotropic Drugs: Fast Facts. New York, W.W. Norton, 1991.
8. Osser D: A systematic approach to the classification and pharmacotherapy of nonpsychotic major depression and dysthymia. J Clin Psychopharmacol 13:133–144, 1993.
9. Prien RF, Kupfer DJ: Continuation drug therapy for major depressive episodes: How long should it be maintained? Am J Psychiatry 143:18–23, 1986.
10. Quitkin FM, et al: Atypical depression, panic attacks, and response to imipramine and phenelzine. Arch Gen Psychiatry 47:935–941, 1990.
11. Tasman A, Goldfinger SM, Kaufmann CA (eds): Review of Psychiatry, vol. 9. Washington, DC, American Psychiatric Press, pp 7–201.

48. ANTIPSYCHOTIC MEDICATIONS

Herbert T. Nagamoto, M.D.

1. What are antipsychotic or neuroleptic medications?

Antipsychotic or neuroleptic medications are used to treat psychotic symptoms in patients with schizophrenia and other conditions. Symptoms may include hallucinations, delusions, paranoia, thought broadcasting, catatonia, bizarre behavior, and associated symptoms such as hypervigilance, agitation, and irritability. Most typical antipsychotic medications also have neurologic side effects, leading to the alternate designation of neuroleptics ("of the neuron"). Antipsychotic medications are sometimes divided into **typical agents**, which basically are similar to chlorpromazine, and **atypical agents**, as exemplified by clozapine, which appear to have different therapeutic and side effect profiles and a different mechanism of action.

2. List the different typical antipsychotic or neuroleptic medications by chemical class, specifying relative potency in chlorpromazine equivalents and typical range of daily oral dose.

Potency and Range of Oral Dose of Neuroleptics

ANTIPSYCHOTIC AGENT: GENERIC NAME (TRADE NAME)	APPROXIMATE AMOUNT (MG) OF DRUG NEEDED TO EQUAL 100 MG OF CHLORPROMAZINE	RANGE OF DAILY ORAL DOSE (MG)
Aliphatic		
Chlorpromazine (Thorazine)	100	25–2,000
Piperazine		
Fluphenazine (Permitil, Prolixin)	2	1–40
Perphenazine (Trilafon)	10	4–64
Prochlorperazine (Compazine)	15	15–150
Trifluoperazine (Stelazine)	5	2–40
Piperidine		
Mesoridazine (Serentil)	50	75–400
Thioridazine (Mellaril)	100	75–800
Butyrophenone		
Haloperidol (Haldol)	2	1–100
Thioxanthene		
Chlorprothixene (Taractan)	100	30–60
Thiothixene (Navane)	4	6–60
Dihydroindolone		
Molindone (Moban)	10	15–225
Dibenzoxazepine		
Loxapine (Loxitane)	10	1–250

From Jenkins S, Gibbs T, Szymanski S: A Pocket Reference for Psychiatrists. Washington, D.C., American Psychiatric Association, 1990, p 134, with permission.

3. What is the mechanism of action of typical antipsychotic medications?

The typical antipsychotic medications are believed to act via central blockade of dopamine receptors, which in limbic areas leads to antipsychotic effects; in basal ganglia, to extrapyramidal side effects; in the brainstem chemoreceptor trigger zone, to antinausea and antiemetic effects; and in the hypothalamus (via blockade of dopamine inhibition of anterior pituitary prolactin release), to increased prolactin release.

4. Name several conditions that are indications for the use of antipsychotic medications.
Antipsychotic medications are used in a number of conditions to treat psychotic symptoms, including hallucinations, delusions, paranoia, combativeness, agitation and hostility, insomnia, catatonia, hyperactivity, and poor grooming and self-care.

Indications for Use of Antipsychotic Medication
- Acute and maintenance treatment of schizophrenia
- Psychosis associated with acute mania and major depression
- Psychosis from any number of medical causes (see chapters on schizophrenia, dementia, and delirium)
- As adjunctive treatment for agitation due to psychiatric conditions, delirium, delirium tremens, and dementia
- Tics due to neurologic conditions such as Huntington's chorea and Tourette's syndrome
- Flashbacks, nightmares, and agitation due to posttraumatic stress disorder
- Nausea and vomiting (prochlorperazine [Compazine], trimethobenzamide [Tigan], metoclopramide [Reglan])
- Gastroesophageal reflux and diabetic gastroparesis (metoclopramide [Reglan])
- Adjunctive use in anesthesia for medical and surgical procedures (droperidol [Inapsine])

5. List the general classes of side effects of typical antipsychotic medications.
Dopaminergic side effects
   *Pseudoparkinsonism
     Cogwheel rigidity
     Shuffling gait
     Parkinsonian tremor
     Masked facies
   *Acute dystonias, such as opisthotonus, torticollis, and †laryngospasm, which may cause
     acute airway obstruction
     Increased prolactin secretion that may lead to galactorrhea
   *Akathisia—subjective or observable restlessness ("thorazine shuffle")
     Tardive dyskinesia, tardive dystonia (see question 12)
   †Neuroleptic malignant syndrome (NMS)
Anticholinergic side effects
   *Dry mouth
   *Blurred vision (accommodation problems or frank blurred vision)
   *Constipation that may lead to †adynamic ileus
   *Urinary hesitancy or †obstruction
     Memory and concentration difficulties, up to †frank delirium
Alpha-adrenergic blockade
   *Hypotension
   *Orthostatic hypotension
Antihistaminergic side effects
   *Sedation, drowsiness
     Weight gain
Others
   †Agranulocytosis
     ECG changes (prolonged QT interval)
     Elevated liver function tests
     Elevated creatine phosphokinase (in the absence of NMS)
     Fetal toxicity
     Photosensitivity

*Common side effects.
†Potentially dangerous side effects.

Pigmentary retinopathy (avoid doses of thioridazine > 800 mg/day)
Seizures (decreased seizure threshold)
*Sexual dysfunction (erectile problems, impotency, delayed, absent, or retrograde
    ejaculation, priapism)
Skin rashes

*Common side effects.
†Potentially dangerous side effects.

6. How is antipsychotic potency related to side effects?

In general, the lower-potency agents, such as chlorpromazine and thioridazine, tend to be high in sedation, orthostatic hypotension, and anticholinergic side effects, whereas the higher-potency agents, such as haloperidol and fluphenazine, tend to be high in pseudoparkinsonian, akathisia, and acute dystonic side effects.

7. Describe the treatment of common side effects of antipsychotic medications.

In general, one should decrease the dose of antipsychotic medications to the lowest effective dose to minimize side effects and avoid polypharmacy whenever possible.

Pseudoparkinsonism and acute dystonias are treated with antiparkinson agents. Benztropine (Cogentin, 1–2 mg up to 4 times/day), diphenhydramine (Benadryl, 25–50 mg up to 4 times/day), and trihexyphenidyl (Artane, 2–5 mg up to 15 mg/day in divided doses) are used for their anticholinergic effects to treat acute extrapyramidal side effects. Prophylactic treatment for approximately the first 10 days of treatment or after dosage increases may be considered for adolescents and other patients who (by history) are highly susceptible to pseudoparkinsonism and acute dystonias. Care should be used to avoid anticholinergic poisoning in combination with other anticholinergic agents, particularly in elderly or medically debilitated patients. The lowest effective doses are prudent, and they should be tapered and discontinued as soon as possible. Amantadine (Symmetrel), which is thought to potentiate dopaminergic neurotransmission, also may be used. In the case of laryngospasm, which may lead to acute airway obstruction, Benadryl, 50 mg intravenously, should be used.

Akathisia usually responds well to dosage reduction, anticholinergic agents, or change to a different class of neuroleptics. Benzodiazepines and beta-adrenergic antagonists such as propranolol are also effective in treating akathisia. It is important to differentiate akathisia due to neuroleptic treatment from agitation due to psychosis. This differentiation may be difficult, but neuroleptic doses may be increased (which improves psychotic agitation but worsens akathisia) or decreased (which improves akathisia but worsens psychotic agitation). Some akathisia treatments (anticholinergics) are unlikely to affect psychotic agitation, whereas others may improve (benzodiazepines) or have differential effects (beta-adrenergic antagonists) on agitation due to psychosis.

Patients often develop tolerance to **anticholinergic side effects**, but they may persist. It is usually best to decrease dosage or switch to a more potent agent if anticholinergic side effects become intolerable. Alternatively, bethanechol (Urecholine, 5–10 mg up to 4 times/day; sometimes 25 mg up to 4 times/day) may be used to decrease dry mouth, blurred vision, constipation, and urinary hesitancy.

Hypotension and orthostatic hypotension are treated with oral hydration, careful instructions to the patient, dose reduction, or change to more potent agents. Occasionally, intravenous hydration is indicated. If a vasoactive agent is required, one should avoid agents with beta-adrenergic agonist properties (such as epinephrine), which may worsen hypotension via vasodilatation and peripheral pooling. In such cases, a selective alpha-adrenergic agonist such as metaraminol (Aramine) should be used.

8. What constitutes an adequate trial of antipsychotic medications?

Antipsychotic medications often induce sedation quickly, but their specific antipsychotic effects may take up to 6 weeks at therapeutic doses to develop fully. Conversely, when a stable schizophrenic patient decides to stop antipsychotic medication suddenly, it may take weeks for psychotic symptoms to return or for patients to decompensate. Therapeutic doses vary widely from patient to patient and within a given patient at various times. In general, maintenance doses range from approximately 100–700 mg/day, averaging 300 mg/day in chlorpromazine equivalents. Acutely ill patients may require higher doses, although the current trend is toward adjunctive use of benzodiazepines in acutely psychotic patients to avoid the side effects often associated with high-dose antipsychotic medications.

In an emergency situation, with a highly agitated or out-of-control patient, many antipsychotic medications can be given intramuscularly. In general, the lower-potency antipsychotics such as chlorpromazine or thioridazine are given in half the amount of oral doses. In some settings, particularly emergency departments, acutely psychotic, out-of-control patients are given intravenous haloperidol, often in very high doses. There is a small chance that intravenous haloperidol will induce the condition known as torsade de pointes, which may lead to ventricular fibrillation and sudden death. Intravenous haloperidol should be used with caution in women and patients with increased QT intervals on electrocardiogram, who are at increased risk for developing torsade de pointes.

9. Delineate an approach to patients who do not respond well to antipsychotic medications.
For patients who do not respond to treatment, one should reassess the diagnosis, particularly in the case of such illnesses as schizophrenia and bipolar affective disorder, which may be quite similar in the acute phases. In revisiting a patient's diagnosis, it is important (1) to rule out occult medical illness that may worsen symptoms or cause the illness under treatment; (2) to rule out alcohol and substance abuse, which may mimic or worsen a number of psychiatric symptoms; and (3) to ensure that the patient is receiving an adequate dosage of neuroleptic for an adequate length of time.

Increasing evidence suggests that antipsychotic medications may have a therapeutic window; thus patients out of the appropriate range may receive too little or too much medication. Plasma levels obtained at steady state help to assess dosage of some neuroleptics (see below; haloperidol and fluphenazine are most studied).

Compliance is a common problem with antipsychotic medications. All too often patients stop medications because of legitimately troublesome side effects and thus experience psychotic decompensation. To ensure acute compliance, one can administer intramuscular injections or observe the patient for 30 minutes after oral ingestion of liquid medications. For long-term maintenance, fluphenazine and haloperidol are available in slow-release depot forms that may be given intramuscularly every 2–4 weeks.

One should also ensure that troublesome side effects do not hinder the effectiveness of treatment, especially akathisia, which may mimic or exacerbate psychotic agitation. Pseudoparkinsonism and oversedation may make patients look artificially depressed, and neuroleptic malignant syndrome may make patients suddenly look worse (e.g., catatonic or delirious). If a schizophrenic patient does not improve, it is also important not to miss a treatable depression. Finally, for patients who cannot tolerate typical neuroleptics, risperidone or clozapine should be considered. For patients who do not respond to adequate trials of different neuroleptics at maximal therapeutic doses, clozapine should be considered. The next few years should see the introduction of a number of clozapinelike agents (see below).

10. How can blood levels of antipsychotic medications be helpful in the clinical management of patients?
As mentioned above, increasing evidence suggests that at least some antipsychotic medications have a therapeutic window of ideal dosage or blood levels. Currently, haloperidol is the most thoroughly studied agent, with best therapeutic effects achieved at plasma levels of 5–12 ng/ml in most patients. Other agents are not as well studied, although plasma levels are useful in ruling out subtherapeutic levels of medication in patients who "hypermetabolize," have poor absorption, or are noncompliant. If a laboratory reports a therapeutic range for a neuroleptic, it is reasonable to inquire how the laboratory arrived at its recommendations.

11. Name possible problematic interactions between antipsychotic medications and other drugs.

Most antipsychotic medications affect a number of neurotransmitter systems, with the notable exceptions of haloperidol and pimozide, which are highly selective for the D2 dopamine receptor. This and other factors may lead to a number of problematic interactions.

Potential Drug Interactions with Antipsychotic Medications

• Anticholinergic agents may place patients at increased risk of anticholinergic delirium.
• Numerous agents may induce or worsen hypotension or orthostatic changes in combination with neuroleptics, including barbiturates and nonbarbiturate hypnotics, narcotics, benzodiazepines, angiotensin-converting enzyme inhibitors, antidepressants, methyldopa, anesthetics, and epinephrine.
• Sedation may be worsened when antipsychotics are used with benzodiazepines, sedatives, narcotics, cimetidine, antidepressants, and antihistamines. In particular, chlorpromazine and meperidine used in combination may lead to hypotension and lethargy.
• Lithium and antidepressants may worsen extrapyramidal side effects (pseudoparkinsonism and acute dystonias). For a more complete listing of drug interactions with antipsychotic medications, including changes in plasma levels, see Watsky and Salzman.[8]

12. What is tardive dyskinesia? Why is it of concern with chronic use of antipsychotic medications?

Tardive dyskinesia is a syndrome of abnormal involuntary movements such as buccolingual masticatory movements, choreoathetoid movements of the limbs or even trunk and neck, and facial grimacing or tics. Long before the advent of antipsychotic medications, such movements were filmed in schizophrenic patients, who probably are at increased risk of developing the syndrome. Tardive dyskinesia tends to develop after months to years of neuroleptic treatment and has been described in patients treated with all available typical agents. It occurs in about 15–20% of patients receiving chronic neuroleptic treatment; the incidence rises significantly in elderly populations. Curiously, it is masked by increased antipsychotic doses and tends to worsen acutely with decreased dosage.

On examination, the abnormal movements are more apparent when patients do not know that they are being observed or when they are concentrating on tasks such as rapid alternating movements. In addition, a syndrome of withdrawal dyskinesias may occur briefly on withdrawal of neuroleptics. Withdrawal dyskinesias are relatively brief and may be confused with true tardive dyskinesia. In a small but significant percentage of cases, tardive dyskinesia becomes permanent and disfiguring. Patients treated with neuroleptics should be examined for abnormal involuntary movements before initiating therapy and every 6 months or with dosage changes or appearance of suspected movements. Patients should be maintained on the lowest effective dosage of medication.

Unfortunately, there are no effective treatments for tardive dyskinesia, although vitamin E (400 IU 3–4 times/day) has been shown to decrease symptoms in some patients, especially those who are young and have had the syndrome briefly. The atypical antipsychotic clozapine appears not to cause this problem and may improve symptoms in patients who develop tardive dyskinesia (see below) and need continued antipsychotic treatment.

13. Define neuroleptic malignant syndrome.

Neuroleptic malignant syndrome (NMS) is a potentially fatal side effect that involves:

1. Fever (up to 42°C) in the absence of infection
2. Rigidity, which may be "lead pipe" and generalized, and other neurologic signs (e.g., akinesia and dyskinesia)
3. Autonomic dysfunction leading to tachycardia, labile hypertension, diaphoresis, and pallor (mix of symptoms varies widely)
4. Changes in mental status ranging from mild obtundation through stupor and coma (in approximately 70% of patients)

5. Other possible symptoms: rhabdomyolysis (with elevated creatine phosphokinase in 40–90%), dysarthria, dysphagia, mutism, Babinski reflex, sialorrhea, opisthotonus

NMS usually occurs within 2 weeks of initiating neuroleptics or increasing dosage but may occur after months of stable-dose treatment. It evolves over 24–72 hours and lasts 5–10 days with oral medications or considerably longer with depot intramuscular medications. NMS has an estimated mortality rate of 15–20%. Prompt diagnosis and discontinuation of neuroleptics are essential. Treatment is primarily supportive, although dantrolene and bromocriptine have been helpful.

14. What is clozapine? Why is it considered the prototypic atypical antipsychotic medication?

Clozapine (Clozaril) is a dibenzodiazepine antipsychotic medication that was synthesized in the 1960s but withdrawn from the market in the U.S. after it led to 13 deaths due to agranulocytosis in Finland in the mid 1970s. It has been continuously used since then in other countries, primarily as an antipsychotic, but also as a hypnotic at low doses in China. In the late 1980s it was reintroduced in the U.S. because:

1. Multicenter trials showed that clozapine was effective in schizophrenic patients who respond poorly to typical neuroleptics. Its superior efficacy occurs in about 30% of treatment-resistant schizophrenics after 6 weeks of treatment and is considerably higher (up to 70%) after longer trials.

2. Careful review of worldwide data established that clozapine probably does not cause tardive dyskinesia or significant acute extrapyramidal symptoms. Patients with preexisting tardive dyskinesia may show considerable reduction in abnormal movements when treated with clozapine.

Clozapine appears to be 1½ to 2 times more potent than chlorpromazine. Average doses are approximately 250–450 mg/day with a range of 100–900 mg/day. It has been designated as an atypical antipsychotic because of its atypical clinical profile and pharmacologic actions. Clozapine requires weekly dispensing and weekly blood monitoring (by FDA mandate) because of the 1–2% incidence of agranulocytosis (vs. approximately 0.1% with typical neuroleptics). Other potentially problematic side effects include seizures (up to 5–10% at doses over 600 mg/day), sedation, orthostatic hypotension, sialorrhea, and significant weight gain. In a number of previously treatment-intolerant or unresponsive patients, however, its use has significantly improved quality of life.

15. What are the possible mechanisms of action of clozapine?

The fact that clozapine affects a large number of neurotransmitter systems has led to various theories about its mode of action. Two of the leading theories involve (1) strong 5-HT2 blockade with relatively weak D2 blockade and (2) strong D4 blockade. Not surprisingly, there is a tremendous rush to duplicate clozapine's therapeutic efficacy and relative lack of motoric side effects without significant risk for agranulocytosis and other problematic side effects.

16. What is risperidone? What are its advantages and indications?

Risperidone is a new antipsychotic with a high affinity for both 5-HT2 receptors (like clozapine) and D2 (like typical neuroleptics). At an optimal dose of 6 mg/day (in divided doses), it has minimal extrapyramidal symptoms in most schizophrenic patients but effectively treats both positive or psychotic symptoms and negative symptoms (e.g., social withdrawal and apathy). Risperidone should be considered in patients who cannot tolerate typical neuroleptics. It is not yet clear whether risperidone is effective in schizophrenic patients who do not respond to typical neuroleptics. It is also unclear whether risperidone causes tardive dyskinesia. At a maximal recommended dose of 16 mg/day, however, risperidone causes extrapyramidal symptoms in a significant number of patients.

17. Why not treat every psychotic patient with clozapine or risperidone?

Although clozapine and risperidone have significant advantages, both cost exponentially more than the typical neuroleptics, which are available relatively cheaply in generic form. Clozapine and risperidone cost several hundred dollars per month for most patients, and clozapine has the added liability of weekly complete blood count testing and prescribing. Clozapine also has a slight mortality risk due to agranulocytosis (12 deaths in over 90,000 patients as of this writing) despite weekly monitoring.

BIBLIOGRAPHY

1. Angrist B, Schulz SC (eds): The Neuroleptic-Nonresponsive Patient: Characterization and Treatment. Washington, DC,. American Psychiatric Press, 1990.
2. Baldessarini RJ: Chemotherapy in Psychiatry: Principles and Practice, 2nd ed. Cambridge, MA, Harvard University Press, 1985.
3. Baldessarini RJ, Frankenburg FR: Clozapine: A novel antipsychotic agent. N Engl J Med 324:746–754, 1991.
4. Janicak PG, Davis JM, Preskorn SH, Ayd FJ: Principles and Practice of Psychopharmacotherapy. Baltimore, Williams & Wilkins, 1993.
5. Jenkins SC, Hansen MR (eds): A Pocket Reference for Psychiatrists, 2nd ed.. Washington, DC, American Psychiatric Press, 1995.
6. Leyyse JE, et al: Risperidone: A novel antipsychotic with balanced serotonin-dopamine antagonism, receptor occupancy profile, and pharmacologic activity. J Clin Psychiatry 55(Suppl):5–12, 1994.
7. Meltzer HY: The mechanism of action of clozapine in relation to its clinical advantages. In Meltzer HY (ed): Novel Antipsychotic Drugs. New York, Raven Press, 1992.
8. Van Putten T, Marder SR, Wirshing WC, et al: Neuroleptic plasma levels. Schizophr Bull 17:197–216, 1991.
9. Watsky EJ, Salzman C: Psychotropic drug interactions. Hosp Community Psychiatry 42:247–256, 1991.

49. MOOD-STABILIZING AGENTS

James L. Jacobson, M.D.

1. What are mood-stabilizing agents?

Mood-stabilizing agents are medications with both antimanic and antidepressant effects. They also may decrease behavioral phenomena related to mood instability, such as impulsivity and episodic violence. Mood stabilizers are sometimes called **thymoleptics**. This term implies the capacity to alter emotional or mental states, once (wrongly) thought to be influenced by the thymus gland. Hence the persistence of terms such as euthymic (normal mood range) and hyperthymic (excessively elevated mood).

Lithium (as a carbonate or citrate salt) is the only medication approved by the FDA as a mood stabilizer. However, the anticonvulsant medications carbamazepine and valproate (valproic acid; divalproex sodium) are now widely used as mood stabilizers.

Dose Ranges and Therapeutic Levels of Mood-stabilizing Agents

MEDICATION	DOSE RANGE (APPROXIMATE)	THERAPEUTIC BLOOD LEVELS*
Lithium	600–1800 mg/day	0.5–1.5 mEq/L
Carbamazepine	600–1600 mg/day	6–12 ng/ml
Valproate acid	750–3000 mg/day	50–100 µg/ml

* Therapeutic blood levels are based on trough values obtained 8–12 hours after the preceding dose of medication.

2. In what conditions are mood stabilizers used?

Bipolar I disorder
Bipolar II disorder
Cyclothymia
Schizoaffective disorder
Intermittent explosive disorder
Mania due to medical conditions (e.g., stroke, temporal lobe syndrome, cancer-related mood disorder)
Major depressive disorder (adjunctive treatment or prophylaxis in recurrent major depressive disorder)

3. What assessment is necessary before initiation of treatment with mood-stabilizing agents?

A general medical assessment, including history, physical examination, and laboratory evaluation focusing on organ systems potentially affected by each agent, is important prior to starting these medications.

Mood-stabilizing Agents: Side Effects and Laboratory Tests

MEDICATION	ORGAN SYSTEM AFFECTED	POTENTIAL SIDE EFFECTS	LABORATORY TESTS
Lithium	Cardiac	Conduction disturbance	EKG
		Sinus node dysfunction	
	Hematologic	Elevated white blood cell count	Complete blood count with differential

Table continued on following page.

Mood-stabilizing Agents: Side Effects and Laboratory Tests (Cont.)

MEDICATION	ORGAN SYSTEM AFFECTED	POTENTIAL SIDE EFFECTS	LABORATORY TESTS
Lithium *(cont)*	Renal	Diabetes insipidus/ development of renal failure	Electrolytes, blood urea nitrogen (BUN), creatinine, urinalysis (specific gravity)
	Reproductive (women)	Fetal abnormalities	Pregnancy test
	Thyroid	Hypothyroidism/goiter	Thyroid-stimulating hormone (TSH)
Valproate	Hematologic	Anemia	Complete blood count with differential
		Leukopenia	Blood count
		Thrombocytopenia	Platelet count/bleeding time
	Hepatic	Hepatic dysfunction or failure	Hepatic enzymes
	Reproductive (women)	Fetal abnormality	Pregnancy test
Carbamaze-pine	Cardiac	Arrhythmia	EKG
	Hematologic	Agranulocytosis	Complete blood count with differential
		Aplastic anemia	
		Thrombocytopenia	Platelet count
	Hepatic	Hepatitis	Hepatic enzymes
		Jaundice	Bilirubin
	Renal	Syndrome of inappropriate secretion of antidiuretic hormone	BUN/creatinine
		Hyponatremia	Electrolytes
	Reproductive (women)	Fetal abnormality	Pregnancy tests

Once treatment is initiated and efficacy is established, periodic blood level monitoring of the mood stabilizer, review of potential side effects, physical examination, and laboratory monitoring for side effects are recommended. The patient's general health and reliability should be taken into account in deciding the frequency of monitoring. For example, in a healthy, reliable 35-year-old patient whose bipolar illness is well controlled, monitoring of medication, blood levels, and laboratory tests screening for side effects every 3 months is probably adequate in the absence of newly developed symptoms attributable to the medication. Some patients may be monitored as infrequently as every 6 months. In a 50-year-old patient with bipolar disorder, a history of alcohol abuse, liver damage, and treatment noncompliance, blood level monitoring and screening laboratory tests may be needed every 2–4 weeks to ensure compliance and to decrease the risk of serious side effects.

4. Discuss the pharmacologic management of an acute manic episode.

The acute manic phase of bipolar illness is heralded by the rapid onset of a persistently elevated, expansive, or irritable mood accompanied by a cluster of symptoms such as inflated self-esteem, grandiosity, decreased need for sleep, increased talking, racing thoughts, easy distractibility, increased motor behavior, increased goal-directed activity, and increased involvement in high-risk, pleasure-seeking activities. The symptoms cause marked impairment in functioning and may have profound effects on others (e.g., intrusive, aggressive behavior, high risk-taking activities, impulsive spending), frank psychotic symptoms may be present (e.g., delusions, hallucinations). Because of potentially life-altering/life-threatening consequences, hospitalization is often necessary.

Medication is the primary mode of treatment. Lithium is the principal treatment for mania, with response rates reported as high as 80% in bipolar I disorder. After appropriate medical and laboratory evaluation, lithium can be initiated at 300 mg orally 3 times/day (no parenteral form is available), then titrated according to side effects, clinical response, and blood level. A blood level of 0.8–1.2 mEq/L is generally required to treat acute mania. A steady-state, stable blood level is generally achieved in about 5 days and is measured 10–12 hours after the lithium dose (e.g., in the morning before the first dose of the day is often convenient). Changes in dosage require monitoring of lithium levels at least every 5–7 days after the change. Some patients require (and tolerate) levels up to 1.5 mEq/L, although higher levels are not advised because of the risk of toxicity. Treatment with lithium alone may have a relatively slow response rate (up to 2 weeks after a therapeutic blood level is established); hence adjunctive medication treatment is usually required.

If psychotic symptoms are prominent, the addition of a neuroleptic (antipsychotic) medication may be essential. Neuroleptics generally result in rapid improvement (days as opposed to weeks) in agitation, thought disorder, and sleep. For example, haloperidol, 5–20 mg/day in divided doses, is a typical regimen. However, bipolar patients are at an increased risk of neuroleptic malignant syndrome and tardive dyskinesia. In addition, neuroleptics may increase the intracellular concentration of lithium and create a syndrome of combined lithium-neuroleptic neurotoxicity (e.g., confusion, encephalopathy, delirium, ataxia, nystagmus, extrapyramidal side effects). Hence, these medications have to be monitored closely.

Benzodiazepines are also widely used in treating acute mania. Both clonazepam and lorazepam have proved effective in decreasing hyperactivity, controlling agitation, decreasing anxiety, and improving sleep during a manic episode. Both are effective orally (clonazepam, 4–20 mg/day; lorazepam, 4–30 mg/day in divided doses). Lorazepam may be given intramuscularly in severely agitated, noncompliant patients who require acute sedation (up to 4 mg IM). Benzodiazepines may decrease the total required dose of neuroleptic medications, resulting in a lowered risk of neuroleptic-related side effects.

In patients with intolerance of lithium, a history of nonresponse, or rapid-cycling or mixed manic and depressive states, valproate or carbamazepine can be used alone or in conjunction with neuroleptics, benzodiazepines and/or lithium. Growing evidence suggests that valproate and/or carbamazepine may be more effective in treating rapid-cycling and mixed-state bipolar disorders. Valproate may be initiated at either 250 mg orally 3 times/day, or an oral loading regimen may be used (e.g., 500 mg orally 3 times/day 3 days; then blood level should be checked). Blood levels should be checked about 10 hours after the previous dose of medication and maintained in the range of 50–100 mg/ml. Valproate has been shown to be as effective as lithium in acute mania, may be more effective in mixed mania or rapid cycling, and is likely to have a more rapid onset of action (e.g., 3–5 days).

Carbamazepine is also effective in acute mania, although it may be slightly less effective than lithium. Treatment is started at 200–600 mg/day in divided doses and titrated as tolerated, usually to 800–1000 mg/day, striving for blood levels of 6–12 ng/ml. Blood levels should be monitored at least weekly initially, with the specimen drawn about 10 hours after the previous dose. Sedation early in treatment may slow the upward titration and attainment of therapeutic blood levels.

Hypomania is generally managed with lithium and benzodiazepines. Doses may be lower than for mania, and treatment may forestall an incipient manic episode.

5. Discuss the pharmacologic management of bipolar depression.

Major depressive episodes in patients with bipolar type I and type II disorders are likely to occur more frequently than manic episodes (see chapter 12). Such episodes are characterized by at least 2 weeks of depressed mood, loss of interest or pleasure in activities, weight loss or gain, insomnia or hypersomnia, psychomotor agitation or slowing, fatigue, loss of energy, feelings of worthlessness, difficulty in thinking, indecisiveness, and recurrent thoughts of death (often with suicidal ideas or attempts). Such patients are significantly distressed, and their functioning is impaired. Bipolar depressions are often characterized by hypersomnia, profound anergy, early age of onset, and/or postpartum onset.

Lithium alone may be used to treat mild-to-moderate bipolar depression with a response rate of 60–70%. However, response may be slow (6–8 weeks). Blood levels may need to be higher (> 1.2 mEq/L) than in mania. Thyroid augmentation (e.g., thyroxine) may be helpful, even if the patient has normal thyroid levels.

Valproate and carbamazepine have not been established as effective in treating or preventing bipolar depression. Carbamazepine may have some advantages over valproate, although this has not been clearly established.

Careful attention is necessary to discern a history of bipolarity in depressed patients, because the course of illness and impact (both positive and negative) of treatment may be quite different. Hypomania in bipolar type II disorder may be especially difficult to document. All antidepressant medications have been reported to induce switching to hypomania or mania in bipolar patients and also may induce rapid cycling from mania to depression and vice-versa. Rates of switching as high as 50% have been reported. However, severe bipolar depression may require the addition of antidepressant medications. When indicated (e.g., severe, life-threatening depression or depression unresponsive to mood stabilizers and psychotherapy), bupropion (75 mg 2 times/day–150 mg 2–3 times/day) and tranylcypromine, a monoamine oxidase (MAO) inhibitor (10 mg 2 times/day–20 mg 3 times/day) may be good choices; some studies have shown decreased rates of switching. Bupropion may induce seizures, hence dosing schedules and total dose must be closely monitored. Tranylcypromine and all MAO inhibitors may interact with other antidepressants, carbamazepine, pressor agents, and food high in the amino acid tyramine to produce a potentially lethal hypertensive crisis; hence it must be monitored closely with particular attention to patient education about diet restrictions. Short half-life serotonin reuptake inhibitors such as sertraline and paroxetine also may be reasonable choices; rates of switching may be relatively lower than with tricyclic antidepressants. Other antidepressants (e.g., tricyclic antidepressants) are clearly effective in treating bipolar depression but may have relatively increased rates of switching. Antidepressants should be used for the briefest period necessary to treat the depression, then gradually withdrawn.

ECT is clearly effective in bipolar depression and at times is the preferred treatment (see below).

Psychostimulants, hypermetabolic doses of thyroid hormone, clozapine (a new atypical antipsychotic agent), and light treatment (2500 watts for 2–4 hours each morning) also may be used. Light treatment also may induce a switch to mania.

6. Why are long-term maintenance strategies important in bipolar disorders?

Bipolar disorder is a chronic, relapsing, and remitting illness. At this time there is no cure. In addition, recurrent episodes predispose toward more frequent and severe episodes (a phenomenon known as kindling). Therefore, long-term management is critical. The goals of maintenance treatment are to decrease the psychosocial impact of the illness (such as job loss, economic ruin, and loss of relationships), suicide risk, and frequency and severity of recurrence; to improve compliance to treatment regimens, and to achieve the most effective treatment regimen with the fewest possible side effects. Many people with bipolar illness also have significant impairment from mood fluctuation and other symptoms between identifiable episodes of illness (subsyndromal symptoms), which also can be improved with continuous pharmacologic intervention and psychotherapeutic efforts.

Lithium maintenance has clearly been shown to decrease the frequency and severity of both manic and major depressive episodes. When lithium is stopped abruptly, more than 50% of patients relapse within 6 months. A slow taper of lithium may decrease the risk of rapid relapse, although this has not been well studied. Maintenance therapy with lithium should focus on maintaining the blood level range that was effective in treating acute illness. Lower-dose maintenance has been associated with an increased relapse rate. Long-term lithium maintenance requires monitoring of lithium blood levels (which may change with age, diet, use of other medications, concurrent illness, and state of hydration) and periodic (e.g., every 6 months) assessment of thyroid (TSH) and renal function (BUN and creatinine; 24-hour creatinine clearance in patients with evidence of altered functioning). Neither valproate nor carbamazepine has been carefully studied in the long-term management of bipolar illness. Some studies (none carefully controlled) suggest that these agents may be useful in decreasing the intensity of recurrent manic episodes. However, when lithium alone is ineffective for maintenance or acute treatment, the addition of either valproate or carbamazepine is often beneficial.

Interepisode management may require intermittent use of benzodiazepines during periods of sleep deprivation (e.g., at times of increased acute stress) for sleep initiation to decrease the risk of precipitating a manic episode.

Antidepressants should be avoided in long-term management, when possible, because of the risk of inducing rapid-cycling disorders.

Neuroleptics also should be avoided because of the increased risk of tardive dyskinesia and neuroleptic malignant syndrome in patients with bipolar disorder. However, some bipolar patients and probably all patients with schizoaffective disorder require neuroleptic medications in maintenance regimens. The lowest effective dose should be established to minimize the risk of side effects. Clozapine may be a good choice, because of lower risk of tardive dyskinesia and emerging reports of mood stabilization. However, clozapine should not be the neuroleptic of first choice because of the risk of potentially fatal agranulocytosis.

Pharmacodynamics of Mood-stabilizing Agents

MEDICATION	PEAK BLOOD LEVEL (HR)	METABOLISM	HALF-LIFE (HR)	PROTEIN BINDING
Lithium	1–2	Renal excretion	14–30	No (distributed in total body water)
Valproate	2	Hepatic	6–16	Yes
(Divalproex sodium)	3–8			
Carbamazepine	4–8	Hepatic	18–55	Yes

7. Describe the clinically pertinent pharmacodynamics of the mood-stabilizing agents.

These pharmacodynamic properties are helpful in understanding various clinically pertinent phenomena. For example, with a patient taking lithium, peak blood levels are more likely to be associated with transient side effects (e.g., tremor), and a decrease in total body water (i.e., dehydration) increases blood level and blood level-sensitive side effects (e.g., diarrhea).

When valproate or carbamazepine is used, competition for protein-binding sites and hepatic metabolic pathways affects the doses of concurrently used medications (see below).

8. Describe the significant drug interactions of the mood-stabilizing agents.

Lithium. Blood levels of lithium are increased by thiazide diuretics and nonsteroidal antiinflammatory agents through renal mechanisms. Intracellular concentrations of lithium are increased by neuroleptic agents. Dehydration also increases lithium levels.

Valproate. Valproate levels are decreased by inducers of microsomal enzymes, such as carbamazepine, and increased by inhibitors of microsomal enzymes, such as fluoxetine and paroxetine. Valproate increases the blood levels of protein-bound drugs, including phenobarbital, phenytoin, tricyclic antidepressants, digoxin, and warfarin.

Carbamazepine. Carbamazepine, an inducer of microsomal enzymes, decreases its own levels (autoinduction) as well as the levels of other drugs, including neuroleptics, benzodiazepines, other anticonvulsants, tricyclic antidepressants, and hormonal contraceptives. However, competition for protein-binding sites may increase blood levels acutely when carbamazepine is added to ongoing treatment regimens.

9. Discuss the clinical presentation and management of lithium toxicity.

Lithium toxicity may occur with blood levels ≥ 2.0 mEq/L. Some individuals may experience toxicity at lower doses. Neuroleptics may increase intracellular lithium; hence toxicity may appear even at therapeutic blood levels. Patients with lithium toxicity may experience lethargy, clumsiness, nausea, vomiting, diarrhea, marked tremulousness, blurred vision, and confusion. Findings on physical exam may include nystagmus, increased deep tendon reflexes, and altered mental status. Such manifestations may progress to include seizures, coma, and cardiac arrhythmias. This progression is more likely to occur in patients with lithium levels > 2.5 mEq/L. Permanent CNS damage may ensue.

Lithium toxicity is a medical emergency and should be managed in an intensive care setting. Fluid and electrolyte monitoring, treatment of arrhythmias and respiratory compromise, and prevention of further gastrointestinal absorption may be required. Hemodialysis is the most effective way of acutely reducing the blood lithium level.

The best treatment of lithium toxicity is prevention, which is often achieved through patient education. Patients need to know the symptoms of lithium toxicity, drugs that may interact with lithium, and the necessity of careful monitoring of blood lithium levels. In addition, they need to be aware that avoidable circumstances (such as dehydration and use of nonsteroidal antiinflammatory agents) may increase lithium levels.

Symptoms and Signs of Lithium Toxicity

SYMPTOMS	SIGNS
Lethargy, fatigue	Nystagmus
Ataxia, clumsiness	Increased deep tendon reflexes
Weakness	Altered mental status
Nausea	Cardiac arrhythmia
Vomiting	
Marked tremor	
Blurred vision	
Confusion	

10. Discuss the management of side effects of mood-stabilizing agents.

Management of Side Effects of Mood-stabilizing Agents

SIDE EFFECT	MANAGEMENT STRATEGY
Lithium	
Gastrointestinal distress (nausea, vomiting diarrhea	Check blood level; decrease dose if clinically possible Take medication with meals Change to slow-release preparation
Poor concentration, confusion, sedation	Give majority of dose at bedtime; decrease if clinically possible
Tremor	As above, and add a beta blocker (e.g., propranolol, 10–20 3 times/day)
Increased white blood count	Monitor, usually resolves with time
Polydipsia, polyuria (nephrogenic diabetes insipidus)	Decrease dose if severe Monitor electrolytes Consider adding nonthiazide diuretic
Renal insufficiency	Nephrology consultation Lower lithium dose; monitor blood level more frequently Consider change to alternate mood stabilizer

Table continued on following page.

Management of Side Effects of Mood-stabilizing Agents (Cont.)

SIDE EFFECT	MANAGEMENT STRATEGY
Lithium *(cont.)*	
Hypothyroidism	Monitor thyroid functions Add T_4
Psoriasis	If moderate-to-severe, consider change to alternate mood-stabilizing agents
Acne	Topical antibiotics and retenoic acid
Weight gain	Advise about diet/exercise; lower dose, if possible
Valproate	
Gastrointestinal distress (change in appetite, nausea, vomiting, diarrhea)	May resolve with time Give drug with meals Change preparations Decrease dose
Sedation	As above Give bulk of dose at bedtime
Tremor	As above Add a beta blocker
Hair loss (usually transient)	B complex vitamins Folic acid Zinc and selenium
Minor hepatic transaminase elevation	Decrease dose Monitor hepatic enzymes
Asymptomatic thrombocytopenia or leukopenia	Decrease dose Monitor platelet and granulocyte counts
Pancreatitis, agranulocytosis, severe transaminase elevation or hepatic failure	Potentially fatal Discontinue valproate Urgent medical consultation
Carbamazepine	
Gastrointestinal distress	Usually transient Decrease dose Give medication with meals Bulk of dose at bedtime
Blurred vision, fatigue, ataxia, sedation, skin rash	As above, may require reduced dose Observe Antihistamines to control itching with mild rash Decrease dose Medical or dermatologic consultation to determine if drug should be discontinued (discontinue if associated with fever, wheezing respiration, or blisterlike skin lesions)
Mild leukopenia	Increase frequency of monitoring white blood cells Discontinue if leukopenia persists or worsens
Mild thrombocytopenia	Increase frequency of monitoring platelet counts Discontinue if thrombocytopenia persists
Hyponatremia	Monitor electrolytes Change mood stabilizers, if hyponatremia persists
Agranulocytosis, aplastic anemia, exfoliative dermatitis, or severe elevation of hepatic enzymes	May be fatal; discontinue drug Urgent medical consultation Discontinue medication

11. When is electroconvulsive therapy (ECT) used in bipolar disorders?

ECT is effective in treating both acute manic and depressive phases of bipolar illness with efficacy rates equal to or greater than those of lithium and often with a more rapid onset of action. Although ECT is generally reserved for cases in which standard agents are not effective, it should be considered as a primary treatment when rapid response is necessary or when standard treatments are contraindicated. Given such considerations, ECT may be the primary treatment in manic delirium (a severe mania with identifiable delirium that may include hyperthermia), mania with neuroleptic malignant syndrome, and mania during pregnancy or other medical contraindications to mood-stabilizing medications (e.g., renal impairment, history of allergy to mood-stabilizing agents). ECT also may be used earlier in the course of treatment in patients with psychotic depression and when the risk of slower response may severely compromise the patient's health (e.g., ongoing serious suicide attempts, deteriorating nutritional status). Lithium is generally discontinued before starting ECT because of an increased risk of delirium and intractable seizures when ECT and lithium are combined.

Indications for ECT as Primary Treatment in Bipolar Illness

Manic delirium
Mania or bipolar depression with neuroleptic malignant syndrome
Medical contraindications to using mood stabilizers
Psychotic bipolar manic or depressive episodes
Severely compromised health (e.g., serious, ongoing suicide attempts)

12. How does age affect the use of mood-stabilizing medications?

Metabolic differences in children, adolescents, and geriatric populations require altered dosing strategies. Because hepatic metabolism is generally less efficient, lower doses of carbamazepine and valproate are used to establish therapeutic blood levels. In elderly patients, renal function is often diminished; hence a lower dose of lithium is typical. In addition, elderly patients often take other medications (hence drug interactions must be reviewed carefully) and are often more sensitive to potential neurotoxic effects (hence blood levels should be maintained at the lower end of the therapeutic range).

13. Are other medications used for mood stabilization?

Although they are not widely used, evidence suggests that calcium channel blockers may be effective as mood stabilizers. For example, verapamil (120–240 mg/day) has been effectively used in bipolar illness. It is probably effective in the same group of patients who respond best to lithium (bipolar type I).

Long-acting depointramuscular injections of neuroleptic medications (e.g., fluphenazine decanoate, haloperidol decanoate) are sometimes the only effective treatment for patients who are not compliant with oral medication and whose illnesses are severe enough to warrant this approach.

In patients whose mood or behavioral instability is caused by an underlying medical condition (e.g., thyroid disease, brain tumor), identification and aggressive treatment of underlying illnesses may cure the secondary mood disorder.

Intermittent explosive disorder and impulsive aggressive behavior in brain-injured patients also may respond to beta blockers (e.g., propranolol in widely variable doses has been used effectively).

14. How do mood-stabilizing medications work?

The mode of action is not yet known for any of the mood-stabilizing medications. A good deal of the current research into the effects of lithium is to determine the basic cellular mechanisms that correlate with clinical processes. For example, lithium attenuates neuronal signal transduction mediated by G-proteins, which may be associated with increasing mood stability. Current research also focuses on lithium inhibition of neurotransmitter-receptor–coupled adenylate cyclase activity, cyclic adenosine monophosphate formation, and metabolism of phosphoinositide in relation to its effect on other significant second-messenger systems. Other research has focused on attenuation of dopamine receptor turnover and function, effects on serotonin synthesis, and function and binding of certain serotonin receptors, interactions with protein kinase C, ion-channel function, and intracellular calcium mobilization.

BIBLIOGRAPHY

1. American Psychiatric Association: Practice guidelines for the treatment of patients with bipolar disorder. Am J Psychiatry 151(Suppl), December, 1994.
2. Bowden CL, et al: Efficiency of divalproex vs. lithium and placebo in the treatment of mania. The Depakote Mania Study Group. JAMA 271:918–924, 1994.
3. Bowden CL, et al (eds): Practical Guidelines for the Management of Bipolar Disorder. Monograph on Treatment. Deerfield, IL, Discovery International, 1992.
4. Gerner RH, et al: Algorithm for patient management of acute manic states: Lithium, valporate, or carbamazepine? J Clin Psychopharmacol 12:576–635, 1992.
5. Goodwin FK, Jamison KR: Manic-Depressive Illness. New York, Oxford University Press, 1990.
6. Jefferson J (Chairperson): Lithium: The present and the future (report on symposium). J Clin Psychiatry 156:41–48, 1995.
7. McElroy SL, et al: Valporate in the treatment of bipolar disorder: Literature review and clinical guidelines. J Clin Psychopharmacol 12(Suppl):42S–52S, 1992.
8. Solomon D, et al: The course of illness and maintenance treatments for patients with bipolar disorder. J Clin Psychiatry 56:5–13, 1995.
9. Suppes T, et al: Risk of recurrence following discontinuation of lithium treatment in bipolar disorder. Arch Gen Psychiatry 48:1082–1088, 1991.

50. ANTIANXIETY AGENTS

John A. Bell, M.D.

1. What is an antianxiety agent?

Antianxiety agents, also known as anxiolytics or minor tranquilizers, are used to treat the protean manifestations of anxiety. To some extent, all drugs used to treat anxiety have sedating properties, but they do not relieve symptoms simply by sedating the anxious patient. In the late 1800s alcohol, bromide salts, chloral hydrate, and paraldehyde were used to sedate and to modify symptoms of tension and anxiety. Barbiturates replaced these compounds as the most favored antianxiety agents through the 1950s. Then concerns about tolerance and drug dependence spurred the development of safer and more effective agents. Meprobamate was widely used in the 1950s and 1960s, but it had many of the same problematic properties as barbiturates. Benzodiazepines, safer and more effective drugs, were discovered in the late 1950s and became the dominant treatment for anxiety in the early 1960s.

2. List benzodiazepines used to treat anxiety.

Benzodiazepines and Their Therapeutic Dose Range

MEDICATION	THERAPEUTIC DOSE RANGE (MG/DAY)*
Chlordiazepoxide	15–40 mg
Diazepam	5–40 mg
Lorazepam	1–6 mg
Clorazepate	15–60 mg
Prazepam	20–60 mg
Oxazepam	10–120 mg
Alprazolam	1–8 mg
Clonazepam	0.5–6 mg
Halazepam	20–120 mg

* Doses in the elderly are often 50%, or less, of those listed above.

3. When should benzodiazepines be used to treat symptoms of anxiety?

Some people have symptoms of anxiety, and others have anxiety syndromes or disorders (e.g., generalized anxiety disorder or panic disorder). Individuals may develop symptoms of anxiety in response to stressful life circumstances (e.g., family illness or financial difficulties), during the course of a medical illness (see chapter 16), or as a manifestation of a psychiatric disorder (e.g., agitated major depression or anxiety about eating in bulimia nervosa). Stressed patients are assisted by finding ways to reduce stress and enhance coping skills. Patients with a medical condition causing symptoms of anxiety or with a psychiatric condition with secondary anxiety should be treated for their primary illness. Short-term use (1–2 weeks maximum) of benzodiazepines often relieves symptoms of anxiety. Patients with a medical condition causing symptoms of anxiety or with a psychiatric condition with secondary anxiety should be treated for their primary illnesses. Benzodiazepines may relieve symptoms of anxiety but also may complicate management because therapeutic effects and appropriate duration of treatment can be difficult to determine when they are combined with other treatments (e.g., lorazepam plus an antidepressant for treating agitated major depression). If benzodiazepines are used during the initial phase of treatment of another disorder, short-term use is recommended. Whether benzodiazepines are prescribed to treat stress-induced anxiety or as an adjunct to a primary treatment, it is crucial to use enough to achieve results. Inadequate dosage is the most common reason for failure to achieve results.

4. What psychiatric disorders are often treated with benzodiazepines?

Psychiatric Disorders Treated with Benzodiazepines

DSM–IV DISORDER	BENZODIAZEPINE DOSING
Generalized anxiety disorder	Diazepam, 5–10 mg 2 or 3 times/day Alprazolam, 0.5 mg 3 times/day Lorazepam, 1.0 mg 2 or 3 times/day
Panic disorder	Alprazolam, 1–2 mg 3 times/day Clonazepam, 0.5–1.0 mg 2 or 3 times/day
Social phobia	Clonazepam, 0.5–1.0 mg 2 times/day
Posttraumatic stress disorder	Lorazepam, 1 mg 2 or 3 times/day

Among benzodiazepines only alprazolam and clonazepam have been shown to be effective in treating panic disorder, and only clonazepam has been shown to be effective in treating social phobia. Any benzodiazepine may be used for generalized anxiety disorder or posttraumatic stress disorder. In addition, benzodiazepines are frequently used to diminish hyperactivity and for sedation in bipolar illness. They often are useful for treating the anxiety symptoms that frequently accompany depression.

5. How do benzodiazepines affect the central nervous system?

The benzodiazepine receptor, discovered in the 1970s, is a locus on a larger complex known as the GABA-benzodiazepine receptor site. Gamma-aminobutyric acid (GABA) is an inhibitory neurotransmitter. Benzodiazepines potentiate the inhibitory effects of GABA by increasing the flux of chloride ions into neurons. It is hypothesized that through their effect on neurons mediated by these receptor complexes benzodiazepines reduce neuronal firing and, therefore, symptoms of anxiety.

6. Describe the metabolism of benzodiazepines.

Benzodiazepines are metabolized by microsomal enzyme systems in the liver. Most undergo transformation of the diazepine ring or hydroxylation followed by conjugation with glucuronic acid. Ring transformation and hydroxylation may be compromised in medically ill patients, especially those with hepatic disease (e.g., cirrhosis or hepatitis). As people grow older, ring transformation and hydroxylation capacities diminish. In ill or elderly patients, benzodiazepines that require 2- or 3-step metabolism (e.g., diazepam or alprazolam) may accumulate to toxic levels as a result of inefficient metabolism. Conjugation with glucuronic acid is not significantly reduced by aging. For this reason, when a benzodiazepine is required, elderly patients should be prescribed lorazepam, oxazepam, or temazepam, which require only conjugation to be metabolized.

7. What are the elimination half-lives of benzodiazepines?

Elimination Half-lives of Benzodiazepines

AGENT	HALF-LIFE (HRS)
Short-acting Agent (6 hrs or less)	
Midazolam (preoperative sedation)	1–2
Triazolam (sedative)	2–4
Intermediate-acting (6–20 hrs)	
Alprazolam	6–10
Oxazepam	5–10
Lorazepam	10–20

Table continued on following page.

Elimination Half-lives of Benzodiazepines (Cont.)

AGENT	HALF-LIFE (HRS)
Long-acting (> 20 hrs)	
Clonazepam	18–50
Chlordiazepoxide	40–80
Clorazepate	50–80
Diazepam	50–100

* Half-lives reflect duration of action of parent compound and active metabolites.

8. Describe the course of treatment with a benzodiazepine.

Treatment begins with an explanation of the symptoms or syndrome to be treated. Treatment approaches, including drug and nondrug interventions, should be discussed, and, as appropriate, choices about treatment should be made by the patient. For example, the patient with generalized anxiety disorder may consider imipramine, lorazepam, or buspirone. Once a benzodiazepine is selected, side effects, especially sedation and risk of physical dependence (habituation), should be reviewed. Target symptoms (e.g., panic attacks in panic disorder or social anxiety in social phobia) should be identified, and an efficient way to monitor symptom change should be established (e.g., diary of anxiety symptoms). Dose titration is necessary. Typical dosing range, tolerance of side effects, and symptom relief should be used to determine a safe and effective dose (see chapter 16). Treatment at the lowest effective dose for the shortest interval of time is desirable because the chance of physical dependence will be lessened. Generally, treatment for 1 month or less is advisable for patients with acute anxiety. Conditions such as generalized anxiety disorder, panic disorder, and social phobia are chronic, often lasting for many years. Longer treatment, even chronic treatment, may be appropriate for patients with panic disorder or social phobia. Pulses of drug treatment (a few months on, then off) may be tried for generalized anxiety disorder.

9. Are benzodiazepines widely abused?

About 95% of all users are prescribed a benzodiazepine for anxiety or insomnia, whereas the remaining 5% abuse drugs and alcohol. Patients in the first category, except those with histories of drug and alcohol abuse, rarely misuse or abuse benzodiazepines. Drug or alcohol abusers have predictable difficulties with benzodiazepines, including misuse, overuse, and use with substances to be avoided (e.g., heavy use of alcohol with benzodiazepines). Overall, benzodiazepines are not widely abused, but abuse is common in confirmed drug or alcohol abusers.

10. What are the characteristics of benzodiazepine dependence?

In most cases, benzodiazepine dependence is not apparent until the regular daily dose is reduced during drug discontinuation. Patients who have taken a daily therapeutic dose (it need not be an excessive dose) of a benzodiazepine for 1 month have a risk of dependence of < 10%, whereas in patients on a benzodiazepine regimen for 4–6 months the risk of dependence approaches 50%. In drug-dependent patients symptoms of withdrawal develop within 24 hours for short-acting agents, within 24–48 hours for intermediate-acting agents, and within 3–7 days for long-acting agents. Onset of withdrawal symptoms due to short- or intermediate-acting benzodiazepines is more rapid, but symptoms have not been shown to be more intense than those due to long-acting agents. Common symptoms of withdrawal include insomnia, agitation, anorexia, sweating, irritability, moodiness, headaches, tremor, nausea, and perpetual disturbances. Withdrawal symptoms usually peak soon after they appear and then gradually dissipate over the next several days. However, some withdrawal symptoms persist and can be remedied only by raising the dose of the benzodiazepine. Discomfort rather than danger characterizes withdrawal; severe reactions such as seizures are rare during a gradual taper of the dose. Abrupt discontinuation may lead to severe withdrawal reactions.

11. How should benzodiazepines be tapered?

When a benzodiazepine is discontinued or tapered, the patient may (1) have no reaction; (2) develop symptoms of withdrawal; (3) experience recurrent symptoms of the underlying disorder; or (4) undergo rebound—an intensification of anxiety symptoms beyond the level before treatment. It is essential to discuss such possibilities with each patient before tapering to enlist the patient's assistance in evaluating the response to discontinuation and to avoid undue concern on the patient's part. Although reactions to discontinuation of a benzodiazepine have been reported after a single dose (rebound insomnia after triazolam), it is safe and prudent simply to stop benzodiazepines that have been taken on a daily basis for 2 weeks or less. A tapering strategy is advisable for patients on a benzodiazepine regimen for 2 weeks or more. If the duration of treatment is less than 4 weeks, the medication usually can be discontinued quickly; e.g., 1.0 mg of lorazepam 2 times/day can be reduced to 0.5 mg 2 times/day for 3 days, then to 0.25 mg 2 times/day for 3 days, and then stopped. For the patient treated for 12 weeks with 1.0 mg twice daily doses of lorazepam, the initial reduction should not exceed 0.5 mg, or 25% of the total daily dose (i.e., 0.75 mg twice daily or 0.5 mg in the morning and 1.0 mg in the evening). One week on the reduced dose is sufficient time to assess the patient's response. Successive decrements in dose should follow a schedule established before discontinuation is started. Adherence to a schedule increases the likelihood of successful discontinuation. An intense response, whether withdrawal or relapse, may alter the schedule. For lorazepam, an intermediate-acting benzodiazepine, an interval of 1 week is selected for dosing changes because a steady state at a new dose is reached in 4 days or less. With a long-acting benzodiazepine (e.g., diazepam) the interval for dosing changes increases to 2 weeks because of the long elimination half-life. When a benzodiazepine has been taken for 6 months or longer (e.g., alprazolam for panic disorder), the tapering schedule may be more gradual, but a schedule should be adopted. Finally, in any tapering scheme, the element of psychological dependence should not be overlooked. Patients who have done well on a medication, even one that, unlike benzodiazepines, is not habit-forming, feel reliant on the medication. Symptoms may recur during discontinuation simply because of psychological factors.

12. What other drugs are used to treat anxiety?

Meprobamate and barbiturates are rarely used now. Antihistamines (e.g., hydroxyzine) and anticholinergic agents are used because of sedating properties; hydroxyzine, however, is not an effective antianxiety agent.

Propranolol, a beta-adrenergic antagonist, reduces autonomic arousal for persons who become anxious in specific phobic situations, such as public speaking.

Buspirone, an azaspirodecanedione that selectively antagonizes the $5HT_{1A}$ receptor, has been shown to be an effective and safe treatment for generalized anxiety disorder but not for panic disorder. Effective doses of buspirone are 5–10 mg 3 times/day. Dependence does not develop, and buspirone does not protect against benzodiazepine withdrawal symptoms.

13. Are antidepressant medications anxiolytic?

Antidepressant medications are effective antianxiety agents. Because antidepressants are not addictive, they are often preferred medications for treating certain anxiety disorders, especially in patients with a history of substance abuse. Antidepressants often need to be started at lower than usual doses and titrated upward more slowly in patients with anxiety disorders because of the potential to increase anxiety symptoms initially. The course of response is slower than the response to benzodiazepines, which are usually rapidly effective. For these reasons, benzodiazepines and antidepressants are sometimes started simultaneously, and the benzodiazepine is then tapered. Although a broad range of antidepressants are often used in clinical practice, research has supported the following usage in treating anxiety syndromes:

Use of Antidepressants for Anxiety Syndromes

ANTIDEPRESSANT	ANXIETY DISORDER
Imipramine	Generalized anxiety disorder, panic disorder
Desipramine	Panic disorder
Fluoxetine	Obsessive compulsive disorder, ?social phobia
Sertraline	?Panic disorder, obsessive compulsive disorder
Paroxetine	Obsessive compulsive disorder
Fluvoxamine	Obsessive compulsive disorder, panic disorder
Phenelzine	Panic disorder, social phobia
Tranylcypromine	Social phobia, panic disorder
Clomipramine	Obsessive compulsive disorder, panic disorder

BIBLIOGRAPHY

1. Rickels K: Antianxiety therapy: Potential value of long-term treatment. J Clin Psychiatry 48(Suppl):7–11, 1987.
2. Salzman C, APA Task Force on Benzodiazepine Dependency: Benzodiazepine Dependence: Toxicity and Abuse. Washington, DC, American Psychiatric Association, 1990.
3. Schnabel T: Evaluation of the safety and side effects of antianxiety agents. Am J Med 82:7–13, 1987.
4. Sellers EM, et al: Alprazolam and benzodiazepine dependence. J Clin Psychiatry 54(Suppl):64–75; discussion, 76–77, 1993.
5. Shader RI, et al: Use of benzodiazepines in anxiety disorders. N Engl J Med 328:1398–1405, 1993.
6. Shorr RI, et al: Rational use of benzodiazepines in the elderly. Drugs Aging 4:9–20, 1993.

51. SEDATIVE-HYPNOTIC DRUGS

Kim Nagel, M.D.

1. What clinical situations provide clearcut indications for sedative-hypnotic drugs?
Transient insomnia and recurrent transient insomnia are the only clearcut indications for sedative-hypnotic drugs. Additional indications and longer-term use require careful clinical assessment and weighing other treatment options.

2. How is transient insomnia defined?
Transient insomnia is a period of insomnia usually 1–14 days in length and often in response to a specific stressor (e.g., loss, illness, hospitalization, long-distance travel). After a duration of 3 months, insomnia is considered to be subacute or chronic and requires further work-up to define underlying etiology. The following example addresses some of these issues:

A 34-year-old woman presents 7 days after the unexpected death of her father. She reports trouble getting to sleep before 2–3:00 AM, difficulty arising for work in the morning, and daytime fatigue. Although sad, she reports few vegetative signs of depression. She is given 20 tablets of zolpidem, 10 mg, to use as needed over the next 3–4 weeks. At follow-up she says that she took the medication nightly with good response and ran out 3 days before her appointment. She has slept only approximately 5 hours for the last 3 nights off medication and feels that continuing it would be helpful. A few times in the last week she woke up early and was unable to return to sleep, but overall she feels that her mood is good. Two additional refills of zolpidem, 10 mg, are given with follow-up as needed. Her next visit occurs in 8 weeks, and she reports that early morning awakening has become more frequent. Occasionally she takes an additional one-half pill to get back to sleep at 3:00 AM. When she ran out of pills, sleep became much more difficult and impairment of concentration at work became more noticeable. She says that she has lost weight and feels less enthusiasm. Major depression is diagnosed, and sertraline is started at 50 mg and increased to 100 mg the next week. Four weeks after starting sertraline, her sleep returns to normal, and she stops zolpidem on her own. At this point she agrees that weekly psychotherapy would be beneficial to deal with issues arising from her father's death and that continuing sertraline is appropriate for an undetermined length of time.

3. What is the recommended treatment for transient insomnia?
A consensus paper published by the National Institute of Mental Health (NIMH) in 1984 stated that benzodiazepines (and closely related compounds) are the first choice of medication for transient insomnia because of safety, efficacy, and side-effect profiles. The consensus recommended use of the lowest possible dose for the shortest period of time until insomnia improves, with a maximum of 20 doses/month for 3 months.

4. Why is it important to avoid long-term use of sedative-hypnotic medication?
Long-term use of hypnotics should be avoided for several reasons. First, many cases of insomnia are truly transient, and patients need to be informed clearly that they most likely can stop medication before long. Some patients develop a habit of use, and others try to stop and are disturbed by brief rebound insomnia, which tells then that they must stay on medication when they may no longer need it. Tolerance, which tends to develop to most sedatives over time, decreases their efficacy and may promote escalation of dosage. All sedative/hypnotics have side effects, which may include decrease in dreaming and deep sleep and increase in brief arousals at night, which make sleep less restful. Even more important is that long-term symptomatic treatment of insomnia may prevent the detection of an underlying medical or psychiatric condition that can be treated with better response.

Although a number of conditions may benefit from long-term sedatives, it is important to diagnose and treat them adequately. In general, nonaddictive agents are preferred to treat chronic insomnias. Of note, an open trial in France of 180 consecutive days of 10–20 mg of zolpidem for insomnia showed little tolerance and virtually no withdrawal or rebound insomnia after discontinuation. Such studies eventually may give additional long-term treatment options.

5. What factors should be considered in deciding which hypnotic is most appropriate for a specific patient?
   1. Assess the form of the patient's insomnia. The four most common types of insomnia are:
      (1) Sleep onset or initial insomnia
      (2) Frequent short awakenings
      (3) One or two long awakenings
      (4) Early morning awakening (early awakening is a common symptom in major depressive disorder).
   2. Assess pertinent characteristics of the sedative-hypnotic:
      (1) Rate of absorption
      (2) Extent of distribution in body and CNS
      (3) Affinity for CNS receptors
      (4) Elimination half-life
      (5) Route of metabolic biotransformation
For single-dose therapy (1), (2), and (3) are more important. For multiple-dose therapy, (4) and (5) assume more importance. For the sake of simplification, rate of absorption and elimination half-life should be raised as guiding factors.

Benzodiazepine-type Hypnotics

	HALF-LIFE (HRS)	ABSORPTION	TYPICAL DOSAGE
Zolpidem (Ambien)	$1\frac{1}{2}$–4	Fast	2.5–10 mg
Triazolam (Halcion)	2–5	Fast	0.125–0.25 mg
Zopiclone	5–6	Fast	3.75–7.5 mg
Temazepam (Restoril)	8–12	Moderate	7.5–30 mg
Estazolam (Prosom)	12–20	Fast	1–2 mg
Oxazepam (Serax)	5–15	Moderate	10–25 mg
Alprazolam (Xanax)	12–20	Fast	0.25–1.0 mg
Lorazepam (Ativan)	10–22	Moderate	0.5–2 mg
Clonazepam (Klonopin)	22–38	Slow	0.5–2 mg
Quazepam (Doral)	50–200	Fast	7.5–15 mg
Flurazepam (Dalmane)	50–200	Fast	15–30 mg

6. What drugs are most helpful for sleep onset or initial insomnia?
If the patient has trouble falling asleep initially, one should think of zolpidem, triazolam, and temazepam as the best choices. In the example in question 2, a 34-year-old woman was given zolpidem, 10 mg, at bedtime. This drug is effective, rapidly absorbed, cleared quickly from the system, and has minimal evidence on memory loss, motor incoordination, tolerance, or withdrawal symptoms. Rare cases of sleepwalking and psychotic reactions have been reported but the major drawback is its price (nearly two dollars/pill).

A number of studies have suggested that triazolam is equivalent in efficacy and side effects (except perhaps rebound insomnia) if not used above 0.25 mg. It is a reasonable second choice at one-third the price.

The third choice is temazepam, 15–30 mg, which is the least expensive of the three. Occasionally the two shorter-acting agents shift the pattern from sleep onset insomnia to early morning awakening after the drug is mostly cleared from the system. Temazepam's longer duration of action may be helpful in this case. As temazepam is slowly absorbed, it may need to be taken $1-1\frac{1}{2}$ hours before bedtime to aid getting to sleep. Elderly patients are generally given one-half the average adult dosage.

7. What drugs are most helpful for nocturnal and early morning awakening?
Temazepam is the first choice for nocturnal and early morning awakenings. It is slowly absorbed, but its peak effect begins about $1-1\frac{1}{2}$ hours after administration and persists for 6–10 hours. This duration of action may be ideal to maintain sleep until morning without leaving the patient groggy the next day. Depending on the patient, shorter-acting (triazolam, zolpidem) or longer-acting (estazolam, oxazepam, lorazepam, clonazepam) may be more suitable.

The long-acting drugs, such as flurazepam, quazepam, and chlorazepate, are quite effective for nocturnal and early morning awakenings, but the patient may have daytime hangover, memory loss, or incoordination. These drugs are best for very anxious patients or for infrequent or intermittent usage.

8. What are the likely side effects of benzodiazepines?
The most common side effects of benzodiazepines are daytime sedation, motor incoordination, slow reaction times, anterograde and retrograde amnesia, confusional states, withdrawal states, rebound insomnia, respiratory depression, tolerance to drug effect, and potential for abuse.

9. With such side effects, why are benzodiazepines the drugs of choice?
Benzodiazepines are easily tolerated by most patients and highly effective in 75–90% of cases. Side effects may be minimized by drug choice and regulation of dosage and dosing schedules. One of the major advantages is their safety in overdose. The lethal dose is so large for all benzodiazepines that one is unlikely to die from even 1 month's supply. A patient merely becomes highly sedated until the drug is cleared from the bloodstream.

10. What is anterograde amnesia? Discuss its cause and prevention.
Anterograde amnesia is the forgetting of new learning after administration of a drug. In contrast, retrograde amnesia is the forgetting of events before use of a drug. Anterograde amnesia may occur when high doses of long-acting or short-acting drugs are used. The mechanism of action is different for the two types of sedatives, but the result is the same. It is generally prevented by using as low a dose as possible and avoiding use of alcohol, which adversely interacts with the hypnotic.

11. What are the guidelines for prescribing to elderly patients or other groups that may suffer from impaired liver metabolism?
For elderly patients or patients with liver impairment, very short-acting drugs such as triazolam or zolpidem or drugs that do not require hydroxylation by the liver are preferred. Temazepam, lorazepam, and oxazepam are excreted by the kidneys without necessity of liver hydroxylation; and therefore their metabolism and excretion are not prolonged by age or liver dysfunction.

Unexpected falls may be an unfortunate consequence of motor incoordination induced by hypnotics used in the elderly. The weakened and brittle nature of their bones makes them highly prone to hip fractures if they fall. The likelihood of hip fracture in the elderly appears to be correlated with the half-life of a regularly used hypnotic. Flurazepam is believed to be twice as likely as triazolam to cause a hip fracture with regular use in elderly patients.

12. What are the effects of benzodiazepine-like sedative/hypnotic drugs on sleep quality?
All effective hypnotics increase total sleep time, tend to suppress and delay REM or dreaming sleep, increase the duration of stage 2 sleep, and decrease the amount of stage 3 and 4 or deep sleep. Most users feel more refreshed and alert in the daytime compared with periods of insomnia but less rested than in periods of normal, unmedicated sleep. Stopping such drugs after short or intermediate term usage may result in REM rebound (increase in REM sleep) and rebound

insomnia for 0–3 days. Some reports on zolpidem indicate that it may slightly increase deep sleep and may not suppress REM or cause rebound.

13. What is the mechanism of action of benzodiazepine-like drugs?

Benzodiazepine-like drugs have an inhibitory effect on the central nervous system that is mediated through the stimulation of benzodiazepine receptors and an agonist effect on the neurotransmitter, gamma-aminobutyric acid (GABA). Benzodiazepine receptors (BZ) are divided into subgroups 1, 2, and 3. BZ-1 receptors seem to mediate sedation, whereas BZ-2 receptors mediate anxiety reduction, anticonvulsant activity and, unfortunately, memory loss and motor incoordination. Most benzodiazepines stimulate both BZ-1 and BZ-2 receptors; therefore, their sedative effect correlates with effect on coordination and memory. BZ-3 receptors are mostly located in the spinal cord and have no relevance to sleep, memory, or coordination.

14. Is it possible to create a drug with fewer side effects by stimulating only the BZ-1 receptors?

Theoretically, yes. Quazepam is apparently BZ-1 selective, but its two long-acting metabolites are approximately 150 times more potent and not BZ-1–selective. Zolpidem is BZ-1–selective and has no significant active metabolites. It has the theoretical advantage of BZ-1 selectivity but has not been shown to have an unequivocal advantage in motor incoordination or effect on memory impairment over non–BZ-1–selective, short-acting benzodiazepines at typical therapeutic dosages. Evidence suggests that zolpidem may offer a more physiologically normal sleep, produce fewer withdrawal symptoms, and be less prone to induce tolerance.

15. In addition to transient insomnia, what other common diagnoses or conditions may benefit from the use of sedative-hypnotic agents?

1. Chronic insomnia due to:
   - Age. One's ability to remain asleep decreases with age. In severe cases, after encouraging physical activity and sleep hygiene, the clinician may give a 2-week trial of zolpidem, 5 mg; triazolam, 0.125 mg; or temazepam, 7.5–15 mg. If the drug is clearly helpful, without side effects, it should be continued with attempts to shift to intermittent dosing if tolerance begins to develop.
   - Chronic pain. Many nocturnal arousals from sleep are caused by pain. Tricyclic antidepressants (e.g., amitriptyline, 10–50 mg, doxepin, 10–50 mg) are first choices in patients with chronic pain, because they reduce pain sensations as well as frequency or duration of awakenings.
   - Chronic medical condition. Congestive heart failure is an example of a chronic medical condition that induces severely fragmented sleep. Temazepam, 15 mg, has been shown to decrease nighttime awakening and arousals and to improve daytime alertness with no compromise of the medical condition.
   - Medication side effects. For example, in a 38-year-old asthmatic woman taking long-acting theophylline (300 mg/day) and using a metaproterenol sulfate inhaler (2 puffs 4 times/day), the stimulating effects of medication may induce severe insomnia and occasional symptoms of anxiety. Flurazepam, 15 mg, is used at bedtime 3–6 times/week to inhibit insomnia and daytime anxiety.
   - Fibromyalgia, chronic fatigue syndrome. First choices are doxepin, 10–50 mg at bedtime; amitriptyline, 10–50 mg at bedtime; or nortriptyline, 10–50 mg at bedtime (if anticholinergic effect of doxepin or amitriptyline is too strong). Studies show that sleep improvement is correlated with improvement in pain or fatigue in some patients. Patients who are intolerant of tricyclic antidepressants may consider trazodone, 25–100 mg, or short-acting benzodiazepines.
2. Major depression
3. Bipolar affective disorder
4. Dysthymic disorder

5. Panic disorder

6. Generalized anxiety disorder

7. Posttraumatic stress disorder

8. Psychophysiologic insomnia. This is a conditioned negative response to one's sleep environment. Sleep hygiene and sleep restriction are usually recommended, but short-term triazolam, 0.25 mg at bedtime, may inhibit bedtime anxiety and help the patient to gain confidence in his or her ability to get normal sleep.

9. Restless leg syndrome. This crawling discomfort in the legs makes one feel a need to stretch or move the legs and causes sleep onset insomnia.

10. Periodic leg movements of sleep. Leg-jerking movements accompany restless leg syndrome but also may occur up to 2–3 times/minute during sleep in patients without restless leg symptoms. The arousals that they cause may make sleep nonrestorative.

Recommended order of treatment for both 9 and 10 is Sinemet (the combination of carbidopa [15 mg] and levodopa [100 mg]), 1–2 tablets at bedtime. (This works about 50% of the time but may induce nightmares.) If it fails try:

- Temazepam, 15–30 mg at bedtime
- Clonazepam, 0.5–2 mg at bedtime
- Percocet (the combination of oxycodone HCl and acetaminophen), 1–2 tablets at bedtime. This may be the most effective treatment, but the addictive nature of the drug requires that the leg movements must be severe and documented by nocturnal polysomnogram. Studies have shown that Percocet and other opiates actually eliminate the leg-jerking movements rather than just allow the patient to sleep through the disturbance of the movement. Dosage can be held steady for many years without significant tolerance to benefits.

11. Circadian/rhythm disturbances

- Melatonin is a hormone created by the pineal gland at night in concert with the calm phase of the body's daily rhythm. Evidence suggests that 1–2 tablets of 2.5-mg Melatonin given in early afternoon help to maintain or reregulate an out-of-sync circadian rhythm.
- Triazolam, 0.125–0.25 mg, or zolpidem, 5–10 mg, also may be used to help reestablish a normal circadian sleep pattern.

16. What changes in strategy may be used in prescribing hypnotics for chronic conditions?

1. Use benzodiazepines on an intermittent basis 1–4 times/week to decrease tolerance and maintain potency.

2. Strictly reinforce daily routine and relaxation techniques to enhance efficacy of medication.

3. In appropriate populations for either primary or adjunctive treatment, consider alternatives, such as:

- Antidepressants (see question 18)
- Mood stabilizers (see question 19)
- Antihistamines (see question 20)
- Chloral hydrate (see question 20)

17. How does one approach the evaluation of the patient who has chronically used benzodiazepines and/or alcohol for treatment of a chronic insomnia?

Because of withdrawal symptoms and tendency to cause arousal and nonrestorative sleep, sedative-hypnotics and alcohol are estimated to be the *cause* of 10–15% of all cases of insomnia. Because alcohol has no place in chronic treatment of insomnia, one first should recommend abstinence. If this is difficult, formal detoxification and enrollment in substance abuse treatment may be needed. More compliant patients can stop alcohol and then reduce their sedative/hypnotic by one therapeutic equivalent/week (e.g., 0.125 mg triazolam, 15 mg temazepam, or 5 mg zolpidem). During this period one should closely evaluate the patient for symptoms beyond the expected mild withdrawal symptoms (e.g., panic attacks, mood instability). The purpose of the taper is to allow better diagnosis of any underlying etiology of the insomnia and potentially to provide more effective treatment.

18. List antidepressant medications that may be used for their sedative properties.

Antidepressant Medications with Sedative Properties*

DRUG	DOSAGE	USES
Amitriptyline (Elavil)	10–100 mg	Chronic pain, peripheral neuropathy fibromyalgia
Doxepin (Sinequan)	10–200 mg	Chronic fatigue syndrome, fibromyalgia, post alcohol withdrawal insomnia, as adjunct with nonsedating selective serotonin reuptake inhibitors (SSRIs).
Trazodone (Desyrel)	25–200 mg	Adjunct to nonsedating SSRI; make sure to warn men about 3% incidence of priapism and potential need for immediate withdrawal from drug; also warn of orthostatic hypotension
Nortriptyline (Pamelor)	10–50 mg	Often helpful for mild-to-moderate anxiety disorder and insomnia
Nefazodone (Serzone)	100–500 mg	New drug in 1995; sedation is much like that of trazodone without risk of orthostatic changes or priapism

* From most sedative to least sedative.

19. How may one use mood stabilizers as hypnotics?

Adequate sleep is essential to stabilize a bipolar affective disorder. Carbamazepine is moderately to highly sedating, and the typical dose is 100–400 mg at bedtime. Valproic acid is mildly to moderately sedating and may be used at doses of 125–1500 mg at bedtime. Both often may be used as adjunctive medicine for sedation or mood stabilization in patients still suffering from insomnia while treated with lithium carbonate. In addition, they may be desired as primary agents in mixed or rapid cycling bipolar disorders with severe insomnia. These show some utility in patients with posttraumatic stress disorder, insomnia, nightmares, night terrors, and agitated drug withdrawal states.

20. What other drugs are of occasional usefulness as sedative-hypnotic agents?

Other Sedative-Hypnotic Agents

DRUG	DOSAGE	USES
Diphenhydramine	25–100 mg	Allergies, mild insomnia, patients at risk to abuse medications, patients on antipsychotic medication with extrapyramidal symptoms such as muscle dystonia or parkinson-like tremor
Cyproheptadine	4–40 mg	Posttraumatic stress disorder, cluster headaches with insomnia
Chloral hydrate	500–1500 mg	Chronic insomnia in elderly patients; little tolerance develops but it is mildly effective and may irritate GI tract and potentiate Coumadin or antiepileptic drugs
Buspirone	5–40 mg	Shown to be effective occasionally for nocturnal agitation in elderly patients

Table continued on following page.

Other Sedative-Hypnotic Agents (Cont.)

DRUG	DOSAGE	USES
Antipsychotics (e.g., haloperidol, thioridazine hydrochloride)	25–800 mg	Best used for patients with psychosis or borderline personality disorder; occasionally low-dose haloperidol is helpful in elderly demented and agitated patients.
Clonidine	0.1–1.2 mg	Opiate withdrawal insomnia, refractory posttraumatic stress disorder, and treatment-resistant bipolar disorder

21. Which agents should not be prescribed for sleep?

Ethchlorvynol, methaqualone, and barbiturates no longer have a place as sedative/hypnotic agents alone. They have greater risk of abuse, dependence, and lethal overdose and tend to lose effectiveness much more rapidly than benzodiazepines. Alcohol is sedating but promotes nocturnal awakenings, and severely impairs sleep quality; tolerance develops rapidly.

22. Are sedative-hypnotics associated with homicidal behavior, psychotic reactions, or agitation?

Short-acting hypnotics have been associated with agitated states, sleepwalking, psychotic reactions, and at least two cases of homicide. Triazolam has been linked with two cases of homicide. It is suspected that the underlying pathology that caused the insomnia may have been a major factor. One patient developed an extensive paranoid delusional system over a number of weeks. Zolpidem has been associated with sleepwalking and psychotic reactions that are unrecallable the next day. With the millions of users of these drugs, it is unlikely that they represent a significant hazard. It is prudent to avoid short-acting sedatives in patients with history of severe agitation, highly anxious states, and impulsiveness.

BIBLIOGRAPHY

1. Ashton H: Guidelines for the rational use of benzodiazepines. When and what to use. Drugs 48:25–40, 1994.
2. Biberdorf DJ, Steens R, Millar TW, Kryger MH: Benzodiazepines in congestive heart failure: Effects of temazepam on arousability and Cheyne-Stokes respiration. Sleep 16:529–538, 1993.
3. Greenblatt DJ, Divoll M, Abernathy DR, et al: Benzodiazepine hypnotics: Kinetic and therapeutic options. Sleep 5:S18–S27, 1982.
4. Kryger M, Roth T, Dement WC (eds): Principles and Practice of Sleep Medicine, 2nd ed. Philadelphia, W.B. Saunders, 1994.
5. National Institute of Mental Health, National Institutes of Health: Drugs and Insomnia. Consensus Development Conference Summary, vol 4, no 10. Bethesda, MD, U.S. Department of Health and Human Services, 1984.
6. Reite ML, Nagel KE, Ruddy JR: Concise Guide to the Evaluation and Management of Sleep Disorders. Washington, DC, American Psychiatric Press, 1990.
7. Roger M, Attali P, Coquelin JP: Multicenter, double-blind, controlled comparison of zolpidem and triazolam in elderly patients with insomnia. Clin Ther 15:127–136, 1993.
8. Shader RI, et al: Appropriate use and regulatory control of benzodiazepines. J Clin Pharmacol 31:781–784, 1991.
9. Vogel G: Clinical uses and advantages of low doses of benzodiazepine hypnotics. J Clin Psychiatry 53(Suppl):19–22, 1992.

52. THE USE OF STIMULANTS IN PSYCHIATRIC PRACTICE

Hubert H. Thomason, Jr., M.D.

1. List the common stimulants prescribed in psychiatric practice.

Trade Name	Generic Name	Molecular Structure
Cylert	Pemoline	
Dexedrine	Dextroamphetamine	
Ritalin	Methylphenidate	

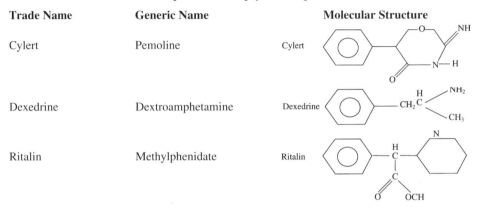

2. Describe the physiologic effects of stimulants.

Stimulants increase catecholaminergic activity in the brain through inhibition of monoamine oxidase (MAO), blockade of neuronal catecholamine reuptake, and direct release of catecholamine from nerve terminals. Serotonin (5HT) activity at the neuronal level is also altered. The resultant physiologic state is characterized on electroencephalography (EEG) by increased power, especially in the alpha range. This finding is related to the clinical state of arousal associated with the use of stimulants. Persons typically report activation, increased motivation, improved mood, and even euphoria (which may be followed by a dysphoric crash when catecholamine stores are depleted in the brain), suppression of drowsiness, and decreased need for sleep. Blood pressure and heart rate may be increased, and appetite suppression is common. Among the unpleasant physiologic effects of stimulants are increased sweating, restlessness and agitation, and stereotypic movements such as teeth grinding, jaw-clenching, and skin picking. Sexual functioning may be impaired with decreased libido in both men and women, inability to maintain an erection in men, and anorgasmia in women.

3. What are the common uses of stimulants in psychiatric practice?

The most common use of stimulants in psychiatric practice is in the treatment of **attention deficit/hyperactivity disorder** (ADHD) in children and occasionally adults. (ADHD is common in children but rare in adults.) The Food and Drug Administration (FDA) sanctions the use of stimulants in this disorder.

Also approved by the FDA is the use of stimulants to treat **narcolepsy**, a rare disorder in which the sufferer is plagued by sleep "attacks."

Important uses of stimulants beyond those approved by the FDA center on the treatment of **mood disorders** and **amotivational states**.

Stimulants may be added to a partially effective **antidepressant regimen** to augment the antidepressant action (see chapters 47 and 49) when it is impractical to increase the antidepressant dose because of adverse effects or because the maximal dose has already been reached without sufficient improvement. Stimulants are not considered to be effective as the primary treatment for depression.

Amotivational states (which may or may not be tied to depression) may respond acutely to the use of stimulants. Such states include **medically compromised patients** who are not participating actively in treatment and therefore are at risk of further deterioration of functioning. The typical scenario involves elderly persons, persons who are having difficulty with weaning from a ventilator, patients infected with the human immunodeficiency virus (HIV), poststroke victims or postoperative neurosurgical patients, and terminally ill patients. Behavioral control and cognition have improved with stimulant treatment in chronic closed-head-injury patients.

In general, weight control and appetite suppression are not clinically appropriate uses for stimulants because of lack of efficacy over time and risk of adverse effects. Behaviorally based treatments are much more useful than stimulants.

Clinical Pearl: Using a stimulant (5 mg of dextroamphetamine) helps to differentiate between depressed and demented patients. Depressed patients are likely to respond with improved mood, cognition, and alertness, whereas demented patients may show increased alertness but cognition is worse.

4. List and discuss some of the common problems associated with prescription of stimulants.

1. **Tolerance**. The sympathomimetic effects of stimulants diminish quickly at a steady dose. Thus persons using stimulants to produce euphoria, appetite suppression, energy, and wakefulness become quickly disappointed and seek to increase the dose to achieve the former level of stimulation. Of interest, tolerance does not develop to the therapeutic benefit of stimulants in ADHD, or to their antidepressant effects when used to augment treatment of depression, or in medically ill patients maintained on stimulants for amotivational states.

2. **Abuse**. Because stimulants are known to produce euphoria, energy, and wakefulness, they have been extensively abused in the past. An historically important form of stimulant abuse occurred during World War II. Allied and Axis forces used amphetamine extensively. Japanese fighter pilots, on suicide missions in the Pacific, used amphetamine. Postwar Japan experienced an epidemic of amphetamine abuse when large stockpiles of amphetamine from the military were placed on the open market. The potential for abuse has caused stimulants to become heavily regulated in the United States.

3. **Adverse effects**. Common or important stimulant-induced side effects include:

Anxiety
Irritability
Insomnia
Dysphoria
Emotional lability
Decreased appetite
Psychological dependence
Physical dependence
Exacerbation of other illnesses such as glaucoma, hypertension, anxiety disorders, psychotic disorders, and seizure disorders
Increased heart rate and blood pressure
Palpitations
Tics and other involuntary movements (teeth grinding/jaw clenching)
Transient growth suppression in children
Paranoia
Hallucinations
Psychosis

4. **Drug–drug interactions**. Stimulants may decrease metabolism (and thus increase plasma level) of certain drugs:

Tricyclic/tetracyclic antidepressants	Phenobarbital
Warfarin (Coumadin)	Phenytoin (Dilantin)
Primidone (Mysoline)	Phenylbutazone (Butazolidin)

Stimulants should be used with extreme caution in the presence of MAO inhibitors because of the possibility of a hypertensive crisis.

5. Summarize governmental regulation of stimulants.
Stimulants are classified by the U.S. Drug Enforcement Agency (DEA) as schedule II, along with certain narcotics. Additional regulations may vary from state to state, including the use of triplicate prescriptions for stimulants (one copy is filed with a state governmental agency). A proper state medical license and DEA certification are required for physicians to prescribe stimulants. Internationally there is much variability in the regulation of stimulants. Sweden has banned stimulants, whereas they are available without prescription in other countries.

6. Summarize practical information about prescribing stimulants.

Prescription of Stimulants*

	CYLERT	DEXEDRINE	RITALIN
How supplied (Tablets)	18.75, 37.5, and 75 mg Chewable: 37.5 mg	5, 10 mg Oral suspension: 5 mg/ml Sustained release: 5, 10, and 15 mg	5, 10, and 20 mg Sustained release: 20 mg
Pretreatment evaluation	Cardiac, liver, and renal function	Cardiac, liver, and renal function	Cardiac, liver, and renal function
Concurrent monitoring	Liver function	None	None
Starting dose (mg) Adults Children	37.5 18,75	2–5–10 2–5 (3–5 yrs) 5 (6 yrs and older)	5–10 5
Increase dose weekly by	18.75 mg	5 mg	5–10 mg
Daily schedule	Once daily in morning	Twice daily divided dose except in sustained release form (once daily)	Twice daily divided dose except in sustained release form (once daily)
Maximal recommended dose	112.5 mg	40 mg	60 mg

* There is no indication for the use of stimulants during pregnancy. Dextroamphetamine (Dexedrine) and methylphenidate (Ritalin) pass into breast milk. It is unknown if pemoline (Cylert) passes into breast milk.

7. What are useful strategies for managing common stimulant-induced adverse effects?

Management of Common Stimulant-induced Adverse Effects in Attention Deficit/Hyperactivity Disorder

ADVERSE EFFECT	MANAGEMENT
Anorexia, nausea, weight loss	Administer stimulant with meals. Use caloric-enhanced supplements. Discourage forcing meals. If using pemoline, check liver function tests.
Insomnia, nightmares	Administer stimulants earlier in day. Change to short-acting preparations Discontinue afternoon or evening dosing. Consider adjunctive treatment (e.g., antihistamines, clonidine, antidepressants).

Table continued on following page.

Management of Common Stimulant-induced Adverse Effects
in Attention Deficit/Hyperactivity Disorder (Cont.)

ADVERSE EFFECT	MANAGEMENT
Dizziness	Monitor blood pressure. Encourage fluid intake. Change to long-acting form.
Rebound phenomenon	Overlap stimulant dosing. Change to long-acting preparation or combine long- and short-acting preparations. Consider adjunctive or alternative treatment (e.g., clonidine, antidepressants
Irritability	Assess timing of phenomena (during peak or withdrawal phase). Evaluate comorbid symptoms Reduce dose. Consider adjunctive or alternative treatment (e.g., lithium, antidepressants, anticonvulsants).
Growth impairment	Attempt weekend and vacation holidays. If severe, consider nonstimulant treatment.
Dysphoria, moodiness, and agitation	Consider comorbid diagnosis (e.g., mood disorder). Reduce dose or change to long-acting preparation. Consider adjunctive or alternative treatment (e.g., lithium, anticonvulsants, antidepressants).

From Wilens TE, Biederman J: The stimulants. In Shaffer D (ed): Pediatric Psychopharmacology: The Psychiatric Clinics of North America. Philadelphia, W.B. Saunders, 1992, with permission.

BIBLIOGRAPHY

1. Arieti S (ed): American Handbook of Psychiatry, 2nd ed. New York, Basic Books, 1986.
2. Evans RW, Gualtieri CT, Patterson D: Treatment of chronic closed head injury with psychostimulant drugs: A controlled case study and an appropriate evaluation procedure. J Nerv Mental Dis 175:106–110, 1987.
3. Fernandez F, Levy JK: Psychopharmacology in HIV spectrum disorders. Psychiatr Clin North Am 17:135–148, 1994.
4. Goodwin K, Jamison KR: Manic Depressive Illness. New York, Oxford Press, 1990.
5. Hales RE, Yudofsky SC: Textbook of Neuropsychiatry. Washington, DC, American Psychiatric Press, 1987.
6. Kaplan HI, Sadock BJ: Pocket Handbook of Psychiatric Drug Treatment. Baltimore, Williams & Wilkins, 1993.
7. Kaplan HI, Sadock BJ: Comprehensive Textbook of Psychiatry, 6th ed. Baltimore, Williams & Wilkins, 1995.
8. Massie MJ, Shakin EJ: Management of depression and anxiety in cancer patients. In Breithart W, Holland JC (eds): Psychiatric Aspects of Symptom Management in Cancer Patients. Washington, DC, American Psychiatric Association, 1994, pp 1–21.
9. Pickett P, Masand P, Murray GB: Psychostimulant treatment of geriatric depression disorders secondary to medical illness. J Geeriatr Psychiatry Neurol 3(3):146–151, 1990.
10. Woods SW, Tesar GE, Murray GB, Cassem NH: Psychostimulant treatment of depressive disorders secondary to medical illness. J Clin Psychiatry 47:12–15, 1986.

53. ELECTROCONVULSIVE THERAPY

Kerry L. Bloomingdale, M.D.

1. Has electroconvulsive therapy (ECT) become a less clinically advantageous psychiatric treatment now that such a wide spectrum of psychoactive medications is available?

ECT dominated the field of somatic treatment of major mental illness until the introduction of the phenothiazines in the 1950s. As neuroleptics, antidepressants, and lithium carbonate were made increasingly available, the market share of ECT naturally diminished. The early 1970s also marked a period when the political pendulum swung away from ECT, in part due to its negative portrayal in film. However, since the mid 1970s, refinement in awareness of not only how but also when to use ECT has given it an established and respected place alongside medications in the armamentarium of somatic treatments for mental illness. Recent research into the dosing of ECT has elaborated dose-response relationships that, although far from exact, have considerably enhanced its user-friendliness. Furthermore, the safety of ECT has improved significantly with the evolution of such techniques as cardiovascular monitoring, pulse oximetry, and anesthesiologic advances (e.g., short-acting barbiturates, modification of treatments [use of muscle relaxation], and short-acting IV beta blockers).

2. Is ECT primarily useful in treating the most severe forms of major depressive disorder, for example, patients with features of psychosis and/or suicidal ideation?

It is a misconception that ECT is useful primarily in severe and/or psychotic forms of major depressive disorders. It is highly effective not only in these disease entities, but also in moderate or even mild forms of bona fide major depressive disorder. Confusion sometimes arises because, compared with antidepressants alone, ECT is much more effective than the antidepressants alone (uncombined with antipsychotic drugs) in treating psychotic depression. Furthermore, even when compared with the combination of antipsychotics and antidepressants, ECT is often preferable in the treatment of psychotic depression; many clinicians find it easier to use than the antidepressant/antipsychotic combination. For instance, the two types of drugs have similar therapeutic and side effects, and the clinician often cannot be certain which drug led to what effect. Moreover, when treating even nonpsychotically depressed patients with significant suicidal ideation, intent, or plan, clinicians generally choose the most expeditious treatment. Although ECT does not work immediately, many clinicians find that it typically works faster than antidepressants.

3. For what psychiatric conditions other than major depressive disorder is ECT useful?

ECT is quite effective for **mania**. It probably is not used more often for this condition because of the rapid effectiveness of neuroleptics, lithium carbonate, and mood-stabilizing anticonvulsants. However, ECT has a particularly appropriate role in the treatment of mania when (1) the patient is in the first trimester of pregnancy (because of concerns about the teratogenicity of lithium carbonate or the mood-stabilizing anti-convulsants) or (2) the patient has a history of neuroleptic malignant syndrome.

ECT is useful, at least transiently, in treating acute forms of **schizophrenic decompensation** with many positive symptoms, such as hallucinations, delusions, or floridly bizarre behavior. Because of the possible brevity of the schizophrenic patient's response to ECT, it may be particularly appropriate in the context of a time-limited stressor, such as loss of a loved one or disruption of a living situation.

ECT is also useful in **lethal catatonia**, a "final common-pathway" disorder probably caused by various affective and psychotic conditions and marked by extreme rigidity. Such rigidity may lead to muscle breakdown, acute renal failure, and death.

ECT also has some utility in a variety of other conditions, including **Parkinson's disease** with significant rigidity and **neuroleptic malignant syndrome**.

Possible Indications for ECT

- Major depression (unipolar or bipolar)
- Mania, especially in the context of first-trimester pregnancy or history of neuroleptic malignant syndrome
- Schizophrenia, especially in the setting of floridly positive symptoms and/or a time-limited stressor
- Organic affective conditions
    Lethal catatonia
    Parkinson's disease
    Neuroleptic malignant syndrome

4. Is ECT useful in depressive conditions marked by features of both axis I major depressive disorder and axis II personality disorders?

To the extent that the clinician can separate the symptoms of major depressive disorder from those of a personality disorder, ECT should be useful in treating the depressive symptoms. However, such discriminations are often difficult to make. In practice, the decision of whether to proceed with ECT in the face of such a combination of symptoms is often better made by using one's clinical sense of whether an autonomous, somatically treatable depressive syndrome exists than by counting cookbook criteria. Moreover, when considering ECT in patients with symptoms of both major depressive disorder and personality disorders, one must consider the patient's post-treatment subjective sense of well-being as well as the treatment team's objective criteria for response. For instance, even if the major depressive symptoms respond to ECT, the patient may experience almost as much dysphoria after ECT as before because of the relatively refractory problems of personality disorder.

5. Should psychoactive medications be stopped when ECT is started?

The combination of psychoactive drugs with ECT has been the subject of much interest in the recent literature. Whereas there has been no conclusive demonstration that any medication or class of medication consistently adds to the therapeutic effects of ECT, reports have documented patients who seemed to do better clinically with ECT and a psychoactive medication than with either alone.

There are, however, reasons to be cautious about the concurrent use of ECT and each class of psychoactive medications. Lithium carbonate, for example, may cause increased neurotoxicity when combined with ECT. Benzodiazepines and anticonvulsant mood-stabilizers, such as carbamazepine and valproic acid, make the elicitation of seizures more difficult. Thus, these medications may be tapered or discontinued (see question 9). Antidepressants generally lower the seizure threshold, which may increase the duration of seizures or the probability of status epilepticus. Certain antidepressants, such as tricyclics, may increase cardiac irritability when combined with ECT. Antipsychotic medications lower the seizure threshold and, when combined with ECT, may cause greater neurotoxicity.

6. Does ECT cause an excessive cardiovascular response (e.g., hypertension, tachycardia) or a diminished cardiovascular response (e.g., bradycardia)?

At different stages in the response to ECT, the procedure may cause either a heightened or an attenuated cardiovascular reaction. Initially, the ECT stimulus may produce a vagally mediated bradycardia, sometimes associated with a sinus pause. This response is replaced, upon elicitation of the seizure, by a catecholaminergically mediated hypertensive and tachycardic reaction. Finally, a compensatory bradycardia may then ensue.

Obviously, each of these stages has different treatment implications. Clinicians concerned about the patient's ability to tolerate a sinus pause and/or bradycardia may pretreat or treat acutely with atropine or a similar anticholinergic preparation. If the patient's vulnerability to the stress of tachycardia and/or hypertension is an issue, pretreatment or acute treatment may consist of a short-acting beta blocker (e.g., esmolol) or short-acting alpha and beta blocker (e.g., labetalol). If the patient is refractory to the electrical stimulus and does not experience seizure, he or she will be particularly susceptible to the original sinus pause and/or bradycardia, because the sinus pause or bradycardia will not be counterbalanced by the seizure-induced, catecholaminergically mediated tachycardia.

Cardiovascular Reactions to ECT and Their Therapy

STAGE OF ECT	CARDIOVASCULAR RESPONSE	PRETREATMENT OR ACUTE THERAPY
Electrical stimulus	Sinus pause and/or bradycardia	Atropine or similar anticholinergic drug
Seizure	Tachycardia and/or hypertension	Beta blocker (e.g., esmolol) or alpha and beta blocker (e.g., labetalol)
Postictal	Compensatory bradycardia	Atropine or similar anticholinergic drug

7. What are the contraindications to ECT?

There are no absolute contraindications to ECT. The major relative contraindications, together with relevant interventions that may allow the use of ECT, are presented in the table below.

Relative Contraindications to ECT

SYSTEM	SIGN, FINDING, OR SYMPTOM	POSSIBLE INTERVENTIONS FOR SAFE AND EFFECTIVE ECT
Cardiovascular	Ischemic heart disease	Reduction in anticipated oxygen consumption by heart (e.g., with preadministration of beta blocker)
	Tachycardia	Reduction of heart rate (e.g., with preadministration of beta blocker)
	Hypertension	Reduction of blood pressure before and/or during ECT
	Ventricular ectopy	Administration before and/or just after induced seizure of antiarrhythmic agents. IV lidocaine should be avoided if possible before the seizure, because it may raise the seizure threshold.
Pulmonary	Gastroesophageal reflux and/or surgical history, either of which may predispose to aspiration.	In addition to standard NPO precaution, preadministration of metoclopramide; intraprocedural pressure on cricoid cartilage; intubation
Orthopedic	Recent fracture, particularly vertebral compression	Use of increased dose of muscle relaxation (e.g., succinylcholine) and/or curare
Neurologic	Space-occupying intracranial lesion (see question 8)	Neurologic and/or neurosurgical consultation indicating that intracranial pressure is not likely to rise to a dangerous level during ECT
	Seizure disorders (see question 9)	Consider lowering dose of anticonvulsant drug in consultation with neurologist

8. Is a space-occupying intracranial lesion a contraindication to ECT?

Yes, but only relatively, not absolutely. At one time space-occupying intracranial lesions were considered absolute contraindications to ECT. Clinicians used to avoid ECT in patients with space-occupying neurologic lesions because of concern over the sometimes already elevated intracranial pressure. They anticipated that the pressure would go even higher with the ECT-induced seizure. However, experience has dictated that such lesions can be compatible with safe and effective ECT; clinicians have administered ECT without complications to patients in whom imaging studies subsequently revealed preexisting space-occupying intracranial lesions.

If space-occupying intracranial lesions are in fact discovered before ECT in patients who are candidates for the procedure (e.g., after work-up for a localizing finding on neurologic examination for ECT), appropriate consultation should be sought. If there is no evidence of a mass effect, such as papilledema on funduscopic examination, or edema and midline shift on imaging studies, and if the lesion appears relatively small, it may be possible to administer ECT safely. In this instance the potential dangers must be balanced carefully against the potential benefits of ECT.

9. Is a patient taking anticonvulsants for seizure disorder a viable candidate for ECT?

Yes, in many cases. The seizure disorder itself is not an absolute contraindication to ECT, although careful consideration should be given to the possibilities that ECT may destabilize an epileptic condition or precipitate status epilepticus. Conversely, of course, ECT may make a patient with epilepsy temporarily more refractory to spontaneous seizures. Anticonvulsants themselves frequently do not interfere with ECT, although they may require higher electrical dosing. If it is impossible to elicit adequate seizures in patients taking anticonvulsants for seizure disorders, the psychiatrist could consider cautious titration downward of the anticonvulsant dose after consultation with the patient's treating neurologist. If the patient is taking anticonvulsants purely for their mood-stabilizing psychiatric effects, the clinician may be more likely to discontinue them before ECT is undertaken.

In addition, before proceeding with ECT, the clinician should consider tapering and discontinuing drugs, such as benzodiazepines, that are not used for anticonvulsant purposes but raise the seizure threshold.

10. Does ECT cause permanent structural or functional brain damage?

No compelling evidence indicates that ECT causes structural brain damage. Data consistent with the absence of structural brain changes due to ECT include animal studies, imaging studies in humans, and postmortem studies of patients who received ECT. When animals are given electroconvulsive shock using parameters analogous to those used in ECT, histopathologic studies reveal no structural neuronal damage. Imaging studies before and after patients have received ECT also reveal no structural brain damage. Moreover, autopsies of patients who received ECT do not suggest a pattern of CNS damage caused by ECT.

It is more difficult to rule out permanent functional CNS damage resulting from ECT. In fact, limited numbers of patients note cognitive changes persisting for extended periods. Studies based on neuropsychological testing of ECT patients show that interference with the ability to form new memories (anterograde amnesia) can persist for at least 3 months after a course of ECT. Patients have difficulty laying down permanent memories of some events that take place just before, during and immediately after a course of ECT. Neuropsychologically documented retrograde amnesia for events that took place more than several weeks before ECT is rare. In general, then, it is difficult to document interference by ECT with memory for events that take place more than a few months before or more than a few months after a course of ECT.

11. Is the suprathreshold approach to dosing in ECT the best way to administer the treatment?

Suprathreshold ECT is defined as the use of electrical charge or energy in excess of the amount minimally needed to elicit a seizure. The parameters for suprathreshold ECT are established by first titrating upward to the minimal electrical charge or energy necessary to elicit a seizure; for subsequent seizures that amount is multiplied by a factor greater than 1, such as 1.5. The universal appropriateness of suprathreshold ECT is not fully clear. Clinical research seems to indicate that higher-than-necessary quantities of charge or energy are often more effective than threshold amounts. It has not yet been firmly established whether the cognitive side effects of suprathreshold ECT are greater than those of threshold ECT.

12. Should electrode placement in ECT be unilateral or bilateral?

The choice of which electrode placement to use for ECT is controversial. In unilateral ECT, one electrode is placed midline and the other over the nondominant hemisphere (generally presumed to be the right). Bilateral ECT involves placement of the electrodes temporally, one over each hemisphere. Bilateral ECT often seems to work more effectively and rapidly than unilateral ECT, but it also may produce more cognitive side effects. Some practitioners believe that bilateral ECT is universally advantageous, if cognitive impairment does not preclude its use. Other clinicians believe that it is appropriate in many cases to initiate ECT treatment with a unilateral approach and then switch to bilateral ECT in patients with poor or sluggish clinical response.

13. What is the optimal number of treatments in a course of ECT?

There is no magic number of ECT administrations per course of treatment. In treating patients who manifest a prompt and full response to ECT for major depressive disorder, a range of experienced practitioners may administer 5–10 treatments, generally at the rate of 3 per week. Alternatively, some clinicians treat the patient until a complete response is achieved and then administer a small number, such as two, additional treatments.

If patients with major depressive disorder do not respond promptly or adequately to ECT, clinicians may give 10–20 treatments, assuming that each treatment results in an adequate seizure of 25 seconds or more. However, in giving such an extended course of treatment, the ECT practitioner is also likely to manipulate various key variables, such as unilateral vs. bilateral electrode approach or increasing the amount of electrical charge or energy used to incremental suprathreshold amounts. If, in fact, the seizure durations are inadequate, the clinician administering the ECT should (1) make sure that the patient is off all drugs that could raise the seizure threshold; (2) adjust the dose or type of anesthetic agent; (3) hyperventilate the patient; and/or (4) use such agents as intravenous caffeine to lower the seizure threshold.

14. How does the clinician know that a patient is responding to ECT?

Generally, objective signs of illness respond before subjective symptoms. For example, if the patient is treated for major depressive disorder, other inpatients on the psychiatric unit or, if the patient is treated on an outpatient basis, the family may report that the patient acts more spontaneously, eats more, or sleeps better before doctors or nursing staff observe changes. Clinical staff may then notice similar neurovegetative changes. Finally, the patient may note improvement in feelings of self-esteem, hopefulness, or physical well-being. Occasionally, the clinician encounters a difficult and awkward period in his or her alliance with the patient, perhaps between approximately the third and seventh treatments, in which objective signs of improvement are relatively clearcut, but the patient is discouraged about the lack of perceived improvement and wants to stop ECT. At such a time, the ECT practitioner's alliance with the patient's family or friends may prove critical in ensuring the continuation of treatment.

15. Is the electroencephalograph (EEG) the best way to assess the duration of a seizure in ECT?

If accessible, an EEG printout readily provides a way to quantify the duration of the seizure. However, a two-lead EEG produced by an ECT apparatus may be difficult to interpret, especially in documenting an exact seizure duration. Accordingly, the EEG printout should be used in conjunction with visual monitoring of seizure duration, especially if the cuff method is used. This technique consists of inflating a blood pressure cuff to a greater than systolic pressure around an extremity before infusion of the muscle relaxant to prevent the extremity from being paralyzed during the seizure. One then uses the visually monitored duration of the convulsion in the extremity as a generally accurate measure of seizure length.

Another way to corroborate seizure duration is to record the rate of change in heart rate. If IV beta blockers are not used, the heart rate will peak in approximate conjunction with the visually and EEG-monitored durations of the seizure.

16. What are continuation ECT and maintenance ECT? Are they always indicated when a patient responds acutely to ECT?

Continuation ECT is generally defined as ECT administered after a successful, acute course of ECT but during the interval when, if unsuccessfully treated, the patient would still suffer from the index episode of illness, in most cases major depressive disorder. Such a period may be presumed to last for several months. Maintenance ECT is defined as ECT administered after the patient may be presumed no longer to suffer from the underlying episode of illness originally treated acutely with ECT. Continuation and maintenance ECT treatments are usually given much less frequently than ECT to treat an acute episode of illness. Preferred schedules of maintenance ECT vary considerably. Some experienced clinicians give follow-up ECT, assuming that the patient remains symptom-free, on a fixed schedule, such as weekly, then biweekly and monthly. Other ECT practitioners plan follow-up ECT on a less frequent basis but increase the frequency of treatments if symptoms recur.

Continuation and maintenance ECT are only one follow-up treatment option for the patient who responds acutely to ECT. If the patient was treated for major depressive disorder, antidepressant or mood-stabilizing medications are typically used for follow-up. Some form of supportive or insight-oriented psychotherapy usually should accompany follow-up ECT or medications.

The decision about the form of follow-up treatment after a successful course of acute ECT is complicated. It should be made on the basis of anticipated safety and efficacy as well as patient preference. One strategy for patients treated effectively with ECT for an episode of major depressive disorder is to consider medication follow-up after the first episode of illness; if the patient breaks through such follow-up, follow-up ECT may be offered. This strategy would be continued if the breakthrough, relapse, or recurrence is treated successfully with further acute ECT.

17. Is ECT too complicated from a medical standpoint to be done on an outpatient basis?

Except in limited cases, ECT may be done safely and effectively on an outpatient basis. In fact, outpatient ECT may be preferable to inpatient ECT, because the patient is able to remain in his or her home environment and the costs are generally much less. Obviously, the severity of a patient's psychiatric condition may preclude outpatient ECT. However, because the periods of greatest physical risk from ECT are the treatment and posttreatment recovery phases, outpatient ECT, assuming that the patient is carefully monitored during these phases, may be considered even for patients with mild-to-moderate medical risk factors. The clinician should give specific pre- and posttreatment suggestions to the patient and responsible family members, such as avoiding oral ingestion and refraining from activities such as driving and operating machinery.

18. Given that many candidates for ECT suffer from diminished cognitive acuity, is the patient's informed consent still an important and necessary prerequisite to initiating the treatment?

Yes. Although the illnesses that respond to ECT commonly affect mental status, it is essential, for legal and ethical reasons, that the patient understand the risks and benefits of ECT before agreeing to the procedure. If the patient is unable to give such informed consent, the clinician should be sure to satisfy the state's legal conditions for alternative means of obtaining permission (see below).

19. If a patient is truly unable to give informed consent for ECT, should the clinician instead get the written informed consent of the patient's nearest relative?

Not necessarily. Inexperienced ECT practitioners may believe that the consent of the nearest relative is automatically an acceptable alternative to informed consent of an incompetent patient. However, the state in which the ECT is to be administered may require court appointment of a guardian (who in fact may be the nearest relative) to make treatment decisions of the patient who is unable to do so. The guardian can give informed consent for ECT.

BIBLIOGRAPHY

1. Abrams R: Electroconvulsive Therapy, 2nd ed. New York, Oxford University Press, 1992.
2. Abrams R, Essman W (eds): Electroconvulsive Therapy: Biological Foundations and Clinical Application. New York, Spectrum Publications, 1982.
3. American Psychiatric Association: The Practice of Electroconvulsive Therapy: Recommendations for Treatment, Training and Privileging. A Task Force Report of the American Psychiatric Association. Washington, DC, American Psychiatric Association, 1990.
4. Coffey C, (ed): The Clinical Science of Electroconvulsive Therapy. Washington, DC, American Psychiatric Association, 1993.
5. Kellner C (ed): Electroconvulsive Therapy. Psychiatr Clin North Am 14(4):1991.
6. Krystal A, Weiner R: ECT Seizure Therapeutic Adequacy. Convulsive Therapy 10:153–164, 1994.
7. Malitz S, Sackein H (eds): Electroconvulsive Therapy: Clinical and Basic Research Issues. New York, The New York Academy of Sciences, 1986.
8. Sackeim H, Pruelic J, Devanand D, et al: Effects of stimulus intensity and electrode placement on the efficacy and cognitive effects of electroconvulsive therapy. N Engl J Med 328:839–846, 1993.
9. Schwartz T, Loewenstein J, Isenberg K: Maintenance ECT: Indications and Outcome. Convulsive Therapy 11:14–23, 1995.

VII. Diagnosis and Treatment of Psychiatric Disorders in Childhood and Adolescence

54. AUTISM SPECTRUM DISORDERS

Loisa Bennetto, M.A., and Sally J. Rogers, Ph.D.

1. What is autism?

Autism is a developmental disability marked by significant impairments in social relatedness, communication, and the quality, variety, and frequency of various activities and behaviors. The onset of autism generally is before age 3, and impairment persists throughout the lifespan. Autism may occur across a range of functioning, and is often associated with mental retardation.

2. What are the main symptoms of autism in childhood and adulthood?

A constellation of symptoms is always seen in autism spectrum disorders, and a variety of other symptoms are often, although not always, associated with the disorder. The presentation of these symptoms varies greatly among individuals, and no single symptom is pathognomonic.

Symptoms of Autism

PRIMARY SYMPTOM CONSTELLATION (PRESENT IN ALL INDIVIDUALS)	ADDITIONAL SYMPTOMS (MAY NOT BE PRESENT IN ALL INDIVIDUALS)
Abnormal social relatedness	Cognitive impairment
Abnormal communicative development	Abnormal sensory responses
Abnormal capacity for symbolic play	Stereotypic behaviors
Restricted and odd behavioral repertoire	Neurologic abnormalities
Onset usually before age 3	Disturbances in sleep and eating patterns
	Extreme behavioral problems

Primary symptoms include the following:

Abnormal social relatedness: Social relatedness is always impaired in autism. The degree of impairment, however, may range from an oddness in social interaction, as in Asperger's disorder, to an almost complete detachment and lack of responsiveness to other's social initiations. Social deficits are most obvious with strangers and with peers; many children with autism show differential preferences for people and some demonstrate evidence of attachment to their primary caregiver. Social abnormalities may include poor use of eye contact, emotional cues, and social smile; lack of social initiation (as opposed to response); and disorganized patterns of reactions to strangers and separations. Children with autism demonstrate a particular inability to imitate others in typical ways, either disregarding the other or, occasionally, inappropriately mirroring the other's behavior.

Abnormal communicative development: Much of the literature on autism has focused on deviance in the development of spoken language. However, the communication deficit is much more profound than impaired language alone. Some children with autism seem to lack the understanding that behavior can be communicative. For example, the most severely affected children do not seem to understand the meaning of a mother's smile, frown, or gesture. Furthermore, they do not use behavior communicatively (e.g., no pointing, showing, seeking to hold the parent's attention with eye contact, or sharing affect with the parent). At the milder end of the spectrum are children who are highly verbal but stilted in their manner of speech. They do not engage in the typical back-and-forth pattern of normal conversation and lack a grasp of humor and irony.

Abnormal capacity for symbolic play: Children with autism are particularly lacking in the pretend play typical of preschool-aged children, including doll play, role play, and dramatic play. For those who have some ability to carry out this kind of play, their play is repetitive and simplistic. Individuals with autism rarely seek out play partners, and symbolic play is not interactive.

Restricted and odd behavioral repertoire: Typical toy play, marked by curiosity, exploration, interest in novelty, and goal directedness is lacking in children with autism. Much time is spent in a very limited range of activities, which may consist of a few highly ritualized or repetitive ways of handling a few objects (e.g., sucking, shaking, arranging, carrying around). When age-appropriate play skills are present, they are often inappropriately repetitive. Water play, watching things move or spin, and watching television commercials or videos are typical interests of young children with autism. For those with well-developed language skills, preferred topics of conversation may be highly ritualized and repetitive, centering around obsessive themes. The interests and activities of older individuals may seem quite restricted and idiosyncratic either in content or in intensity of involvement. Finally, changes in familiar routines or aspects of the environment may be very upsetting.

Onset usually before age 3: Children with autism usually have symptom onset within the first 3 years of life. In the first year of life, symptoms most often reported include either passivity or unusually difficult behavior (e.g., irritability, poor feeding and sleeping patterns), and a lack of imitative mother-baby games. However, a number of children do not show specific symptoms in the first year of life. For those with apparent onset after 12 months, deviance in language development is often the symptom parents first report. These children display a pattern of normal onset of words at 12–14 months, but do not develop further language or lose already acquired words. This is usually accompanied by decreased social engagement and interest. Additional symptoms, often including stereotypic and repetitive behavior and rituals, and intense emotional reactions may develop in the third and fourth years.

In addition, the following symptoms are often, but not always, present in individuals with autism:

Cognitive impairment: Mental retardation, ranging from mild to severe, is present as an additional primary handicap in approximately 75% of children with autism. General cognitive ability, or IQ, tends to be stable across the lifespan and is predictive of long-term outcome. Children with autism often show a distinct pattern in the development of cognitive abilities. Language and social development are the slowest areas to develop and demonstrate the most deviance. Some facets of development, such as gross and fine motor development, are the least delayed.

Abnormal sensory responses: Children with autism often display either hyper- or hyperactivity to sensory stimulation of all types (e.g., visual, auditory, tactile, pain). Some experts on autism consider this a primary, not associated, feature of the disorder.

Stereotypic behaviors: Children with autism often display the following repetitive actions, which have no meaning and appear to provide sensory stimulation: finger and hand movements, teeth grinding, jumping and flapping, rocking, and peculiar movement patterns when excited or anxious.

Neurologic abnormalities: Abnormal muscle tone and movement patterns are common in children with autism. In addition, 25–35% of children with autism develop seizures during adolescence or early adulthood. Abnormal neuroanatomic features (e.g., ventricular enlargement on MRI scans) have been reported in some patients with autism.

Disturbances in sleep and eating patterns: These symptoms occur in some patients with autism.

Extreme behavioral problems: A minority of children with autism exhibit extreme behavioral difficulties such as self abuse, high levels of aggression and destruction, and difficult to manage behavior.

3. What is pervasive developmental disorder (PDD)? How is it related to autism?

PDD is a term that engenders some confusion among parents and others trying to understand diagnoses. It is sometimes used interchangeably with autism, particularly with higher functioning or milder cases. It is also sometimes incorrectly interpreted as a qualitatively different diagnosis than autism.

PDD is actually a broader category in which autism is one diagnosis. PDD refers to a number of disorders that begin in infancy or early childhood and are characterized by qualitative impairment in social interaction, impairment in communication skills, and the presence of stereotyped behavior, activities or interests. Autism is the most familiar of the PDDs. The other disorders in this category all have different features and courses. They include Asperger's disorder, Rett's disorder, and childhood disintegrative disorder.

The diagnostic criteria for **Asperger's disorder** are, in general, similar to those for autism. Individuals with Asperger's disorder have severe and sustained impairments in social interaction, which are particularly marked in interactions with peers, and a restricted and repetitive range of activities, behaviors, and interests. In contrast to autism, there are no clinically significant delays in language and no clinically significant delays in cognitive development. However, individuals with Asperger's disorder do tend to show pragmatic abnormalities in language (e.g., poor conversational skills) and impairments in nonverbal expressiveness (e.g., gestures, facial expression). The symptoms of Asperger's disorder often lead to significant difficulties in personal and occupational functioning.

Asperger's disorder is usually not diagnosed as early as autism. Prevalence estimates indicate that Asperger's disorder occurs in 1-3 per 1,000 school-aged children, with a higher rate in boys than girls. Young children may be identified for significant motor delays or motor clumsiness, but their perseverative tendencies and odd way of relating to others is less noticeable. By school age, however, impaired social interaction skills become more of a handicap and children may have few or no peer friendships. These children also often develop idiosyncratic or circumscribed interests. These interests are often pursued quite perseveratively through reading, collecting, or memorizing facts.

Many researchers and practitioners consider Asperger's disorder to be a milder form of autism. In fact, the differential diagnosis may be difficult to make for very young children. By later childhood and adolescence, however, these children can be distinguished from those with autism by their relatively intact language skills, their cognitive profile, and the presence of perseverative interests.

Rett's disorder is a progressive neurologic disorder that occurs only in females. It is quite rare, occurring in 1 to 1.5 per 10,000 live female births. Early in development, these girls may show many autistic characteristics including withdrawal, social isolation, impaired communication, and cognitive delays. They often receive an early diagnosis of autism. However, Rett's disorder can be distinguished from autism by its degenerative course and certain striking characteristics.

Girls with Rett's disorder show normal development until between 6 and 18 months, at which point their development appears to stop or regress. Most notably, they show loss of purposeful hand movement, decelerated head growth, severely impaired expressive and receptive communication skills, severe cognitive deficits, and loss of social interaction skills. Loss of hand use is replaced by characteristic stereotypic midline movements, including hand wringing, hand washing, and hand biting. As girls with Rett's disorder grow older, their overall motor skills deteriorate, with about half losing independent walking abilities altogether. The autistic features of social isolation and withdrawal may improve somewhat with age. Other symptoms associated with Rett's disorder include scoliosis, abnormal gait (in those who can walk), feeding difficulties, and abnormal breathing patterns including hyperventilation and breath holding.

Childhood disintegrative disorder is characterized by a significant regression in two or more areas of functioning, after a period of at least two years of normal development. The onset of the regression can be gradual or abrupt. Loss of previously acquired abilities can affect social skills, expressive or receptive language, motor skills, play, toileting, and other adaptive behaviors.

Typically, these children's regressions reach a developmental plateau, at which point some further learning can occur.

Like children with autism, those with childhood disintegrative disorder exhibit qualitative impairments in social interaction and communication, have a restricted range of behaviors, and tend to exhibit motor stereotypes. This disorder can be differentiated from autism by its course: children with autism tend to show significant delays within the first year or two of life.

Finally, some children with mild autism, or autistic-like features, are given a diagnosis of **Pervasive Developmental Disorder Not Otherwise Specified**. This diagnosis is used if a child's behavior does not meet the full range of diagnostic criteria for *Autistic Disorder*. While these children may be functioning at a higher level than most children with autism, the nature of their symptoms still constitutes a significant impairment and often necessitates intervention.

4. How do you diagnose autism?

There is no specific medical test for autism. Diagnosis is based on parental report of history and current functioning, and on observations of the child's behavior. In making a diagnosis, all other explanations for the presenting symptoms must be ruled out (e.g., Rett's disorder, mental retardation). A comprehensive medical workup must be done to check for the presence of medical conditions that are sometimes associated with autism. Gillberg and Coleman[6] provide recommendations for an appropriate medical workup when a diagnosis of autism is being considered.

Several standard interview formats have been designed for making a diagnosis of autism.[15] Behavior checklists also help the clinician to organize observations. Two such checklists that are helpful and easy to use are the ABC checklist[8] and the Childhood Autism Rating Scale.[13] Ehlers and Gillberg[5] have developed a checklist specifically designed for diagnosing Asperger's disorder.

After the clinician has gathered information, however, the diagnostic gold standards of the DSM-IV or the ICD-9 definitions of autism must be applied to make an accurate diagnosis.

For children who may be autistic, the differential diagnosis must rule out the presence of severe language disorder, nonverbal learning disability, mental retardation (within autism), deafness, and reactive attachment disorder as alternative explanations for the difficulties with social, communicative, and play behavior. For adults, the differential diagnosis must rule out schizoid or schizotypal personality disorder, mental retardation (without autism), nonverbal learning disabilities, and neurologic disorder. Clinicians must have experience in the field of autism, since the disorder is unique and varies considerably among individuals and over time in the same individual.

Whereas the purpose of diagnosis is to determine the existence of autism, assessment is the process of identifying the individual's strengths, weaknesses, and needs. This information is used to develop appropriate therapeutic and educational programs, as well as to judge their effectiveness. For children with autism, assessment is best done from a variety of perspectives: adaptive functioning, cognitive ability, speech/language skills, and motor development. A full interdisciplinary assessment is helpful in making the initial diagnosis and in planning treatment approaches. The assessment team ideally involves psychology, psychiatry, occupational therapy, and speech and language pathology (neurology and physical therapy are also often included, depending on the presenting medical symptoms).

A complete assessment during the elementary school years is recommended to aid in optimal educational planning and curriculum development. Adolescents with autism may also benefit from a comprehensive assessment as issues of vocational training, further education, and planning for independence from the parental home arise. A tertiary facility such as a university hospital or children's hospital, or a university-affiliated program for developmental disabilities, can provide comprehensive interdisciplinary assessments and recommendations.

5. What causes autism?

The precise pathogenesis of autism is unknown. We do know, however, that autism has a biological basis, related to neurologic or neurophysiologic factors. Historical theories about psychosocial etiologies (such as inadequate or poor parenting) have been rejected empirically.

Autism is associated with several genetic conditions and prenatal and perinatal risk factors. Compared to the general population, there is a higher incidence of autism in individuals with fragile X syndrome, phenylketonuria, neurofibromatosis, and tuberous sclerosis. Identified prenatal risk factors include maternal rubella and cytomegalovirus infection; postnatal risk factors include herpes simplex encephalitis and mumps.

Neuroanatomic and neuropathologic studies using brain imaging and autopsy have revealed various abnormalities, although no consistent pattern has emerged. The most common finding has been ventricular hypertrophy. Additional abnormalities include hypoplasia of the cerebellar vermis, increased cell packing density in the limbic system, occipital horn dilation, and asymmetry of the parietal-occipital region.

Neurochemical and neurophysiologic studies are also somewhat inconclusive. Abnormalities in serotonin and catecholamine metabolism have been reported, although findings are not always consistent. Recently, positron emission tomography (PET) studies have found elevated glucose metabolic rates in diffuse brain regions.

6. How common is autism?

The prevalence of autism in the general population is approximately 4–5 per 10,000 live births. In the broader diagnostic category of all children within the entire spectrum of autistic conditions (e.g., Asperger's disorder, pervasive developmental disorder not otherwise specified), the prevalence rises to over 20 per 10,000.

Autism occurs more often in boys than girls; the gender ratio is approximately 4:1 males to females. The etiology of this gender ratio has not been identified but is likely related to biologic factors.

Research in behavioral genetics indicates that autism is both familial and heritable. No candidate genes have been identified, however, and the mode of inheritance is still unknown. Autism occurs more often in families in which there is already one child with autism. For parents who already have one child with autism, the risk of having a second affected child increases 50 times (which translates to a prevalence rate of 1–2%). Research on nonautistic siblings of individuals with autism has revealed a slightly higher rate of social abnormalities, as well as specific cognitive and language difficulties in the siblings. There does not appear to be a familial relationship between autism and mental retardation.

7. Discuss the different levels of severity in autism.

Each of the main and the related symptoms of autism varies in severity, making this disorder quite different from one individual to the next. Similarly, the level of intellectual impairment may vary from severe to profound mental retardation to normal or superior intelligence. Individuals at the ends of the spectrum often are the most difficult to diagnose accurately. Those with severe autistic symptoms and severe mental retardation may be hard to differentiate from those with severe to profound mental retardation alone. Similarly, those with the mildest symptoms may appear similar to individuals with social problems due to personality disorders, nonverbal learning disabilities, pragmatic language disorders, and social anxiety.

8. Is there treatment for autism?

Autism is generally considered a lifelong, chronic disability. Nevertheless, specific educational and therapeutic interventions are critical for stimulating development in all areas and improving the person's adaptive functioning in all settings (home, school, work, and community).

For children, intervention needs to begin as early as the diagnosis is made, in the toddler and preschool period. Specific interventions should focus on developing language, appropriate behavior, cognitive skills, and social responsiveness. There is some evidence that interventions delivered in the preschool period are maximally effective in promoting development.

The school-aged child with autism needs a curriculum that is tailored to individual strengths and needs. With appropriate educational approaches, virtually all children with autism can be expected to make clear, measurable progress in learning. The kinds of programs that are helpful vary from individualized instruction in regular school classrooms to special schools for children with autism. There is an array of educational choices for families, but all effective education programs are highly individualized, using well-structured, systematic teaching routines, consistency and repetition, and concrete, functional learning objectives.

Adolescents and adults with autism frequently need specific help in negotiating the complexities of life demands. Social skills groups, recreational activities, individual psychotherapy, and vocational coaching and assistance can help them acquire skills necessary for a satisfying adult life. Participating in typical community activities with nondisabled peers is an important part of community life for adults with autism.

People with autism often have areas of strength that must be supported through further teaching and extracurricular activities, since they may represent an ability that will be respected and valued by peers or be important in establishing a vocation or an avocation in adult life. These areas of talent may also develop into activities around which the person with autism may participate in typical community events.

Interventions that are particularly helpful for treating the core symptoms of autism include cognitive/behavioral approaches, systematic instruction, and concrete, pragmatic approaches to life's challenges. Speech and language therapy is important in helping individuals with autism develop their communicative capacities to their fullest. Augmentative communications strategies are crucial for nonverbal individuals. One highly controversial strategy is facilitated communication. Although this strategy has received considerable attention, empirical studies have not been consistently supportive. Finally, occupational therapy and physical therapy are often important in treating motor abnormalities involving both motor development and sensory processing dysfunction.

Less common approaches to treatment include nutritional and vitamin supplementation, vision therapy, and auditory training. There is almost always a "new cure" for autism being discovered and publicized, but these approaches have failed to demonstrate consistently positive effects.

9. What medications are helpful in autism?

At present, no pharmacological treatment can "cure" autism. However, several classes of medications have been used to treat specific associated behavioral problems.

Stimulant medications, such as methylphenidate and amphetamines, have been used to control the hyperactive behaviors sometimes seen in children with autism. These medications may decrease the activity levels and improve the attention span of some children, which then may lead to a better response to behavioral and educational treatments. While anecdotal reports have suggested some effectiveness in certain children with autism, a review of the research on stimulant medications suggests little or no clinical improvement. Furthermore, some studies report a worsening of behavior in some children.

Neuroleptics have also been considered in treating some of the symptoms of autism. The preponderance of the research has been done with haloperidol, which has been reported to improve hyperactivity, aggression, agitation, stereotypic behaviors, and mood lability in some studies of children with autism. Other symptoms such as abnormal relatedness, social withdrawal, and cognitive functioning were less affected. Although haloperidol does appear to have some limited clinical effectiveness in autism, the serious side effects of this drug warrant extreme caution.

Fenfluramine has recently received attention in the treatment of some symptoms of autism. This medication, which was originally used as a weight-control drug, was found to decrease the sometimes elevated blood serotonin levels in children with autism. Early studies reported behavioral improvements in attention, communication, and responsiveness. Unfortunately, continued trials with fenfluramine have not been very successful. These equivocal findings, and the significant side effects of this drug, suggest that it may not be an ideal treatment at this time.

Antidepressants, such as fluoxetine, imipramine, desipramine, and the mood stabilizing agent, lithium, have been used in treating individuals with autism with some success. These drugs may be particularly helpful in addressing depressed mood, anxiety, and obsessive-compulsive symptoms that are sometimes evident, particularly in high-functioning individuals with autism or Asperger's disorder.

Antianxiety medications such as buspirone and propranolol have also been used, particularly in children who display a great deal of anxiety or agitated behavior.

Clonidine has been used in some children with autism to reduce high levels of hyperactivity, impulsivity, distractibility, and acting-out behaviors. At present, however, little empirical work has been done to establish the effectiveness of this medication in treating these symptoms in children and adolescents, and no studies have addressed its use in autism.

Anticonvulsants, such as phenytoin and carbamazepine, are used to treat children with autism who suffer from seizures. These medications may also be effective in decreasing aggressive behavior and episodic behavioral outbursts, particularly in children with seizure disorder.

10. What is the prognosis for children with autism?

With appropriate educational and treatment services, children with autism will show some improvements. The preschool years are typically the most difficult, because children with autism tend to be the least social, least communicative, and have the most difficulties behaviorally. IQ remains stable across the lifespan, but the severity of the social and communicative deficits tends to diminish as children grow older. Learning continues throughout childhood and adolescence, as long as children are receiving appropriate services. Adolescence can be a difficult time for some individuals with autism, because of increased sexual behavior and aggressiveness. Others' behavior improves during this time. In addition, some high-functioning adolescents with autism, and particularly Asperger's disorder, may experience depressed mood which may improve with specific treatment for depression.

A number of follow-up studies have been conducted with individuals with autism. These studies are typically based on samples of individuals who did not receive the intensive treatment services that are more prevalent today. Therefore, some of the commonly cited statistics may underestimate positive outcomes. These studies suggest that 5–17% of individuals with autism will work and live independently as adults. The most important positive prognostic indicators are functional (i.e., useful) language before age 5, and cognitive abilities above the mentally retarded range (i.e., IQ > 70). Another 30% are reported as achieving some degree of partial independence in adulthood. Finally, roughly 25% of children with autism develop seizures beginning in adolescence or early adulthood. The seizures are typically grand mal or psychomotor seizures, and usually respond well to anticonvulsant medication.

11. How is autism related to other mental disorders?

Individuals with autism may demonstrate symptoms of other psychiatric disorders. Treatment of comorbid conditions is likely to improve the response to interventions aimed at symptoms of autism. Some of the more common comorbid conditions include:

Attention deficit–hyperactivity disorder (ADHD): ADHD is present in some, but certainly not all, children with autism. Many children with autism display some of the characteristic symptoms of ADHD, such hyperactivity and distractibility.

Tourette's syndrome: Tourette's syndrome appears to share some genetic loading with autism spectrum disorders. It is sometimes difficult to discriminate between the motor tics of Tourette's syndrome and the motor stereotypies of autism. Likewise, the obsessive and compulsive symptoms that can accompany Tourette's syndrome may appear similar to the repetitive behaviors in autism. It has been suggested that these two disorders may have some similar neurobiologic impairments perhaps involving the basal ganglia.

Depression and anxiety: These disorders coincide with autism with some frequency. Depression is known to be associated with Asperger's disorder, particularly in adolescence. Anxiety can be seen at all ages and levels of functioning. Anxiety can be responsible for some of the behavioral outbursts, resistance to change, and need for repetitive routines that are often a part of autism. Because many people with autism are not verbal enough to describe their symptoms, the clinician must be sensitive to vegetative signs and other nonverbal markers of these conditions.

Mental retardation: Mental retardation frequently co-occurs with autism. However, it is quite important that psychological testing be conducted by clinicians who are familiar with autism, and that the intelligence tests used are appropriate to the individual's abilities and understanding. For example, nonverbal intelligence tests or nonverbal adaptations of tests are appropriate for younger children with autism and those who have limited verbal skills.

For individuals with autism who do not have mental retardation, there is a common pattern of cognitive strengths and weaknesses, in which visual perceptual skills are often significantly better than verbal abilities, and concrete problem solving is better than abstract knowledge. Thus, in high-functioning individuals with autism, there is often a learning disability profile, which necessitates individual approaches to education.

For individuals with **Asperger's disorder**, the pattern of cognitive strengths and weaknesses is often reversed, with verbal skills stronger than nonverbal skills, and significant problems with math and handwriting. This pattern of performance is also known as **nonverbal learning disability**, and is often accompanied by social problems. Thus, this can led to a complicated differential diagnosis. There are probably many children with Asperger's disorder for whom only the nonverbal learning disability profile has been diagnosed. These learning profiles are not just important in childhood; they have important implications for adult life and vocational adjustment.

Finally, there has been some confusion in the past regarding the distinction between autism and **schizophrenia**. Initially, autism was considered to be a form of childhood schizophrenia. Labels such as "infantile psychosis" and "symbiotic psychosis" were often applied to children with autism spectrum disorder. Current thinking, however, separates autism from all psychotic disorders.

BIBLIOGRAPHY

1. Cohen DJ, Donnellan AM (eds): Handbook of Autism and Pervasive Developmental Disorders. Silver Spring, MD, V.H. Winston, 1987.
2. Dawson G (ed): Autism: Nature, Diagnosis, and Treatment. New York, Guilford Press, 1989.
3. Diagnostic and Statistical Manual of Mental Disorders, 4th ed. Washington, DC, American Psychiatric Association, 1994.
4. Frith U (ed): Autism and Asperger Syndrome. Cambridge, Cambridge University Press, 1991.
5. Ehlers S, Gillberg D: The epidemiology of Asperger syndrome. A total population study. J Child Psychol Psychiatry, 34:1327–1350, 1993
6. Gillberg D, Coleman M: The Biology of the Autistic Syndromes, 2nd ed. London, MacKeith Press, 1992.
7. Grandin T, Scariano MM: Emergence: Labeled Autistic. Novato, CA, Arena Press, 1989.
8. Krug D, Arick J, Almond P: Behaviour checklist for identifying severely handicapped individuals with high levels of autistic behavior. J Child Psychol Psychiatry 21:221–229, 1990.
9. Lindberg B: Understanding Rett's Syndrome. Toronto, Hogrefe and Huber, 1991.
10. Maurice C: Let Me Hear Your Voice. New York, Alfred A. Knopf, 1993.
11. Powers MD (ed): Children with Autism: A Parents' Guide. Rockville, MD, Woodbine House, 1989.
12. Rutter M, Schopler E (eds): Autism: A Reappraisal of Concepts and Treatment. New York, Plenum, 1976.
13. Schopler E, Reichler RJ, Renner BR: The Childhood Autism Rating Scale (CARS) for Diagnostic Screening and Classification of Autism. New York, Irvington, 1986.
14. Schreibman L: Autism. Developmental Clinical Psychology and Psychiatry, Volume 15. Newbury Park, Sage Publications, 1988.
15. Stone W, Hogan K: A structured parent interview for identifying young children with autism. J Autism Devel Disord 23:639–652, 1993.
16. Volkmar FR (ed): Psychoses and pervasive developmental disorder. Child Adolesc Psychiatr Clin North Am January 1994.

55. ATTENTION DEFICIT-HYPERACTIVITY DISORDER

Frederick B. Hebert, M.D.

1. What is attention deficit-hyperactivity disorder?

Attention deficit-hyperactivity disorder (ADHD) has been described for at least 50 years. It is characterized by persistent activity or inattention. In the past, hyperactivity was a requirement for the diagnosis, but it is now recognized that inattention is the core disturbance. Thus either attention deficit or hyperactivity is required for the diagnosis.

2. What are the signs of inattention?

Children with attention deficit fail to give attention to details or make careless mistakes in school; they also have difficulty paying attention during play. Frequently, they seem not to have heard, even when they maintain eye contact. They also repeatedly lose items such as pencils, books, jackets, or sports equipment.

3. What are the signs of hyperactivity?

Overall, hyperactive children are more active than peers of similar age and same gender. They fidget with their hands or their feet and squirm in their seats. In the classroom they get out of their seat (e.g., go to the pencil sharpener) and touch and intrude on other students. Their peers report that children with ADHD are "all wound up like rubber bands." If there is no gross motor activity, both girls and boys often talk incessantly without getting to the point.

4. When children with ADHD are not hyperactive, are they impulsive?

Yes. Impulsive behavior is usually most apparent in the classroom, where children with ADHD blurt out answers before the teacher can finish the question. Hyperactive children cannot wait in lines and wander around, loosing their place. They may butt into others' games or conversations without thinking or even being aware of their social faux pas.

5. How is ADHD diagnosed?

DSM–IV requires six or more symptoms of hyperactivity or inattention, such as those listed above. The common symptoms of ADHD have been collected into a checklist. The Teacher's Checklist (see page 318) is commonly used. Ten critical items are scored in one of four categories: not at all (0), just a little (1), pretty much (2), or very much (3). The maximal score is 30 points. Scores for children with ADHD vary with age, but a score of 18 for boys or 15 for girls supports the diagnosis of ADHD. DSM–IV also requires the onset of symptoms before age 7 years to rule out recent traumatic problems. Hyperactivity may occur because of the child's adjustment to a recent traumatic event. A careful history for physical or sexual abuse may need to be elicited to rule out posttraumatic stress disorder. The Parent's Checklist (see page 319) is given first to the parents; if they score all 48 questions as "pretty much" or "very much," the checklist should be considered invalid; the parents probably are angry at the child for another reason. Concurrently the Teacher's Checklist is sent to school. In families where one or more of the parents appear disorganized, the checklist may have to be mailed directly to the school to ensure that it will be returned to the physician.

6. What laboratory tests are helpful?

None. Although certain parts of IQ tests, such as the digits span performance test on the Wechsler Intelligence Scale for Children–Revised, can measure attention indirectly, the standardized

This modified form of Conner's Checklist is widely available. On the parent's questionnaire, the following items are scored: 4, 10, 11, 13, 19, 25, 30, 31, 33, 37. On the teacher's questionnaire, the following items are scored: 1, 3, 7, 8, 14, 15, 21, 22, 26, 28.

Teacher's Questionnaire

Name of Child_____ Grade_____

Date of Evaluation_____

Please answer all questions. Beside *each* item, indicate the degree of the problem by a check mark (✓)	Not at all	Just a little	Pretty much	Very much
1. Restless in the "squirmy" sense.				
2. Makes inappropriate noises when he shouldn't.				
3. Demands must be met immediately.				
4. Acts "smart" (impudent or sassy).				
5. Temper outbursts and unpredictable behavior.				
6. Overly sensitive to criticism.				
7. Distractibility or attention span a problem.				
8. Disturbs other children.				
9. Daydreams.				
10. Pouts and sulks.				
11. Mood changes quickly and drastically.				
12. Quarrelsome.				
13. Submissive attitude toward authority.				
14. Restless, always "up and on the go."				
15. Excitable, impulsive				
16. Excessive demands for teacher's attention.				
17. Appears to be unaccepted by group.				
18. Appears to be easily led by other children.				
19. No sense of fair play.				
20. Appears to lack leadership				
21. Fails to finish things that he starts.				
22. Childish and immature				
23. Denies mistakes or blames others.				
24. Does not get along well with other children.				
25. Uncooperative with classmates.				
26. Easily frustrated in efforts.				
27. Uncooperative with teacher.				
28. Difficulty in learning.				

Parent's Questionnaire

Name of Child _____ Date _____

Please answer all questions. Beside *each* item, indicate the degree of the problem by a check mark (✓)	Not at all	Just a little	Pretty much	Very much
1. Picks at things (nails; fingers; hair; clothing).				
2. Sassy to grown-ups.				
3. Problem with making or keeping friends.				
4. Excitable, impulsive.				
5. Wants to run things.				
6. Sucks or chews (thumb; clothing; blankets).				

Parent's Questionnaire *(Cont.)*

7. Cries easily or often.				
8. Carries a chip on his shoulder.				
9. Daydreams.				
10. Difficulty in learning.				
11. Restless in the "squirmy" sense.				
12. Fearful (of new situations; new people or places; going to school).				
13. Restless, always up and on the go.				
14. Destructive.				
15. Tells lies or stories that aren't true.				
16. Shy.				
17. Gets into more trouble than others the same age.				
18. Speaks differently from others the same age (baby talk; stuttering; hard to understand).				
19. Denies mistakes or blames others.				
20. Quarrelsome.				
21. Pouts and sulks.				
22. Steals.				
23. Disobedient or obeys but resentfully.				
24. Worries more than others (about being alone; illness or death).				
25. Fails to finish things.				
26. Feelings easily hurt.				
27. Bullies others.				
28. Unable to stop a repetitive activity.				
29. Cruel.				
30. Childish or immature (wants help he shouldn't need; clings; needs constant reassurance).				
31. Distractibility or attention span a problem.				
32. Headaches.				
33. Mood changes quickly and drastically.				
34. Doesn't like or doesn't follow rules or restrictions.				
35. Fights constantly.				
36. Doesn't get along well with brothers or sisters.				
37. Easily frustrated in efforts.				
38. Disturbs other children.				
39. Basically an unhappy child.				
40. Problems with eating (poor appetite; up between bites).				
41. Stomach aches.				
42. Problems with sleep (can't fall asleep; up too early; up in the night).				
43. Other aches and pains.				
44. Vomiting or nausea.				
45. Feels cheated in family circle.				
46. Boasts and brags.				
47. Lets self be pushed around.				
48. Bowel problems (frequently loose; irregular habits; constipation).				

questionnaires are easier and more accurate. Complicated electronic devices (e.g., the Gordon Performance Test) that measure attention directly are expensive and unnecessary. Recently a computer feedback of EEG rhythms showed promise of providing diagnosis and definitive treatment without need for further intervention. This method is not validated in the general literature and should not be used for the typical patient with ADHD.

7. What is the differential diagnosis of ADHD?

The most important behavior to rule out is age-appropriate behaviors of normal children; for example, running around on the playground, squirming at the dinner table, and difficulty with staying quiet in the car are normal behaviors in younger children. ADHD is not diagnosed if another disorder accounts for the hyperactivity. Hyperactivity associated with psychotic disorders is often peculiar; e.g., spinning objects or tearing paper for hours. In most other disorders the onset of hyperactivity occurs after the age of 7 years. Many conduct-disordered children are misdiagnosed with attention deficit-hyperactivity disorder because of their intrusive behavior. However, conduct-disordered children violate basic rights of others intentionally, whereas children with ADHD do so by accident (e.g., bumping into other children because of their high activity level). Anxious children may fidget and appear hyperactive but do not demonstrate the impulsivity of ADHD. In addition, they are often timid and withdrawn instead of intrusive.

Differential Diagnosis of ADHD

Age appropriate behavior	Posttraumatic stress disorder
Oppositional (defiant disorder)	Psychotic disorder
Mood disorder	Substance abuse
Anxiety disorder	Conduct disorder

8. Is the cause of ADHD known?

The cause remains unknown. Recent evidence demonstrates that patients with ADHD have metabolic deficiencies of adrenergic amines in the central nervous system, but the cause of such changes is unknown.

9. Discuss the incidence, comorbidity, and long-term prognosis.

ADHD has a 3% incidence. Of children with ADHD, 30–50% or more have an associated learning disability. Although one-third of patients with aDHD have a greater than average number of auto accidents, divorces, and job changes during adulthood, two-thirds become normal adults. Only 1% of adults with ADHD continue to show hyperactivity. Although as many as 50% of children referred for ADHD evaluations are diagnosed instead with oppositional disorders, many patients with ADHD also have associated behavior problems. When ADHD is associated with aggression at an early age or with low IQ, the prognosis is poor. Children with Tourette's disorder frequently have associated ADHD.

10. What are the treatments for ADHD?

The treatment for ADHD includes interventions at home and school as well as biologic treatment. Home should be organized to give the child a predictable environment. Bedtime, mealtimes, homework, and even playtime can be scheduled to help the child organize his or her day. A simple reward system of stars glued to a calendar or other daily charting as a reward for good behavior is often helpful. Help is also necessary in school. A range of structures from a special class (1 hour/day) to a completely self-contained classroom should be available. Frequently the child should be evaluated for appropriate classroom placement by the local school district. Schools are required to educate students under federal law but often try to divert help to medical or social caregivers to contain costs.

11. Can behavior therapy be used to modify hyperactivity?

In most scientific reports behavior therapy is helpful. However, when behavior therapy and medications are compared in the same study, most of the improvement appears to result from medication.

12. What medications are helpful? How should they be given?

Medication is best given by targeting the patient's symptoms over 4-hour periods. Almost all patients need morning medication, most an early afternoon dose, and some a late afternoon or early evening dose.

Methylphenidate (Ritalin) is usually started at about 0.25 mg/kg, and the dose is gradually increased to an effective level (usually < 1 mg/kg). Methylphenidate is also available in an extended-release form that lasts for 8 hours or more. The extended-release tablet cannot be split, because the medication will not be evenly absorbed; regular tablets (5, 10, and 20 mg), however, are scored and can be divided. Although some studies show that higher doses cause a detriment in learning, most studies have shown a straight-line response with increased doses and increased effectiveness.

Side effects are rarely serious. Insomnia is common early in treatment or if the last dose is given late in the day; some children may need medication to go to bed. Stomachaches, probably secondary to decreased motility from the sympathomimetic effect, usually resolve if the medication is given with food, which is no longer believed to interfere with absorption. In addition, all children on stimulants suffer some initial weight loss from the anorexic effect of the medication, but this effect usually diminishes in the first month. Recent studies have shown that the growth inhibition previously reported is only a delay. However, it is still reasonable to maintain height and weight charts over the longer term to demonstrate that children continue to follow their own growth curve. Each summer or during extended school breaks, the patient should receive a 2-week trial off medication to evaluate continued need. Eventually the patient's family and physician no longer notice a change when the medication is discontinued.

Dextroamphetamine (Dexedrine) is twice as potent as methylphenidate and is more often used for children. Spansules have been shown to be erratically absorbed and less effective than regular tablets. **Pemoline** (Cylert), which is about one-fourth as potent as methylphenidate, has been effective in clinical trials in doses from 75–112 mg/day. Compared with methylphenidate and dextroamphetamine, pemoline has a long duration of action. Patients started on pemoline frequently have initial problems going to sleep. Benefits may not be seen for up to 3 weeks, reflecting a gradual increase in effectiveness and the fact that any stimulant at too low of a dose may initially increase the patient's activity levels. If there is concern about substance abuse or an overriding need to give medication only once a day, pemoline is a good alternative. At a minimum, baseline serum glutamate oxaloacetate transaminase (SGOT) should be assessed to monitor for rare cases of liver toxicity. An increase in tics as well as lip-licking and biting has also been reported in children taking pemoline.

13. What are the alternatives to stimulant medication?

Patients with ADHD who are depressed or anxious may do better on tricyclic antidepressants (TCAs). Both imipramine and desipramine have been effective in total doses of 2–4 mg/kg, given once or twice a day. Clinicians sometimes note a decreased effect over time. Because TCAs can be dangerous to the myocardium, a baseline EKG is necessary before treatment is started. Because several children have died while taking desipramine, clinicians are cautious about its use. Bupropion, an antidepressant structurally related to the stimulants, has been used to treat ADHD in two studies. The doses ranged from 150–250 mg/day in divided doses. In one study decreased hyperactivity and global improvement were significant, but no effect was seen on conduct. In a Canadian study, 70% of 17 boys showed improvement. Primary side effects from bupropion are nausea and stomachache. Bupropion may be useful in treating patients with ADHD who have become depressed. Two recent studies have used fluoxetine, a specific serotonin reuptake inhibitor, as an adjunct in the treatment of ADHD in patients who are not responsive to stimulants alone; about 70% showed improvement.

14. Does ADHD have the same signs and symptoms in adolescents and adults?
About one-half of children with ADHD lose their hyperactivity in adolescence. However, the attention problems often persist into adulthood. Diagnosis of adult ADHD requires input from another adult who has lived with the patient. Asking the patient's mother to fill out a checklist describing the patient during ages 6–10 is ideal, but a spouse or roommate may be helpful. Diagnosis of adult ADHD requires childhood and current symptoms with onset before adolescence. One checklist also requires adult patients to have at least two of the following: (1) affective lability, (2) task incompletion, (3) short-lived outbursts, (4) impulsivity, and (5) stress intolerance. Adult patients with high checklist scores were more likely to respond to stimulant treatment. Medication is frequently discontinued but resumed under stress.

BIBLIOGRAPHY

1. Biederman J, et al: Patterns of psychiatric comorbidity, cognition, and psychosocial functioning in adults with attention deficit disorder. Am J Psychiatry 150:1792, 1993.
2. Biederman J, et al: Diagnoses of attention-deficit hyperactivity disorder from parent reports predict diagnoses based on teacher reports. J Am Acad Child Adolesc Psychiatry 32:315, 1993.
3. Casat C, et al: Buproprion in children with attention-deficit disorder. Psychopharmacol Bull 25:198, 1989.
4. Conners CK: A teacher rating scale for use in drug studies with children. Am J Psychiatry 126:884–888, 1969.
5. DuPaul G, Rapport M: Does methylphenidate normalize the classroom behavior of children with attention deficit disorder? J Am Acad Child Adolesc Psychiatry 32:190, 1993.
6. Fischer M, et al: The adolescent outcome of hyperactive children: Predictors of psychiatric, academic, social, and emotional adjustment. J Am Acad Child Adolesc Psychiatry 32:324, 1993.
7. Gadow K, et al: Methylphenidate in hyperactive boys with comorbid tic disorder. II: Short-term behavioral effects in school settings. J Am Acad Child Adolesc Psychiatry 31:462, 1992.
8. Garfinkel BD, et al: Tricyclic antidepressant and methylphenidate treatment of attention deficit disorder in children. J Am Acad Child Adolesc Psychiatry 22:343, 1983.
9. Handen B, et al: Effects and non-effects of methylphenidate in children with mental retardation and ADHD. J Am Acad Child Adolesc Psychiatry 31:455, 1992.
10. Hunt RD, et al: Clonidine benefits children with attention deficit disorder and hyperactivity: Report of a double-blind placebo-crossover therapeutic trial. J Am Acad Child Adolesc Psychiatry 24:617, 1985.
11. Kemph JP, et al: Treatment of aggressive children with clonidine: Results of an open pilot study. J Am Acad Child Adolesc Psychiatry 32:577, 1993.
12. Klein RG, Mannuzza S: Hyperactive boys almost grown up. III: Methylphenidate effects on ultimate height. Arch Gen Psychiatry 45:1131, 1988.
13. Porrino LJ, et al: A naturalistic assessment of the motor activity of hyperactive boys. I: Comparison with normal controls. Arch Gen Psychiatry 40:681–687, 1983.
14. Rapport M, et al: Methylphenidate and desipramine in hospitalized children. I: Separate and combined effects on cognitive function. J Am Acad Child Adolesc Psychiatry 32:333, 1993.
15. Sleator EK, Ulmann RK: Can the physician diagnose hyperactivity in the office? Pediatrics 67:13, 1981.
16. Spencer T, et al: A double-blind, crossover comparison of methylphenidate and placebo in adults with childhood-onset attention deficit disorder. Arch Gen Psychiatry 52:434, 1995.
17. Sprague RL, Sleator EK: What is the proper dose of stimulant drugs in children? In Gittleman-Klein R (ed): Recent Advances in Child Psychopharmacology. New York, Human Sciences Press, 1975, pp 79–108.
18. Steingard R, et al: Comparison of clonidine response in the treatment of attention-deficit hyperactivity disorder with and without comorbid tic disorders. J Am Acad Child Adolesc Psychiatry 32:350, 1993.

56. CONDUCT DISORDER

Paula DeGraffenreid Riggs, M.D.

1. Define conduct disorder.

Conduct disorder is a psychiatric disorder of children and adolescents characterized by a persistent and repetitive pattern of behavior that violates the basic rights of others or major age-appropriate societal norms or rules. According to the specific diagnostic criteria in DSM IV, three (or more) characteristic behaviors must have been present during the past 12 months, with at least one behavior present in the past 6 months (criterion A). Such behaviors generally are present in various settings and cause clinically significant impairment in social, academic, or occupational functioning (criterion B).

The diagnostic criterion behaviors of conduct disorder fall into four main groupings:

1. **Aggressive conduct** that causes or threatens harm to other people or animals (bullying, fighting, use of weapons, physical cruelty to people or animals, stealing with confrontation of victim, forced sex)

2. **Nonaggressive conduct** that causes property loss or damage (deliberate destruction of property or fire-setting)

3. **Deceitfulness or theft** (breaking and entering, "conning" others, theft of nontrivial items without confrontation of victim)

4. **Serious violations of rules** (staying out late at night despite parental prohibitions before age 13, running away from home overnight at least twice, truancy from school before age 13).

Conduct disorder is subdivided into two main subtypes:

1. **Childhood-onset type**—defined by onset of at least one criterion characteristic of conduct disorder before age 10. Youths with this type of conduct disorder are usually male and aggressive, with disturbed peer relationships, and meet full criteria for conduct disorder before puberty; they are more likely to have persistent antisocial behaviors into adulthood, ultimately meeting criteria for antisocial personality disorder.

2. **Adolescent-onset type**—defined by the absence of any criterion of conduct disorder before age 10. Patients are generally less aggressive than those with childhood-onset conduct disorder and have more normative peer relationships. Youths with adolescent onset are less likely to have persistent conduct disorder evolving into antisocial personality disorder; thus they more often have adolescence-limited conduct disorder. Girls with conduct disorder are more likely to have this type.

2. How common is conduct disorder?

Conduct disorder is the most common reason for referral of children for psychiatric evaluation and treatment. It appears to be more prevalent in urban than rural settings. It is about 3 times more common in boys than in girls. The prevalence rates for boys under the age of 18 is 6–16%; for girls, rates range from 2–9%.

3. What causes conduct disorder?

There is no single cause of conduct disorder. Generally factors associated with and contributing to conduct disorder can be categorized as intrinsic and extrinsic.

Intrinsic factors include the following:

1. Genetic studies demonstrate greater concordance for antisocial behavior in monozygotic than dizygotic twins.

2. Some data support that conduct-disordered youths may have autonomic hyporeactivity, possibly making them difficult to condition with positive reinforcement.

3. Diminished serotonin levels in the cerebrospinal fluid are associated with impulsivity, aggression, and violence—all characteristics of conduct-disordered youths.

4. Soft neurologic signs (such as awkward rapid alternating movements, inability to skip, choreiform movements) are prevalent among conduct-disordered youth, as are verbal learning difficulties.

5. Early aggression (before age 7) is a robust predictor of later aggression and is associated with the development of conduct disorder.

Extrinsic factors include the following:

1. Parental factors such as (1) low maternal affection; (2) father's deviance (alcoholism or criminality); (3) substance use disorders in parents or parental surrogates; (4) parental aggression or violence and/or physical or sexual abuse of children; (5) inability of the parents to provide adequate supervision, structure, and limits; and (6) lack of consistent parental emotional investment, support, and affection.

2. Sociocultural factors, such as low socioeconomic status and living in areas with easy access to antisocial or deviant peer groups.

4. What is the differential diagnosis of conduct disorder?

Oppositional defiant disorder includes some features of conduct disorder but does not include the persistent pattern of more serious deviant behavior in which the basic rights of others or age-appropriate societal norms or rules are violated. According to DSM IV, when an individual meets criteria for both conduct disorder and oppositional defiant disorder, the diagnosis of conduct disorder takes precedence.

Children with **attention deficit-hyperactivity disorder** (ADHD) often exhibit hyperactive and impulsive behavior and low frustration tolerance, which may be disruptive. Yet this behavior does not violate age-appropriate societal norms and does not usually meet criteria for conduct disorder. The key features of ADHD are inattentiveness, motoric hyperactivity, and poor concentration. Such features distinguish ADHD from conduct disorder.

The irritability and impulsivity of a manic or hypomanic episode, characteristic of **bipolar disorder**, may contribute to behavioral problems. These features usually are distinguished from the disruptive behavioral pattern of conduct disorder based on episodic course and other symptoms, such as pressured speech, reduced need to sleep, and racing thoughts.

The diagnosis of **adjustment disorder** (with disturbance of conduct and emotions) should be considered if clinically significant conduct problems, not meeting criteria for another specific disorder, develop in clear association with the onset of a psychosocial stressor.

For individuals over the age of 18 years conduct disorder may be diagnosed only if the criteria for **antisocial personality disorder** are not met. The diagnosis of antisocial personality disorder cannot be given to individuals under the age 18 years. On the other hand, the diagnosis of antisocial personality disorder requires evidence of conduct disorder before age 15 (DSM IV).

Aggression, impulsivity, and behavioral problems may be manifestations of various **neurologic problems**, including seizures. Usually such disorders are easily distinguished from conduct disorder by considering longitudinal course and associated features. The same is true for **chronic psychotic disorders**. However, both psychosis and neurologic disorders may be separately comorbid with conduct disorder.

Because many different kinds of psychiatric disorders may present as behavior problems and because the diagnostic criteria for conduct disorder are broad, it is essential for the clinician to perform a detailed comprehensive neuropsychiatric evaluation before making the diagnosis of conduct disorder. It is equally essential to assess thoroughly for comorbid disorders.

5. What other disorders are associated with conduct disorder?

Substance use disorders and conduct disorder are highly associated both in adolescence and later adulthood. Although the exact prevalence of substance abuse or dependence with conduct disorder in adolescence is not clear, the Epidemiologic Catchment Area study demonstrated that 84% of individuals with antisocial personality disorder (vs. 17% of the general population) had diagnoses of a substance use disorder in adulthood and all had conduct disorder as youths. Most antisocial adults with substance use disorders begin substance abuse in adolescence. As the number of conduct symptoms increases, so does the incidence of associated substance use disorder.

ADHD occurs in 30–50% of cases of conduct disorder in both epidemiologic and clinically referred samples. Although both conduct disorder and ADHD are classified as disruptive behavior disorders and may have some symptoms in common, recent studies support that they are separate disorders and that ADHD does not "cause" conduct disorder. If the diagnostic criteria for both disorders are met, both should be diagnosed and treated.

Depressive disorders occur with conduct disorder in 15–24% of cases in both epidemiologic and clinically referred samples.

Anxiety disorders are also more prevalent among youths with conduct disorder (15–24%) than among those without conduct disorder (5–11%).

There are no good estimates of the incidence of **bipolar disorder** with conduct disorder, partly because of the low prevalence of bipolar disorder in adult populations (approximately 1%). The incidence of a manic or hypomanic episode with prior depression presenting before age 15 is even more rare. Large community-based or multicenter studies will be necessary to address this comorbidity more adequately.

Learning disabilities are comorbid with conduct disorder in 10–90% of cases. The broad range is most likely due to differences in assessment and diagnosis of learning disorders. Nevertheless, the literature supports high rates of comorbid learning disabilities with conduct disorder overall. Most conduct-disordered children are not severely retarded but tend to score in the low normal or borderline ranges of intelligence. Language deficits may contribute to inability to express feelings and attitudes verbally rather than physically.

6. Are there gender differences in conduct disorder?

As mentioned, conduct disorder is about 3 times more common in boys than in girls. Boys are also more likely to have the childhood-onset type of conduct disorder and associated ADHD than girls. Boys are more likely to have persistence of conduct disorder, evolving into antisocial personality disorder in adulthood. Girls may be more likely to have associated depressive disorders than boys.

Gender differences are also found in specific types of conduct problems. Boys with a diagnosis of conduct disorder frequently exhibit fighting and other aggressive acts, stealing, vandalism, and school discipline problems. Girls with a diagnosis of conduct disorder are more likely to exhibit lying, truancy, running away, and prostitution. Both boys and girls with conduct disorder have a high prevalence of comorbid substance use disorders.

7. Are there effective treatments for conduct disorder?

Offord and Bennett[8] recently reviewed the four major intervention strategies used to treat conduct disorder: (1) parent- and family-targeted programs, especially parent management training; (2) social-cognitive programs; (3) peer- and school-based programs; and (4) community-based programs.

Parent management training (PMT) is aimed at redirecting interactional processes between the parent and child or within the family that may inadvertently develop and sustain aggressive and antisocial behavior. PMT has been demonstrated to have short-term effectiveness in clinically referred populations. A serious problem, however, with PMT is that parents of conduct-disordered children are often not able to participate because of their own psychopathology, substance abuse, marital discord, or family dysfunction.

Social-cognitive and problem-solving skills training assume that changing cognitions and affects will lead to changed or enhanced behavioral adjustment. Children and adolescents with conduct disorder have been shown to have deficits in problem-solving skills, perceptions, self-statements, and self-attributions. For instance, aggressive children are more likely to interpret the intentions and actions of others as hostile and to have poor social relations with peers, teachers, and parents. They often have a limited verbal and behavioral repertoire from which to draw their reactions to strong affects or situations. Thus, a cognitive-behavioral therapeutic approach is aimed at enhancing and broadening this repertoire to help conduct-disordered youths deal better with anger-provoking situations as well as their own impulsive behaviors. The success of these interventions is difficult to interpret because of the heterogeneity of studied children. Reports of the effectiveness of such interventions are therefore somewhat mixed. Overall, the effective translation of cognitive change into behavioral change has not been demonstrated in conduct-disordered samples.

Peer- and school-based interventions are focused on the role of peer relations and schools in the development of conduct disorder and antisocial behavior. Its theoretical basis is that parental factors are more important in the development of conduct disorder in the preschool years, but that school and peer factors may become ascendent in the early to middle school years. Forty percent of peer-rejected children are aggressive and at high risk to develop antisocial behavior in adolescence. Thus, this treatment focuses on prosocial skills training aimed at reducing aggressive behavior, improving peer and teacher relations, and preventing the development of antisocial behavior. Some evidence supports the short-term effectiveness of this intervention, but no long-term benefit has been demonstrated.

Community intervention strategies are generally developed from existing community-based programs and are aimed at strengthening the ability of the community to promote prosocial behavior and to deter antisocial and delinquent behavior through changing or enhancing existing systems. Community-based programs have been demonstrated to be effective in the short-term when interventions (often using highly structured, behaviorally focused treatments) were initiated at an early age (preschool to early grade school). However, no long-term benefit has been demonstrated.

Treatment of comorbid disorders such as substance use disorders, depression, ADHD, and learning disorders is essential. Specific treatment modalities for comorbidities must be used in conjunction with the behavioral management of the conduct problems; treatment of the comorbid disorder(s) may affect the effectiveness of management and treatment of conduct disorder.

Overall the available literature provides limited evidence for the effectiveness of either primary or secondary prevention of conduct disorder, and no treatment has demonstrated long-term efficacy. Further research is needed to determine the effectiveness of interventions that use broad-based multimodal neuropsychiatric assessments and long-term treatment for conduct disorder and also thoroughly assess and treat comorbid disorders.

8. Is there evidence for a specific neurochemical abnormality in conduct disorder and its associated features?

Yes. A growing database supports abnormalities of serotonin (low 5HIAA in cerebrospinal fluid) in the modulation of brain functions in the disruptive behavior disorders of childhood. A low serotonin syndrome has been associated with early onset of impulsive violent behavior, chronic impulsivity, aggression, and substance abuse—all clearly associated with conduct disorder. Depression and suicidality (both with and without a concurrent diagnosis of major depressive disorder) occur at high rates among conduct-disordered youth and are associated with reduced 5-hydroxyindoleacetic acid (5-HIAA), the major metabolite of serotonin. Current data are insufficient to determine whether serotonergic agents are helpful in the treatment of conduct disorder. Data indicate that lithium, a nonselective serotonergic agent enhancing 5HT function, is better than placebo in improving the behavior of children with aggressive conduct disorder as well as aggression in adult felons. Additional studies are needed.

BIBLIOGRAPHY

1. American Psychiatric Association: Diagnostic and Statistical Manual of Mental Disorders, 4th ed. Washington, DC, American Psychiatric Association, 1994.
2. Bukstein OG, Brent DA, Kaminer Y: Comorbidity of substance abuse and other psychiatric disorders in adolescents. Am J Psychiatry 146:1131–1141, 1989.

3. Crowley TJ, Riggs PD: Adolescent substance use disorder with conduct disorder, and comorbid conditions. In Adolescent Drug Abuse: Clinical Assessment and Therapeutic Interventions. NIDA. Research Monograph Series, 1995.

4. Kaminer Y: Adolescent Substance Abuse. A Comprehensive Guide to Theory and Practice. New York, Plenum, 1994.

5. Lewis DO: Conduct disorder. In Lewis M (ed): Child and Adolescent Psychiatry: A Comprehensive Textbook. Baltimore, Williams & Wilkins, 1991.

6. Moffitt TE: The neuropsychology of conduct disorder. Dev Psychopathol 5:135–151, 1993.

7. Moffitt TE: Adolescence—limited and life-course-persistent antisocial behavior: A developmental taxonomy. Psychol Rev 100:674–701, 1993.

8. Offord DR, Bennett KJ: Conduct disorder: Long-term outcomes and intervention effectiveness. J Am Acad Child Adolesc Psychiatry 33:1994.

9. Riggs PD, Baker S, Mikulich SK, et al: Depression in substance-dependent delinquents. J Am Acad Child Adolesc Psychiatry 34:1995.

10. Robins LN, Regier DA (eds): Psychiatric Disorders in America. The Epidemiologic Catchment Area Study. New York, Macmillan, 1991.

11. Zubieta JK, Alessi NE: Is there a role of serotonin in the disruptive behavior disorders? A literature review. J Child Adolesc Psychopharm 3:1993.

57. OBSESSIVE COMPULSIVE DISORDER IN CHILDREN AND ADOLESCENTS

Frederick B. Hebert, M.D.

1. Define obsessive compulsive disorder.

Obsessive compulsive disorder (OCD) was formerly thought to be rare and to have a poor prognosis. It is now known to be one of the most treatable of psychiatric disorders. OCD is a lifelong condition that waxes and wanes and is often complicated by depression and anxiety. Defined as a type of anxiety disorder, the symptoms of OCD consist of obsessions or compulsions and sometimes both.

2. What are obsessions?

Obsessions are demonstrated by recurrent and persistent ideas, thoughts, impulses or images that are felt as intrusive and recognized as senseless. The person attempts to ignore, suppress, or neutralize the obsessions with some other thought or action. The obsessions are recognized as the product of the person's own mind rather than imposed from without (except perhaps in children). If another disorder is present, the content is not related (i.e., the obsession is not about guilt or depression). Typical themes are aggression, fear of contamination, doubting, or ordering of objects.

3. What kinds of behavior demonstrate compulsions?

Compulsions consist of repetitive, purposeful, and intentional behaviors performed in response to an obsession or according to certain rules in a stereotyped fashion. The behavior is designed to neutralize or prevent discomfort or some dreaded event; however, the activity is not connected in a realistic way or is clearly excessive. The person recognizes that the behavior is excessive or unreasonable (children may not). Common compulsions are hand-washing, checking, counting, hoarding, or touching performed in a rigid manner.

4. Since almost everyone has a few obsessions or compulsions, does everyone have OCD?

No. The obsessions or compulsions must cause marked distress and take more than 1 hour/day or significantly interfere with occupational or social functioning to meet DSM IV criteria for diagnosis.

5. How often does OCD occur? What is the prognosis?

OCD occurs frequently in most ethnic groups with a 2.5% prevalence rate. The onset is in childhood in 33–50% of the cases, with an average onset at age 15. Onset over age 40 is rare. In most cases the onset is gradual or follows some trivial precipitant. The family may have a scrupulous religious background; the disorder is recognized among all major religions and is known as scrupulosity. Girls are actually afflicted more frequently, but boys have an earlier onset. In families with one affected member, 20% of relatives meet OCD criteria and another 20% meet criteria for compulsive personality disorder. A patient's prognosis worsens with concurrent cluster A personality traits (schizoid, schizotypal, paranoid), but a patient's prognosis is not worsened with compulsive personality or passive traits.

As an example, an 11-year-old boy became depressed. When he gradually became obsessed with the idea that his mother would be harmed and simultaneously had suicidal thoughts, he was hospitalized. On the ward, he would pace around the perimeter of the day room. At each corner, he would stop for a ritual of hand wringing. This ritual decreased when it was interrupted by staff, and an antidepressant was started. Although one of his siblings also suffered from obsessive thoughts, the mother was quite organized in her work and suffered no disabling rituals.

6. What's the cause of OCD?

The underlying mechanism causing OCD is unknown. Recent biologic, clinical, radiologic, and physiologic evidence of problems in the caudate nucleus or connections from the caudate to pre-frontal area of the brain point to an ultimate organic or biologic cause. Self-grooming problems in dogs, particularly canine acral lick disorder, suggest overstimulation of parallel CNS pathways from a disturbed serotonin balance. Canine acral lick dermatitis (ALD) is helped by use of selective serotonin reuptake inhibitors (e.g., fluoxetine).

7. What other disorders are frequently associated with OCD?

Depression is frequently associated with OCD; a significant number of children with OCD have a major depression. As many as one-half have suffered from some other anxiety disorder; 20% have tics, and 5% have Tourette's disorder, which is otherwise rare among the general population.

8. How does OCD present to other health care practitioners?

OCD is often initially seen by physicians other than psychiatrists, such as family practitioners, pediatricians, and dermatologists. Pediatricians see parents exhausted by the stress of the cleaning or checking rituals of their children. Sometimes a child will use an entire roll of toilet paper for a single bowel movement. If the child cannot attend school or is repeatedly late to school, truancy officials may make the first intervention. Family practitioners or dermatologists may see OCD presenting as nonspecific dermatitis. In children and adolescents OCD often takes the form of multiple daily showers, an otherwise uncommon behavior in this age group. Children are sometimes noticed when they erase and reerase until they have worn holes in their school papers. Pediatric neurologists may see OCD when consulting for children with repetitive movements after a streptococcal infection. Sydenham's chorea may thus present as a compulsion in the form of repetitive leg movements. Such patients often have radiologic evidence of dysfunction. Surgeons frequently are asked by patients with OCD to perform cosmetic surgery for minimal disfigurement; this obsessive demand for bodily perfection is especially seen in adolescent performing artists. Dentists may be the first to see children with OCD when they present with bleeding gums secondary to repetitive brushing.

9. What is the differential diagnosis of OCD?

In generalized anxiety disorder, the patient has anxiety must of the time, but it is not focused on one area. In specific phobias the patient is symptom-free except from a particular stimulus that causes anxiety. In OCD, the patient seems focused on the symptom, yet the patient is also upset by it. Adolescents with OCD know their symptoms come from their own mind. Children with OCD may not know that their symptoms are the product of their own thinking, making the diagnosis more difficult. It is necessary to rely instead on a history of time-consuming rituals from the parents. Patients with OCD are generally not considered psychotic. Major depressive episodes may present with concurrent obsessional thinking; however, the mood disturbance dominates the clinical picture with obsessing occurring later and remitting with successful treatment of depression.

10. What are the so-called OCD spectrum disorders?

Several disorders that may be related to OCD are called spectrum disorders. Compulsive hair pulling or trichotillomania, urinary and bowel obsessions, and body dysmorphias (obsessive concern that one part of the body is misshapen) are most likely variants of OCD and are referred to as spectrum disorders. Ritualistic vomiting associated with bulimia is under active debate as a variant, because the vomiting often continues without significant weight loss or obvious personal gain. All of these disorders may have their onset in childhood or adolescence.

11. Are there different types of OCD?

OCD comes in several varieties. Most patients (up to 85%) are cleaners at some time in their illness. Some are checkers, endlessly testing whether they have shut doors or turned off a switch.

Other children classify baseball cards in endless ways or count ceiling tiles over and over. Some patients must have a special symmetry, such as lining up pencils, colored crayons, or shoes; others balance everything that they do or say, such as reading until the number of pages is divisible by two. Far less commonly, the patient cannot enter a doorway without ritual or taps out a rhythm on a fence while repeatedly walking a certain route. A common presentation in children is to ask questions over and over. Adolescents who need to have the last word may have an obsessive fear that things will not be evened out if they do not.

12. What are the nonmedication treatments?
OCD is particularly interesting among psychiatric disorders, because research indicates an overall low response to either placebo or psychotherapy. In behavior therapy successes and failures have been noted. Systematic desensitization techniques (gradual increase in the presentation of a feared stimulus) were tried first, but failed. Other behavioral techniques also have been tried; they reduce anxiety but not obsessions. Another form of behavior therapy, exposure in vivo (stimulus exposure), has been known to be effective for some time. This technique requires the patient to come in contact with the obsessive stimulus, such as door handles or toilet seats. Response prevention (interrupting or interfering with the patient's response after the obsessive stimulus) keeps the patient from performing the usual cleaning ritual. Several studies, both controlled and uncontrolled, have demonstrated 70–80% rates of effectiveness. Individuals who receive both imagined (fantasied) and actual exposure tend to maintain their gains more successfully over time. Patients with prolonged stimulus exposure do better than those with less exposure, but in response prevention, there were no differences between patients who received 24-hour supervision and patients with minimal supervision. A cotherapist, including a family member, who works with the practitioner has improved results. One author found that about 60% of patients could be treated overall as outpatients with assigned homework, which stressed an opportunity to learn new strategies. He also found that most of the treatment needed to be carried out in the patient's immediate environment where the rituals take place. However, up to 25% of patients drop out of behavior therapy, and many refuse to follow through with the treatment. The 75% success rate is obtained in the 75% of patients who complete treatment–for an overall response rate of 50%. Persistent reductions in compulsive rituals over time have been seen most often with behavior therapy, but it is less effective with obsessions, because it is impossible to deal with them in vivo. For such patients, particularly those with severe obsessions, medications are indicated.

13. What medications should be used?
Antianxiety agents, neuroleptics, and antidepressants have been tried for patients with obsessional thoughts. Infrequently patients respond to imipramine or clonidine, a medication first found useful in Tourette's syndrome. Monoamine oxidase inhibitors (MAOIs) have been noted to reduce OCD behavior in patients who also had panic attacks. Clomipramine was first noted to reduce obsessions in 1968 in a European study. Many studies, including several double-blind comparisons with other medications, have substantiated earlier results. In one early study combining clomipramine and behavior therapy, medication improved depression, anxiety, social adjustment, and rituals as well as compliance with behavior therapy. In other studies, clomipramine in lower doses reduced obsessive thoughts, but lower doses had no effect on rituals. Clomipramine has a typical tricyclic antidepressant side-effect profile; dry mouth, constipation, and tremor are frequent. Less often, dizziness, sedation, headache, and fatigue occur. Sometimes sweating, weight increase, and ejaculation failure are seen. All side effects are reported less frequently by children and adolescents, so clomipramine remains the drug of choice.

14. All of the medications are antidepressants. Does the patient have to be depressed?
No. The antiobsessive effect is independent of antidepressant effect and is usually maintained with treatment. Most studies do report no correlation with serum levels, but a dose of clomipramine over 100 mg/day is usually needed. Onset of action is in 2–4 weeks with final improvement over 8–10 weeks. The dose is up to 200 mg/day or 3 mg/kg for children or adolescents.

Overall, symptoms are reduced by 70%. Less than 10% of children can be expected to drop out of treatment, but children and adolescents include a greater number of placebo responders; thus children actually may not respond as well as adults. Patients with OCD and an avoidant style or sexual themes in their obsessions have poorer response. The antiobsessional action of clomipramine has been related to its inhibition of serotonin reuptake, and the selective serotonin reuptake inhibitors (SSRIs) have been most successful in OCD. In addition to clomipramine, fluoxetine and fluvoxamine have demonstrated efficacy in children and adolescents with OCD and are available in the U.S. as Anafranil, Prozac, and Luvox, respectively.

15. What if the patient does not respond in 8–10 weeks?

If behavior therapy and clomipramine are not effective, augmentation of the medication with lithium, fenfluramine, or buspirone may be effective. If side effects limit use of clomipramine, fluoxetine may be administered after tapering clomipramine over 1 week. Fluoxetine is long-acting and frequently competes with other plasma bound medications for receptor sites; thus care must be taken if other drugs are given. Fluoxetine alone often works well; only 16% of patients report insomnia or anxiety. Stomachaches are frequent if the drug is taken without food. It is best not to start with fluoxetine, because treatment failure may require a drug-free period of up to 5 weeks. Sertraline has a shorter duration of action and may interact less with drugs than fluoxetine because of its cytochrome P-450 metabolic pathways. Patients with tics and OCD often need an additional neuroleptic or clonidine for sustained response. Neuroleptics may increase the blood levels of clomipramine significantly as does the concomitant use of cimetidine (Tagamet). All SSRIs have sexual side effects, of which anorgasmia is the most common but in practice they are not reported by children or adolescents. Cyproheptadine (Periactin), 4–8 mg, may be taken 3 hours before sex to avoid anorgasmia.

16. Do all patients with OCD need hospitalization?

Overall treatment of OCD has progressed to the point that usually it can be accomplished on an outpatient basis with a combination of behavior therapy and medication.

BIBLIOGRAPHY

1. Flament MF, et al: Obsessive compulsive disorder in adolescence: An epidemiological study. J Am Acad Child Adolescent Psychiatry 27:764–771, 1988.
2. Geller DA, et al: Similarities in response to fluoxetine in the treatment of children and adolescents with obsessive-compulsive disorder. J Am Acad Child Adolescent Psychiatry 34:36–44, 1995.
3. Insel TR, Akiskal HS: Obsessive-compulsive disorder with psychotic features: A phenomenologic analysis. Am J Psychiatry 143:1527–1533, 1986.
4. Jenike MA, et al: Obsessive-compulsive disorder: A double-blind, placebo-controlled trial of clomipramine in 27 patients. Am J Psychiatry 146:1328–1330, 1989.
5. Kirk JW: Behavioral treatment of obsessional-compulsive patients in routine clinical practice. Behav Res Ther 21:57–62, 1983.
6. Marks I, O'Sullivan J: Drugs and psychological treatment for agoraphobia/panic and obsessive-compulsive disorders: A review. Br J Psychiatry 153:650–658, 1988.
7. Perse T: OCD: A treatment review. J Clin Psychiatry 49:48–55, 1988.
8. Reynynghe deVoxrie VG: Anafranil in obsession. Acta Neurol Belg 68:787–792, 1968.
9. Rapoport JL: The Boy Who Couldn't Stop Washing. New York, Plume, 1989.
10. Rasmussen SA: Obsessive compulsive disorder in dermatologic practice. J Am Acad Dermatol 13:965–967, 1985.
11. Zak JP, et al: The potential role of serotonin reuptake inhibitors in the treatment of obsessive compulsive disorder. J Clin Psychiatry 49(Suppl):23–29, 1988.

58. ENCOPRESIS AND ENURESIS

Benjamin P. Green, M.D.

ENCOPRESIS

1. Define encopresis. How common is it?

As defined by the Diagnostic and Statistical Manual–IV (DSM–IV), encopresis is the repeated involuntary or intentional passage of feces into inappropriate places, such as into clothing or onto the floor, at a frequency of at least monthly for a duration of 3 or more months. To qualify for this diagnosis, the patient must be at least 4 years old (corrected for mental and developmental age), and the condition must not be due to a medication (e.g., laxative) or caused by a general medical (somatic) condition other than constipation.

Although encopresis may occur at any age—especially among individuals with severe organic brain disease—it is primarily an affliction of childhood. Approximately 15% of 8 year olds and 0.8% of 11-year-olds suffer from this disorder; the male:female ratio is 3:1. Although historically much has been made of the distinction between primary encopresis (in which bowel continence has never been achieved) and secondary encopresis (in which incontinence has been established but then lost), the most useful clinical subtyping is organized around the presence or absence of constipation with overflow incontinence. Constipated or retentive encopresis is usually associated with small, soft, poorly formed stools that leak out both day and night. When constipation is absent, the stools tend to be large, well-formed and intermittently deposited, often in particularly offensive places. The nonretentive type is more likely associated with oppositional and defiant behavior.

2. Which causes encopresis—psyche or soma?

Throughout the psychiatric literature subsequent to Freud, much has been written about anality and encopresis. A good deal of theorizing focused on psychosexual arrests and deviations, instinctual forces, superego prohibitions, and even the "anal character," whose traits included punctuality, an obsessive insistence on orderliness, stinginess, and stubbornness. This body of work brilliantly illuminated one facet of human nature, but its clinical utility has been somewhat marginalized by subsequent empirical research and the evolution of more practical treatments.

Over the past several decades, writings from the field of behavioral pediatrics have increasingly defined thinking about encopresis. This is not to say that psychosocial variables are not significant risk factors; children ranked by parents' questionnaire in the top decile for behavioral problems are five times more likely to soil. The direction of causality—if any—between encopresis and emotional/behavioral problems is less certain, however (e.g., one may soil because of angry obstinacy, or one may become angry and defiant because of bowel failure and the consequent interpersonal conflicts and social rejection).

By contrast, the temporal primacy of physiologic variables is all but undeniable in many cases. Infantile "early colonic inertia" and an imperforate or stenotic anus and/or rectum strongly predispose a child toward later fecal difficulties. Rather than to assert causality per se, however, it is more rigorously correct to assess the relative etiologic weighting of the various predisposing, potentiating, precipitating, and perpetuating factors.

The muscular ability to defecate a rectal balloon (an approach commonly used in experiments to quantify rectal mobility) evaluates one of the primary somatic, constitutional aspects of encopresis. It has been used to predict both the presence of encopresis and the likely response to treatment. In one study, 43% of encopretic boys, compared with 10% of controls, could not extrude a distal rectal balloon because of tightening of the muscles near the anal canal. Furthermore, failing at balloon defecation lowered the probability of treatment success from 63% to 15%.

Ultimately, most authorities conclude that causality is best explained in terms of both psyche and soma. The most elegant pathogenic models are interactive, contemplating the ways in which constitutional and acquired physiologic factors influence outcome in conjunction with individual and familial psychosocial variables. One conceptualization describes the interaction in terms of developmental stages:

	Physiologic Factors	**Psychosocial Factors**
1. Infancy and toddler (0–2 years)	Simple constipation Early colonic inertia Congenital anorectal problems Other anorectal condition	Parental overreaction Overzealous anal manipulations
2. Early childhood (3–5 years)	Painful or difficult defecation	Idiosyncratic toilet fears Psychosocial stresses during training period Coercive or extremely permissive toilet training
3. Early school years (6–11 years)	Prolonged or acute gastro-enteritis Food intolerance, lactose deficiency	Attention deficit/task impersis-tence Frenetic life style Psychosocial stresses Avoidance of school bathrooms

For the sake of completeness, several rare pediatric conditions that can—in and of them-selves—cause colonic encopresis should be mentioned: Hirschsprung's disease (and the still con-troversial variant known as ultrashort segment Hirschsprung's), hypothyroidism, spinal cord lesions, Crohn's disease, malnutrition, and disorders of voluntary muscle function, such as amy-otonia congenita, infectious polyneuritis, and cerebral palsy.

3. What data should a competent evaluation include?
Resources permitting, a full pediatric and psychiatric evaluation should be undertaken.

The **history of present illness** should begin with the child's and then the parents' description of the problem and their explanations of causality. Often, surprising issues are raised that may help to focus and prioritize the treatment plan.

A **developmental history** should be taken of the child's bowel habits and the environment's response to same over time. Particular attention should be paid to the timing, characteristics, and outcome of initial toilet training efforts and to subsequent epochal events, such as relapses, exac-erbations, or progressions. For each significant period, data should include biomedical, social/contextual, and individual psychological factors.

Biomedical questions should cover the frequency, chronology, volume, viscosity, and cal-iber of stooling as well as the presence or absence of defecatory pain.

Social/contextual data should include the health and stresses of the caretakers, marriage and family, parental history for elimination disorders, expectations of the child, attempts at teach-ing continence, response to successes and failures, utilization of help (from both professional and lay sources), and the variability of caretakers' behaviors across different settings (e.g., grandpar-ents, day care providers, school staff).

Individual psychological evaluation should emphasize the assessment of global develop-mental projectory, acquisition of adaptive intelligence, quality of relatedness generally and with primary caretakers specifically, negativism, oppositionality, dependence and counterdependence, inattention, forgetfulness, self-monitoring, depression, guilt, peer relationships, and self-esteem.

While taking the history of present illness and developmental history, the clinician should observe carefully the interaction between child and caretakers with regard to empathy, ability to discuss difficult subjects openly, degree of agreement regarding the encopresis, conflict resolu-tion skills, interdependence, intimacy, demoralization, anger, shame, guilt, and frank potential for violence and abuse.

The **physical exam** should evaluate the child's general health, thyroid, lower limb neurologic status, abdomen, and the perianal area to evaluate, respectively, for (the wasting of) Hirschsprung's disease, hypothyroidism, neuromuscular disorders, retained stool, and perianal fissures, sores, or group A streptococcal cellulitis. Impactions may not be detected by a rectal exam; experienced practitioners know that the midline suprapubic area is the most frequent location of retained stools.

Barium enemas and manometric evaluation of sphincter function are seldom contributory, but a **plain film** of the abdomen should be ordered routinely to assess for fecal retention. Rectal or colonic biopsies should be considered only for extreme cases. Radiographic studies should be repeated after the initial bowel clean-out, because 30% of the disimpacted patients once again will be found to have retained stools.

4. When and how should toilet training be carried out?

Many health care professionals have a minimal understanding of optimal toilet training. This knowledge is critical for both prevention and treatment of disorders of elimination. Developmentally, toilet training is anything but trivial. Successful training is a source of pride and of a growing sense of developmental mastery for both child and family. Conversely, problems in this area may result in intense conflicts, low self-esteem, and even violence; in one study, toilet training failure was the second most common precipitant of fatal child abuse.

Crosscultural studies demonstrate that the ability for self-initiated toileting can be consolidated by 10½ months of age! The timing of training is primarily influenced by social values and assumptions. Surveys in the United States, for instance, document that in 1947, 95% of children had completed toilet training by 33 months of age, whereas by 1975 this figure had fallen to 58%. A child who can crawl or walk is probably neurologically ready for training. The usual recommendations for parents include the following:

1. Children are usually ready for toilet training between 18 and 24 months (corrected for mental age). Signs of readiness include verbal awareness of "poop" and "pee," understanding the "potty chair" and how its use can prevent being wet or soiled, expressed preference for being dry (which should be encouraged by the parents), and a demonstrated ability to postpone elimination.

2. The parental approach should be characterized by praise, patience, and encouragement. Punishment and pressure should be avoided. Parents are teaching a skill, not attempting to subjugate an adversary.

3. Helpful equipment includes a floor-level potty chair offering good foot support, training pants, food rewards, stickers or stars, and an educational picture book to make the process more friendly and familiar.

4. The potty chair should be selected by the child and parent together and then decorated and individualized. It can be used outside the bathroom as a chair (with clothes on) during enjoyable activities (e.g., watching television) for a week or so before being used for its designated function.

5. "Practice runs" should be used to rehearse the interrupting of play activities, going to the bathroom, undressing, sitting, waiting, wiping, and redressing. Reading stories or watching television on the potty can make the process more pleasant. Such sessions should not exceed five minutes, but they should happen several times a day, especially right after meals (thus taking advantage of the gastrocolonic reflex).

6. Rewards of praise, food, stickers, stars, or even money should be given for compliance with practice runs, for successful toileting, and especially for self-initiated toileting.

It is important to assess whether the parent understands this basic approach to toilet training. If not, parental education and support should be the first order of business. Sometimes, of course, the problem may be more serious than lack of knowledge. Any child over 2½ years of age who is not continent after several months of training can be assumed to be resistant rather than undertrained. Intermittent minor underwear wetting or small fecal smears should be considered as an expected part of the learning process and not as pathological resistance unless the frequency or degree is extreme.

Entrenched power struggles over toileting may occur. Parental behaviors that exacerbate such a conflict include repeated nagging, long periods of enforced toilet sitting, use of shame-inducing techniques, excessive physical punishment, and inappropriate use of enemas and/or digital disimpaction. Suggestive behaviors on the part of the child may involve daytime incontinence, refusal to sit on the toilet, wetting and soiling immediately after enforced toilet sitting, and apparent indifference to the problem. When such an impasse is detected, referral should be made to a mental health professional or to a pediatrician specializing in behavior disorders.

5. When and how should pharmacologic treatments be used?

Despite a few anecdotal reports of successful treatment with imipramine, pharmacotherapeutic agents of established efficacy include only enemas, laxatives, and stool softeners. Before any of these are used, however, it is imperative that nonretentive soiling be distinguished from retentive, constipated soiling; the treatment of the former is behavioral, not chemical.

The use of **enemas** to treat retentive encopresis carries a certain degree of psychological stress, but it is absolutely necessary to ensure initial bowel emptying. Fleet's hyperphosphate enemas should be used, 1 ounce for every 20 pounds of body weight, up to a maximal dose of 4 ounces. A second dose should be given 1 hour later. An optional third enema may be administered after another 12–24 hours if continued soiling or persistent abdominal mass suggests incomplete evacuation. Ultimate treatment failure is inevitable unless the fecal impaction is cleared from the onset. Once this is accomplished, however, subsequent enemas should be unnecessary (unless severe reimpaction occurs) and may even be countertherapeutic. It is wise to have the child drink 1–2 glasses of water before an enema to minimize dehydration.

Once the impaction has been treated, relapse can usually be prevented with **stool softeners.** Mineral oil is most commonly used; it tastes best when refrigerated and chased by the fruit juice of choice. A vitamin pill should be given each day that mineral oil is used to prevent nutritional leeching. The alternatives to plain mineral oil are the better tasting emulsified oils such as Retrogalas, plain Agoral, Metamucil, and Kondremul. Because of the risk of aspiration and pulmonary complications, none of these oils should be given to children who have gastrointestinal reflex vomiting or who are not yet walking.

If stool softeners prove inadequate in promoting daily evacuations, **laxatives** may be used to stimulate colonic motility. Laxatives can be prescribed with relative impunity; "laxative dependence" is an unfounded concern. Recommended products include Senokot, Fletcher's Castoria, Milk of Magnesia, Haley's M-O, and Ducolax.

Definitive treatment in all but the mildest cases requires a minimum of 6 months. The relapsing of symptoms and the lapsing of therapeutic compliance are more the rule than the exception; persistent, gentle support and redirection from the physician are usually necessary.

6. Should the child be reminded to toilet?

Normal children and adults perceive when their rectum is full, but chronic constipation causes stretching and desensitization of the lower gastrointestinal tract. Psychological reluctance and constitutional inattention also may contribute to the child's failure to initiate trips to the bathroom. It is therefore recommended that the child be gently reminded to adhere to scheduled sittings on the toilet after breakfast and dinner either until a bowel movement has occurred or until 10 minutes have expired. To take full advantage of the gastrocolic reflex, 5–30 minutes after eating is optimal. Bending forward while sitting, relaxing the anus and buttocks, and pushing gently with the abdomen may help. For shorter children, a foot stool is recommended to enhance pushing leverage and to provide a greater sense of security. If recurrent soiling occurs (indicating a full rectum) or if the child complains of stomachache, cramping, or feeling blocked up, a more intensive program of sitting on the toilet is indicated. On weekends and after school, 10 minutes of every hour should be dedicated to sitting on the toilet until a large bowel movement has been produced.

Individuals in the child's other significant environments (e.g., school, day care, family relatives) should be advised to allow unfettered access to bathrooms and to offer gentle reminders when the child evinces flatulence, abdominal cramping, or frank soiling. Lectures, harsh criticism, and shame induction should be avoided.

7. How should one respond to soiling?

Evidence (either olfactory or visual) of soiling should be met with an immediate, firm but restrained request that the child clean him- or herself and put on fresh clothing. Spare undergarments should be available at school or at day care. The child should be involved in scraping off (e.g., with a spatula or spoon) solid waste and then washing the soiled underwear in the toilet. A bucket of water with bleach and a lid can be left for this purpose in the bathroom. This procedure reinforces the message that soiling is not catastrophic but neither is it to be tolerated.

8. Is diet important?

Absolutely. Milk products and cooked carrots tend to be constipating, whereas fruits and vegetables—especially raw ones—promote healthy defecation. Particularly recommended are figs, dates, raisins, peaches, pears, apricots, celery, cabbage, broccoli, cauliflower, peas, and beans. The cereal food groups also provide much fiber, including popcorn, nuts, bran flakes, bran muffins, shredded wheat, oatmeal, brown rice, and whole wheat bread. Copious consumption of water and fruit juices also should be encouraged, although—as with all of these items—in a manner gentle enough to avoid conflict.

ENURESIS

9. Define enuresis.

DSM–IV defines enuresis as the intentional or involuntary voiding of urine into clothes or any other inappropriate place by a child at least 5 years old (corrected for mental and developmental age). The condition cannot be caused by a substance (e.g., a diuretic) or by a medical condition (epilepsy), and the frequency must equal or exceed 2 times/week for a duration of at least 3 consecutive months. Finally—as with any disorder of clinical significance—the symptoms must result in significant subjective distress and/or dysfunction (e.g., social failures). Subtypes include nocturnal, diurnal, and combined. Another distinction is primary vs. secondary enuresis. Primary enuresis denotes life-long incontinence, whereas in secondary enuresis continence was achieved for at least 1 year but then lost. Among school-age children primary and secondary enuresis are roughly equal, but three times as many children have nocturnal rather than diurnal enuresis. Daytime and secondary enuresis are more likely to be related to emotional and behavioral problems and times of psychosocial stress; ages 5–7 and the onset of adolescence are developmental periods at highest risk for these subtypes. The total incidence of enuresis by age is roughly as follows:

Age	Percentage of the Population
3	40
4	30
5	20
8	7
12	3
18	1

10. What is known about the cause of enuresis?

As with encopresis, causality is best explained by simultaneous consideration of both psychosocial and physiologic factors and their interactions. Enuretic children appear to suffer from developmental delays across multiple domains; they tend to have small bladders, immature bone-age scores, learning disabilities, and disturbances of behavior. The presence of enuresis doubles the risk for an additional psychiatric diagnosis, although the association is not specific to any particular concurrent disorder. The numerous sleep stage and sleep arousal theories are at present more suggestive than definitive. Genetic predisposition is significant; having one enuretic parent increases the life-time risk to 45%, whereas having two afflicted parents increases the likelihood to 75%. In the general population, the male:female ratio is 2:1.

Among the numerous organic causes that should be ruled out, the most important is urinary tract infections. Also to be considered are diabetes mellitus and insipidus, constipation, ectopic ureter, lower urinary tract obstruction, neurogenic bladder, bladder calculi (or other foreign bodies), epilepsy, and sleep apnea due to enlarged adenoids. However, in the absence of such phenomena as a weak or dribbly urinary stream, excessive urine production, or manifestations of convulsive diathesis, a simple urinalysis is the only laboratory evaluation recommended to augment the routine history and physical exam. More intrusive studies (e.g., intravenous pyelography) tend to be expensive, traumatizing, and noncontributory.

11. How similar to encopresis is enuresis?
Very similar. To avoid redundancy, the reader is referred to the section about encopresis for discussion of the psychosocial factors to be assessed in an evaluation, the psyche-soma controversy, toilet training procedures, and behavioral management. Apart from the obvious differences in physiologic factors, the major phenomenologic difference between the two disorders of elimination is the propensity of enuresis to be nocturnal. The behavioral management of diurnal enuresis is virtually identical with that described for encopresis. The pharmacologic treatments of enuresis—as one would expect—are also quite different.

12. What are the behavioral treatments for nocturnal enuresis?
The fundamental problem causing nocturnal enuresis is the combination of a small bladder and an inadequate capacity for self-arousal during sleep. Either or both traits can be heritable.

Bladder capacity is measured by asking the child to try on three separate occasions to hold his or her urine for as long as possible and then to void into a container. The maximal quantity should equal in ounces a child's age; a smaller quantity suggests small bladder size. In such cases it may well help to prescribe bladder-stretching exercises, which encourage the child to hold his or her urine for as long as possible during the day. Whenever the urge to void is felt, self-distracting techniques should be used in an effort to override the bladder spasms for a minimum of 10 seconds. Physiologically, this exercise may increase the functional bladder capacity while psychologically the child is learning to resist and postpone the first urge to urinate. Parents are encouraged to challenge the child playfully to try to break the record for maximal single-void volumes.

Several strategies also may be used to address the child's **inability to self-awaken** in response to bladder fullness. First, fluid intake should be gently discouraged for the 2 hours prior to bedtime; however, heated arguments over a few swallows are unwarranted. Secondly, the bladder must be emptied just before the child goes to sleep. The majority of nocturnal urine is produced in the first third of the night. One implication of this fact is that parents who stay up several hours later than their child may routinely wake the child for a second voiding just before their own bedtime. Even small bladders may then be adequate to contain the urine produced during the remainder of the night. If this technique is used, it should be carefully discussed with the child in advance and the child's cooperation should be rewarded with praise, stickers, stars (put on a chart or calendar), or even small food treats or toys (to avoid over-stimulating the child, these rewards should be given the next morning). Optimally, the child should learn to self-awaken. An alarm clock can be set for 3 hours after bedtime; in many ways, this approach is preferable because it encourages more autonomous functioning.

Another helpful approach focuses on **teaching the child to attend and respond** to nocturnal bladder sensations. The child and parent(s) practice three times each night before bedtime the sequence of lying down, closing eyes, pretending to perceive bladder fullness in the middle of the night, feeling the ache, getting up, running to the bathroom, urinating, and then returning to bed. This sequence should be rehearsed physically as if one were practicing for the theater. It is more realistic if the child voids a small amount during each repetition before finally emptying his or her bladder completely before being tucked in. Appealing to the child's developmentally appropriate magical thinking, one can personify the bladder and describe it as trying to wake up the child "before it's too late." Another helpful metaphor is to suggest that the child is a fireman or firewoman who needs to respond to the alarm and get up in time to put out the fire with their urinary stream. Both compliance with practicing and nocturnal successes should be rewarded. Also, putting a nightlight or flashlight in the child's room and/or in the bathroom may add a measure of safety and control.

13. When and how should a nocturnal alarm be used?

Enuresis alarms should be used when the simpler behavioral techniques have been unsuccessful and when the child is sufficiently motivated and mature to cooperate. This approach tends to work best when the child is at least 8 years of age and when the prescribing physician is comfortable with and knowledgeable about the treatment. Caveats notwithstanding, it is the opinion of many experts that nocturnal alarms are the most definitive therapy for nocturnal enuresis. Compared with imipramine treatment, the use of enuresis alarms is associated both with a higher cure rate (70% vs. 60%) and a dramatically lower relapse rate (10–15% vs. 50–100%); it is therefore curious that less than 5% of physicians recommend nocturnal alarms. The newer alarms are lightweight, comfortable to wear, inexpensive, and widely available. (If local pharmacies do not stock them, the Nyton Alarm can be ordered from Nyton Medical Products, 2424 South 900 West, Salt Lake City, UT 84119, or the Nite Train'r Alarm can be ordered from Koregon Enterprises, 9735 SW Sunshine Court, Beaverton, OR 97005.)

These alarms fit into or clip onto underwear and generally do not impede sleep. Parents and children should be encouraged to experiment with the alarm before putting it into use; it is important to demonstrate that a few drops of fluid result in an auditory signal but not—as some may imagine—any form of shock or pain. The child should be encouraged to feel ownership for both the alarm and the treatment program. Again, practicing before sleep helps to make the requisite response to the alarm more automatic. The child can rehearse by setting off the alarm with a few drops of water, getting up, voiding, putting on dry underwear, resetting the alarm, and returning to bed. The goal of awakening before wetting should be underscored; it can become a game to "beat the buzzer." Parents should be told to wait several seconds after the alarm has begun before trying to awake their child (e.g., by stroking the face with a cold washcloth) and to let the child turn off the alarm. The child's participation should be maximized. The alarm should be used until a month has elapsed without incontinence—usually after 2–3 months of treatment. Relapses, if they occur, usually respond to a few additional months of the program.

14. What are the pharmacologic treatments for enuresis?

If the more benign nonpharmacologic methods have failed, imipramine and desmopressin (DDAVP) should be considered.

Several dozen studies since 1960 have demonstrated the efficacy of **imipramine** as a treatment for enuresis. The initial starting dose is 25 mg/day; low-dose responders should not be overmedicated. If necessary, the dosage should be increased at a rate of 25 mg/week until therapeutic success is realized, adverse side effects (e.g., anticholinergic symptoms) become intolerable, or the maximal daily recommended dose of 5 mg/kg of body weight is reached. The usual therapeutic daily dose is 75–125 mg. For children who wet early in the night, the total dose may be divided into a midafternoon dose and another dose 1 hour before bedtime; for children with other enuretic patterns, the entire dose should be given 1 hour before sleep. An electrocardiogram (EKG) should be obtained during the baseline period and for every dosage increase over 3.5 mg/kg of body weight. Although various EKG parameters may be monitored, the primary concern is that the quinidinelike effect of imipramine will result in cardiac dysrhythmia if the corrected (for heart rate) QT duration (i.e., the QTc) exceeds 450 ms. Several studies suggest that successful treatment is most likely when the combined imipramine plus desipramine serum level is at least 80 ng/ml. Some children seem to respond transiently to imipramine (e.g., for 2–3 weeks) but then demonstrate tolerance to each successive dosage increase up to and including the maximal recommended daily dose. As many as 60% of enuretic children are successfully treated with imipramine; however, the relapse rate is 50–100% once the medicine is discontinued. Imipramine has a rather narrow therapeutic index; numerous pediatric tragedies have resulted from accidental tricyclic overdoses, many related to lack of precaution regarding medication storage.

Desmopressin is a more recent addition to the therapeutic armamentarium. Supplied as a nasal spray, DDAVP has efficacy and relapse rates similar to imipramine without the concomitant unpleasant side effects and the risk of cardiac conduction delays. Treatment with DDAVP, however, costs 3–6 dollars/night.

Both medicines have their pros and cons. Some clinicians believe that successful treatment (e.g., for 3 months) results in permanent cures at rates greater than one would expect from spontaneous remission alone. Others point to the lack of empiric support for this claim. Temporary use of either medicine—e.g., for summer camp or overnight stays with a friend—are much less controversial and may well be a real boon to a child's social life. For a number of patients, the risks and costs of these medicines given continuously may be more than offset by the psychosocial benefits; in such cases, drug tapering every 3 months should be scheduled to detect as soon as possible maturationally driven remissions.

15. How should one respond to bed wetting?

1. The child should be encouraged to try to stop the urinary flow as soon as he or she realizes that wetting has begun. At this juncture, the child should hasten to the toilet to eliminate whatever urine remains.

2. The child should change into dry nightclothes and place a dry towel over the wet part of the bed; to encourage the child's independence, clean pajamas and a towel should be laid out the night before on a chair near the bed.

3. In the morning the child should wash him- or herself and the pajamas.

4. As with soiling, pains should be taken to avoid criticism, humiliation, or punishment by parents or siblings. Support and encouragement for attaining developmental mastery minimize psychological trauma and accelerate the learning process.

A few more practical recommendations may help to reduce the family's aggravation and frustration. Extrathick underwear may be provided for nighttime use. Sheets and bedding may be protected with a towel placed under the child's buttocks and a plastic mattress cover. Sheets may be allowed to air dry and then laundered twice weekly. One also may remind the parents that the problem is esthetic, not sanitary (i.e., urine is sterile). To discourage infantilization, diapers and plastic pants should be discontinued by age 4 years (corrected for mental age).

ACKNOWLEDGMENT

The author acknowledges the contributions of Carol Green, Janet Nakata, and Bart Schmitt.

BIBLIOGRAPHY

1. Aladjem M, Wohl R, Boichis H, et al: Desmopressin in nocturnal enuresis. Arch Dis Child 57:137–140, 1982.
2. Bemporad JR, Hallowell E: Advances in the treatment of disorders of elimination. In Noshpitz JD, Call JD, Cohen RL, et al (eds): Basic Handbook of Child Psychiatry, vol. 5. New York, Basic Books, 1987, pp 479–483.
3. Fergusson DM, Horwood LJ, Shannon FT: Factors related to the age of attainment of nocturnal bladder control: An 8-year longitudinal study. Pediatrics 78:884–890, 1986.
4. Foxman B, Valdez RB, Brook RH: Childhood enuresis: Prevalence, perceived impact and prescribed treatments. Pediatrics 77:482–487, 1986.
5. Kaplan SL, Breit M, Gauthier B, et al: A comparison of three nocturnal enuresis treatment methods. J Am Acad Child Adolesc Psychiatry 28:282–286, 1989.
6. Levine MD, Bakow H: Children with encopresis. A study of treatment outcome. Pediatrics 58:845–852, 1976.
7. Levine MD: Encopresis: Its potentiation, evaluation and alleviation. Pediatr Clin North Am 29:315–330, 1982.
8. Nrgaard JP, Hansen JH, Wildschitz G, et al: Sleep cystometrics in children with nocturnal enuresis. J Urol 141:1156–1159, 1989.
9. Schmitt BD: Toilet training refusal: Avoid the battle and win the war. Contemp Pediatr 4(12)32–50, 1987.
10. Schmitt BD: Your Child's Health, 2nd ed. New York, Bantam Books, 1991.
11. Rapoport JL, Mikkelsen EJ, Zavadil A, et al: Childhood enuresis. II: Psychopathology, tricyclic concentration in plasma, and antienuretic effect. Arch Gen Psychiatry 37:1146–1152, 1980.
12. Watanabe H, Azuma Y: A proposal for a classification system of enuresis based on overnight simultaneous monitoring of electroencephalography and cystometry. Sleep 12:257–264, 1989.

59. ADOLESCENT DRUG ABUSE

Frederick B. Hebert, M.D., and Gordon K. Farley, M.D.

1. How common is adolescent substance abuse?

Use or abuse of alcohol and other drugs by adolescents in the United States is a common, serious, and sometimes life-threatening problem. In a study of consecutive appearances at a large city psychiatric emergency room, 35% of the adolescent admissions were for suspected or confirmed drug abuse. About one-third of eighth graders and about two-thirds of twelfth graders use alcohol. Over one-half of twelfth graders report that they drive after drinking. Over one-half of fatal car crashes involving drivers under 20 are alcohol-related. Well over one-half of twelfth graders report marijuana use. Cocaine and crack use are reported to be high among teenagers. Overall, it is estimated that 10–15% of all teenagers will develop serious problems with drug and alcohol abuse. With the frequent use of psychoactive substances by adults to change their moods and emotions, it is not surprising that substance abuse is among the most common problems of adolescents. Adults use substances to wake up in the morning, to sleep at night, to enjoy sex more, to improve their alertness, and to self-medicate their inner selves. By the time an adolescent is 15, he or she will have had thousands of experiences of seeing respected and admired adults smoking, ingesting, and perhaps even injecting psychoactive substances, both in person and in the media.

2. What are the most frequently abused drugs?

Commonly abused drugs in rough order of frequency include:

Alcohol, still the most commonly used drug by adolescents.

Marijuana, known as dope, grass, stash, hash, Mary Jane, M.J., pot, reefer.

Stimulants, including amphetamines (speed, dexedrine, bennies, white crosses), methylphenidate (Ritalin), cocaine (coke, cocoa, paste, snow, powder, crocks, quarter rock, crack), and anorectic drugs either by prescription (Preludin, Tenuate) or over the counter, such as phenylpropanolamine and pseudoephedrine.

Hallucinogens, including lysergic acid diethylamide (LSD, acid), psilocybin (magic mushroom, boomers, shrooms), ecstasy, mescaline (peyote, cactus), phencyclidine (angel dust, PCP).

Narcotic analgesics, such as morphine (morf, Miss Emma), codeine, and heroin (smack, stuff, horse, junk).

Volatile substances (inhaled), including solvents (gasoline, paint thinner, benzene, acetone), toluene (Rustoleum Clear paint, plastic and rubber cement), aerosol sprays (paint, hair spray, cooking oil), and cryogenic chilling fluids (Freon).

Sedative hypnotics, including barbiturates (reds, yellows, rainbows) and barbiturate-like drugs, such as methaqualone (soapers), even though now only illegally manufactured.

Benzodiazepines (e.g., Librium, Valium, Xanax, Halcion).

Anticholinergic drugs, such as atropine, scopolamine (scope) and some antihistamines, antiparkinsonian medications (Artane, Kemadrin).

3. What are the general concerns in treating acute intoxication with any drug?

Obviously, the major concern in the acute drug abuser is to maintain life-support systems until it is known what specific drug has been ingested. The acute treatment of intoxication or acute drug abuse is a highly specialized activity and best done in inpatient medical or psychiatric settings where medical support is readily and immediately available.

4. What makes alcohol intoxication more dangerous?

Alcohol intoxication often occurs in combination with other substances, most frequently sedative hypnotics. The symptoms vary with route of administration, amount used, specific substance, previous history of use and addiction, and period of time over which the substance has been consumed. Because alcohol is rapidly absorbed through the gastric mucosa, when one observes or hears a history of rapid change in mental status, alcohol intoxication should be suspected. Laboratory confirmation of alcohol use is easily obtained; however, behavioral symptoms correspond only roughly to blood alcohol levels. Nystagmus on extreme lateral gaze, mild dysarthria, and mild ataxia are relatively early signs. The most important part of treatment is to follow the patient carefully to avoid coma. Some adolescents have died from high alcohol blood levels when their breathing stopped; apparently, levels were high enough to block the medullary breathing centers.

5. What about hallucinogens?
Psychotomimetics include marijuana, LSD, psilocybin, and phencyclidine (PCP). These agents cause a cognitive disorder with illusions ("trails" with marijuana), frank visual hallucinations (color and shape changes with LSD), and disordered thinking (body image changes progressing to thought blocking and delirium with PCP). What is not generally known is that all hallucinogens produce anxiety, ranging from mild transient dysphoria with marijuana to anxious irritability with PCP and genuine panic with LSD (bad trips). Physical changes are few with the exception of PCP. Injected conjunctivae are seen with marijuana, and dilated but reactive pupils are seen with LSD and psilocybin. Only euphoria and physiologic changes are seen with ecstasy, the newest member of the group. PCP, however, always produces physical signs. Paresthesias in the limbs, initially or at low doses, progress to analgesias (cigarette burns are common), then muscular rigidity, myoclonus, or even convulsions and coma. When seen in the emergency department, the patient taking PCP may be mute or amnestic with catatonic posturing; ptosis and nystagmus may be the only clues to diagnosis. Lab tests are not helpful, except for urine screens for marijuana, which may be positive for several days after a single dose.

6. Is "glue sniffing" dangerous?
Solvents produce a giddy delirium that may progress to coma with prolonged inhalation. Despite newspaper reports, few youth have died from acute inhalation, but many have suffered long-term brain damage by repeated use. Usually this damage takes the form of dementia but sometimes presents as pure cerebellar degeneration. The diagnosis is suspected when a patient has a ketone breath and body odor and swollen mucous membranes but no other cold symptoms. Poverty and depression are frequently associated with solvent abuse. Initial medical treatment is supportive.

7. Why is abuse of stimulant drugs harder to treat?
Stimulants are known as "body" drugs for their ability to produce physiologic changes. Cocaine in its many forms is now the best known illicit stimulant, but even caffeine produces many symptoms if sufficient amounts are taken. Symptoms include dilated but reactive pupils with a host of Ts: tremor, tachycardia, tachypnea, talkativeness, temperature, and tension (muscular and nervous). Grand mal convulsion and high temperatures may lead to shock. Deaths have been related to strokes, cardiac irregularities, and delirium. Initial euphoria is followed by anxiety and irritability, then anger and rage with higher doses. Speeded-up thinking may become maniacal acutely or paranoid over prolonged periods. In this case a urine toxicology screen or hospitalization is the only method for distinguishing chronic stimulant abuse from schizophrenia. Acute treatment for mild reactions requires only general support or, at most, single-dose neuroleptics (e.g., haloperidol, 5 mg intramuscularly) to calm the patient, but serious toxicity requires major supportive measures in a structured medical setting with ice packs and diazepam (Valium) to control temperature and seizures. Physical and mental depression frequently follows withdrawal; thus the tendency to increase the dose of the drug is high. With the advent of lower melting point cocaines through freebasing and high-tech marketing (pagers and crack houses), the drug has come into widespread use. Cocaine, particularly in its newer form as coca paste, is a highly concentrated and dangerous drug.

8. Do adolescents who take drugs have other problems?
The danger to youth is often less the drug itself than the associated criminal activity. There are only three methods of supporting one's habit—theft, prostitution, or distribution—and none is legal. Current methods of distribution emphasize use of youngsters on the front lines, because they face less severe penalties when caught. Although most adolescents do not become addicts, the U.S. leads all industrialized nations in percentage of young people involved with illicit drugs.

9. Can drugs be detected without blood or urine tests?
Cocaine recently has been shown to be excreted in saliva at levels parallel to plasma levels. It may be possible to develop a saliva screening test using a dipstick method.

10. What are the basics of long-term treatment for drug abuse?
Because no one method is more effective than others, treatment reflects a plethora of methods. Basic approaches emphasize the goals of acceptance, education, and, usually, abstinence. More recently approaches have emphasized addiction as a family disease and focused on sexual abuse as a common theme. Inpatient programs emphasize a stepwise approach, last 4–6 weeks, and make frequent use of videos and films. Patients are taught to increase self-esteem and to recognize their individuality; return to the community is gradual. Codependency and adult children of alcoholics have been described by Black, who points out the family's attitude toward substance abuse: "Don't talk, don't trust, don't feel." This attitude leads to specialized roles in the family and frequently results in emotional abuse and passage of substance abuse to the next generation.

11. What factors predict adolescent drug abuse?
A number of contributors to adolescent drug abuse have been identified by workers in the field:

Social sanction	Family patterns
Previous risk-taking behavior	Family dysfunction
Abuser personality characteristics	Modeling
Economic feasibility	Peer influences
Anxiety	Alienation
Depression	Reinforcing chemical properties of the substance

Any comprehensive treatment program must take such factors into consideration and attempt to alter or influence them in some way.

12. What stages of drug abuse have been identified by various groups?
The National Commission on Marijuana and Drug Abuse describes the following patterns or stages:

1. Experimental drug use	4. Intensified drug use
2. Social or recreational use	5. Compulsive drug use
3. Circumstantial or situational drug use	

The American Medical Association describes the following patterns of drug use:

1. Drug experimentation	3. Drug abuse
2. Drug use, first recreational, then regular	4. Drug dependency

A common pattern of cocaine use and abuse by groups includes the following steps:

1. Curiosity	7. Psychopathic behavior
2. Initiation	8. Ritualistic behavior
3. Pleasure	9. Dependency tolerance
4. Group identification	10. General physical deterioration
5. Group prestige	11. Severe sociopathic personality destruction
6. Family isolation	

Despite the different labels, each of these progressions notes a movement from curiosity and controlled casual use to uncontrolled obligatory use (addiction).

13. How can the stages help to identify at-risk adolescents?

To treat adolescent drug abuse effectively, many experts believe that the stage of the abuser or potential abuser must be recognized. Many questionnaires purportedly reveal adolescents who are at risk for or already in the early stages of drug abuse. The questions revolve around parent and peer relations, school adjustment, and observed drug use.

Drug abuse by teenagers is believed by many to be seriously underestimated because of numerous factors, including denial by physicians, mental health people, and family members as well as the often episodic nature of drug abuse. The use of routine questions about family and individual patterns of drug abuse and use can aid in detection.

14. Can treatment during early stages be helpful?

During the early stages of drug curiosity and experimentation, parental attitudes and peer attitudes are crucial. Parents must present appropriate guidelines and expectations to the adolescent and let the adolescent know what their actions will be if drug use is discovered. Because adolescents are susceptible to peer influences, the use of group sessions to explore attitudes toward drug use and anticipated consequences and alternatives may be helpful.

15. How successful is treatment during the middle stages?

During middle stages of adolescent drug use and abuse, traditional mental health approaches have been relatively unsuccessful. By contrast, many different kinds of self-help and peer-support groups claim remarkable success. Examples include Parents, Peers and Pot; Palmer Drug Abuse Program (PDAP), Channel One; Alcoholics Anonymous (AA); Al-Anon Family Groups; Families Anonymous; Narcanon Family Groups; and Narcotics Anonymous. Often a traditional psychotherapeutic approach combined with chemically enforced abstinence and a self-help peer-support group leads to the best results.

BIBLIOGRAPHY

1. Bachman JG, Johnston LD, O'Malley PM: Smoking, drinking, and drug use among American high school students; correlates and trends, 1975–1979. Am J Public Health 71:59–69, 1981.
2. Galanter M, Gleaton T, Marcus CE, McMillen J: Self-help groups for parents of young drug and alcohol abusers. Am J Psychiatry 141:889–891, 1984.
3. Johnson LD, O'Malley PM, Bachman JG: Use of Licit and Illicit Drugs by American's High School Students, 1975–1984. Rockville, MD, National Institute of Drug Abuse, 1981.
4. Kandel DB: Epidemiological and psychological perspectives on adolescent drug use. J Am Acad Child Psychiatry 21:328–347, 1982.
5. Kandel DB: Marijuana users in young adulthood. Arch Gen Psychiatry 41:200–209, 1984.
6. Khaiawall AM, Erickson TB, Simpson GM: Chronic phencyclidine abuse and physical assault. Am J Psychiatry 139:1604–1606, 1982.
7. Larson R, Csikszentmihalyi M, Freeman M: Alcohol and marijuana use in adolescents' daily lives: A random sample of experiences. Int J Addict 19:367–381, 1984.
8. Lewis JD, Moritz D, Mellis LP: Long-term toluene abuse. Am J Psychiatry 138:368–370, 1981.
9. Macdonald DI: Drugs, Drinking and Adolescents. Chicago, Year Book, 1984.
10. Polich JM, Ellickson PL, Reuter P, Kahan JP: Strategies for Controlling Adolescent Drug Use. Santa Monica, CA, Rand, 1984.
11. Riggs PD: Depression in substance-dependent delinquents. J Am Acad Child Adolesc Psychiatry 34:764–771, 1995.

60. PRINCIPLES OF CHILD AND ADOLESCENT PSYCHOPHARMACOLOGY

Frederick B. Hebert, M.D.

1. Why are physicians concerned about child and adolescent medications?

Practitioners sometimes avoid giving medications to children and adolescents because they are concerned about unusual responses or dosage requirements. Except for the lack of a euphoric response to stimulants in children, there are few qualitative differences between children and adults in their response to medication. Children's younger organs frequently clear medications more quickly, whereas adolescents generally need adult doses.

2. What are major issues for the family practitioner?

Families sometimes focus all difficulties on unlikely organic causes or past injuries and expect that medications either will not work at all or will work miracles. Medications may allow a seriously ill child to be treated as an outpatient; this is an important point but hardly a miracle. Medications are part of a total treatment plan. Parents and practitioners need to be supportive, never using medications as a punishment. Children and adolescents need to remember that medications do not excuse them from the need to work on their problems. Below are specific principles for treatment of attention deficit-hyperactivity disorder, depression, psychosis, conduct disorders, and anxiety disorders.

ATTENTION DEFICIT-HYPERACTIVITY DISORDER

3. Why is so much attention paid to attention deficit–hyperactivity disorder?

Attention deficit–hyperactivity disorder (ADHD) is a common and well researched childhood disorder. The central notion of a short attention span and hyperactivity has been around since a German poet wrote about "Fidgety Phil" a hundred years ago. In the ensuing years over 10,000 articles have been published in the scientific literature. Although stimulant medications have been used for over 50 years, from time to time splinter groups have raised questions about their use. From the standpoint of the scientific community, stimulants remain one of the safest and most effective of all psychotropic medications. The increase in use of stimulants is probably the result of an increased recognition that 15% of patients with ADHD continue to show signs and symptoms in adolescence. Girls suffer from ADHD only one-fourth as often as boys. In the differential diagnosis, mood disorders are most difficult to rule out. A positive family history of mood disorder and lack of learning disability are more likely in bipolar patients.

4. Are stimulant medications still the mainstay of the medication treatment for ADHD?

Absolutely (see chapter 55).

5. What can we tell parents about ADHD?

Because only 20% of children show signs of ADHD in the office, the physician must take a careful history and have parents and teachers fill out checklists. Historical factors in ADHD known to be associated with the mother's pregnancy include heavy metal exposure, chronic drug abuse, moderate alcohol use, or smoking more than 4 cigarettes/day. Once the diagnosis is made and before medication is started, an explanation to the parents will be helpful. If one compares the brain to a machine, parents can be told that the medication lubricates the system and makes it run more smoothly; it does not offer a cure. Physician and parents can tell the child that the medication is like a baseball glove: if the child takes the medication, it will help him or her, but the child must still try to play the game.

6. What is the role of clonidine in the treatment of child and adolescent behavior disorders?

Clonidine is useful in treating patients with ADHD and oppositional defiant disorders who have not responded to more conservative treatment with stimulants and school and behavioral therapy. Clonidine is a centrally acting drug that inhibits release of norepinephrine and acts centrally to reduce brain arousal; its effects on attention are indirect. Its antihypertensive effects are not clinically evident in children and adolescents, despite a 10% decrease in measured blood pressure. Clonidine reduces arousal and irritability, improving frustration tolerance. Parents noted improvement in doing chores, and teachers saw a reduction in classroom aggression. Clonidine is rapidly absorbed, peaking in 60–90 minutes. If inactive, such as sitting on a school bus, patients may fall asleep for up to 30 minutes afterwards. When active, patients are alert and not sedated. The clinical effects last only 3–4 hours because of rapid metabolism by both liver and kidneys. The dose ranges from 4–6 µg/kg/day. A typical starting dose is one-half of an 0.1-mg tablet at bedtime for 3 days. Another half tablet is added in the afternoon or morning, increasing gradually to a total dose of 2–4 tablets given 2–3 times/day. Clonidine has been used as a test for growth hormone release, but it is not clear whether it actually increases growth. It increases appetite, however, and this effect is helpful in reducing weight loss when clonidine is combined with methylphenidate hydrochloride (Ritalin). Clonidine also reduces energy and stamina, and these effects, along with blood pressure, should be monitored. Clonidine is available in the form of a skin patch (Catapres TTS) in doses of 1, 2, and 3 mg; the patch lasts about 5 days. Young patients adapt easily and wear the patch on their back. The patch tolerates brief exposure to water (as in the shower), but if submerged or pulled at, it loosens. An overlay patch, which comes with each medication patch, may be used. A new area of the back should be chosen each week. From 25–50% of patients react with local irritation, itching, and erythema. The reaction is more commonly to the gum in the patch than to the medication itself. Older children and adolescents frequently want to demonstrate their own control by moving or removing the patch. Some adolescents explain its presence as a way of staying off nicotine, although clonidine was not effective for this indication in adult trials.

7. Can clonidine be combined with methylphenidate hydrochloride?

For patients with both oppositional or conduct disorders and ADHD, clonidine may be combined with methylphenidate hydrochloride. Such children are often highly distractible and explosively aggressive; combined medication helps to avoid institutional placement. Often patients take high (> 1 mg/kg) does of methylphenidate hydrochloride in the morning and at noon and are difficult to control in the afternoon and evening. The addition of clonidine allows an afternoon nap for younger children and more controlled bedtime behavior. In the evening, clonidine should be given at bedtime; otherwise, some patients awaken later in the evening and cannot return to sleep. Frequently, the dose of methylphenidate hydrochloride can be reduced by one-third or more. Side effects such as anorexia and insomnia are relieved whether clonidine is given concurrently or separately later in the day. Clonidine also has been combined clinically with tricyclic antidepressants (TCAs) and neuroleptics. In one case report a patient with only a 1-day wash-out from propranolol had a serious reduction in heart rate when clonidine was started. Heart rate rebounded when clonidine was discontinued. Propranolol and clonidine should not be given simultaneously.

8. Can Tourette's disorder (TD) in children be treated with clonidine?

It is important to establish the correct diagnosis. Many children have motor tics, but the diagnosis of TD requires additional vocalizations (grunts, yelps, explosive sounds or words). TD in adults is most often treated with haloperidol, but child psychiatrists often start with clonidine. Clonidine has a slower onset of action and lower response rate than haloperidol or pimozide but a lower incidence of side effects and no risk for tardive dyskinesia.

DEPRESSION

9. Do children become depressed like adults?

Depression is now recognized in children, although it may not be the same disorder as in adults. Because larger numbers of children respond to placebo, it is difficult to tell whether medications are effective. Symptoms of depression in children include self-deprecation, inhibition, sleep disturbance, morning tiredness, decreased activity, difficulty in concentrating, and poor school performance. But they also may exhibit aggression, enuresis, and hypochondriasis—symptoms not predicted from an adult model. TCA doses have ranged from 1–5 mg/kg, usually of imipramine, after an initial EKG. Blood levels and serial EKGs are performed weekly when patients take doses > 4 mg/kg to monitor the quinidinelike effect of imipramine. Responders had higher plasma levels (about 150 ng/ml) than nonresponders, with optimal response at levels about 200 ng/ml of imipramine and its metabolites. Higher levels were associated with decreased efficacy and delirium on some occasions.

10. Is monitoring of blood levels necessary in every child?

It is important to measure blood levels routinely in children, because there is no relationship between dose and clinical response; a 40-fold difference may exist in plasma concentration of different patients receiving the same dose. Because children differ from adults in body fat nd percent of total body water with protein-binding characteristics and have more active enzyme systems, they may create and accumulate more metabolites than adults. Available studies indicate that both beneficial and serious side effects of TCAs are related to plasma concentration and that the therapeutic range is relatively narrow; thus monitoring of plasma levels is necessary in the treatment of childhood depression. All children should be given a 1-week baseline period before treatment; 20% will no longer be depressed after this interval.

11. What about adolescent depression?

Although scientific evidence is lacking, most clinicians agree that adolescents whose depression resembles adult endogenous depressions respond to TCAs. Adolescent depressions are characterized by gradual onset, anorexia, weight loss, middle- and late-night insomnia, psychomotor disturbance, and family history of serious depression. Early morning wakening is so strikingly different from the usual "stay-up late and sleep-in" style of adolescents that it should raise the clinician's suspicion. The dexamethasone suppression test is not a reliable tool for diagnosis. Many adolescents also no longer appear depressed after a 2-week hospital stay without medication.

12. Are adolescents at risk for overdosing on medications?

The adolescent's ability for rapid behavior change necessitates caution. Adolescents attempt suicide more than other age groups, many by drug overdose. This fact emphasizes the need for careful follow-up of adolescents taking medications with a high potential for lethal overdose.

13. What is the first step in treatment of adolescent depression?

After confirming that the adolescent patient has no cardiovascular problems, one begins with imipramine, 1 mg/kg, and increases the dose to 2 mg/kg by the end of the first week. If the adolescent has not responded in 3 weeks, the serum level is assessed. The clinician must be certain that blood levels are adequate and that the patient is taking the medication. The dose is then adjusted to achieve levels of 150–250 ng/ml (allowing 5 days between adjustments to achieve a steady state). When a dose > 4 mg/kg is required to achieve therapeutic blood levels, daily pulses and weekly EKGs to check for arrhythmias are in order until significant cardiac side effects have been ruled out. Unless agitation requires divided doses, the majority of patients take their medication at bedtime. Improved sleep is often the first sign of response, and its absence should raise questions about diagnosis or dose. Irritability and frank mania have been reported in adolescents taking TCAs. This response should raise strong suspicions of bipolar disorder, and TCAs should be discontinued. Side effects are largely the results of anticholinergic activity. Dry mouth, blurred vision, and, less often, orthostatic hypotension may require a change to desipramine at equivalent doses. Any use of desipramine justifies preliminary EKGs because it has led to sudden cardiac death in several patients. Nortriptyline at half the dose of imipramine also may be used; blood levels are available for both these medications. Sixty days after a positive response the medication often can be reduced to about one-half the therapeutic dose, but adult studies support use of full therapeutic dose for 6 months.

14. What about outpatient follow-up?

When the patient is ready for outpatient follow-up, only small amounts of TCAs are prescribed at one time; thus the patient must be seen frequently or a responsible adult must be in control of dispensing. In follow-up visits, the patient is asked routinely about sleep disturbance. If middle or late insomnia recurs, the patient should resume therapeutic doses and may be on maintenance treatment for 1 year. Such long-term therapeutic regimens are extrapolations of prescribing patterns for adults; there are no comparable adolescent studies. To date drug studies in adolescents do not demonstrate the superiority of antidepressant over placebo in the treatment of depression, but practitioners continue to see clinical improvement after careful diagnostic screening for major depression.

15. Are other medications safer?

Newer antidepressants, fluoxetine and trazodone, have been used clinically with adolescents. Fluoxetine is the selective serotonin reuptake inhibitor (SSRI) that has been used most often with adolescents who are depressed as an extrapolation of its wide use in adults. Trazodone also has been successfully used clinically in doses about twice that of TCAs (up to 400 mg/day). Because trazodone is initially quite sedating and may cause light-headedness, it was originally given in divided doses after meals. Now it is most often used as an adjunct to fluoxetine to help the patient sleep. It is given at bedtime after a snack. Anticholinergic and cardiac effects are unlikely, but priapism shortly after initiating treatment has been reported; this side effect is a relative contraindication for adolescent boys. Like all currently known antidepressants, trazodone is excreted in breast milk and should not be given to nursing mothers; it is considered a category C drug because of increased fetal absorption in rats.

16. Do all cases of depression in adolescents look like depression in adults?

Although major depressions respond to regular antidepressants, many depressed adolescents do not meet criteria for major depression. Atypical depressions present with dysphoric mood, but patients maintain mood reactivity while depressed; that is, they respond to comments by the interviewer with a change in mood. In addition, patients may have a history of sensitivity to rejection. Instead of weight loss and inability to sleep, they may show increased appetite or weight gain and sleep over 10 hours/day. Any sleep disturbance in adolescents needs to be distinguished from the common habit of staying up late and sleeping in with overall adequate sleep time. Patients also may complain of severe fatigue, sometimes manifested by complaints of leaden weights in arms or legs.

17. What medications are useful in atypical depression?

Earlier studies demonstrated that for atypical depression in young adults, monoamine oxidase inhibitors (MAOIs) were better than TCAs. Of adolescents unresponsive to TCAs, 75% responded to phenelzine in one study. Side effects were numerous, but dietary compliance was a problem for less than one-third. Most patients had no significant effects, even with indiscretion. Later studies concluded that atypical depression may reflect primarily the age of the patient. A more recent study found that adolescents who fail to respond to treatment with TCAs often improve when lithium carbonate is added. At therapeutic doses of lithium, adolescents took up to 2 weeks to respond, but improvement persisted.

18. Can newer medications be used for atypical depression?
Concern over lethal overdose led to a search for treatments of adolescent depressions of all types with agents that are less likely to be harmful. Fluoxetine has gained wide use in adults, but few studies are available in adolescents. Bupropion, which is unrelated to both TCAs and SSRIs, has been effective in atypical depression in adults. It has shown stimulant effects and was withheld from introduction because of seizures in bulimic patients who took the drug. Overall risk is low if the dose is below 400 mg. The usual dose is 75–100 3 times/day; a typical dose in adolescents is 250 mg/day or less. Menstrual irregularities were seen infrequently with buproprion. Both medications are safer in overdose than TCAs, MAOIs, or lithium carbonate.

PSYCHOSIS

19. What kinds of psychosis are seen in children and adolescents?
Psychosis in children and adolescents may be either organic or functional. Acute organic psychosis or delirium is usually the result of drug ingestion, either accidental in children or recreational in adolescents. In either case treatment is directed to the underlying cause, but delirium-induced agitation may need separate treatment.

20. How is delirium treated in children and adolescents?
Treatment usually takes the form of a structured and locked setting, including the use of a seclusion room or restraints if necessary. Delirium-induced agitation also may require judicious medication. A child who is thrashing about may need to be sedated for brain scan, EEG, or radiograph. Adolescents who have taken hallucinogens usually can be talked down. Patients who have taken phencyclidine (PCP), on the other hand, may become agitated if a therapeutic encounter is attempted. Such patients may seriously harm themselves and others because the anesthetic properties of PCP keep them from knowing that they have painful injuries. Agitated and delirious patients can be sedated with haloperidol, 0.1–0.3 mg/kg, over the space of 1 hour; dystonia is the only likely side effect. This side effect frequently is more frightening to the patient and family than the original delirium. Any child or adolescent given haloperidol should be observed closely for 24 hours so that dystonic reactions can be treated. Benadryl (diphenhydramine), 25–50 mg orally or intramuscularly, and reassurance once the dystonia subsides are usually the only treatments needed for dystonias.

21. What about chronic organic disorders such as autism and head injuries?
More recently, clomipramine has been used to treat the obsessive-repetitive behaviors in autistic children. Clomipramine and now fluoxetine have reduced stereotypic behaviors. Patients with chronic organic psychoses due to head injury, autism, or pervasive developmental disorders respond to low doses of haloperidol, which reduce stereotyped and aggressive behavior.

22. Can short-term use of neuroleptics cause dyskinesia?
A major concern is the potential for movement disorders, especially tardive dyskinesia (TD). Children and adolescents may develop a time-limited form of TD after taking neuroleptics only 6 months. Symptoms appear in the extremities as choreiform movements or as ataxia and usually disappear 2 weeks after the medication is discontinued, but movements may persist from 3–12 months. Many organically ill children and adolescents may need to be on neuroleptics for years and, like adults, are at risk for long-term oral-buccal tardive dyskinesia.

23. What are the functional psychoses in youth?
Functional psychoses include mania and schizophrenia and possibly depression. Psychotically depressed children and adolescents have more auditory hallucinations than adults; these can be treated by adding neuroleptics to the antidepressants. Hallucinations usually remit in less than 1 month, and the neuroleptics can be discontinued. Adolescents and children with psychotic

depressions are at risk for bipolar disorder. Although mania is quite uncommon in children, 20% of all bipolar disorders have their onset before the age of 20, most often presenting initially as major depression.

24. How is mania treated?
Mania in children and adolescents presents more commonly with irritability than euphoria and also has a high incidence of hallucinations, making differentiation from schizophrenia difficult. Clinicians should err in favor of the least disabling diagnosis; thus the diagnosis frequently is mania, even if not all hallucinations are related to mood. Agitation and hallucinations respond to neuroleptics, but the grandiosity usually requires lithium carbonate. Baseline kidney and thyroid function studies are done to conform the patient's ability to clear lithium and euthyroid status. Lithium carbonate is begun at up to 30 mg/kg in divided doses. Lithium carbonate, 300 mg in sustained-release form, avoids the gastric upset and dizziness associated with regular lithium. Within 5 days the patient should be in range of 0.8–1.2 mEq/L. Children and many adolescents need to reach levels of 1.5 mEq/L for a good response. The usual convention of waiting 12 hours after the last dose allows assessment of trough serum levels. Once the mania subsides, the dose can be reduced so that the serum range is 0.8–1.2 mEq/L. The serum level is followed at gradually greater intervals; after a certain period, a trial off medications is appropriate. Thyroid studies should be repeated at 6-month intervals, because a few patients become hypothyroid.

25. What are the alternative medications for mania?
Because 30–40% of adult manic patients do not respond to or cannot tolerate lithium carbonate, both carbamazepine and valproic acid have been used as alternatives. The use of carbamazepine is less common in children than in adults. Sodium divalproex is used for dysphoric mania, rapid cyclers, and patients whose presentation includes psychotic symptoms or substance abuse in addition to mania. Because many adolescents present with psychotic symptoms, sodium divalproex is often added to lithium carbonate but also may be used alone.

After baseline liver and platelet studies, sodium divalproex is given in divided doses of 20 mg/kg. It is rapidly absorbed with a peak action at 4–6 hours. The dose is gradually increased until levels of 50–120 mg/ml are reached. Patients frequently respond in 5–10 days. The most common side effect is GI upsets, mild tremor, and initial lethargy. A decrease in platelets and an increase in liver function values are dose-related. An increase of liver function values to 300% of baseline is acceptable, and thrombocytopenia is usually not seen until blood levels exceed 100 mg/ml of valproate. Hair thinning is transient and dose-related but may be particularly disturbing to adolescents. Sodium divalproex also is available in pull-a-part capsules as a sprinkle that can be used in soft foods with younger children or patients who cannot take capsules by mouth. Unlike lithium, sodium divalproex is 80–95% protein-bound and thus competes with other protein-bound medications, such as carbamazepine or fluoxetine. As a result of the interaction, the less tightly bound drug is displaced and its side effects are increased. Although sodium divalproex and carbamazepine have been used in combination in adults, their interaction is complex. Because little experience is available in adolescents, it is safer to use one or the other by itself. Sodium divalproex is a recent addition to the child psychiatry armamentarium and, if polypharmacy is avoided in younger children, a safe alternative to lithium.

26. How is schizophrenia treated?
Schizophrenia frequently begins in adolescence. A gradual decline in functioning with the onset of suspiciousness and auditory hallucinations that comment on one's behavior are ominous signs. A baseline CT scan is done to check ventricular size. Atrophy is associated with poor prognosis. Treatment with neuroleptics requires a minimal dose of 300 mg of chlorpromazine or 5 mg of haloperidol. Chlorpromazine and thioridazine cause problems with sexual side effects (retrograde ejaculation or galactorrhea) and general inhibition of movement (akinesia). The potent neuroleptics tend to induce dystonias, particularly if large doses are given early in treatment.

Akinesia, which may appear later with any neuroleptic, requires a reduction in dose or the addition of propranolol, 40–120 mg/day. If the patient's agitation or perplexity persists, the dose of neuroleptic is gradually doubled, and the patient is observed for approximately 1 week before increasing the dose again. Over a period of approximately 6 weeks the patient's hallucinations and psychosis gradually come under control. The dose then may be reduced slowly to the previously mentioned minimums; after 6 months the medication may be discontinued. A significant portion of functional psychoses in adolescents seem to result from severe external stresses and remit without further recurrence. Mania and schizophrenia, on the other hand, are considered life-time diagnoses.

BEHAVIOR OR CONDUCT DISORDERS

27. Is there a practical way of classifying behavior disorders?
Behavior disorders can be divided into "good kid" and "bad kid" styles. The good kid has discrete episodes of anger, usually with little or no precipitant. Adolescents trash their rooms, throw things, or hit whoever happens to be close. Once over this episode, they are contrite and apologetic. An EEG may be helpful, because some patients have an epileptic focus, usually in the temporal lobe. However, up to 40% of EEGs are false negatives, and nasal pharyngeal leads are not well tolerated. Sometimes diagnosed with explosive disorders, such patients do better on carbamazepine. A baseline CBC with reticulocyte count is necessary, because carbamazepine usually reduces the WBC initially. If carbamazepine is started at a low dose of 200 mg/day and increased by 200 mg each week with weekly blood counts for the first month, there are few problems. If the dose is increased too quickly, the patient often complains of upset stomach. In almost all cases, the reticulocyte count decreases, with a later decrease in the overall white cell count. A petechial rash rarely appears. The goals are a carbamazepine level of 0.8–1.2 µg/ml and a reduction in outbursts after 1 month with adequate drug serum levels. If the white cell count drops below 4000, the clinician may consider the trial a failure. Patients who respond need regular white counts with gradually decreasing frequency. As in adults, blood levels may drop over time because of enzyme induction. Clinically, some adolescents show increased irritability on carbamazepine, particularly those with an associated affect disorder.

28. Are the "bad kids" more commonly diagnosed?
The "bad kids" are difficult to deal with for parents, peers, and practitioners and are classified as conduct disorders. DSM-IV lists 15 symptoms of conduct disorder, requiring at least three for the diagnosis:
1. Often bullies, threatens, or intimidates others
2. Often initiates physical fights
3. Used a weapon that can cause serious physical harm to others
4. Has been physically cruel to people
5. Has been physically cruel to animals
6. Has stolen with confrontation of victim
7. Forced sexual activity on someone
8. Deliberately engaged in fire setting with intention of serious damage
9. Deliberately destroyed others' property
10. Has broken into someone else's property
11. Often lies, to obtain favors or avoid obligations (cons)
12. Has stolen without confrontation of victim more than once
13. Stays out at night, with onset before age 13
14. Has run away from home overnight at least twice
15. Often truant from school, with onset before age 13

Because only three symptoms from the list above are required for the diagnosis of conduct disorder, it is much more common than explosive disorder ("good kid").

29. What other diagnosis should be considered?

Even when the patient meets the criteria for diagnosis of conduct disorder, a careful review for the possibility of ADHD and affective disorders should be performed. ADHD is commonly associated with conduct disorder and worsens the overall prognosis. It is worthwhile to consider a trial of clonidine if the aggression is mostly verbal and ADHD is prominent; clonidine seems to reduce irritability in patients with ADHD. Of delinquent populations, 23–30% meet the criteria for major depression and deserve treatment. In one study of depressed conduct-disordered male adolescents, behavior improved as the depression lifted after treatment with imipramine. Bipolar disorder also should be ruled out, with particular attention to family history. Clinicians have increasing awareness of bipolar disorder in adolescents with the understanding that the offspring of bipolar parents are at risk for mania also. Because mania in adolescents frequently presents as irritability and underlying irritability frequently accompanies conduct disorder behavior, lithium was tried in the treatment of conduct disorder. One study comparing lithium with haloperidol found both to be equally effective, but lithium caused fewer side effects, including no detrimental effect on learning. Although responsiveness to lithium does not prove a bipolar diagnosis, it is reasonable to give a conduct-disordered adolescent a trial of lithium if other treatable disorders are unlikely. Only one controlled study has shown that youth with affective symptoms are more responsive to lithium.

30. What are the general principles of treating conduct disorder with medication?

Treatment for conduct disorder with lithium follows the regimen for bipolar disorder with kidney and thyroid studies and with gradual increase in the lithium level to the range of 1.0–1.5 mEq/L. An EEG should be obtained before lithium is started, because lithium in the system creates EEG artifacts. Hand tremor and gastric distress are common but mild. Sustained-release lithium may be used to reduce gastric distress, and beta blockers may reduce tremors. Medications are frequently necessary for conduct disorder but never sufficient. Structure and control during inpatient care and follow-up are always necessary. Many, if not all, patients with conduct disorders need remedial education for reading and learning disabilities.

GENERAL ANXIETY AND OBSESSIVE COMPULSIVE DISORDER

31. Why were childhood anxiety disorders not treated in the past?

Child psychiatrists have traditionally not treated anxiety disorders with medications because of a belief that anxiety was part of the developmental process and a concern that medication may interfere with the process. Until recently medications used to treat anxiety also carried some potential for addiction or at least psychological dependence among adults. The introduction of buspirone allows the treatment of anxiety disorders with a medication that has no addiction liability and does not produce sedation. There are few reports of its use in children or adolescents. Case reports have found it useful in treating anxiety in adolescents. Additional reports have shown it to be a useful adjunct in reducing aggression in autistic adolescents. Currently the indications are clinical; its efficacy has not been established for general use.

32. Does increasing evidence suggest that obsessive compulsive disorder (OCD) is an organic medical problem?

One specific type of anxiety associated with obsessions and compulsions has responded to agents that increase serotonin in the CNS. Such agents markedly reduce behaviors associated with this particular anxiety. Although the cause is unknown, recent biologic, clinical, radiologic, and physiologic evidence strongly implicates problems in the caudate or connections from caudate to the prefrontal area of the brain. Patients with Sydenham's chorea and postencephalitic patients have OCD more often than the general population, and both disorders have obvious organic causes. OCD is much more common than previously thought. As much as 2–3% of the U.S. population is estimated to be affected—more than 4 million people. Clues in children include erased school papers (sometimes so repeatedly that holes are worn through the paper) and/or retraced letters.

33. What treatments have been used for OCD?

Many treatments have been tried. Psychotherapy is ineffective. Behavior therapies have been variably effective. Stimulus exposure with response prevention is effective, but 25% of patients drop out and many do not follow through on exposure-response prevention. Antianxiety agents, neuroleptics, and antidepressants have been tried without much success. Infrequently child patients respond to imipramine and sometimes clonidine. Clomipramine is a strong serotonin reuptake blocker and was discovered to be helpful in OCD; it is the only agent approved for use in children. Clonipramine has a typical tricyclic side-effect profile of dry mouth, constipation, tremor, dizziness, somnolence, headache and fatigue, but such effects are seen less often in children. As much as 200 mg/day or as little as 3 mg/kg may be used for children or adolescents. Behavior therapy with parental assistance helps (see chapter 57).

BIBLIOGRAPHY

1. Bloomingdale LM (ed): Attention Deficit Disorder: Identification, Course, and Rationale. New York, Spectrum, 1985.
2. Campbell M, et al: Lithium in hospitalized children with conduct disorder: A double-blind and placebo-controlled study. J Am Acad Child Adolesc Psychiatry 34:445–453, 1995.
3. Conners CK, Wells KC: Hyperkinetic Children: A Neuropsychosocial Approach. Beverly Hills, CA, Sage, 1986.
4. Cowart VS: The Ritalin controversy: What's made this drug's opponents hyperactive? JAMA 259:2521–2523, 1988.
5. Farley GK, Hebert FB, Eckhardt LO: Handbook of Child and Adolescent Psychiatric Emergencies and Crises, 2nd ed. New York, Elsevier, 1986.
6. Gualtieri CT, et al: Tardive dyskinesia and other clinical consequences of neuroleptic treatment in children and adolescents. Am J Psychiatry 41:20–23, 1984.
7. Hunt RD, Minderaa RB, Cohen DJ: Clonidine benefits children with attention deficit disorder and hyperactivity: Report of a double-blind placebo-crossover therapeutic trial. J Am Acad Child Adolesc Psychiatry 24:617–629, 1985.
8. Mattes JA: Psychopharmacology of temper outbursts: A review. J Nerv Ment Dis 174:464–470, 1986.
9. Satterfield JH, et al: Multimodality treatment: A two-year evaluation of 61 hyperactive boys. Arch Gen Psychiatry 37:915–918, 1980.
10. Satterfield JH, et al: Therapeutic interventions to prevent delinquency in hyperactive boys. J Am Acad Child Adolesc Psychiatry 26:56–64, 1984.
11. Simeon JG, Ferguson HB: Recent developments in the use of antidepressants and anxiolytic medications. Psychiatr Clin North Am 8:893–9-7, 1985.
12. Weller EB, Weller RA: Major Depressive Disorders in Children. Washington, DC, American Psychiatric Press, 1984.

VIII. Disorders Associated with Pregnancy and Menstruation

61. PREMENSTRUAL SYNDROME (PMS)

Carol S. Birnbaum, M.D.

1. Describe PMS.

PMS is a recurrent constellation of symptoms experienced by women of reproductive age at some point between ovulation and the onset of menstrual flow. The symptoms experienced include those of mood and behavior, such as depression, irritability, rejection-sensitivity, and somatic complaints such as bloating, breast tenderness, and headache. Although the symptoms themselves are not specific, their timing and severity indicate the presence of PMS. Both clinical and research criteria require that the symptoms occur at some point between ovulation and the onset of menstrual flow and that they be severe enough to cause significant disruption of performance at work, of social relationships, or of home life.

The Premenstrual Syndrome

Symptoms: Any combination of:
    Mood, i.e., depression, lability
    Behavior, i.e., interpersonal conflicts, rejection sensitivity
    Physical complaints, i.e., breast tenderness, swelling, headache
Timing
    Symptoms occur between ovulation and the onset of menstrual flow
Severity
    Symptoms are severe enough to disrupt social or occupational functioning

2. How common is PMS among the general population?

Originally, assessments placed the prevalence of PMS complaints in the general population as high as 20 to 90%. It has been found, however, that when women actually maintain prospective rating scales, a large number of them either have symptoms which are not limited to the premenstrual phase of their cycles, or are not consistent throughout two or more cycles. Thus a movement was made toward a more precise diagnosis, beginning a decade ago when a National Institute of Mental Health (NIMH) workshop recommended that the diagnostic criteria for PMS include prospective documentation of a 30% increase in symptom intensity from the follicular to the late luteal phase of the menstrual cycle for at least two consecutive months. These guidelines do not specify the precise symptoms to be measured. DSM–IV proposes a disorder called premenstrual dysphoric disorder (PMDD) as a diagnostic category needing further study. The criteria include a list of symptoms (affective, behavioral, and somatic), require prospective daily self-ratings during at least two symptomatic cycles, and specify that symptoms must be present during the last week of the luteal phase and remit within a few days of the onset of the follicular phase. The diagnosis of PMDD requires the presence of one affective symptom, although somatic symptoms need not be present. Approximately 2.5 to 8% of reproductive age women meet these criteria. In this chapter, the term PMS includes women without affective symptoms or women with premenstrual worsening of affective disorder who would not meet criteria for PMDD, but who form a large percentage of women who present for treatment.

3. What about women with other known psychiatric disorders; can they also have comorbid PMS?

The DSM–IV criteria for PMDD allow for the presence of comorbid disorders, although most research criteria currently exclude women with comorbid psychopathology in an effort to eliminate heterogeneity, which may confound both attempts to clarify etiology and to assess empiric treatment responses. This remains a point of controversy: is PMS an exacerbation of an underlying condition or a separate entity? Studies have shown that the incidence of comorbid psychiatric disorders in women meeting criteria for PMS is high, particularly for affective disorders. Researchers have found the lifetime prevalence of axis I disorders to be 70 to 85% in women with prospectively confirmed PMDD, with most women reporting a history of depressive disorder. The incidence of axis II disorders among these women has been found to be approximately 10%, which is similar to rates estimated for the general population. Because the incidence of comorbid depressive disorders appears to be quite significant, it is difficult to determine whether PMS is an autonomous disorder or a depressive disorder somehow linked to, or triggered by, the menstrual cycle.

4. How do you diagnose PMS?

The clinician must answer several questions to evaluate premenstrual complaints:

Is the Patient Ovulating?

PMS symptoms occur during the luteal phase. This implies that successful ovulation has occurred, and that the hormonal milieu is dominated by progesterone secretion from the corpus luteum. Patients taking oral contraceptive pills must be excluded from research protocols as their hormonal profile is altered. These women may, however, experience a similar complex of symptoms prior to menses. For the clinician not concerned with a rigorous research protocol, adequate evidence of ovulatory cycles may be obtained by a history of spontaneous menstrual cyclicity. If there is any question about ovulation or if cycles are irregular, a basal body temperature chart can be obtained or a urine LH surge predictor kit can be used. Clinically, there is no need to obtain serum gonadotropin or hormone levels, which are quite costly.

Does the Patient Have an Underlying Medical Disorder?

A past medical history should be taken with careful consideration of any syndromes that could mimic or suggest PMS. For example, endometriosis can cause significant pelvic discomfort before the onset of menses. Migraine, epilepsy, herpes, and allergies can occur with a premenstrual pattern and may cause subsequent behavioral or affective symptoms that confuse the patient and the practitioner. A careful physical exam should be performed by an internist or gynecologist with this differential in mind.

What Should be Included in the Psychiatric Assessment of the Patient?

Taking the past psychiatric history should include a careful review of responses to past pregnancies. Patients with a history of post-partum depression are more likely to develop subsequent PMS. Past psychiatric pathology should be reviewed carefully, as a known tendency toward any axis I disorder may suggest premenstrual worsening of that disorder and could affect treatment decisions. Two separate psychiatric evaluations should be performed. Careful mental status exam, including questions regarding current drug or alcohol use, should be obtained separately for the follicular phase and the luteal phase in order to allow the clinician the best opportunity to pick up undiagnosed axis I pathology and to assess objectively the degree of change that occurs within the cycle. Patients who look and feel quite well when initially evaluated in the follicular phase are often relieved to be asked back just before their expected period "so you can see what I'm really like!" Obvious axis I pathology should be treated until the patient is without symptoms in the follicular phase before continuing the prospective search for either comorbid PMS or premenstrual worsening of an underlying disorder.

Differential Diagnosis of PMS

• Cyclic recurrence of medical disorders
  Seizures
  Migraines
  Herpes
  Allergies
	• Dysmenorrhea
	• Endometriosis
	• Psychiatric disorder with or without
	  premenstrual exacerbation

How Should Prospective Daily Rating Scales be Used?

Once it is determined that the patient is not suffering from a medical or psychiatric disorder, or once that disorder has been adequately treated and a complaint of luteal phase symptoms persist, the patient should be asked to keep prospective daily rating scales for two consecutive cycles. This will allow the clinician to assess the type of symptoms suffered, their pattern of timing, and the level of symptom severity. Rubinow and colleagues reported that fewer than 50% of women presenting with an apparent history of PMS show a cycle-dependent pattern prospectively. This illustrates the importance of prospective, longitudinal ratings when making the diagnosis. A commonly used form is the Daily Record of Severity of Problems developed by Endicott and Harrison, which uses a six point scale, breaks symptoms down into clusters of the most commonly reported symptoms of PMS, and includes items assessing level of dysfunction in terms of productivity, recreational and social activities, and interpersonal relationships. Patients describe that lack of acknowledgment by physicians of PMS symptoms makes them feel "crazy" or accused of being "a typical complaining female." Prospective documentation can thus help build a treatment alliance: patients often feel they are checking-in every day when charting and appreciate having a careful record of their symptoms that clarifies their monthly experience. Persistent follicular symptoms without sharp luteal phase worsening should convince clinician and patient that something other than PMS is the problem.

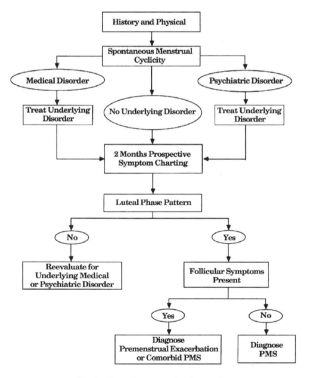

Evaluation of premenstrual symptoms.

5. What is the pathophysiology of PMS?

Although it is well known that women with PMS who are placed in premature menopause either surgically or medically experience a dramatic resolution in their symptoms, a precise dysregulation in the menstrual cycle which may be associated with PMS has yet to be clarified. Therefore, the earliest theories of the etiology of PMS postulated abnormal levels of gonadal steroids in affected women. The most popular of these for many years was that women with PMS suffer from a deficiency in luteal phase progesterone. Although this was never confirmed, it resulted in women with the complaint of premenstrual symptoms being treated with progesterone suppositories, a treatment both costly and cumbersome. Subsequently, several prospective, double-blind studies of progesterone have found this therapy to be no more effective than placebo. The importance of ovarian steroids in the pathophysiology of PMS was first clearly demonstrated in 1984 by Muse and colleagues, who administered a gonadotropin-releasing hormone (GnRH) agonist to women with PMS, causing a cessation of ovarian stimulation and a dramatic reduction in premenstrual symptoms. Despite this significant finding, no difference in level of ovarian steroids, estrogen-to-progesterone ratio, gonadotropins, or ovarian steriod–binding globulin have been consistently detected between patients with PMS and controls. Therefore, no consistent evidence supports earlier hypotheses that PMS was caused by abnormal levels of circulating ovarian steroids or abnormal gonadotropin release. Thus, women who manifest PMS have been thought to be biologically predisposed to manifest an exaggerated response to normal ovarian steroid fluctuations. This is further substantiated by the finding that women with PMS may be nearly twice as likely to develop postpartum depression as those in the general population. Both genetic and environmental origins for this predisposition have been postulated, leading some investigators to propose a multifactorial etiology which may account for the heterogeneous presentation of the syndrome.

Other nonreproductive neuroendocrine markers that have been considered in depression have also been examined in PMS. The cortisol secretory pattern of symptomatic women appears to be the same as in asymptomatic controls. Thyroid-stimulating hormone response to thyroid-releasing hormone has been found to be similar in symptomatic women and controls in one study, and then abnormal in symptomatic women in another. Serum circadian malatonin profiles were found to be similar to those in depressed individuals; however, some of the women in the PMS group also met criteria for major depression, leaving these results in question.

6. What about nonbiologic or environmental factors?

The primary environmental factors investigated as predisposing variables for PMS have been stress and diet. Early studies which found an association between stressful life events and PMS have been criticized for using retrospective assessments of stressful life events. Later, prospective studies of women with disabling PMS found that the amount of stress experienced during a given menstrual cycle has a negligible role in determining the severity of PMS symptoms. When women with PMS without comorbid Axis I disorders are compared with volunteer controls, few significant demographic differences exist.

7. Do certain foods exacerbate the condition?

Dietary factors have long been postulated as contributing to PMS symptoms. The elimination of sweet and salty foods is frequently suggested, although to date no scientific evidence supports this. Chocolate has been associated with PMS, although no evidence suggests chocolate consumption as a causal agent. Consuming a carbohydrate-rich, protein-poor evening test meal during the late luteal phase may improve premenstrual mood symptoms in women with PMS. The consumption of carbohydrates without protein causes the insulin-driven increase in availability of the serotonin precursor, tryptophan, to the brain, thus ultimately enhancing serotonin levels. Some investigators have speculated that women who complain of carbohydrate binges premenstrually may be self-medicating a mood disturbance.

Although nutritional supplementation has been widely used as a treatment for PMS, there has been no consistent documentation of either deficiency or excess of vitamins or minerals in affected patients when compared with controls. Studies have suggested that treatment with vitamins A, B_6, and E, evening primrose oil, zinc, magnesium and calcium, among others, has relieved symptoms. Many of these studies have been criticized for methodologic flaws involving the lack of rigorous subject selection and valid and reliable prospective rating scales with which to measure improvement of symptoms. Additionally, the doses of vitamins and minerals administered in these studies often dramatically exceeded recommended daily allowances for these substances. Responses to such doses may represent a pharmacologic response rather than a correction of a deficiency state.

8. Does the link between PMS and depressive disorder suggest a possible role for central neurotransmission in the etiology of PMS?
The most recent addition to existing etiologic hypotheses for PMS is the suggestion that ovarian sex-steroid flux causes a dysregulation in central neurotransmission in susceptible individuals. Estrogen and progesterone and their metabolites are known to alter function in the opioidergic, noradrenergic, serotonergic, and the gamma-aminobutyric acidergic systems. Their effects are thought to occur through three separate mechanisms: the classic genomic interaction leading to altered protein production, a direct effect on monoamine turnover and metabolism, and the direct effect of the steroid or its metabolite on the nerve cell membrane. Progesterone metabolites are known to have both stimulatory and inhibitory effects on gamma-aminobutyric acid receptors in laboratory mice. Most recently interest has turned to the effects of estrogen and progesterone on the serotonergic system, as patients have responded dramatically to the serotonin reuptake-inhibitor, fluoxetine, as a treatment for PMS symptoms. Diminished whole blood serotonin and platelet serotonin uptake have been found in the luteal phase of women with PMS. Still, much of the evidence suggesting a serotonin dysregulation hypothesis in PMS has not been consistently reproducible, and much work remains to be done to explore the effects of ovarian sex steroids on this and other central neurotransmitter pathways. Dysregulation of these CNS modulators is also implicated in the development of mood and anxiety disorders, both of which have significant symptoms in common with PMS. Researchers are thus faced with the task of identifying subgroups of women who may be vulnerable to changes in the female reproductive hormonal milieu and who consequently develop mood and anxiety symptoms at these vulnerable points.

9. Could PMS represent an autonomous mood disorder?
Over the years one of the most solidly held premises has been that symptoms are related to luteal phase estrogen and progesterone flux, as luteal changes in ovarian steroid levels correspond temporally to symptom manifestation. This premise was called into question by a recent important study by Schmidt et al. In this study, women with prospectively confirmed PMS experienced a "truncated" luteal phase due to administration of the antiprogesterone mifepristone (RU 486). The startling finding of this study was that these women with abbreviated luteal phases experienced their characteristic premenstrual mood state after the mifepristone-induced menses, whereas they had peripheral endocrine profiles consistent with the follicular phase. The authors concluded that either PMS symptoms result from hormonal events that occur before the late luteal phase, or that PMS represents an autonomous, cyclic disorder that is linked to the menstrual cycle but can become dissociated from it.

10. How does one select an appropriate treatment for PMS?
As the etiology of PMS remains unknown, available treatments are primarily directed toward its symptoms. Over the years, numerous treatments for PMS have been suggested, including changes in diet, exercise, vitamin supplementation, diuretics, hormones, medical and surgical oophorectomy, and various psychotropic agents, but few of these were proven efficacious through rigorous prospective study. With the advent of more stringent diagnostic criteria and the development of reliable prospective daily rating scales, this is beginning to change. The initial choice of treatment should be based on a careful assessment of symptoms and their severity, beginning with the least invasive measures available.

11. What are the least invasive treatments?
If the patient is highly motivated and symptoms are mild or of brief duration, a course of psychoeducation, either individually or in a group, may be all that is needed. Psychoeducation should focus on explaining what is currently known about the disorder to the subject and her family members as well as prescribing certain lifestyle changes, such as frequent small meals to prevent hypoglycemia and an enhanced exercise regime during the luteal phase. Psychoeducation can be offered either in a group or individual format depending on both available resources and the preferences of patient and clinician.

The specific effects of dietary modifications on PMS symptoms have not been well studied. The anecdotal reports from women who have implemented these modifications indicate some symptom improvement and are discussed in question 7.

12. What is the role of exercise?
No prospective assessments of exercise as a treatment for PMS have been made. However, aerobic exercise is known to improve mood; the mechanism for this response is believed to derive from enhanced endorphin levels. A program of moderate regular aerobic exercise may therefore be helpful in treating mood-related symptoms and will certainly create overall health benefits. Women who already exercise on a regular basis should be instructed to increase their activity throughout the luteal phase of their cycles.

Alterations in circadian rhythm have also been implicated in PMS. One pilot study found that sleep deprivation, which has been shown to reduce symptoms of major depression, reduced premenstrual symptoms in eight of ten women with PMS. Another pilot study found a reduction in luteal phase depressive symptoms of six women treated with evening bright light therapy.

13. Describe the current view regarding vitamin and mineral supplements.
Although these are frequently recommended to women suffering from PMS, few solid scientific studies have demonstrated their efficacy. Optivite (Optimox) is a high-potency multiple vitamin preparation marketed for PMS which has yielded beneficial results in two placebo-controlled trials. However, this preparation contains potentially unsafe levels of both vitamins A and B_6. Calcium and magnesium supplementation both have been shown to be useful in reducing PMS symptoms in well-designed clinical trials, although there is less scientific support for other supplements, including vitamin B_6. In cases of mild to moderate premenstrual symptoms, a trial of calcium (1,000 mg q.d.) and magnesium (360 mg q.d.) along with the dietary and exercise changes recommended above should be attempted before going to a more aggressive or expensive form of treatment.

14. How does one treat specific physical symptoms?
The most common physical complaints of PMS include bloating, weight gain, and swelling. For most women these symptoms are annoying, but do not require treatment with prescription diuretics. I begin by recommending a low-salt diet. In the above-mentioned studies of calcium and magnesium, fluid retention diminished, so these supplements are also recommended. If these fail, and if significant weight gain is documented during the luteal phase for more than one cycle, diuretics may be tried. Spironolactone is a reasonable choice because it is a low-potency, potassium-sparing agent associated that is thought less likely to produce diuretic dependence or rebound cyclic edema when discontinued than the thiazides do. When dramatic cyclic edema is noted throughout the cycle, the patient should be referred to an internist for the evaluation of idiopathic cyclic edema, a renal disorder that can be aggravated by improper use of diuretics.

Breast tenderness is another frequent somatic complaint in PMS. Initial management should include the use of a support bra throughout the day. Anecdotal evidence also suggests that elimination of caffeine from the diet can be helpful. When breast tenderness is severe and does not respond to these measures, bromocriptine has been shown to reduce premenstrual breast tenderness significantly, although it may cause side effects, including nausea and constipation. A starting dose of 1.25 mg/day should be initiated and titrated, according to symptom severity and toleration of side effects.

15. Does hormonal therapy play a role in PMS treatment?

For many years a prominent treatment for PMS was the luteal phase administration of progesterone by vaginal suppository, usually given in doses of 200 to 400 mg/day. As already discussed, there have been more recent double-blind, placebo-controlled studies indicating that progesterone provides no more relief from PMS symptoms than placebo, thus there is clearly no scientific evidence to suggest the efficacy of this cumbersome treatment. Oral micronized progesterone has been shown to improve symptoms much more than placebo; however, its use is not currently approved by the Food and Drug Administration for any indication, and it is not currently marketed in the United States. Given the many alternatives to both natural progesterone and progestin therapy, and the lack of solid scientific evidence suggesting their efficacy, these agents are best not used in the treatment of PMS.

A small number of studies have assessed the chronic administration of estradiol in the treatment of PMS, based on the hypothesis that symptoms may be related to late luteal phase estrogen withdrawal. These studies have generally found chronic administration of estrogen to be more effective than placebo in the treatment of premenstrual symptoms; however, long-term treatment is complicated by PMS-like side effects from oral progestins required to prevent endometrial hyperplasia. Additionally, the long-term effects of chronic estradiol administration are not known. Further investigation of estradiol therapy is required before this treatment can be widely recommended.

Oral contraceptive pills have also been tried as a potential treatment of PMS, based on the principle that they replace endogenous menstrual cyclicity with constant levels of estrogen and progestin throughout the cycle. The only placebo-controlled studies of oral contraceptive pills in PMS did not use the lower-dose pills currently available, therefore no definitive judgment can be made about their efficacy. What can be gleaned from the literature is that oral contraceptive pills do improve symptoms of dysmenorrhea, yet PMS symptoms or pretreatment depression can occasionally be precipitated or worsened by oral contraceptive pill use. This treatment should therefore be reserved for women for whom the chief complaint is dysmenorrhea, and an alternative form of contraception should be used in women with significant affective premenstrual symptoms.

16. When are psychotropic agents indicated?

One often encounters premenstrual worsening of an underlying disorder of mood or anxiety rather than a pure case of PMS. When this is the case, the treatment should focus on the underlying condition. Women with a history of an anxiety or a panic disorder with premenstrual worsening may be treated by increasing the benzodiazepine dosage or adding a benzodiazepine to an existing agent for the last 10 to 14 days of the menstrual cycle. When symptoms of mania or of complex partial seizures appear to break through previously adequate treatment during the last few days of the menstrual cycle, one may aim to increase levels of the mood-stabilizing agent or antiepileptic to prevent this breakthrough. The same holds true for premenstrual worsening or recrudescence of major depression; the antidepressant dosage should be increased or augmented as one would normally do in a case of treatment-resistant depression. The question of augmentation for only part of the cycle proves tricky, as the experiment by Schmidt and associates indicated that the provocative event of the hormone cycle that triggers premenstrual symptoms may in fact occur much earlier in the cycle than currently thought. Therefore, augmentation should probably be continuous throughout the cycle. Only two psychotropic agents have been demonstrated through rigorous double-blind studies to be efficacious in women with PMS and with no comorbid disorder. The first is alprazolam, but a recent attempt at reproducing these results found this agent no more effective than placebo. Alprazolam was given in doses of 0.25 mg q.i.d. as needed during the luteal phase. The discrepancy in results between these two studies could be explained by the existence of a subgroup of women with PMS who have an anxiety or panic diathesis. The obvious advantage to treatment with alprazolam is that it can be given only during the symptomatic period because of its direct anxiolytic properties. The major side effect reported was drowsiness, and in one sample withdrawal anxiety was experienced in 13% of treated subjects. Therefore the clinician should be alert for symptoms of withdrawal or dependence.

The second treatment proven efficacious in prospective, double-blind, independently reproducible studies is the serotonin-reuptake inhibitor called fluoxetine. Fluoxetine has been found to reduce dramatically the affective and behavioral symptoms of PMS, with less definitive improvement in somatic symptoms. In one study, 20 women who were established prospectively to have PMS and did not respond to placebo were subsequently randomized to receive either 20 mg fluoxetine/day or placebo for two consecutive menstrual cycles. Nine of ten subjects receiving fluoxetine had a significant decrease in symptoms compared to only two of ten in the placebo group. Some side effects such as nausea, change in appetite, sexual dysfunction, headache, and dizziness were reported, although all responders elected to continue on fluoxetine following the completion of the study. Other studies looking at serotonergic agents have also shown promising results. Clomipramine has been more effective than placebo in a few smaller trials.

When patients are unable to tolerate treatment with a serotonin-reuptake inhibitor because of the side effects of headache, jitteriness, or nausea, a tricyclic antidepressant should be tried. Women who have not responded to another medication may have a good therapeutic response to a variable dose of nortriptyline. Women with premenstrual anxiety and irritable bowel syndrome respond quite well to tricyclic antidepressants.

17. What are the risks and benefits of inducing menopause as a treatment for PMS?

The most definitive treatment for PMS is stopping menses. This can be done medically with the use of a GnRH agonist, usually administered intranasally or in depot form. Danazol has also been used successfully to suppress ovulation in PMS treatment, but its high rate of side effects make it a less desirable choice. The obvious drawback of ovarian suppression is that it exposes women to the known risks of menopause such as osteoporosis and coronary artery disease. (The agents themselves are also expensive.) In patients with severe PMS that had proved refractory to any of the treatments suggested above, a temporary suppression of ovarian function will have initial diagnostic value, as persistent symptoms in the absence of ovarian steroid function must preclude a diagnosis of PMS. Therapeutic ovarian suppression can only be maintained for a 6 month course, however, because of the risk of osteoporosis, and patients should be counseled regarding calcium supplementation and appropriate exercise to minimize bone loss as much as possible. A recently published study has provided preliminary evidence that combining the GnRH agonist with postmenopausal doses of estrogen and progestin "added back" will relieve menopausal symptoms and prevent bone loss while maintaining efficacy in the treatment of PMS. Because of the ease of administration of the GnRH agonists, a total hysterectomy is no longer necessary in severe cases of PMS and should be reserved for women with comorbid gynecologic disease such as fibroid tumors or endometriosis.

Treatments for Premenstrual Symptoms

TREATMENT	APPROPRIATE FOR	WHEN TO USE
Psychoeducation	Patients with mild to	Initial treatment
Cognitive and behavioral therapy	moderate symptoms	Luteal phase
Lifestyle changes		
Calcium 1000 q.d.	Patients with mild to	Initial treatment
Magnesium 360 mg q.d.	moderate symptoms	Luteal phase
Diuretics	Patients with severe bloating only	After trying sodium restriction Luteal phase

Table continued on following page.

Treatments for Premenstrual Symptoms (Cont.)

TREATMENT	APPROPRIATE FOR	WHEN TO USE
Bromocriptine	Patients with severe mastalgia only	After trying a support bra, xanthine restriction Luteal phase
Nonsteroidal antiinflammatory drugs	Patients with arthralgias, myalgias, headache	When symptomatic Luteal phase
Anxiolytics Benzodiazepines Buspirone	Patients with prominent premenstrual anxiety, panic, or irritability	Following less invasive treatment failure, or as initial treatment if symptoms are severe Luteal phase
Antidepressant Selective serotonin reuptake inhibitors Trycyclic antidepressants	Patients with prominent premenstrual mood disturbance	Following less invasive treatment failure, or as initial treatment if symptoms are severe Throughout cycle
Gonadotropin-releasing hormone agonists Danazol	Patients with severe treatment refractory symptoms	Following less invasive treatment May be used to induce amenorrhea for a maximum of 6 months unless low-dose HRT is added back

18. Are there any other management considerations that the clinician should consider when treating a patient with PMS?
When advising a patient about potential pharmacologic treatment for PMS, she should be informed that none of the drugs currently used have been approved by the FDA for this purpose. When considering a pharmacologic treatment, one should always establish that the patient is using a reliable form of contraception in order to prevent fetal intrauterine exposure to psychotropic agents, the long-term effects of which are unknown. Additionally, because most women require long-term treatment, thoughtful consideration of both side-effect profile and cost should be made. Once a successful program has been established, the frequency of follow-up depends on the patient's needs. She should be counseled to expect occasional greater severity of symptoms. The daily rating scales should be reinstituted whenever a treatment regime requires alteration.

19. What will the future bring in terms of understanding the etiology and treatment of PMS?
The constant struggle to develop more sophisticated models for the etiology of PMS has brought us closer to understanding the multifactorial nature of the occurrence of psychiatric disorders. Future research is thus being directed toward uncovering the complex interactions in genetic predisposition toward mood and anxiety disorders, the potential triggering events of the ovulatory cycle, and the environmental factors present in women with this syndrome. These women may, in fact, represent a heterogeneous group, differing from one another in which axis, or axes, contain the primary dysregulation. These differences need to be explored and may reveal differences in response to treatment as well. The risks for recurrent psychopathology throughout the female reproductive life cycle, including puerperal illness and recurrence at the time of menopause, should also be investigated through rigorous longitudinal studies that will help to further clarify the nature of the complex interrelationship between mood and female reproductive hormonal flux.

BIBLIOGRAPHY

1. Blackstrom T, Hansson-Malmstrom Y, Lindhe B, et al: Oral contraceptives in premenstrual syndrome: A randomized comparison of triphasic and monophasic preparations. Contraception 46:253–268, 1992.
2. Chuong CJ, Dawson EB: Critical evaluation of nutritional factors in the pathophysiology and treatment of premenstrual syndrome. 35(3):679–692, 1992.
3. DeJong R, Rubinow D, Roy-Byrne P, et al: Premenstrual mood disorder and psychiatric illness. Am J Psychiatry 142:1359, 1985.

4. Freeman E, Rickels K, Sondheimer SJ, Polansky M: Ineffectiveness of progesterone suppository treatment for premenstrual syndrome. JAMA 264:349, 1990.

5. Harrison WM, Endicott J, Nee J: Treatment of premenstrual depression with nortriptyline: A pilot study. J Clin Psychiatry 50:136, 1989.

6. Harrison WM, Endicott J, Nee J, et al: Characteristics of women seeking treatment for premenstrual syndrome. Psychosomatics 30:405, 1989.

7. McEwen BS, Parsons BS: Gonadal steroid action on the brain: Neurochemistry and neuropharmacology. Annu Rev Pharmacol Toxicol 22:555–558, 1982.

8. Mortola JF, Girton L, Fischer U: Successful treatment of severe premenstrual syndrome by combined use of gonadotropin-releasing hormone agonist and estrogen/progestin. J Clin Endocrinol Metab 71:252A–F, 1991.

9. Muse KN, Cetel NS, Futterman LA, Yen SSC: The premenstrual syndrome: Effects of "medical ovariectomy." N Engl J Med 311:1345, 1984.

10. Parry BL, Mahan AM, Mostofi N, et al: Light therapy of late luteal phase dysphoric disorder: An extended study. Am J Psychiatry 150:1417–1419, 1993.

11. Pearlstein T, Rivera-Tovar A, Frank E, et al: Nonmedical management of late luteal phase dysphoric disorder. J Psychother Pract Res 1:49–55, 1992.

12. Pearlstein TB, Frank E, Rivera-Tova A, et al: Prevalence of axis I and axis II disorders in women with late luteal phase dysphoric disorder. J Affect Disord 20:129, 1990.

13. Rubinow D, Roy-Byrne P, Hoban C, et al: Prospective assessment of menstrually related mood disorders. Am J Psychiatry 141:684–686, 1984.

14. Schmidt PJ, Grover GN, Rubinow DR: Alprazolam in the treatment of premenstrual syndrome: A double-blind placebo controlled trial. Arch Gen Psychiatry 50:467–473, 1993.

15. Schmidt PJ, Nieman LK, Grover GN, et al: Lack of effect of induced menses on symptoms in women with premenstrual syndrome. N Engl J Med 324:1174, 1991.

16. Severino SK, Moline ML: Premenstrual Syndrome: A Clinician's Guide. New York, Guilford Press, 1989.

17. Smith S, Rinehart JS, Ruddock VE, Schiff I: Treatment of premenstrual syndrome with alprazolam: Results of a double-blind, placebo-controlled, randomized crossover clinical trial. Obstet Gynecol 70:37, 1987.

18. Stone AB, Pearlstein TB, Brown WA: Fluoxetine in the treatment of late luteal phase dysphoric disorder. J Clin Psychiatry 52:290, 1991.

19. Stout AL, Steege JF, Blazer DG, George LK: Comparison of lifetime psychiatric diagnoses in premenstrual syndrome clinic and community samples. J Nerv Ment Dis 174:517, 1986.

20. Wurtman JJ, Brzezinski A, Wurtman RJ, Laferrere B: Effect of nutrient intake on premenstrual depression. Am J Obstet Gynecol 161:1228–1234, 1989.

21. Yonkers KA, White K: Premenstrual exacerbation of depression: One process or two? J Clin Psychiatry 53:289–292, 1992.

62. PSYCHIATRIC DISORDERS AND PREGNANCY

Doris C. Gundersen, M.D.

1. Describe hyperemesis gravidarum.

Hyperemesis gravidarum is a psychosomatic illness with both organic and psychological components. Social and cultural factors also contribute to its development. The disorder typically begins between the eighth and twelfth weeks of pregnancy, during the peak incidence of morning sickness. The vomiting is of such severity as to require hospitalization for treatment of dehydration and electrolyte disturbances. Cross-cultural studies have repeatedly demonstrated an incidence of 0.05–1%. In 40% of cases, past histories of gastric disorders, including vomiting, are present.

Early psychoanalytic writers believed that the nausea and vomiting of pregnancy represented a rejection of femininity or a wish not to be pregnant. Others viewed the illness as a manifestation of intrapsychic conflict. The vomiting represented the defense mechanism of "undoing." Nausea and vomiting occurred when the woman attempted to throw off something that she wished had not happened. Whatever the specific psychological causes, psychosocial factors play an important causative role. Hyperemesis gravidarum is associated with below-average intelligence, strong dependency, and immature personalities, including histrionic personality disorder. Women with hyperemesis appear to receive less support from spouses and parents. Hyperemesis gravidarum is often viewed as a maladaptive coping behavior to express dysphoria related to unmet needs. The literature supports this theory. In the vast majority of cases, symptoms resolve when the woman is hospitalized and supportive care is available.

Treatment for hyperemesis gravidarum is supportive. Brief hospitalization, intravenous fluids, and antiemetics are used. Psychotherapy to address conflictual relationships is encouraged. Social work assistance to identify additional community supports also may be appropriate.

2. How are pregnant women with eating disorders diagnosed and managed?

Few reports of anorexia nervosa associated with pregnancy are found in the literature. To some extent, the two conditions are mutually exclusive. The endocrine abnormalities associated with anorexia nervosa substantially diminish fertility. The paucity of published information on bulimia in pregnancy may reflect the failure of physicians to identify the problem, despite an incidence of up to 13% in women of childbearing age.

The possibility of an eating disorder should be considered in any woman whose pregravid weight is subnormal or who fails to gain appropriate weight as pregnancy progresses. Any patient who casually mentions that she has an eating problem should be carefully questioned. An eating disorder should be suspected in patients who are excessively preoccupied with weight gain and body image during pregnancy. A history of persistent vomiting before or during pregnancy should be investigated. A psychosocial history may reveal comorbidity with other psychiatric conditions such as depression or chemical dependency in bulimic women.

Psychological conflicts thought to be important in the development of eating disorders concern adult sexuality, body image, autonomy, dependency, and relationships with parents. Because such issues become highlighted during pregnancy, exacerbations of eating disorders are likely. Women with active eating disorders at the time of conception typically experience many difficulties during pregnancy. They gain less weight and have smaller babies with lower Apgar scores. Serious complications of bulimia include acid-base disturbances, electrolyte imbalances, and disruption of normal intestinal motility. Anorexic women with reduced weight gain during pregnancy have associated intrauterine growth retardation. In one Danish study of 50 pregnant women treated for anorexia nervosa, 7 perinatal deaths were reported, with 6 attributed to prematurity.

Hospitalization is recommended for the eating disordered pregnant patient with excessive weight loss, severe metabolic disarray, or prominent symptoms of depression. Psychotherapy and nutritional counseling should complement standard prenatal care. Enlisting the support of families to monitor weight gain and nutrition is helpful. Ideally, eating disorders should be identified before conception. The afflicted woman should be advised to delay pregnancy until the eating disorder is truly in remission.

3. What risks do illicit substances, tobacco, and alcohol pose to the child exposed in utero?
The incidence of substance abuse in women of childbearing age is high. The risk for developmental abnormalities in the fetus of a drug abusing mother is significant.

Cocaine-abusing women have a significantly higher rate of spontaneous abortion, abruptio placentae, and stillbirths. Peripherally, cocaine causes a marked rise in maternal catecholamines with concomitant increases in blood pressure and heart rate. Acute myocardial infarction or cardiac arrhythmias may result. Maternal brain hemorrhage has been reported. Prolonged administration of cocaine results in depletion of presynaptic intraneuronal neurotransmitters, which is associated with profound depression. Increased levels of circulating catecholamines also lead to increased uterine vascular resistance and decreased uterine blood flow. Fetal hypoxia is produced by the diminished placental perfusion. Cocaine freely crosses the placenta. Fetal hypertension and tachycardia are direct effects of the cocaine. The cocaine-exposed fetus risks hemorrhagic cerebral lesions. Intrauterine growth retardation is common.

Neonates of cocaine-abusing mothers demonstrate low birth weight and low Apgar scores. They have a higher than expected rate of genitourinary tract malformations and cardiac anomalies. An increased frequency of sudden infant death syndrome (SIDS) is reported. Neonates with in utero exposure to cocaine exhibit transient neurobehavioral symptoms, including tremulousness, hyperreflexia, and hypertonicity. They are irritable and less consolable and have abnormal sleep patterns. They are at high risk for abuse and neglect. Cocaine appears in significant quantities in breast milk. Long-term administration of cocaine may result in irreversible decreases in dopamine, persistent mood dysfunction, and an inability to experience pleasure.

Infants of **opiate-dependent mothers** face greater perinatal morbidity and mortality. In the first trimester, a common complication is spontaneous abortion. A 30–50% increased risk for growth retardation is observed.

The majority of drug-dependent pregnant women must rely on the street supply of narcotics. Because of the irregularity with which they receive opiates, intermittent withdrawal may occur, leading to uterine irritability. The incidence of premature labor is increased. Meconium aspiration is a common complication. Infants born to drug-addicted mothers often suffer from septicemia, hyperbilirubinemia, intracranial hemorrhage and hypoglycemia. They demonstrate a withdrawal syndrome, characterized by irritability, poor feeding, respiratory difficulties, and tremulousness. Such infants are difficult to console and, like cocaine-exposed babies, are at high risk for abuse and neglect.

Heavy tobacco use doubles the rate of spontaneous abortion. Smoking is linked to intrauterine growth retardation, premature labor, and low birth weight. One study assessed over 700 children of mothers who smoked during pregnancy. At the age of 3 years, the children demonstrated decreased height and weight compared with unexposed 3-year-old controls. Statistically significant cognitive impairment in the tobacco-exposed children persisted, even after controlling for environmental variables.

Cannabis abuse is also associated with negative effects on fetal growth. Delta-9-tetrahydrocannabinol elevates carbon monoxide levels in the mother, resulting in poorer oxygenation in the fetus. Elevations in maternal heart rate and blood pressure reduce placental blood flow to the fetus. Finally, delta-9-tetrahydrocannabinol freely crosses the placenta and is exceptionally fat-soluble, requiring up to 30 days for the fetus to excrete.

Alcohol and its metabolite acetaldehyde have direct toxic effects on cellular growth and metabolism. Five to six drinks of hard liquor per day are associated with the most serious teratogenicity, called "fetal alcohol syndrome." Abnormalities include mental retardation, cardiac defects, growth retardation, and facial and limb deformities. Irritability in infancy and attention deficit symptoms during childhood are characteristic findings. The severity of the syndrome depends on the amount of alcohol exposure, the gestational age of exposure, and the genetic constitution of the infant. No safe level of alcohol consumption has been determined.

Summary of Major Risks of Drug Use During Pregnancy

Cocaine	Maternal depression, cerebrovascular accident Fetal cerebral hemorrhage Spontaneous abortion Low birth weight Increased rate of sudden infant death syndrome Neurobehavioral problems in neonates
Opiates	Increased perinatal morbidity and mortality Spontaneous abortion Fetal growth retardation Premature labor Neonatal septicemia, liver damage, cerebrovascular accidents Neonatal addiction and withdrawal
Cannabis	Slowed fetal growth Fetal hypoxia
Tobacco	Spontaneous abortion Slowed fetal growth Low birth weight Premature labor
Alcohol	Fetal alcohol syndrome includes • Mental retardation • Cardiac defects • Growth retardation • Facial and limb deformities

4. How should a substance-abusing woman be managed during pregnancy?

Clinical management of substance-abusing women during pregnancy can be challenging. Drug-abusing women commonly neglect health care in general. Up to 75% fail to seek prenatal care. Drug abuse should be suspected in women who present late for prenatal care or have poor weight gain or other signs of compromised health. The patient also should be screened for other psychiatric conditions that predispose to substance abuse, such as anxiety and depression. Most pregnant women will disclose a history of drug or alcohol abuse if questioned in a nonjudgmental, straightforward manner. Authoritarian moralizing leads to an avoidance of prenatal care altogether. Providing an opportunity for treatment is the most effective strategy.

The first intervention should be to educate the patient about the hazards of drug use during pregnancy. Some will discontinue use on their own in response to the counseling. They should be offered prenatal care in conjunction with treatment for substance abuse. Outpatient care is usually indicated, but hospitalization may be needed for more severe cases, such as mothers addicted to tranquilizers or barbiturates in addition to opiates. In some cases, it is necessary to pursue involuntary commitment to protect the fetus.

Treatment goals should include developing a strong support system to allow the woman to break ties with the drug culture. Social stressors such as poor housing and inadequate income must be remedied. Emotional problems, including depression, low self-esteem, and poor coping skills, should be addressed in individual as well as group therapy. Urine toxicology screening detects relapse.

Pharmacotherapy during pregnancy may be used to prevent or lessen withdrawal symptoms, to diminish cocaine craving, and/or to treat comorbid psychiatric disorders. The benefits of using a particular drug must be carefully weighed against the risks posed to the fetus. If possible, medication should be avoided in the first trimester. It should be administered in the lowest effective doses for the briefest periods possible.

Dopamine agonists decrease acute cocaine craving. Bromocriptine has been used in pregnancy to treat hyperprolactinemia and pituitary adenomas. Multiple studies show no increase in pregnancy complications or untoward effects in the fetus. For severe cocaine craving, bromocriptine, 2.5 to 10 mg/day, may be a reasonable short-term intervention to facilitate abstinence after acute withdrawal. The tricyclic antidepressant desipramine also reduces cocaine craving and appears to be effective in facilitating longer-term abstinence. It should be avoided in the first trimester and during the few weeks before delivery.

Detoxification from opiates during pregnancy is possible but extremely difficult and fraught with possible hazards of abortion in the first trimester and fetal distress in the third. If detoxification is requested, it should be attempted from the fourteenth to twenty-eighth weeks of gestation and should not exceed a taper of more than 5 mg/week.

The absolute safety of methadone during pregnancy is uncertain. Infants have a lower birth weight, shorter length, and smaller head circumference. They suffer from a greater incidence of SIDS. However, methadone likely poses less risk to the fetus than do severe withdrawal, infectious diseases contracted by the mother from contaminated needles, and absence of prenatal care. Research suggests that the results for patients receiving methadone maintenance along with good prenatal care and counseling are comparable to those for nonaddicted mothers.

A vulnerable period for relapse is in the postpartum period. Treatment and supportive measures should continue. Finally, the pediatrician must consider relapse in the mother of any infant exhibiting signs of neglect and/or abuse. Child protective services should be notified.

5. Describe the potential hazards of in-utero exposure to mood stabilizers.

In most industrialized nations, about 0.1% of the population receives maintenance lithium therapy for bipolar illness; 50% are women, many in the fertile age range. Of all the psychotropic agents, lithium warrants the most caution during pregnancy. It should be avoided altogether if possible because of the potential risks to the developing fetus and neonate.

Lithium is a known teratogen in the first trimester. An increased rate of cardiovascular abnormalities is observed. The most recent epidemiologic data suggest a risk of 0.1% for Ebstein's anomaly. The risk for any congenital abnormality in lithium-exposed infants is estimated to be between 4 and 12%, a rate 2–3 times greater than that in untreated comparison groups. Stillbirth and Down's syndrome are associated with lithium exposure during the first 12 weeks of pregnancy.

In the last trimester, lithium inhibits hormone release from the thyroid gland of the developing fetus, thereby stimulating increased TSH production and resulting in goiter. Lithium exerts an insulinlike effect on carbohydrate metabolism, leading to macrosomia. Premature delivery and increased perinatal mortality are potential complications.

Neonates exhibit decreased renal clearance. The half-life of lithium is generally prolonged, increasing the risk for toxicity. Lithium toxicity in the newborn is characterized by hypothermia, bradycardia, shallow respiration, and cyanosis. Hypotonia and feeding difficulties are not uncommon. Such effects are presumed to be reversible, but conclusive studies are lacking.

Animal studies suggest that behavioral teratogenicity may result from in-utero exposure to lithium. In one study, rats with in-utero exposure demonstrated significant impairment in performance on T-mazes.

A large Scandinavian study of lithium-exposed children who were born without physical malformations and had reached the age of 5 years or older revealed no significant neurobehavioral differences compared with unexposed but genetically similar siblings. The study does not rule out the possibility of behavioral teratogenicity in humans but suggests that, if present, the changes are subtle. Finally, it is not clear whether in-utero exposure to lithium increases the risk for behavioral or affective abnormalities later in life.

Despite such risks, lithium is the safest mood-stabilizing agent currently available. Carbamazepine is associated with craniofacial abnormalities (11%), developmental delay (20%), and digital hypoplasia (26%). The risk of spina bifida and other neural tube defects with valproic acid is between 1 and 4%. The use of these anticonvulsants during pregnancy is not justified except perhaps in the clinical setting of nonresponse to other treatment modalities and severe, life-threatening illness. Clonazepam, a benzodiazepine with anticonvulsant and antimanic properties, proved to be the least teratogenic of six anticonvulsant agents in mice. Whether this holds true for humans is yet to be determined.

6. What is known about the safety of antidepressants in pregnant women?

Tricyclic antidepressants have been studied the most extensively. Early reports in the 1970s suggested that use of tricyclic antidepressants in the first trimester of pregnancy was associated with limb reduction deformities. This conclusion was based largely on sporadic case reports. Subsequently, large-scale evaluations in a number of different countries failed to identify a link between tricyclic use and congenital malformations of any kind. Animal studies give conflicting data. It is recommended that this class of medication be avoided in the first trimester.

During the final six months of pregnancy, the tricyclics are considered relatively safe. Because they readily cross the placenta, the developing fetus is vulnerable to anticholinergic side effects, including tachyarrhythmias. Thus the less anticholinergic compounds, nortriptyline and desipramine, are recommended for pregnant women needing somatic treatment for depression.

After delivery, the neonate no longer has the support of maternal circulation to metabolize drugs. Toxicity may result, characterized by respiratory distress, cyanosis, hypertonia, irritability, and even seizures. In addition, a tricyclic withdrawal syndrome has been described, consisting of colic, irritability, difficulty with feeding, and tachypnea. The argument is made for gradually withdrawing the medication several weeks before the estimated date of delivery to provide a washout period for the fetus and to lessen the risk for anticholinergic complications. If necessary, the antidepressants may be reinstated immediately after delivery.

The effect of tricyclic compounds on the developing central nervous system of humans is not known. Neurobehavioral sequelae have been documented in animals. Studies have revealed decreased exploratory responses, delayed reflex development, and changes in hypothalamic dopamine levels in rats exposed to imipramine. The changes in behavioral response persist into adulthood. No human studies have clarified this issue. In one study, 23 children were followed until the age of 2 years after in-utero exposure to tricyclic antidepressants. No neurobehavioral abnormalities were identified.

Monoamine oxidase inhibitors (MAOIs) are known teratogens in animals. Preclinical studies suggest that this teratogenicity may also apply to humans. Given the risk of an MAOI-precipitated hypertensive crisis and the availability of safer alternatives, MAOIs are contraindicated in pregnancy.

Less is known about the newer antidepressant agents. Of 500 women taking Prozac during the first trimester of pregnancy, no predominant malformations were reported in their infants. Even fewer data are available for Zoloft, Paxil, Wellbutrin, BuSpar, and Desyrel. These agents should generally be avoided during pregnancy until a more substantial database is established to support their safety.

7. What is known about the safety of antipsychotic agents during pregnancy?

Animal studies have not demonstrated teratogenicity with the use of neuroleptics in the period of organogenesis, even when they are administered in toxic doses. Early studies examining children exposed to neuroleptics before 10 weeks of gestation suggested an increased occurrence of congenital anomalies compared with unexposed controls. However, many confounding factors, such as maternal age, gravidity, previous miscarriage or pregnancy complications, alcohol or tobacco use, polypharmacy, and timing of exposure, were not considered. More contemporary reviews of the literature, including several prospective studies of tens of thousands of women exposed to neuroleptics in the first trimester, do not support an increased rate of malformations.

Neuroleptics, like the tricyclic antidepressants, readily cross the placenta. Toxicity is similar to that seen in adults. Extrapyramidal symptoms, including hypertonicity, restlessness, and tremor, are observed in neonates of mothers taking antipsychotic agents at the time of delivery. Tachycardia, urinary retention, and functional bowel obstruction are seen in infants of mothers taking low-potency (and therefore strongly anticholinergic) antipsychotic drugs. Maintaining pregnant women on high-potency neuroleptics such as Haldol, with gradual discontinuation 5–10 days before delivery, minimizes complications in the newborn.

Postnatal behavioral changes, including poor performance in maze learning and shock avoidance, has been demonstrated in animals, whether or not exposure occurred before or after the completion of organogenesis. Rats exposed to Haldol have decreased dopamine receptor activity.

Data about long-term behavioral consequences in humans are lacking. One study of 14 children exposed to antipsychotics in utero failed to reveal memory or learning deficits by age 4 years. Another study of 52 children exposed prenatally to thorazine failed to identify behavioral abnormalities or changes in IQ scores compared with controls. A cohort of 3,056 infants exposed to phenothiazines at various times during gestation showed no statistically significant differences in IQ scores by age 4 years. More prolonged prospective follow-up studies are needed to establish the possible relationship between such drugs and subtle long-term behavioral or cognitive abnormalities

Little is known about the safety of atypical antipsychotic drugs such as clozapine and risperidone. They should be avoided during pregnancy.

Prophylaxis against extrapyramidal symptoms (dystonias, tremor, akathisia) is not recommended. Although not implicated as frank teratogens, anticholinergic agents used to treat the side effects of antipsychotic drugs are best prescribed on an as-needed basis and withdrawn at the earliest possible time to avoid complications in the neonate.

8. What is known about the effects of benzodiazepines on the developing fetus?

Little is known about the effects of lorazepam, alprazolam, or clonazepam on the developing fetus. The largest amount of data exists for diazepam. Increased rates of oral clefts in infants exposed to diazepam in utero were reported in the 1970s. However, several large prospective studies failed to demonstrate an increased risk of craniofacial or other malformations, even with the first-trimester exposure. Despite the increased use of benzodiazepines over the last several years, investigators have not observed a concomitant rise in the incidence of cleft lip or palate abnormalities.

Pregnant women should be advised that even with early exposure, the risk of cleft malformation is approximately 0.4%. As with all drugs, benzodiazepines should be withheld in the first trimester of pregnancy or at least until after the tenth week of gestation when palate closure is complete. In addition to cleft palate abnormalities, a syndrome reminiscent of fetal alcohol syndrome has been reported in fetuses with in-utero exposure to benzodiazepines. However, the most recent prospective data are contradictory.

The literature suggests that use of benzodiazepines in the second and third trimesters is probably safe. However, with prolonged administration, cord plasma concentrations in the fetus may become greater than in the maternal circulation. Transient neurologic deficits, hypotonia, and respiratory depression have been reported in neonates born to mothers medicated in the later stages of pregnancy. In addition, neonates are at risk for withdrawal symptoms within a few days to 3 weeks after birth. Gradual discontinuation of diazepam several weeks before delivery is recommended.

Abnormalities of motor and arousal processes in rodents exposed to diazepam in utero have been demonstrated. The significance of these findings in humans is not known.

Similar affects on the fetus to those found with benzodiazepines have been reported in mothers taking barbiturates during pregnancy.

Finally, infants born to mothers who are dependent on barbiturates are at risk for serious toxicity and withdrawal symptoms.

9. What legal considerations must be kept in mind in prescribing medication for a pregnant woman with psychiatric illness?

Clinicians must keep in mind that they are treating two patients, the psychiatrically impaired pregnant woman and her unborn child. The literature about psychotropic drug use in pregnant women is primarily retrospective and to some extent anecdotal. Thus the decision to prescribe such medications during pregnancy must be made based on a thoughtful risk-benefit analysis. It is of paramount importance to document the specific benefits that justify the risk. In documenting consent, it is important to indicate the patient's competence to understand the specific risks, benefits, and alternative treatments, including no treatment. Ideally, a course of action should be agreed upon before conception when the woman is psychiatrically stable and documented clearly in treatment records. If the woman deteriorates during the course of pregnancy and becomes incompetent to participate in treatment decisions, temporary guardianship must be pursued so that appropriate psychiatric care can proceed.

10. Describe the management of the bipolar patient who desires pregnancy.

Bipolar disorder (manic-depressive illness) has a mean age of onset in the early twenties, coinciding with childbearing years. The advice offered to bipolar women desiring pregnancy is based on the most recent literature. Bipolar women need prenatal counseling to be advised of the risk of fetal anomalies associated with psychotropic medication. The prospective mother also must be made aware of her risk for manic decompensation when somatic therapy is withdrawn.

Ideally, psychotropic medications should be discontinued several weeks before conception. For the woman who has had a single episode of mania with complete recovery and a long period of stability, slowly tapering medication before attempting to conceive is a reasonable course of action. When a woman taking lithium conceives unknowingly, the drug should be gradually discontinued, because abrupt withdrawal is associated with manic relapse. Close observation should follow. With early and mild relapse, hospitalization with structure, reduced environmental stimulation, and elimination of exacerbating stressors may avert worsening of symptoms. If conservative measures fail, low-dose antipsychotics should be instituted to ameliorate the most severe symptoms, for example, insomnia. An adjuvant benzodiazepine such as clonazepam may reduce the total required dose of either medication used alone. If such measures fail to stabilize the patient, lithium may be reinstated in the second trimester after morphogenesis is complete.

A more difficult decision must be made for women with brittle illness, which is characterized by high relapse risk in the absence of mood-stabilizing medication. The potential morbidity associated with the drugs must be weighed against the likelihood of severe psychiatric symptoms and the associated danger to the mother and her developing child. The decision to continue psychotropic medication throughout pregnancy must be made jointly by the physician and the carefully informed couple wishing to conceive. The consent process, which outlines risks, benefits, and alternative treatments as well as the planned course of action, should be documented carefully in the patient's records.

For women maintained on lithium in the first trimester, fetal ultrasound should be obtained at 18 weeks to rule out cardiac malformations. Women need to understand the prognosis of Ebstein's anomaly. The literature suggests that up to 50% of affected infants die in the first week of life.

If lithium is used during pregnancy, it must be administered in several small doses to decrease the risk of toxicity associated with peak serum levels. Lithium levels should be monitored frequently. In the second trimester, higher doses may be necessary because of the increased glomerular filtration rate in the mother. Minimal effective serum levels should be maintained. The dosage should be reduced by at least 50% at the onset of labor to avoid toxicity due to abrupt falls in renal filtration rates and pronounced fluid shifting.

Bipolar patients are 4–5 times more likely to develop mania in the postpartum period than at any other time. Clinicians should follow such women closely. Extending the postpartum hospital stay for longer observation is warranted. Provisions for continued monitoring and support by family or professional agencies should be arranged before discharge.

11. Describe the management of women who develop depression during pregnancy.

Several recent prospective studies have demonstrated an incidence of depression during pregnancy as high as 10–20%. Symptoms are generally of less severity than those observed with postpartum mood disorders. Risk factors for developing depression during pregnancy include a history of elective abortion, ambivalence about the pregnancy, and unrelated bereavement. Women prone to depression during pregnancy do not appear to differ from nondepressed women in regard to stressful life events, level of marital satisfaction, or personal and/or family histories of mood disorders.

Despite the relatively high number of women who develop depression during pregnancy, not all require pharmacotherapy. Many women develop minor depressive symptoms in the first trimester of pregnancy that are more consistent with an adjustment disorder. They usually respond to support, reassurance, and efforts to minimize psychosocial sources of distress. Pharmacotherapy is generally reserved for the most severe depressions characterized by neurovegetative dysfunction, including poor appetite and sleep disturbance. As with all psychotropic medications, the risks associated with pharmacotherapy must be weighed against the risks of withholding treatment.

Tricyclic antidepressants are the drugs of choice for women requiring treatment. The less anticholinergic secondary amines, desipramine and nortriptyline, are preferred. Nonbiologic interventions, such as hospitalization with supportive psychotherapy, should be used to eliminate the need for initiating medications in the first trimester. Blood levels of the antidepressant should be monitored frequently as the pregnancy progresses and maternal fluid shifts occur. The medication should be tapered and withdrawn before the onset of labor to avoid adverse effects in the newborn.

A severely depressed woman expressing suicidal intent and/or showing signs of nutritional or physical deterioration represents a psychiatric emergency. Electroconvulsive therapy is the treatment of choice in such patients, who require rapid response.

12. Describe the management of women with psychotic illnesses during pregnancy.

Women with schizophrenia are at high risk for exacerbation during pregnancy. For each month medication is withheld, approximately 10% of schizophrenics will relapse. It is estimated that 65% of unmedicated schizophrenics and 26% of those maintained on psychotropics will relapse during pregnancy.

Schizophrenia is the most difficult psychiatric disorder to deal with both during pregnancy and in the postpartum period. Psychotic women often have exaggerated and distorted responses to the somatic changes associated with pregnancy. Not infrequently, psychotic denial of the pregnancy prevents participation in prenatal care. Health professionals caring for them may develop intense and conflicting feelings toward the patient, ranging from anger to sadness.

When pregnancy is confirmed, if the patient is stable, a trial of no medication in the first trimester, with a plan to reinstitute treatment at the first sign of psychosis is recommended. A woman who first becomes psychotic during pregnancy should be thoroughly evaluated to identify reversible organic causes. Hospitalization or intense case management is desirable to ensure compliance with prenatal care and perhaps to reduce the total amount of medication required for adequate stabilization.

High-potency neuroleptics, such as perphenazine or haloperidol, should be given at the minimal effective dose for controlling the most disabling symptoms. As with other psychiatric disorders, complete amelioration of symptoms is not the goal in managing a pregnant woman with schizophrenia. Maintenance of self-care and moderately good functioning are more realistic achievements. Antiparkinson agents, such as Cogentin or Artane, should be given in the smallest effective dose on an as-needed basis.

A close obstetric-psychiatric liaison must be established and maintained throughout the pregnancy and postpartum period. When the patient is transferred to the obstetrics department for labor and delivery, she should be accompanied by psychiatrically trained nursing staff.

During the postpartum period, schizophrenic mothers often demonstrate limited ability to attend to the infant or to recognize its needs. This should be anticipated by making provisions for supervised feedings and visits with the infant. The decision must be made about the appropriateness of a referral to child protective services for ongoing evaluation and monitoring of the mother's ability to care for her infant. If the mother shows gross inability or severely impaired reality testing, it may be necessary for the infant to be temporarily placed in foster care.

Schizophrenic patients have an increased risk of postpartum psychotic decompensation. Extended hospitalization should be planned. Many schizophrenic mothers are unmarried and have impoverished support systems. Before discharge, arrangements for a visiting nurse and involvement of social agencies should be made.

Finally, contraception should be strongly encouraged to prevent a close succession of pregnancies in vulnerable women. Noncompliance with oral contraceptives and barrier methods is common. The patient should be informed of the availability of long-acting injectable preparations such as Depo-Provera and Norplant. The option of tubal ligation should be discussed.

13. How is the patient with anxiety disorder managed during pregnancy?

Anxiety disorders are common in women and tend to aggregate in those of childbearing age. Historically, it was believed that pregnancy was a time of quiescence for women with pregravid histories of anxiety. More recent literature contradicts this assumption. Such conditions tend to worsen during pregnancy. For example, several studies have associated the onset of obsessive compulsive disorder (OCD) with pregnancy and childbirth. Preexisting disease is typically exacerbated by pregnancy. Women with panic disorder also experience a worsening of symptoms during pregnancy, especially in the last trimester and postpartum period.

A considerable volume of literature supports the finding that women with moderate to severe symptoms of anxiety during pregnancy and delivery experience more complications. Preterm labor, preeclampsia, placental abruption, stillbirths, and fetal hypoxia have been reported. Such complications may be related to increases in catecholamine secretion, which result in transient elevations in blood pressure and vasoconstriction of the fetoplacental unit.

The goal of managing anxiety disordered women during pregnancy is to minimize risk to the mother and infant, not to achieve complete control of symptoms. Before instituting pharmacologic treatment, behavioral techniques such as progressive relaxation or biofeedback should be attempted. Such measures, in addition to supportive psychotherapy, may prevent the need for medication or at least minimize the required amount.

If psychotropic medication is required, a tricyclic antidepressant such as nortriptyline is recommended for panic. Benzodiazepines should be avoided if possible. If used, the smallest effective dose for the shortest amount of time is the goal. Gradual tapering and discontinuation should occur before the estimated date of confinement to avoid toxicity and/or withdrawal in the neonate.

14. Is electroconvulsive therapy safe for pregnant women?

Electroconvulsive therapy (ECT) is an underutilized treatment modality in pregnant as well as nonpregnant patients. It is an excellent therapeutic alternative when psychotropic medications have failed or are contraindicated. ECT is considered the first-line treatment in pregnant women requiring a rapid therapeutic response. Studies suggest that ECT is safe for women in any stage of pregnancy. Mortality associated with ECT is less than that observed for inadequately treated depression during pregnancy. The ECT complication rate of 5–6% is less than that for untreated pregnant psychotic women and pregnant women without psychiatric illness. Finally, the rate of miscarriage in the general population is considerably higher than that observed in pregnant women undergoing ECT, suggesting that ECT does not increase the likelihood of miscarriage.

15. Describe the management of the pregnant patient undergoing ECT.

Several steps are taken to decrease potential risk to the mother and fetus:

1. Pelvic examination to rule out vaginal bleeding or cervical dilation is performed before a course of ECT.

372   Psychiatric Disorders and Pregnancy

2. The prolonged gastric emptying time in pregnant women increases the risk of aspiration. Nonessential anticholinergic medications are discontinued to avoid further slowing of gastric transit. A nonparticulate antacid, such as sodium citrate, is administered to raise gastric pH, and thus to minimize the risk of aspiration pneumonitis. After the first trimester, some anesthesiologists recommend intubation.

3. Fetal circulation may be compromised if the gravid uterus is large and heavy enough to compress the inferior vena cava when the patient is in a supine position. Elevating the patient's right hip to displace the uterus to the left can prevent this complication. Pretreatment intravenous hydration is also recommended.

4. Excessive hyperventilation, usually done to lower the seizure threshold, is not recommended. Respiratory alkalosis in the mother hinders oxygen unloading from maternal to fetal hemoglobin. Fetal hypoxia is a real risk.

5. Transient hypertension during a seizure may increase the risk for placental abruption. Intravenous Labetalol is recommended to control blood pressure.

6. Self-limited fetal cardiac arrhythmias may occur during the seizure. External fetal cardiac monitoring is performed throughout the procedure and recovery period.

7. An anticholinergic agent is administered before ECT to prevent excessive vagal bradycardia and to decrease oropharyngeal and tracheal secretions. Atropine, which quickly crosses the placental barrier, may produce fetal tachycardia. Glycopyrrolate has a more limited rate of transfer across the placenta and thus reduces risk to the fetus; it is the preferred anticholinergic drug for pregnant patients undergoing ECT.

8. Adequate relaxation in the mother is essential to prevent injury to the fetus. Fortunately, succinylcholine in ordinary doses does not cross the placenta.

16. Should women taking psychotropic medications breastfeed their infants?

The benefits of breastfeeding are well documented. Human milk possesses antimicrobial and unique trophic properties that benefit the infant. Breastfeeding enhances the process of maternal bonding. Unfortunately, the literature contains little information about psychotropic drug excretion in breast milk. However, all major classes of psychotropic drugs have been isolated in breast milk. Concentrations vary depending on the properties of the individual compound. Drugs that have high protein binding tend to remain in the mother's plasma. Lower molecular weight compounds and compounds with high lipid solubility diffuse into breast milk. Weak bases undergo ion trapping in the relatively acidic milk.

Lithium concentration in breast milk is about 30–50% of that in the mother's serum. Because an infant's regulatory and excretory mechanisms are not fully developed, toxicity is a real risk. Breastfeeding is contraindicated for women requiring maintenance lithium treatment.

In general, **benzodiazepines** should not be given to breastfeeding mothers because of the risk of prolonging physiologic jaundice in the infant. In addition, withdrawal syndromes have been observed in nursing infants exposed to benzodiazepines.

Antidepressants should be used with caution in the nursing mother. Imipramine, nortriptyline, and desipramine are not excreted in breast milk in appreciable quantities. If a mother taking these medications insists on nursing her infant, care should be taken to minimize the infant's exposure. This can be accomplished by having the mother take medication immediately after the breastfeeding that precedes the infant's longest period of sleep. The infant should be observed for signs of drug effect such as sedation or inexplicable irritability. Newer antidepressant agents should be avoided until more data attest to their safety. If a mother requires antipsychotic medication, she is best advised to bottle-feed her infant.

Even when obvious drug effects in the infant are absent, advances in neurobehavioral teratogenicity raise the question of long-term harm to the infant's immature nervous system. More research is needed to determine whether infants exposed to such agents via breast milk risk physical or mental impairment. Lactating women who require psychotropic medication should be encouraged to defer breastfeeding until the potential risks to nursing infants are better understood.

BIBLIOGRAPHY

1. Brandt KR, MacKenzie TB: Obsessive-compulsive disorder exacerbated during pregnancy: A case report. Int J Psychiatry Med 17:361–365, 1987.
2. Calabrese JR, Gulledge DA: Psychotropics during pregnancy and lactation: A review. Psychosomatics 26:413–426, 1985.
3. Chasnoff IJ, Burns WJ, Schnoli SH, Kayreen AB: Cocaine use in pregnancy. N Engl J Med 313:666–669, 1985.
4. Cohen LS: The use of psychotropic drugs during pregnancy and the puerperium. Curr Affect Illness 11:9, 1992.
5. Feingold M, Lyons K, Kaminer Y, et al: Bulimia nervosa in pregnancy. Obstet Gynecol 71:1025–1027, 1988.
6. Hawkins DR, Casiano ME: Major mental illness and childbearing. Psychiatr Clin North Am 10:33–51, 1987.
7. Haynes JS: An update on psychotropic drugs in breastfeeding. Psychiatr Times June 1994.
8. James ME: Cocaine abuse during pregnancy: Psychiatric considerations. Oral presentation, 1990.
9. Katon WJ, Ries RK, Bokan JA, Kleinman A: Hyperemesis gravidarum: A biopsychosocial perspective. Int J Psychiatry Med 10:151–160, 1980.
10. Kerns LL: Treatment of mental disorders in pregnancy: A review of psychotropic drug risks and benefits. J Nerv Ment Dis 174:652–659, 1986.
11. McCance-Katz EF: The consequences of maternal substance abuse for the child exposed in utero. Psychosomatics 32:268–274, 1991.
12. Miller LJ: Clinical strategies for the use of psychotropics during pregnancy. Psychiatr Med 2:275–298, 1991.
13. Milner G, O'leary MM: Anorexia nervosa occurring in pregnancy. Acta Psychiatr Scand 77:491–492, 1988.
14. Miller LJ: Use of electroconvulsive therapy during pregnancy. Hosp Community Psychiatry 45:444–450, 1994.
15. Nurnber HG, Prudic J: Guidelines for treatment of psychosis during pregnancy. Hosp Community Psychiatry 35:67–71, 1984.
16. Oates MR: The treatment of psychiatric disorders in pregnancy and the puerperium. Clin Obstet Gynecol 13:385–395, 1986.
17. O'Hara MW: Social support, life events, and depression during pregnancy and the puerperium. Arch Gen Psychiatry 43:569–573, 1986.
18. Pastuszak A, et al: Pregnancy outcome folowing first trimester exposure to fluoxetine. JAMA 269:2246–2248, 1993.
19. Repke JT, Berger NG: Electroconvulsive therapy in pregnancy. Obstet Gynecol 63:39–41, 1984.
20. Roberts RJ, Blumer J, Gorman R, et al: Transfer of drugs and other chemicals into human milk. Pediatrics 84:924–936, 1989.
21. Robinson GE: The rational use of psychotropic drugs in pregnancy and postpartum. Can J Psychiatry 31:183–190, 1986.
22. Robinson L: Cognitive-behavioral treatment of panic disorder during pregnancy and lactation. Can J Psychiatry 37:523–626, 1992.
23. Schou M: Lithium treatment during pregnancy, delivery and lactation: An update. J Clin Psychiatry 51:410–412, 1990.
24. Sitland-Marken PA, Rickman L, Wells B, et al: Pharmacologic management of acute mania in pregnancy. J Clin Psychopharm 9:78–87, 1989.
25. Spielvogel A, Wile J: Treatment of the psychotic pregnant patient. Psychosomatics 27:487–492, 1986.
26. Stewart DE, Raskin J, Garfinkel P, et al: Anorexia nervosa, bulimia and pregnancy. Am J Obstet Gynecol 157:1194–1198, 1987.
27. Stoudemire A, Fogel B (eds): Obstetrics and Gynecology. Oxford, Oxford University Press, 1993.
28. Susman VL, Katz JL: Weaning and depression: Another postpartum complication. Am J Psychiatry 145:498–501, 1988.
29. Varan AR, Gillieson M, Skene D, et al: ECT in an acutely psychotic pregnant woman with actively aggressive (homicidal) impulses. Am J Psychiatry 30:363–367, 1985.
30. Willis DC, Rand CS: Pregnancy in bulimic women. Obstet Gynecol 71:708–710, 1988.
31. Wise MG, Ward S, Townsend-Porchman W, et al: Case report of ECT during high-risk pregnancy. Am J Psychiatry 141:99–100, 1984.

63. POSTPARTUM PSYCHIATRIC DISORDERS

Doris C. Gundersen, M.D.

1. What psychiatric disorders are seen in the postpartum period?

Maternity blues, postpartum psychosis, and postpartum depression are the psychiatric diagnoses most often made after delivery.

2. Define maternity blues.

Maternity blues, or baby blues, is a term used to describe a self-limiting, relatively mild mood syndrome experienced by 30–80% of all postpartum women. Symptoms include lability of mood, anxiety, sadness, crying spells, insomnia, and fatigue. The onset of maternity blues is usually 3–10 days after parturition. The symptoms typically remit within 2 weeks.

3. Which risk factors predispose women to maternity blues?

Because of its frequency and spontaneous remission, many regard maternity blues as a normal postpartum phenomenon. However, some women appear to be at higher risk. Major predictive factors include primiparous pregnancy, history of late luteal phase dysphoria (PMS), personal history of depression, or first-degree relative with depression.

4. What causes maternity blues?

The precise cause of maternity blues is unknown. Because the condition is common in all cultures and races and appears to occur independently of psychosocial factors, a biologic cause is likely. Studies have demonstrated that estrogen and progesterone influence the sensitivity of neurotransmitter-binding sites much like chronic administration of antidepressant drugs. With the delivery of the placenta, the elevated estrogen and progesterone levels maintained throughout pregnancy fall precipitously, and pregravid serum concentrations are reached within 3 days, coinciding with peak symptoms of maternity blues. It is hypothesized that this rapid decline in reproductive hormones after delivery destabilizes neurotransmitter mechanisms involved in mood regulation.

5. Describe postpartum psychosis.

Postpartum psychosis is sometimes called peurperal psychosis or postpartum psychotic depression. It develops in 1–2 per 1000 postpartum women worldwide. In the majority of cases, the symptoms are manifest within the first 2 weeks after delivery. However, a second peak has been observed 1–3 months after delivery.

A common prodrome for postpartum psychosis is worsening insomnia in the absence of a crying infant or physical discomfort in the mother. Psychomotor agitation may precede the psychosis. Women experience confusion, memory impairment, irritability, and anxiety. Intrusive thoughts, usually about harming the infant, are not uncommon. Paranoid and religious delusions, auditory hallucinations, thought insertion, thought withdrawal, and thought broadcasting have been reported. Faulty interactions with the infant, either misreading cues or blatant disinterest, also may be manifestations.

A unique feature of postpartum psychosis is the mercurial changeability of the symptoms. A brief period of elation characterized by incessant talking, increased energy, and euphoric mood may shift rapidly to profound, inexplicable sadness or rage. Lucid intervals are common and may give a deceptive impression of recovery. Abrupt episodes of floridly psychotic behavior may resurface after weeks of calm. Postpartum psychosis may resolve abruptly, but more often it evolves into serious, protracted depression. Postpartum psychosis frequently resembles mania and may prove to be a variant of bipolar affective disorder.

6. How frequently do women with postpartum psychosis harm their infants?
The level of infant morbidity correlates well with the severity of psychiatric symptoms in the mother. Infants of mildly to moderately impaired mothers may demonstrate difficulty with feeding or bonding. Infants of more severely afflicted mothers present with failure to thrive or evidence of frank physical abuse. Infanticide occurs in an estimated 4% of cases. Approximately 80–120 infanticides are committed by psychotic new mothers in the United States each year. At least 50% of the infant deaths take place weeks to months after the acute symptoms have subsided. Such numbers emphasize the importance of continuous monitoring of the mother's behavior, well beyond the initial psychotic episode. The capacity for the psychosis to recur after lucid periods must always be kept in mind.

7. Are there specific risk factors for postpartum psychosis?
Hereditary factors and prior history of affective episodes confer the greatest risk. A woman with a history of depression unrelated to pregnancy has a 20–25% risk of developing postpartum psychosis. This risk is higher for women with bipolar mood disorders than for women with a history of unipolar depression. If a bipolar woman develops postpartum psychosis, she carries a 50% risk for recurrence with subsequent deliveries. Women with a history of postpartum psychosis have a 1 in 3 chance of recurrence with future deliveries. The same women have a 38% risk for developing nonpsychotic postpartum depression. The need for careful prenatal screening and counseling is obvious. Other risk factors include single or primiparous women, history of incest, cesarean section, or perinatal death. Postpartum psychosis peaks between ages 25–29 and 30–34 years, which coincide with vulnerable times for the development of PMS. A relationship between the two disorders has yet to be established.

8. What is the cause of postpartum psychosis?
Postpartum psychosis is regarded as an organic syndrome. Psychological and social variables are considered secondary to organic factors. After delivery of the placenta, a large source of hormone production is lost. As with maternity blues, the sudden and dramatic decline in serum estrogen may initiate a sequence of neuroendocrine events that produce serious psychiatric symptoms in susceptible women. Estrogen has antidopaminergic properties. It is hypothesized that the abrupt withdrawal of estrogen exposes sensitive postsynaptic receptors in the brain; this may be the triggering event for development of psychosis. The propensity for relapse at the time of menses further implicates sex hormones in development of this disorder.

A decline in serum estrogen also leads to a fall in serum binding proteins, including transcortin. Cortisol levels are elevated during pregnancy. A surge of cortisol at labor is followed by an accelerated decline to second trimester levels within 72 hours. Acute psychotic reactions have been reported with adrenal insufficiency and/or steroid withdrawal. Small doses of the cortisol analog given to women with postpartum illness appear to decrease the severity and duration of symptoms. Unfortunately, no controlled studies of this regimen have been conducted.

Finally, women with postpartum illness have a high incidence of thyroid abnormalities. T3 levels are significantly lowered in women with postpartum psychosis compared with controls. The absolute values often fall within the normal range, with no overt physical signs of hypothyroidism. Perhaps it is the slope of the T3 decline rather than the specific serum concentration that influences the development of psychosis.

9. Describe postpartum depression.
Between the extremes of maternity blues and postpartum psychosis lies postpartum depression, which develops in 10–20% of women after delivery. Unlike the blues or psychosis, postpartum depression tends to develop insidiously 3 or more weeks after delivery. The mood symptoms are more sustained, and the course of the illness is typically prolonged. Symptoms include crying spells, poor concentration, indecisiveness, and profound sadness. Thoughts are characterized by themes of failure and inadequacy. Suicidal ideation is common. Postpartum depression is characterized by physical signs and symptoms resembling moderate-to-severe hypothyroidism. Cold

intolerance, fatigue, dry skin, slowed mentation, constipation, and fluid retention are commonly reported.

10. What are the risk factors for postpartum depression?
As with the blues and psychosis, hereditary factors and a history of previous psychiatric illness are identified as significant risk factors for postpartum depression. Women with previous episodes of depression unrelated to reproduction have a 10–40% chance of developing postpartum depression. Women with a history of postpartum depression have a 50% rate of recurrence with subsequent pregnancies. Several psychosocial risk factors have been identified, including marital discord, stressful life events during pregnancy, ambivalence about motherhood, low socioeconomic status, isolation from extended family or friends, and single status. Unrealistic expectations or romanticized ideas about motherhood, which inevitably clash with reality, may predispose a woman to depression. High prenatal scores on neuroticism scales are associated with postpartum depression.

11. Is postpartum depression considered to be primarily a biologic illness?
Not entirely. Ethnographic literature about childbirth suggests that the depressive reaction is at least partly attributable to cultural patterning of the postpartum period. Postpartum depression is not expressed globally; it appears rarely in non-Western cultures in which a new mother is absolved of all responsibilities beyond self-care and feeding her infant. Rituals practiced in third-world countries include provisions of social support for the new mother and clearly define her role. With modern birthing practices in Western society, there is less social structuring of postpartum events and a lack of clear role definition and social support for new mothers.

12. Are there endocrine or biologic correlates for postpartum depression?
Postpartum depression is often accompanied by symptoms related to hypothyroidism, and research points to varying degrees of pituitary dysfunction and related thyroid abnormalities as contributing factors in development of the illness.

After normal delivery, blood supply to the pituitary gland wanes. Trophic hormone secretion is reduced to prepregnancy quantities. If the delivery is complicated by shock (e.g., massive hemorrhage), the anterior pituitary may be damaged by infarction. In this scenario, secretion of trophic hormones ceases. Targeted endocrine glands fail. The patient develops profound apathy, cold sensitivity, loss of libido, memory impairment, lethargy, and thinning of axillary and pubic hair. Psychosis and eventually coma develop in untreated cases. This is known as Sheehan's syndrome.

It is hypothesized that postpartum depression is an intermediate condition. A sluggish pituitary may compromise endocrine functioning. After delivery thyroxine levels tend to decline and remain at values below the nonpregnant average for up to 1 year. Although depressed, the thyroxine level tends to overlap with the normal range, possibly masking hypothyroidism. The level of thyroid-stimulating hormone (TSH) usually is normal in hypothyroidism of pituitary origin (secondary hypothyroidism).

Case studies support the link between subclinical hypothyroidism of pituitary origin and postpartum illness. Antidepressant and antipsychotic medications, alone or in combination, frequently fail to treat adequately the symptoms of postpartum depression. With the addition of thyroid hormone, some patients experience rapid alleviation of psychiatric symptoms.

Further support for partial pituitary dysfunction or damage is suggested by the heightened sensitivity to sunburn or diminished capacity to tan reported by several postpartum women. This finding suggests reduced or absent melanin production by the pituitary gland. Finally, 5–30% of postpartum cases become chronic, implying some degree of residual damage.

Primary hypothyroidism, which originates in the thyroid gland, is also diagnosed in the postpartum period. Painless autoimmune thyroiditis, characterized by positive thyroid antibodies, occurs in 2–9% of postpartum women, surpassing the number observed in nonpregnant controls. Thyroxine may rise briefly with the inflammation. This rise is followed by a reduction in thyroid hormone and a corresponding rise in TSH. One study revealed persistent thyroid abnormalities 3 years after delivery in 50% of women.

In summary, postpartum depression often includes symptoms identical to moderate-to-severe hypothyroidism. Routine laboratory screening may fail to identify the abnormality if it is of pituitary origin. Such subclinical hypothyroidism may render postpartum depression refractory to treatment.

13. Can postpartum disorders be prevented?

Postpartum illnesses are notoriously difficult to treat. For this reason, efforts should be made to prevent their onset by eliminating or at least reducing known risk factors. High-risk patients can be identified early in the course of pregnancy through the use of risk assessment checklists, ideally at the first prenatal visit. When significant vulnerability is identified, interventions may include reducing environmental stress, enlisting the aid of family members, and mobilizing additional sources of support. Prenatal anticipatory guidance prepares a new mother for maternity blues and helps her to distinguish the blues from more ominous symptoms that warrant professional attention. Women with past histories of depression or psychosis should be followed more closely. The earlier a postpartum illness is identified, the greater the opportunity for secondary prevention.

14. What are the barriers to diagnosis?

Early detection of postpartum illness is rare, in part as a result of modern obstetric practices. In the United States, postpartum women are discharged from the hospital within 48 hours. The symptoms of postpartum illnesses are usually manifest after the third postpartum day, when the expert observation of nursing staff and physicians is no longer available. Six weeks pass before the next professional contact is made, resulting in a window of extreme vulnerability for new mothers.

The stigma placed by American culture on mental illness creates another barrier to early diagnosis. Patients and their families may conceal the severity of the problem out of shame, guilt, or embarrassment. Furthermore, depression after delivery contradicts the cultural expectation of "parental bliss."

The prodrome for serious postpartum pathology often mimics the blues. Women who voice concerns about such symptoms may be reassured without further investigation. Finally, the focus of the first postnatal visit is the reproductive health of the mother; her emotional well-being is not routinely addressed.

15. What biologic treatment strategies are available?

Maternity blues is a mild, transitory mood syndrome that typically resolves within a few days. Reassurance, observation, and occasionally a short-acting sedative are the primary interventions. It is important, however, to take the patient's complaints seriously. This increases the likelihood of her reporting symptoms that linger or become more severe.

Postpartum psychosis usually merits hospitalization because of the level of dysfunction and grave risk for both infanticide and suicide. The symptoms of postpartum psychosis are predominantly affective. Lithium or other mood-stabilizing medications are often helpful. Antipsychotic doses are typically lower than those required for other psychotic disorders. Electroconvulsive therapy (ECT) is indicated for severe, pharmacologically refractory cases.

For **postpartum depression** antidepressants, especially those that are selective for serotonin, appear to have some efficacy in targeting symptoms. Low doses of antipsychotic medications should be included if symptoms of psychosis are present. As with postpartum psychosis, some women may respond preferentially to ECT.

Thyroid screening should be performed routinely. For all postpartum cases, levels of serum thyroxine, TSH, and autoimmune antibodies should be assessed. Weekly thyroxine levels should be obtained. If a downward trend is identified, thyroxine replacement therapy should be initiated. A typical starting dose is 0.05 mg per day.

In women at **risk for recurrence**, psychotropic drugs to prevent or mitigate serious psychiatric symptoms should be given serious consideration. Women with histories of postpartum psychosis should receive lithium immediately after delivery. Rapid achievement of therapeutic blood levels is the goal. Care must be exercised to prevent toxicity. Lithium excretion may be impaired by fluid and electrolyte changes in the immediate postpartum period. Low-dose antipsychotic medications are also recommended for at least 2–3 weeks after delivery. In women with previous nonpsychotic postpartum depressions, antidepressant medication may be initiated somewhat earlier than onset of the previous episode.

Postpartum disorders that develop a more **chronic course** warrant endocrinology consultation to rule out more subtle disorders of the hypothalamic–pituitary–thyroid axis.

16. Which psychosocial interventions are effective?
Psychotherapy is crucial for preventing psychological scarring. Most patients have not experienced prior mental illness and may have difficulty with accepting the need to participate in treatment. It is often helpful to emphasize the biologic aspects of postpartum illness, which should be considered a complication of pregnancy—a medical illness with psychiatric symptoms related to physiologic changes after childbirth. Opportunities for eliminating feelings of failure and guilt become obvious. Group therapy is particularly helpful for postpartum women. It is important to convey that postpartum illness has an excellent prognosis.

New fathers are often the silent victims of postpartum disorders. They benefit from supportive outreach and education. Studies demonstrate that a father's support positively influences his partner's recovery.

Extended family must be recruited to support a postpartum woman during recovery. Providing literature and directing them to local support groups are often helpful.

17. What areas are the focus of current research?
Depressed levels of **tryptophan** and a slower than normal rise in tryptophan levels after delivery predict the blues. Attempts to avert the blues through tryptophan loading have failed, leading to speculation that a defect in metabolism rather than an absolute deficiency in tryptophan may be causally related to maternity blues.

Pyridoxine is a cofactor required for neuronal utilization of tryptophan. With oral administration for 28 days after delivery, an experimental group of high-risk women demonstrated a recurrence rate of the blues several times lower than the rate in a control group receiving placebo. A tryptophan study including pyridoxine supplementation may yield valuable information.

Another highly experimental strategy for preventing more severe postpartum disorders involves administering **long-acting estrogen** to high-risk women at delivery. It is theorized that the supplementation of estrogen cushions the fall of the hormone after the placenta is delivered. In a series of 50 high-risk women receiving estrogen at delivery, none had recurrences. Because of concerns about the risk of thromboembolic phenomena, this strategy is not currently recommended.

BIBLIOGRAPHY

1. Bluglass R: Infanticide. Bull R Coll Psychiatrists August:130–141, 1978.
2. Federman DD (ed): The Thyroid. New York, Scientific American, 1988.
3. Gitlin MJ, Pasnau RO: Psychiatric syndromes linked to reproductive functioning in women: A review of current knowledge. Am J Psychiatry 146:1413–1419, 1989.
4. Hamilton JA, Harberger PN (eds): Postpartum Psychiatric Illness: A Picture Puzzle. Philadelphia, University of Pennsylvania Press, 1992.
5. Hamilton JA: Postpartum psychiatric syndromes. Psychiatr Clin North Am 12:89–102, 1989.
6. Harkness S: The cultural mediation of postpartum depression. Med Anthropol Q 1:194–209, 1987.
7. Nikolai TF, Turney SL, Roberts RC: Postpartum lymphocytic thyroiditis. Arch Intern Med 147:221–224, 1987.
8. O'Hara MW: Social support, life events, and depression during pregnancy and the puerperium. Arch Gen Psychiatry 43:569–573, 1986.

9. O'Hara MW, Schlechte JA, Lewis DA, Wright EJ: Prospective study of postpartum blues. Arch Gen Psychiatry 48:801–806, 1991.
10. O'Hara MW, Zekowski EM: Postpartum depression: A comprehensive review. In Kumar R, Brockington IF (eds): Motherhood and Mental Illness, vol. II. London, Butterworth, 1988.
11. Paffenbarger RS: Epidemiological aspects of mental illness associated with childbearing. In Kumar R, Brockington IF (eds):Motherhood and Mental Illness, vol. I. London, Academy Press, 1982.
12. Parry BL (ed): Women's disorders. Psychiatr Clin North Am 12:207–220, 1989.
13. Prange AJ, Garbutt JC, Loosen PT: The hypothalamic-pituitary-thyroid axis in affective disorders. In Psychopharmacology: The Third Generation of Progress. New York, Raven Press, 1987.
14. Rosenblatt JE, Rosenblatt NC (eds): Currents in Affective Illness, vol 11. Bethesda, MD, Currents Publications, Ltd., 1992, pp 5–11.
15. Rosenblatt JE, Rosenblatt NC (eds): Currents in Affective Illness, vol 12. Bethesda, MD, Currents Publications, Ltd., 1993, pp 1–2.
16. Steiner M: Postpartum psychiatric disorders. Can J Psychiatry 35:89–95, 1990.
17. Stewart DE, Addison AM: Thyroid function in psychosis following childbirth. Am J Psychiatry 145:1579–1581, 1988.

IX. Geriatric Psychiatry

64. DEVELOPMENTAL ISSUES IN LATE LIFE

Roberta M. Richardson, M.D.

1. What are some of the central themes of development in the later years of adulthood?

According to Nemiroff and Colarusso,[9] a central theme of adult development is "the normative crisis precipitated by a growing awareness of the finiteness of time and the inevitability of personal death." This normative crisis leads to thoughts and questions about the meaning of one's life, accomplishments, and mark on the world and may underlie such psychiatric presentations as the depression that sometimes accompanies retirement and anxiety about a decline in personal health, or illness and death of friends and loved ones.

Erikson defines the developmental task of late life as integrity vs. despair. He refers to the task of reviewing life and integrating experiences into a value system that leads to a feeling of fulfillment and satisfaction. If this task is not accomplished, the emotion associated with this stage of life is most likely to be despair, caused by the conclusion that one did not accomplish what is perceived as necessary and no longer has the time to do so.

Jung noted that in the second half of life, men become more aware of their "feminine" side and women of their "masculine" side.

Another central theme of late life involves repeated injury to self-esteem as the older adult is displaced at work, loses physical and possibly sexual prowess, and must accept a degree of dependence on others. The realities of aging undermine defenses in some individuals, leading to intense feelings of envy, rivalry, rage, and, subsequently, loneliness. Psychotherapy may be especially useful in such patients by assisting them to accept the changes of aging and refocusing their attention on positive feelings about themselves.

2. How can changes in relationships stimulate developmental crises in older adults?

The aging and death of one's parents are major events in life. If parents become feeble, roles are often reversed. This reversal involves at least some degree of difficulty for most adult children. Psychologically adult children can no longer maintain the fantasy that their parents will take care of them. This may be particularly difficult if psychological separation has not fully occurred and feelings about the adequacy of parenting received in childhood remain ambivalent. Thoughts of mortality are strongly stimulated by the death of parents, which brings the realization that one's own generation is the next to pass.

Changes in relationships with grown children also may precipitate developmental crises in parents. The classic "empty nest" syndrome occurs later in life as childbearing is delayed and adult children stay longer in the home. Some parents may be reluctant to lose the parenting role as they face other losses and changes in their bodies. They may feel envy of their own children as they watch them start out with "their whole lives ahead of them."

3. Discuss the compensating aspects of relationships with grandchildren.

In most cases, relationships with grandchildren are idealized and mutually gratifying. Through grandchildren the displaced parent may recapture unqualified love and admiration. The grandparent may identify with the grandchild and act out frustrated, self-indulgent impulses through "spoiling" of the child. This process also may compensate for possible envious feelings toward adult children, the parents of the grandchild.

Grandchildren also represent immortality. It may be tremendously gratifying and reassuring to notice inherited genetic features in a grandchild when one is struggling with questions about one's legacy and asking, "Will I be remembered when I'm gone?"

4. How does late life development affect psychotherapy?

The older patient's experience of the therapist may be influenced by any number of important relationships in life, such as parent, spouse, sibling, or child. When the therapist is young, a transference related to the patient's relationship with his or her own children is more easily stimulated. Themes of unresolved expectations and disappointments with children may arise early. The therapist may be idealized as the "good" child who offers what the patient's own children do not or become the focus of angry feelings about abandonment.

The therapist's reactions to the psychotherapeutic relationship with an elderly patient may color which themes and reactions emerge. The therapist may be uncomfortable, for example, with sexuality in an older person or with the patient's dependency needs. If the patient is experienced as a parent, the therapist's unresolved wishes to control the parent or fears of domination may interfere with the therapy. Ongoing problems with parents in real life may make it particularly difficult for some therapists to work with older patients.

5. Do sex and sexuality continue to be a concern for people over the age of 60 years?

In 1974 the Duke Longitudinal Study on Aging found that 70% of men at age 63 and 25% of men at age 78 were still sexually active. Pearlman[10] found that 25% of men in their 60s and 10% of men over 70 reported sexual intercourse at least once a week. Data for older women are fewer. Christenson and Gagnon[4] found that 50% of married women over age 65 reported regular coitus. For women the availability of a socially sanctioned partner is a significant factor in the frequency of sexual activity, whereas for men this factor is not as important. For example, it is culturally more acceptable for an elderly man than an elderly woman to date a younger partner. Single women in their later years, however, remain interested in sex, and many compensate for the lack of a partner by masturbation.

Many doctors do not recognize the importance of sex and the prevalence of sexual dysfunction in older patients because they do not ask. Doctors who routinely ask about sex estimate that 50% of geriatric patients have sexual complaints, whereas doctors who do not routinely ask place the estimate at less than 10%.

6. What normal changes in sexual functioning occur with aging?

For men aging brings fewer spontaneous erections. Direct stimulation is usually required to obtain full erection, and the process takes longer. The force of ejaculation is decreased, along with the volume of seminal fluid. Ejaculatory control is improved, but the refractory period is longer (i.e., a longer period is necessary before another erection is possible).

For women late middle age often brings an increase in sexual desire, which gradually declines with old age. Lubrication decreases postmenopausally, and a longer period is required to achieve adequate lubrication. The vaginal vault decreases in size, with thinning walls. The orgasmic phase is shorter, and orgasmic uterine contractions may cause pain in the lower abdomen.

7. Discuss the causes of male impotence.

According to Hackett,[7] "Achieving a normal erection is a complex event requiring an adequate blood and nerve supply to the penile area and appropriate psychological conditions." Although it used to be thought that psychological factors were primarily responsible for the great majority of cases of male impotence, it is now believed that at least 50% have an organic basis. As would be expected, the incidence of organic factors increases with age.

Vasculogenic impotence is probably the most common organic type. It usually appears around age 50 and is characterized by partial erections and retained ability to achieve orgasm, which is neurologically controlled. **Neurologic impotence** occurs when diseases such as Parkinson's disease, multiple sclerosis, spinal cord injury, diabetes, alcoholism, or tumor interfere with the functioning of the nerves involved in developing and maintaining an erection. **Endocrinologic impotence** occurs when testosterone levels are low. Finally, many **prescription drugs** may decrease libido, reduce potency, or interfere with the ability to ejaculate.

Psychological factors are the primary cause in about one-half of the cases of male impotence. Depression, both as a primary major affective disorder and as a mood associated with bereavement or other losses, is by far the most common psychological cause of impotence and other sexual dysfunction. Another major category of psychological impotence involves medical illnesses unrelated biologically to sexual function, including common fears of sexual activity after myocardial infarction and fears of hurting oneself or one's partner when diseases such as arthritis or chronic lung disease are present.

Psychological factors often play a significant role in cases of impotence in which an organic cause is primary. Low self-esteem and performance anxiety may result from recognition of diminished sexual prowess.

8. What are the common complaints and causes of sexual dysfunction in elderly women?

Dyspareunia (painful intercourse) is a common complaint after menopause because of decreased lubrication and/or narrowing of the vagina. The vaginal mucosa also atrophy. Such problems can be overcome with systemic estrogen or estrogen creams applied to the vagina. Nonhormonal vaginal lubricants also may be helpful.

Psychological factors are equally important in the sexual functioning of older women and older men. Women may suffer from feelings of unattractiveness that makes them recoil from sexual activity. Such feelings may be caused or compounded by an apparent decrease in interest on the part of a spouse or partner who is having his own difficulties with sexual functioning. Often partners do not discuss the problem with each other, and the woman may assume that the cause is her loss of attractiveness.

Mastectomy often leaves many women feeling disfigured and reluctant to pursue sexual activity. Fortunately, more and more hospitals anticipate this problem and address it immediately after or even before surgery. The partner often needs to be involved in the counseling. Involving the partner in surgical aftercare and rehabilitation is a good way to desensitize and address such issues. Wearing of a prosthesis during intercourse is not a good solution, because it tends to perpetuate denial and self-doubt.

9. How can the physician assist older patients with problems related to sex and sexuality?

The most important intervention is to incorporate questions about sexual functioning into the routine history. Many people are uncomfortable bringing up such issues, even to the doctor. Often allowing the patient to air concerns and educating the patient about normal changes in sexual functioning with aging make all the difference.

Once sexual difficulties are described, the physician first should consider the patient's medical history, including medications, to see whether a physical factor is involved, especially one that can be corrected. Inquiries about alcohol and over-the-counter medications are also important. Referral to a urologist or gynecologist may be appropriate for further evaluation of specific problems.

The patient also should be screened for depression, and inquiries should be made about relationship difficulties and sexual functioning of the partner. Pharmacologic treatment for depression may be appropriate, but the high incidence of sexual dysfunction caused by antidepressants should be kept in mind. A mental health referral may be appropriate.

10. Discuss grief and its role in the evaluation and treatment of older adults.

Grief is the emotional suffering experienced in reaction to loss. Late life is characterized by increasing numbers and severity of losses. The death of a spouse is perhaps the best known cause for grief in older people—and one of the most devastating. However, many other major losses are also common. Parents, siblings, and, as more people live to a more advanced age, children also die. Friends may die in fairly quick succession.

Death of loved ones is not the only cause of grief. Older people lose relationships through retirement, changes in residence (by themselves or others), and inability to congregate for social activities because of loss of transportation or failing health. Grief also may be triggered by material loss, such as loss of home and possessions (when one must move to a smaller place). A move also may necessitate loss of a beloved pet. Finally, one may grieve for loss of body parts or functions, such as eyesight, hearing, or mobility. Avid readers, for example, may feel desperate when they no longer can see. Loss of hearing isolates one from others as communication becomes more and more difficult.

The symptoms of grief are varied. Loss is often instrumental in precipitating major depressive episodes. Although antidepressant medications are often helpful and may be necessary, psychotherapy may be at least as important. Sometimes a depressive episode represents the culmination of a series of losses so close together that one is not dealt with before the next comes along, overwhelming individual coping capacity.

Anger and resentment are also common reactions to loss, especially losses that undermine the sense of self-esteem, such as loss of physical function and opportunities. Anxiety and fear may underlie the anger or be frank expressions of loss. Suicide may be considered or threatened as a way of gaining a feeling of control over one's body and life.

The deficit model of loss and grief is helpful in guiding intervention. A loss leads to deficits in the sufferer's life. Grief will not be eased until other resources are found to compensate for such deficits. For example, loss of a spouse leads to loss of help with basic activities of living (e.g., "he always balanced the check book"), validating responses that enhance self-esteem, and emotional supports. It also leaves a deficit in social identity. Older people with a greater number of social contacts and a diversity of roles fare better than those who functioned mainly as a spouse, with few outside contacts.

11. What are the tasks of the therapist in assisting grief-stricken older patients?

The therapist helps patients by encouraging them to talk about the loss of the loved one. Although listening may seem like a cliché, the therapist may be the only person who is willing to sit quietly with patients while they cry, express their feelings, and repeat painful stories. Some therapists may be too quick to jump in with reassurances, platitudes, or distractions, giving the message that they do not want to hear the pain. The therapist must tolerate intense affect and let patients know that avoiding the pain often only prolongs grief or causes it to remain unresolved.

Education about grief and loss is important, because many people had abnormal models or were taught myths about the grieving process. Grieving alone, keeping a stiff upper lip, and not feeling sorry for oneself are among the myths that many people have learned. Validating feelings of all kinds, including anger, relief, and guilt, is important.

Assistance with problem solving also helps to replace the deficits left by loss. In the case of bereavement, the survivor must adjust to an environment from which the deceased is missing and reinvest emotional energy in other relationships. The bereaved may need concrete guidance and instructions for moving on to other people and activities.

According to Taylor, effective work with grief must involve a search for meaning in the experience, an attempt to regain mastery over one's life, and an effort to enhance self-esteem. These guidelines are particularly helpful in assisting with losses of function and role that are almost inevitable in the elderly. For example, the man who is forced to retire at age 65 may not feel ready to leave his job, which may be his primary source of self-esteem and the area in which he feels most capable and in control. He may feel helpless and frustrated. The therapist's task is to help the man look beyond his job for meaningful activity, self-esteem, and fulfillment.

12. Discuss the common fears about death and dying in older adults.

Attitudes toward death are grounded in culture. North American culture tends to deny death and to stigmatize the notion of vulnerability. Independence, self-control, and autonomy are highly valued. Thus many adults come to old age with fears and conflicts about death with which they must struggle alone.

Most people in North America do not die suddenly but become progressively ill with one or more diseases that eventually kill them. Most of these diseases are chronic and ambiguous. Increasingly, even cancer is a diagnosis that may or may not be terminal. Thus older people are fated to ponder the circumstances of their death.

The most common fears center on the dying process, specifically on isolation or abandonment and loss of dignity and control. Fortunately, we seem to have passed the heyday of high-tech death, but many people still have great fears of dying alone in a hospital room with tubes in every orifice and hisses and beeps for company. Many fear humiliating exposure in the presence of strangers as they struggle with terrible physical suffering and possible loss of mental capacities.

Older people must have the opportunity to discuss such issues with their loved ones and doctors. They need assurances that they will be cared for with courtesy, concern for their dignity, and attention to alleviation of suffering. Most people also want reassurance that every effort will be made not to allow them to die alone. In addition, efforts should be made to clarify specific wishes for medical interventions near the end of life, before circumstances render the individual incompetent to choose. Such efforts should include choosing and executing some form of formal advance directive for health care, according to the various laws in the different states.

13. Discuss common characteristics of people most likely to have a debilitating fear of death.

People who have unresolved religious questions about death and dying may develop severe anxiety in late life. They may fear that they will die before resolving their doubts and suffer after death as a consequence; for example, by spending eternity in hell. Or they may have been raised in a tradition that promises a blissful afterlife but fear they instead will find an eternal unbearable nothingness.

For some, the realization of personal death arouses intense separation anxiety. Such individuals have struggled with separation anxiety in their relationships throughout life. They may envision death as an agonizing aloneness. A resurgence of clinging, regressive behavior may be the manifestation of this unspoken fear.

People with lingering guilt for hostile or impulsive acts and an immature ego structure may view death as a punishment and thus develop debilitating fears in late life. Such people continue to struggle with anger over their lot, feelings of mistreatment, and subsequent guilt over having and/or expressing such feelings. They present with mixed and alternating emotions of hostility, depression, and anxiety.

On a more concrete level, people who live alone are more likely to develop debilitating fear of death, because they are afraid they will become ill or injured and die alone before they are able to get help.

14. What interventions are helpful to older people facing death?

Assistance in clarifying beliefs and feelings about death and end-of-life issues may be helpful. Such issues may be discussed with the physician, a religious leader, family and friends, or a counselor or psychotherapist. The family may need assistance in knowing how to help a dying relative. The quality of close relationships strongly influences the reactions to dying.

If problems are sufficiently debilitating to require professional therapy, the therapist can help the person to develop a "fantasy of immortality." It is soothing for most people to feel that they will continue to live in a positive way through their children, creations, or even possessions. The life review is also therapeutic at this stage. The therapist guides the person through a review of the facts and accomplishments of his or her life to assist in developing a feeling that life has had meaning and purpose. This technique is not advised for patients suffering from major depression. The nature of depression leads patients to recall selectively and to dwell on negative life events and deeds, which is more harmful than helpful.

BIBLIOGRAPHY

1. Atchley RC: The aging self. Psychother Theory Res Pract 19:388–396, 1982.
2. Baum N, Sakauye K: What's causing your patient's impotence? Senior Patient Oct:21–26, 1990.
3. Butler RN: The life-review: An unrecognized bonanza. Intl J Aging Hum Dev 12:35–38, 1980.
4. Christenson CV, Gagnon JG: Sexual behavior in a group of older women. J Gerontol 20:351–356, 1965.
5. Feinberg MR, Feinberg G, Tarrant JJ: Leavetaking: How to Successfully Handle Life's Most Difficult Crises. Lexington, MA, Ginn Press, 1978.
6. Fry PS: Depression, Stress, and Adaptations in the Elderly. Rockville, MD, Aspen, 1986, pp 323–347.
7. Hackett TP: Sexual activity in the elderly. In Jenicke MA (ed): Clinical Perspectives on Aging. Philadelphia, Wyeth-Ayerst Laboratories, 1985.
8. James JW, Cherry F: The Grief Recovery Handbook. New York, Harper & Row, 1988.
9. Nemiroff RA, Colarusso CA: The Race Against Time. New York, Plenum Press, 1985.
10. Pearlman CK: Frequency of intercourse in males at different ages. Med Aspects Hum Sex 6:92, 1972.
11. Weisman A: On Dying and Denying. Behavioral Publications, 1972, pp 137–157.

65. PSYCHOPHARMACOLOGY FOR ELDERLY PATIENTS

Roberta M. Richardson, M.D.

1. Discuss pharmacokinetic changes in the aging body as they relate to use of psychotropic medications.

It is useful to imagine the passage of a medication through the body from the time it is swallowed until the time it is excreted and to consider age-related changes at each point along the way.

The changes in absorption of oral medications that occur with aging have little effect on psychotropic medications. Changes in the distribution of the medication after it is absorbed, however, are significant. The aging body shows a significant decrease in lean body mass, corresponding increase in total body fat, and a decrease in total body water. Thus water-soluble drugs may have a greater concentration per unit dose because of the apparent decrease in the size of the reservoir. The most important example, although it is not used therapeutically, is alcohol. The older one becomes, the higher the blood alcohol level per drink. Thus an elderly person who has been drinking two martinis every day for 50 years may develop problems without an increase in intake. Fat-soluble drugs, on the other hand, have a greater volume of distribution. They are stored in the fat, released gradually, and therefore show a prolonged half-life in the elderly. The most important examples are the highly fat-soluble benzodiazepines, particularly diazepam. Antipsychotic medications are also fat-soluble and clearly affected by this phenomenon.

Changes in drug metabolism that occur with aging are also important. It is important to know by which route a drug is primarily metabolized. Most drugs are metabolized primarily through the liver. In general, hepatic blood flow and size decrease significantly with aging. However, individual variation in overall hepatic metabolizing ability is vast. For example, there is as much as a 20-fold difference in appropriate dose of certain antidepressants among patients of the same advanced age. This fact leads to two common mistakes in prescribing: overdosing and underdosing. The rule is to start low and go slow—but not to stop too soon. Blood levels, when they are known, are very useful. Otherwise, one must prescribe cautiously and increase the dose as tolerated, watching for toxicity, until therapeutic efficacy is reached. One also must take into account other medications that may interfere with the metabolism of the psychotropic medication and the effects of other illnesses, such as liver congestion secondary to congestive heart disease.

Medications metabolized by the kidney are more predictable. Creatinine clearance decreases steadily with age, according to the following formula:

$$\frac{(140 - \text{age}) \times \text{body weight (kg)} \times 0.85 \text{ (women only)}}{72 \times \text{serum creatinine}}$$

The older and smaller the patient and the higher the serum creatinine, the lower the level of creatinine clearance per unit time. This equation correlates directly with the clearance time for any drug metabolized by the kidneys. Lithium is the psychotropic medication most influenced by this phenomenon. Dosages must be drastically reduced in elderly patients to avoid toxicity. Some of the benzodiazepines are also metabolized renally and have a slower clearance in elderly patients.

2. How are changes in receptor sensitivity and neurotransmitters relevant?

Aging brings reduced sensitivity to some pharmacologic agents and increased sensitivity to others. The most important consideration in prescribing psychotropics, however, is the cholinergic neurotransmitter system. Several of the commonly used psychotropic agents have significant anticholinergic properties. But in the aging brain, cholinergic binding sites are decreased; choline acetyltransferase, vital for making acetylcholine, is decreased; and acetylcholine is even more decreased in the brains of patients with Alzheimer's disease. Therefore, the elderly are predisposed to central anticholinergic toxicity in the form of confusion, delirium, and psychosis.

Whenever prescribing psychotropic medications for the elderly, therefore, one should choose the least anticholinergic agent in each class and avoid combining two or more highly anticholinergic medications. For example, among the tricyclic antidepressants, the secondary amines nortriptyline and desipramine are preferred. Amitriptyline is highly anticholinergic and should be avoided. Among the antipsychotics, the high-potency agents such as haloperidol are preferred over the more anticholinergic thioridazine or chlorpromazine.

Note: Central anticholinergic toxicity may occur without peripheral manifestations in older patients.

Summary of Changes in the Aging Body and Their Effect on Psychotropic Drugs

CHANGE	EFFECT	EXAMPLE
Increased body fat	Fat-soluble drugs stored longer, released slowly	Diazepam
Decreased body water	Water-soluble drugs show higher concentration	Ethanol
Decreased liver size and blood flow	Drugs metabolized in liver cleared more slowly, but individual variation is great	Antidepressants
Decreased creatinine clearance	Drugs metabolized renally cleared more slowly; predictable	Lithium
Decreased acetylcholine in brain	Anticholinergic drugs more likely to cause central toxicity	Amitriptyline Chlorpromazine

3. What are the major considerations in choosing an antidepressant for older patients?
Consider first the various classes of antidepressants available:
1. Tricyclics (TCAs)
2. Selective serotonergic reuptake inhibitors (SSRIs)
3. Monoamine oxidase inhibitors (MAOIs)
4. Bupropion
5. Trazodone
6. Psychostimulants
7. Electroconvulsive therapy (ECT)

Setting aside psychostimulants and ECT, which are discussed separately, none of the antidepressants is statistically more effective than the others. In choosing, therefore, one considers first contraindications, then side effects, and finally cost and convenience.

For example, one may too quickly dismiss a tricyclic antidepressant in patients with heart disease, even though TCAs may be considerably less expensive than the newer agents. However, if there are no contraindications to TCAs and cost is of any concern, one should consider the less expensive antidepressants before immediately prescribing sometimes prohibitively expensive newer agents. If the TCA proves intolerable or ineffective, one may need to prescribe other classes and to assist the patient in dealing with the cost.

4. Why should one always check the electrocardiogram before prescribing a TCA in patients over the age of 40?
The TCAs have quinidinelike effects on cardiac conduction; i.e., they slow conduction across the atrioventricular node. Clinically relevant problems at therapeutic blood levels are limited to patients with preexisting conduction disease. However, only severe disease absolutely contraindicates use of TCAs. Stoudamire and Atkinson reported that "asymptomatic patients with right bundle branch block, isolated left anterior fascicular block, and left posterior fascicular block usually can be treated safely with TCAs if dosage is increased gradually and ECGs obtained

following each dosage increase."[9] Note the word "asymptomatic." Syncopal attacks suggest an intermittently higher degree of block, and TCAs should not be used unless a pacemaker is in place. The same applies to patients with bifascicular or trifascicular block.

TCAs are also contraindicated for at least 6 weeks after an acute myocardial infarction. In patients who develop persistently long Q-Tc intervals, the risk for fatal ventricular fibrillation is increased. If TCAs must be used, they should be used cautiously, in association with ECG monitoring and consultation with a cardiologist about the acceptable upper limit of Q-Tc intervals for the particular patient.

5. List contraindications to the use of TCAs.

Other contraindications to TCAs are due to their anticholinergic effects: These include (1) narrow-angle glaucoma, (2) significantly enlarged prostate, and (3) marginally compensated congestive heart failure (because tachycardia may precipitate failure). The possibility of (4) orthostatic hypotension, which increases the risk of falling, should also be considered.

6. Is it safe to prescribe MAOIs to elderly patients?

MAOIs can be tricky in elderly patients. The biggest concern is the need for compliance with dietary restrictions, because ingestion of food high in tyramine may cause a hypertensive crisis. MAOIs should not be prescribed for patients who cannot be relied on to understand and follow this diet. Certain concurrent medications must also be avoided. Most significant are the sympathomimetics, which include medications used to treat asthma; therefore, patients with asthma should not receive MAOIs. The same applies to patients with a history of anaphylaxis, because the epinephrine required for treatment may precipitate a hypertensive crisis in the presense of MAOIs. Orthostatic hypotension is also a common side effect.

7. Are the newer antidepressants preferable?

Bupropion is a relatively new antidepressant in a class by itself. It was released and then withdrawn when an unacceptably high incidence of seizures was reported. After further study, bupropion was re-released with guidelines for maximal dosage and the caveat that patients with a history of seizure should not take it. In addition, patients with active bulimia have an increased incidence of seizures. With these restrictions in mind, bupropion can be a safe and effective antidepressant for elderly patients. The most common side effects are stimulation, insomnia, and constipation.

To date, SSRIs are the safest of the antidepressants; there are no absolute contraindications to their use. They should be used cautiously in patients with Parkinson's disease because of the possibility of worsening parkinsonian symptoms. SSRIs also may cause increased agitation, which may resemble the akathesia observed with antipsychotics. In addition, older patients frequently experience postural instability early in the course of treatment with SSRIs. Although the instability resolves within a few weeks, it may cause falls, which often have severe consequences in elderly patients. Other significant and common side effects include nausea, anorexia, diarrhea, and headache. Fluoxetine has an extremely long half-life, which is even longer in the elderly. Therefore, side effects such as headache, diarrhea, or agitation may develop 2 or more weeks after the medication is initiated. Many an unsuspecting clinician has instituted a GI work-up for unrelenting diarrhea that in fact was caused by fluoxetine. For this reason, the newer SSRIs such as paroxetine and sertraline may be preferable. The newer agents, especially sertraline, are also less likely to interfere with the metabolism of commonly prescribed medications such as coumadin, phenytoin, and cimetidine.

8. What are the treatment options if none of the above antidepressants is safe, tolerated, and/or effective?

Psychostimulants, such as methylphenidate, may be helpful in very old, frail patients with apathetic depression; for example, medically ill patients who are not participating in their care or rehabilitation or not eating. In spite of their reputation for suppressing appetite, in this setting the stimulants generally increase appetite, energy, and interest. The stimulants are rarely contraindicated; even patients with heart disease usually tolerate them. A careful approach, beginning with a low dose and monitoring vital signs after each dose, is recommended.

Electroconvulsive therapy is another possibility for frail elderly patients who are depressed. Despite its scary reputation, ECT is one of the safest treatments for certain older people. Intracranial masses should be ruled out, and consultation with a cardiologist is necessary for patients with significant heart disease. In addition, patients with a history of retinal detachment should have a consultation with a knowledgeable ophthalmologist, because the sudden increase in blood pressure may cause problems.

9. How should one approach the treatment of anxiety in elderly patients?
The first step is to make a careful diagnosis. In many older people who present with anxiety as their chief complaint, the actual diagnosis is major depression. Anxiolytics do not treat such patients adequately. In fact, the sedative-hypnotics may worsen depression. The appropriate response is to prescribe an antidepressant, which often provides sufficient treatment even in the short term while waiting for the antidepressant to take full effect.

If an anxiolytic medication is needed, consider low doses of the benzodiazepines lorazepam and oxazepam, both of which are metabolized in the blood through oxidation. Because this process does not change appreciably with aging, lorazepam and oxazepam, unlike other anxiolytic agents, do not accumulate in the aging body as a result of slowed metabolism. This unique method of metabolism, however, does not mean that older people should receive the same dosages as younger people. Older people are much more susceptible to postural instability and memory loss. In all cases, the lowest possible dosage should be used, and signs of toxicity should be monitored carefully.

Buspirone is not a substitute for benzodiazepines, because the patient will feel no immediate relief. Buspirone may be helpful with generalized anxiety over time, and some evidence suggests that it may have antidepressant effects. However, it is not very helpful as an early treatment of depression or as treatment for situational anxiety.

Do not neglect nonpharmacologic means of anxiety control, such as relaxation exercises, deep breathing, and manipulation of the environment.

10. Discuss important considerations in the treatment of psychosis in elderly patients.
As always, the first consideration is diagnosis. Elderly schizophrenics need and usually tolerate higher doses than demented or delirious patients. Patients with affective illness show a wide range of need and tolerance.

The high-potency agents are preferred for geriatric patients because of their side effect profile. The minimal advantage of increased sedation with the low-potency medications, such as chlorpromazine and thioridazine, is far outweighed by the disadvantages of increased anticholinergic side effects and higher incidence of orthostatic hypotension. This point cannot be overemphasized: do not choose thioridazine because the patient is agitated or sleeping poorly. Haloperidol works probably as well for treatment of agitation and perhaps as well for treatment of insomnia.

The main problem with haloperidol and other high-potency antipsychotics is the likely occurrence of extrapyramidal symptoms. Acute dystonia is extremely uncommon in the elderly. Parkinsonism, however, is quite common and contributes significantly to the risk for falling. Its onset may be insidious. One month after hospital discharge, for example, the patient may be found to be stooped, shuffling, stiff, and possibly tremulous. For these reasons, the physician must be very cautious, using the lowest effective dose and monitoring the patient closely for a few months if he or she is to stay on the antipsychotic medication. Prophylactic anticholinergic medications such as benztropine are no substitute; they increase the risk of mental confusion and other side effects of anticholinergics in general.

The physician must evaluate elderly patients for symptoms of parkinsonism before starting an antipsychotic. Patients with Parkinson's disease or similar syndromes may deteriorate clinically, and antipsychotics should be avoided in such patients if at all possible. The only currently available antipsychotic that does not worsen Parkinson's disease symptoms is clozapine, which is quite useful in treating psychosis associated with Parkinson's disease. The required dosages are much lower than those used to treat schizophrenia—25–50 mg/day is often sufficient. Weekly blood counts are needed because of the risk of agranulocytosis.

Although not free of extrapyramidal side effects, the new antipsychotic agent, risperidone, carries a lower incidence and may be better tolerated by elderly patients. Because it is the only antipsychotic agent that acts as an antagonist of both dopamine and serotonin, risperidone may be effective in some patients who do not respond to the more traditional antipsychotic medications.

The risk of tardive dyskinesia increases with age. The incidence is higher in women and in patients treated with antipsychotics for indications other than schizophrenia. Thus elderly women with psychotic depression are at particular risk for developing tardive dyskinesia; antipsychotic medications should be prescribed only with informed consent and close follow-up. With frequent and careful examination for early signs, tardive dyskinesia can be detected and the offending agent stopped before a debilitating condition develops.

11. Name one of the most common and serious, yet overlooked, complications of psychotropic medication in elderly patients.
Most of the psychotropics in current use increase the risk of falling in older patients. Despite the well-known commercial featuring the woman who has "fallen and can't get up," this is no laughing matter. Because osteoporosis is endemic among elderly women, it does not take much to cause serious fractures. A fractured hip may lead to all of the morbidity and mortality associated with prolonged immobility and possible surgery, including pulmonary embolus, pneumonia, urosepsis, decubitus ulcers, and lengthy and expensive rehabilitation efforts after the bone has healed. Subdural hematomas may result from relatively minor blows to the head in older people. The elder who lives alone and cannot get up after a fall may develop muscular necrosis and even dehydration if not found for some time. For many elderly people the prospect of falling is so frightening that, especially after one fall has occurred, activity may be significantly limited. Such limitation may lead to increasing depression and declining health.

Psychotropic medications can contribute to falling through various mechanisms, and the physician must be alert for symptoms in several areas. TCAs, MAOIs, and some of the antipsychotics commonly cause orthostatic hypotension. Patients must be warned and then asked about a feeling of faintness upon rising from a lying or sitting position. If the reply is positive, blood pressure should be measured in recumbent and standing positions. A drop of 20 points or more in systolic pressure is usually considered significant. Asymptomatic findings may be tolerated; symptomatic findings should not. Fainting is one of the most dangerous reasons for a fall, because the victim has no control over the landing.

Unfortunately, the SSRIs are not foolproof in this regard. Sertraline causes significant postural instability in many older people early in the course of treatment. Fortunately, this symptom seems to resolve within a few weeks, and the risk may be minimized by more gradual titration of the dose. Although not yet supported by research, other SSRIs are likely to have similar effects. Dizziness is a relatively common side effect of the new antidepressant venlafaxine at all ages. Elderly patients taking these medications should be asked if they feel dizzy or unsteady on their feet. If so, the dosage should be lowered or special precautions taken to increase safety, depending on the frailty and dependability of the patient as well as the severity of the depression and dizziness.

Benzodiazepines also cause postural instability. The effect may be subtle, but the risks are not. When geriatric patients are prescribed doses that are too high or a long-acting agent that accumulates over time, frank intoxication may lead to a fall as long as 2 weeks after the drug is started. The classic example is the patient who is prescribed flurazepam in the hospital and discharged with instructions to continue the drug at home. Two weeks later, when this particularly long-acting medication reaches peak blood level, the patient falls—or falls asleep at the wheel of a car. Nystagmus is a sign of excessive levels of benzodiazepine and indicates cerebellar dysfunction.

Antipsychotics also are commonly associated with falls among elderly patients because of the induction of parkinsonism. One of the cardinal features of this syndrome is postural instability. If the more obvious signs of parkinsonism are present (i.e., pill-rolling tremor, cogwheel rigidity, shuffling gait, masked facies, inhibited arm swing), postural instability is present too. Steps should be taken either to decrease, discontinue, or change the medication or to treat the parkinsonism with anticholinergic agents (with attention to possible attendant complications).

BIBLIOGRAPHY

1. Friedman JH: A role for clozapine in Parkinson's disease. Neurol For 3:3–15, 1992.
2. Jenike MA: Geriatric Psychiatry and Psychopharmacology: A Clinical Approach. Chicago, Year Book, 1989.
3. Jenike MA: Tardive dyskinesia: Special risk in the elderly. J Am Geriatr Soc 31:71–73, 1983.
4. Laghrissi-Thode F, Pollack BG, Miller MW, et al: Comparative assessment of postural stability in elders treated with antidepressants [unpublished abstract]. 1994.
5. Nakra BRS, Grossberg GT: Lithium use in the elderly. J Geriatr Drug Ther 2:47–63, 1987.
6. Salzman C: Recent advances in geriatric psychopharmacology. In Tasman A, goldfinger SM, Kaufmann CA (eds): American Psychiatric Press Review of Psychiatry, vol 9. Washington, DC, American Psychiatric Press, 1990, pp 279–293.
7. Salzman C, Lebowitz BD (eds): Anxiety in the Elderly. New York, Springer, 1991.
8. Stanislav SW, Fabre T, Crismon ML, et al: Buspirone's efficacy in organic-induced aggression. J Clin Psychopharmacol 14:`126–130, 1994.
9. Stoudemire A, Fogel BS, Gulley LR, et al: Psychopharmacology in the medical patient. In Stoudemire A, Fogel BS (eds): Psychiatric Care of the Medical Patient. New York, Oxford University Press, 1993, pp 155–206.
10. Tune LE, Steele C, Cooper T: Neuroleptic drugs in the management of behavioral symptoms of Alzheimer's disease. Psychiatr Clin North Am 14:353–373, 1991.
11. Yudofsky SC, Silver JM, Hales RE: Pharmacologic management of aggression in the elderly. J Clin Psychiatry 51:22–32, 1990.

X. Consultation–Liaison Psychiatry

66. PSYCHIATRIC CONSULTATION IN THE GENERAL HOSPITAL

Michael K. Popkin, M.D.

1. When is psychiatric consultation indicated or advisable?

Most general hospital psychiatric consultation services see 3 to 5% of all admissions to the medical-surgical units of the hospital. Consultation may be requested for a wide range of reasons: disturbances in behavior; changes in cognition, thinking, or mood; maladaptive responses to the physical illness process or hospitalization; legal issues, such as competency, informed consent, desire to leave against medical advice; and problems in the doctor-patient relationship.

Psychiatric disorders are common in the general hospital population. Various studies have reported that 20% to 30% of medical-surgical inpatients have current depressive disturbances. An equal percentage manifest anxiety disorders, and between 5 and 10% of medical-surgical patients experience an episode of delirium during hospitalization. Collectively these data suggest high rates of psychiatric disorders in the general hospital; only select patients are referred for psychiatric consultation.

Although certain issues may routinely prompt referral (e.g., violence or profound noncompliance), difficulties in the interaction between the patient and physician often seem crucial to the decision. Hard and fast rules do not apply here, but consultation is advisable whenever first-line or standard psychiatric remedies have not resolved the issue; when diagnostic expertise is required; when the primary physician is "at bay" in the engagement and management of the patient; or when an objective, external review may be needed to weigh a proposed course of action.

2. What are the consultation psychiatrist's goals in the initial dialogue with the referring physician or nurse?

Direct dialogue with the referring physician is crucial to the consultation process; seldom does a written request suffice. In this first exchange, the consultant's principal task is to identify a *specific* consultation question or questions. The consultant's ability to assist is largely a function of pinpointing the concern or issues generating the referral. Surprisingly, physicians are often reluctant to explain their reasons for consulting a psychiatrist. The consultant may need to ask, "What would you like to have done?" The more precise the question, the better the chance that the consultant's answer may render a service. (The phrase "Please evaluate" is unlikely to yield the desired endpoint.) Next, the consultant must ensure that the request for psychiatric consultation has been discussed with the patient. The unexpected arrival of the psychiatric consultant is usually regarded with hostility. The consultant's final goal in the first dialogue is to inform the referring physician of the proposed consultative steps, including when impressions and recommendations will be conveyed and how further communication will be achieved.

3. How should the consultation interview be conducted?

At the outset, the consultant should inquire whether the patient has been advised of the consultation and its purpose. A negative answer usually requires postponing the interview. Once the primary physician has informed the patient of the request for consultation and the objectives in this step, the consultant may proceed. It is best to begin the interview with basic questions concerning age, place of origin, family, education, marital status, and number of children. These constitute important background information and together with a careful review of the medical situation, offer nonthreatening areas with which to develop rapport. In the first meeting, the goal is to facilitate an alliance and maintain neutrality.[2] The patient should be encouraged to tell his or her own story and the consultant should pay attention to the style of presentation. Generally the consultant should be friendly and tolerant, but signal clearly if the patient's interpersonal conduct is inappropriate or "out-of-bounds." The interview must be flexible in timing and format, less formal than that conducted in the office or clinic setting. The consultant should strive to maintain privacy; this may require asking a roommate to depart for a time or herding away direct care personnel. The patient must be advised at the start how much time will be needed; similarly, at the close, the patient deserves a summary statement regarding observations and the plan of action. It is important that follow-up be specified. Although its goal is largely investigatory, the initial interview can, and should, be therapeutic as well. Even humor can have its place in the sometimes all-too-serious medical setting.

Often in conducting the consultation interview, pursuit of specific content or data will be frustrated. Either intentionally or unwittingly, the patient will obstruct or blockade the consultant's efforts to secure information. When this occurs repeatedly and threatens to disrupt the sequence, it is useful to consider "changing gears" and to address the process of the interview. For example, "I'm here to try to be of assistance, but for the last 10 minutes you've refused to allow me to understand what you are feeling or experiencing. How will this be helpful to you?" The theme is *not* necessarily confrontation, rather it is shifting focus to the *process* unfolding between the consultant and the patient (as opposed to the pursuit of *data* per se).

4. What is the role of corroborative history in the consultation setting?

The elderly and cognitively impaired comprise a significant percentage of patients referred for psychiatric consultation. Histories and accounts provided by these patients may be marred or jeopardized by questionable reliability, altered levels of consciousness, and cognitive dysfunction (in an otherwise clear sensorium). Accordingly, corroborative or alternative histories are often vitally important in the consultation-liaison (CL) setting. The consultant is obligated to review carefully the available medical records and to elicit the input of direct care personnel familiar with the patient. Corroborative reports from family members and significant others should be gathered after the patient is interviewed; contact before engaging the patient can make the consultant the agent of that family member. This, in turn, may disrupt the consultant's link to the patient.

5. What should be included in the consultation report?

The consultation report is a legal document which should concisely address (and hopefully, answer) the original consultation questions. Lengthy reports often are not read by consultees; rather, the tendency is to skip to the conclusions and recommendations. One strategy, now common with psychiatric consultation services, is to present resultant diagnoses and recommended actions first, followed by the case synopsis or summary and the mental status examination (MSE). The consultant must convey an awareness of the patient's medical/surgical issues, but it is not necessary to reiterate the full chronology of the medical situation. Psychiatrically, the focus should be on the history of the present illness, rather than a lengthy reconstruction of early childhood or adolescent trauma. In most cases, no more than a page of synopsis of the problem is indicated, in addition to the MSE, differential diagnosis, and recommendations.

Elements of the Consultation Report and Suggested Sequence of Presentation

Resultant psychiatric diagnosis (per DSM–IV) in order of reason for the consultation
Recommendations, prioritized and specific
One page synopsis of the psychiatric problem
  History of presenting complaint(s)
  Pertinent psychiatric history, including familial and medical history
  Mental status examination
  Psychiatric differential diagnosis

6. What psychiatric disorders are most commonly encountered by the consultation psychiatrist?

Formal studies of the distribution of psychiatric diagnoses assigned by psychiatric consultation services show clustering into a relatively brief list. Teaching consultation-liaison services diagnose a cognitive impairment disorder in approximately 25% of patients; these diagnoses include delirium and dementia. Another 25% of the consultation-liaison population are diagnosed as suffering from a mood disorder, whether primary or secondary to a medical condition. Approximately 15% are given a diagnosis of adjustment disorder, signalling a maladaptive response to identified stressors (including medical illness). Less than 10% of consultation-liaison patients receive a diagnosis of anxiety disorder, somatoform disorder, or psychological factors affecting a nonpsychiatric medical condition. Data on the distribution of Axis II disorders in consultation-liaison are limited. The interface of psychiatry and medicine has long posed problems with regard to psychiatric diagnosis and nosology. This is most readily exemplified in the problem of depression emerging in the context of medical illness. The usual guideposts for the diagnosis of major depression are sleep, appetite, energy, libido, and the like; such "vegetative" parameters are often confounded in the medical-surgical patient with a disseminated malignancy or poorly controlled diabetes. Substitute criteria and guidelines for judgments regarding the relative contributions of the medical illness have not achieved strong consensus to date. Those drafting DSM–IV labored with these issues, and some changes have been instituted. Clinicians now can identify "Depressions Due to a Medical Condition," putting Axis III directly in the Axis I diagnosis. The same holds true for psychotic disorders and anxiety disorders which are seen in consultation.

Commonly Reported Distribution of Psychiatric Disorders Seen by a General Hospital Psychiatric Consultation Service

• Affective disorders (primary and those resulting from a general medical condition)	25%
• Delirium, dementia, amnesia and other cognitive disorders	25%
• Adjustment disorders	25%
• Somatoform disorders, anxiety disorders, and personality disorders	each < 10%

7. To what extent do consultees follow the recommendations of consultation psychiatrists?

Traditionally, psychiatric consultants offered their recommendations without the benefit of data concerning the likelihood that such recommendations would be followed. However, studies with specific concordance criteria published in the last decade provide some guidance to the psychiatric consultant. These studies indicate a hierarchy in which more than two thirds of consultants' recommendations for psychotropic medications are implemented, but only half the directives for diagnostic steps are instituted. Referring physicians are also unlikely to demonstrate an interest in, or an appreciation for, the consultant's psychiatric diagnoses: fewer than 50% of these diagnoses are accurately represented in discharge summaries of the hospitalization.

Thus, the psychiatric consultant can expect heightened receptivity to management suggestions, but less concern for proposals that involve further assessment and matters of diagnostic classification. The data suggest that consultees are largely concerned with practical or empiric steps to control behavior or improve mood. In the busy medical-surgical setting, the pursuit of psychiatric diagnosis or clarification of psychiatric factors is often overlooked or set aside. Most strikingly, some data from the concordance studies suggest that the medical work-up and management of patients with comorbid psychiatric conditions are more often abbreviated than are those of patients without psychiatric issues.

8. What factors govern concordance with consultants' recommendations?

When concordance studies were first initiated, it was expected by investigators that a major factor in achieving concordance would be the individual consultants. As some consultants are more skilled, more articulate, more compelling, it seemed logical that consultants' identities and the particular pairings with referring physicians would be crucial to the outcomes achieved. The data from the studies have been quite clear: concordance is not a function of the identities of the consultants or consultees. Concordance rates are surprisingly consistent no matter who performs the two roles. Equally surprising have been the data which show that concordance with recommendations for psychotropic drugs or diagnostic actions is not a function of which class of drug (antipsychotic, anxiolytic, or antidepressant) or which diagnostic measure (laboratory test, procedure, or consultation) is advised. What does explain concordance? There is no single or simple answer. The variables influencing concordance differ by the various areas studied, however. Best concordance rates seem to be achieved when recommendations are *brief, prioritized, and unequivocal.* It appears that conditional recommendations (i.e., do "A" if the following things happen) are often perceived as a sign of an indecisive or uncertain consultant. Most consultees want a pragmatic set of directives, not a lengthy academic discussion of possibilities.

9. What changes will DSM–IV bring to consultation-liaison psychiatry?

From a consultation-liaison perspective, the extensive revision of the Organic Mental Disorders section of the manual is the major impact of DSM–IV. Gone is the title, Organic Mental Disorders and in its place is Delirium, Dementia and Other Cognitive Disorders. To many, an *organic* section of the manual implied that the remainder must be *nonorganic.* Removal of the functional-organic dichotomy should help to remind clinicians that both factors need to be explored in all instances of psychiatric symptoms.

DSM–IV has also returned Organic Mood, Organic Anxiety, Organic Delusional, and Organic Personality Syndrome to their phenomenologic home bases. For example, a depression caused by a stroke will be classified as Mood Disorder, Depressive Type Due to a Cerebrovascular Accident. Axis III is directly incorporated in the Axis I diagnosis. The clinician confronted with a patient exhibiting depression now has to think routinely of Axis III in the differential diagnosis.

Multi-infarct dementia has been retitled Vascular Dementia and a fuller roster of behavioral subtyping has been added. Finally, the diagnostic criteria for many formerly termed Organic Mental Disorders have been reworked.

10. What are the usual interventions provided by the consultation psychiatrist?

A primary task of the psychiatric consultant is to help the medical-surgical patient cope with the demands of hospitalization. Consultation work is pragmatic. It is based in the present. Its objectives are to identify and strengthen the patient's own defensive constellation and proclivities in the short-term; consultation-liaison is seldom confrontational. Consultation-liaison work favors an active approach in which establishing a direct personal linkage with the patient is vital.

Many regard supportive intervention as the psychiatric consultant's principal function. By various actions and gestures, the consultation-liaison psychiatrist reassures, comforts, listens, and coordinates. At the heart of the intervention are genuine concern for the patient's plight, and a willingness and an ability to empathize. The consultation-liaison psychiatrist must be attuned to themes of uncertainty, fear, and abandonment. The repertoire must include skills in grief work, engaging the spouse and family, and anticipating the likely progression of events in the hospitalization and medical course.

In addition to psychotherapy skills, the consultation-liaison psychiatrist must be conversant with a range of psychopharmacologic interventions. This includes the management of agitation, delirium, depression, anxiety, drug-induced psychotic disorders, and psychiatric presentations "due to a general medical condition." Regrettably, the use of psychotropics in the medically ill has had limited systematic study. The consultant often assumes liaison or educational functions with referring physicians and nursing staff; psychosocial interventions are emphasized by some consultation-liaison clinicians (especially in Europe). Cognitive and behavioral interventions are occasionally used in consultation-liaison. Finally it should be noted that 5 to 10% of consultation-liaison interventions result in a psychiatric hospitalization/transfer. The number of patients referred for outpatient treatment or follow-up is presently undefined but is growing.

11. Is depression in the medically ill a discrete entity? (Are these depressions generic or specific to the given physical illness?)
The idea that depression arising in the patient with a medical illness might differ from depression found in patients without physical disease has only lately gained a measure of acceptance. Because physical illness confounds many of the vegetative signs by which depression is routinely diagnosed, investigators have generally avoided the nosologic and diagnostic complexities of "medical depression." Many have found it simpler to assume that medical depression is the same as primary depression. However, some data suggest this is not so. For example, the prevalence of primary depression in women is twice that of men, but medical depression is equally prevalent in both genders. Primary depression has strong genetic loading; medical depression appears independently of familial affective history. A shortened REM latency in sleep electroencephalographic studies is a useful biologic marker of primary depression. Studies exist which suggest that depression in the medically ill (predominantly pathophysiologic rather than reactive) responds less favorably to antidepressant medication than does primary depression.

In several major neurologic illnesses (Parkinson's disease, Huntington's disease, stroke, Alzheimer's), lifetime prevalence rates of major depression are surprisingly consistent, ranging from 30% to 50%. Multiple sclerosis is an exception. In multiple sclerosis, the prevalence of depression in patients with only spinal involvement is less than 10%; for those with cortical disease, the rate of occurrence of depression exceeds 30%. Lifetime prevalence rates of depression in systemic medical illnesses are more variable, ranging from 5% to 8% in end-stage renal disease to 33% to 67% in Cushing's disease.

Collectively, evidence argues that depression occurring in the medically ill is a discrete entity which has features all its own. Whether these depressions are specific to the given physical illness or generic in their presentation and features remains to be further clarified. It is currently thought that there may be a commonality to those depressions emerging in the setting of loss of structural integrity of the central nervous system. For those encountered in systemic medical conditions, the picture appears less consistent.

12. How should a *medical depression* be treated by the psychiatric consultant?
This remains an area of controversy. Literature indicates that electroconvulsive therapy may be the intervention most likely to benefit the patient with marked medical depression. However, such data are retrospective rather than prospective. In the medically ill, traditional tricyclic antidepressants have questionable efficacy (at least less than usual) and carry substantial side effects. Selective serotonin reuptake inhibitors (SSRIs) await formal study in populations of medically ill patients, but hold some potential (combined with the benefits of single daily dosing without increments and a more tolerable side effect profile). The combination of an SSRI and supportive psychotherapy is a reasonable first step in the face of medical depression. Subsequent steps may be necessary as the medical illness waxes and wanes, hospitalization concludes, and additional stressors emerge.

BIBLIOGRAPHY

1. Fava GA, Sonino N, Wise TN: Management of depression in medical patients. Psychother Psychosom 49:81, 1988.
2. Hackett TP, Cassem NH: Handbook of General Hospital Psychiatry. Littleton, MA, PSG Publishing, 1987.
3. Hales RE: The benefits of a psychiatric consultation-liaison service in a general hospital. General Hosp Psychiatry 7:214–218, 1985.
4. Huyse F: Systematic Interventions in CL. Amsterdam, Free University Press, 1989.
5. Levenson JL, Hammer RM, Rossiter LF: Relation of psychopathology in general medical inpatients to use and cost of services. Am J Psychiatry 147:1498, 1990.

6. Pasnau RO: Consultation-liaison psychiatry: Progress, problems and prospects. Psychosomatics 29:1, 1988.

7. Popkin MK, Mackenzie TB, Callies AL: Consultation-liaison outcome evaluation system: Consultation-consultee interaction. Arch Gen Psychiatry 40:215, 1983.

8. Popkin MK, Tucker GJ: "Secondary" and drug-induced mood, anxiety, psychotic, catatonic and personality disorders: A review of the literature. J Neuropsychiatry Clin Neurosci 4:369–385, 1992.

9. Seward LN, Smith GC, Stuart GW: Concordance with recommendations in a consultation-liaison psychiatry service. Aust N Z J Psychiatry 25:243–254, 1991.

10. Stoudemire A, Fogel BS: Psychiatric Care of the Medical Patient. Oxford, Oxford University Press, 1993.

11. Thompson T (ed): Research advances in consultation-liaison psychiatry. Psychiatr Med 9:506–648, 1991.

12. Wells KB, Golding JM, Burnham MD: Psychiatric disorder in a sample of the general population with and without chronic medical conditions. Am J Psychiatry 145:976, 1988.

67. PSYCHIATRIC DISORDERS IN PRIMARY CARE SETTINGS

Steven Kick, M.D., M.S.P.H.

1. How common are psychiatric disorders in primary care settings?

The primary care sector has been labeled a de facto mental health care system because almost two-thirds of all patients with psychiatric illnesses in the U.S. are seen exclusively in primary care settings. Prevalence studies in primary care clinics have consistently shown rates of up to 30% for psychiatric disorders meeting DSM–III–R criteria; this probably will not change using DSM–IV criteria. It is probable, however, that significant psychiatric illness exceeds this rate because of so-called mixed or minor disorders that do not meet full diagnostic criteria. In any case, primary health care settings carry the burden of patients with psychiatric disorders in the U.S.

2. Which disorders are seen most frequently in primary care settings?

Anxiety, mood disturbance, and psychoactive substance abuse are the most common disorders in primary care settings. The following table lists the disorders by decreasing lifetime prevalence rates:

Disorder	%
Major depression	17.1
Alcohol dependence	14.1
Social phobia	13.3
Simple phobia	11.3
Alcohol abuse	9.4
Drug dependence	7.5
Dysthymia	6.4
Agoraphobia	5.3
Generalized anxiety disorder	5.1
Panic disorder	3.5
Manic episode	1.6
Nonaffective psychosis	0.7

3. How do persons with psychiatric disorders present to the clinician?

Patients with psychiatric disorders often present to primary care providers with somatic complaints referable to their underlying disorder. For mood disorders, the most frequent complaints are fatigue, alteration in sleep, and chronic pain. Among anxiety disorders, panic disorder has been the most thoroughly studied for association with medically unexplained symptoms. The following table lists the prevalence of panic disorder among patients with medically unexplained symptoms:

SYMPTOMS	PREVALENCE OF PANIC DISORDER (%)
Chest pain with negative angiogram	33–43
Irritable bowel	29–38
Unexplained dizziness	13
Migraine headache	4.9 (panic)
	1.6 (agoraphobia)
Chronic fatigue	13–30
Chest pain in emergency department	18

In patients with 5 more more medically unexplained symptoms, the odds of having panic disorder were 204 to 1.

Frequently, patients have a number of nonspecific symptoms that frustrate both patient and provider. For example, a young man with lightheadedness and atypical chest pain came to our clinic after having a magnetic resonance imaging (MRI) scan of the brain, electroencephalogram, Holter monitor testing, exercise treadmill, echocardiogram, cerebral angiography, and numerous blood tests. A careful history revealed that he had panic disorder. In this case, a good history may have saved thousands of unnecessary dollars in testing.

4. What medical conditions are associated with psychiatric disorders?

A number of medical conditions are associated with symptoms that may mimic psychiatric disorders. Illnesses with significant functional impairment or mortality may be associated with anxious or depressed moods. Usually, medical conditions can be diagnosed with a careful history, physical exam, and prudent laboratory tests, as demonstrated with the differentiation between panic disorder and pheochromocytomas. Panic disorder is associated with intense fear, apprehension, and often avoidant behavior, whereas pheochromocytomas present with recurrent bouts of hypertension, palpitations, and sweating; fear and apprehension develop later in the episode. Establishing causal relationships between medical and psychiatric disorders can be difficult, especially when the prevalence of both is high. Such is the case with depression and hypothyroidism. Although it is popular to do a variety of tests, the history and physical exam should guide the clinician. For example, computed tomography or MRI scanning of the brain is generally helpful only if the patient has a dementia or focal neurologic findings; brain scans are not helpful for the diagnosis of other psychiatric disorders.

Medications also may result in symptoms that mimic psychiatric disorders. In particular, sedative-hypnotics and centrally acting antihypertensive agents, such as reserpine and clonidine, may produce a depressed mood. Contrary to popular belief, beta-adrenergic blocking agents do not generally cause depressive symptoms. Several agents may cause sleep disturbances and agitation or anorexia, such as pseudoephedrine and thyroxine. A careful medication history with diminution or cessation of the drug may reveal the cause and treat the apparent psychiatric disorder.

5. How common are substance abuse problems in primary care?

Substance abuse and dependence are quite common in primary care settings and carry significant morbidity and mortality. It is estimated that 10% of the adult population and 30–50% of persons in primary care may have alcohol abuse or dependence. The cost to society for medical care and lost productivity was estimated to be $115 billion in 1983. Alcohol abuse and dependence, the most common disorder, may aggravate a number of medical problems, including sleep disturbances, hypertension, diabetes, peptic ulcer disease, anemia, and mood disorders. Often such aggravations or laboratory abnormalities (elevated aspartate aminotransferase, alanine aminotransferase, gamma glutamyl transpeptidase, mean corpuscular volume) may alert the clinician to the possibility of alcohol use. Similarly, alteration in daily activities such as work delinquency and/or legal problems may suggest alcoholism.

Screening instruments such as the CAGE questionnaire are easy to use and may have diagnostic sensitivities of 85–89%:

1. Are you **C**oncerned about your drinking?
2. Have others **A**ngered you about your drinking?
3. Have you felt **G**uilty about your drinking?
4. Have you ever had an **E**ye-opener (e.g., morning drink)?

Unfortunately, clinicians often do not inquire about a history of substance use or use readily available screening tools.

Finally, alcohol and other psychoactive substances are strongly correlated with other psychiatric disorders, particularly major depression, bipolar disorder, panic disorder, social phobia and posttraumatic stress disorder.

6. Which psychiatric disorders can the primary care provider treat?

The type of psychiatric disorder that a primary care physician can treat varies with the severity of the disorder, expertise of the physician, availability of treatment options, and desires of the patient. Disorders marked by psychosis, severe behavioral changes (such as avoidant behavior), and lethality (suicide or homicide) should be treated by or with a mental health professional. Because psychiatric disorders occur so commonly in general medical settings, the primary care provider must be confident in assessing such patients. Indeed, patients often feel more comfortable and less stigmatized with primary care physicians. Often, treatment may be initiated and the patient closely followed. If improvement in symptoms does not occur in 6–8 weeks, the patient may then be referred.

7. Why should the primary care provider not treat every depressed patient with the newer antidepressants such as fluoxetine, which appear safe?

It is certainly easy for the primary care physician to prescribe the newer antidepressants, as evidenced by the overwhelming increase in the number of prescriptions. Such drugs are attractive because they are simple to dose, do not require monitoring of serum levels, and are generally well-tolerated. Nonetheless, because they are easy to give does not warrant their use outside approved indications. It is not known whether such agents are effective for mixed or minor disorders. In addition, they may precipitate agitation or mania and are therefore to be used cautiously or not at all in persons with a history of hypomania, mania, or agitation. Likewise, they are not free from side effects and are not inexpensive. Therefore they should be used prudently by the primary care provider. In addition, research demonstrates the need for psychotherapy in many depressed patients. Combining psychotherapy with pharmacologic treatment is likely to provide better results. Hence, providing medication alone may treat a depressive illness only partially.

8. How useful are screening instruments for psychiatric case-finding?

Currently several screening instruments are available to the primary care provider, ranging from self-administered questionnaires to more formal interviewer-rated instruments. All have the advantage of suggesting a disorder when the provider faces time constraints. However, even the best instruments have predictive values of only 70–85%, and unfortunately, few have been adequately validated against standard structured interviews. Such instruments should be used only for case-finding and not for definitive diagnosis.

Commonly Used Screening Instruments

DISORDER	PATIENT-RATED	INTERVIEWER-RATED
Depression		
CES-D	X	
Beck	X	
Hamilton		X
MOS	X	
HADS	X	
Anxiety		
Zung	X	
Hamilton	X	
Sheehan	X	X
Beck Cognition	X	
HADS	X	
Both		
SDDS-PC	X	X
Prime-MD	X	X

CES-D = Center for Epidemiologic Studies—Depression, MOS = Medical Outcomes Study, HADS = Hospital Anxiety and Depression Scale, SDDS-PC = Symptom-Driven Diagnostic Schedule—Primary Care

BIBLIOGRAPHY

1. Kessler RC, McGonagle KA, Zhao S, et al: Lifetime and 12-month prevalence of DSM-III-R psychiatric disorders in the United States: Results from the National Comorbidity Survey. Arch Gen Psychiatry 51:8–19, 1994.
2. Kessler LG, Cleary PD, Burke JD: Psychiatric disorders in primary care. Arch Gen Psychiatry 42:583–587, 1985.
3. Lustman PJ: Anxiety disorders in adults with diabetes mellitus. Psychiatr Clin North Am 11(2):419–431, 1988.
4. Von Korff M, Shapiro S, Burke JD: Anxiety and depression in a primary care clinic. Arch Gen Psychiatry 44:152–156, 1987.
5. Walker EA, Katon WJ, Jemelka RP: Psychiatric disorders and medical care utilization among people in the general population who report fatigue. J Gen Intern Med 8:436–440, 1993.
6. Yingling KW, Wulsin LR, Arnold LM, Rouan GW: Estimated prevalences of panic disorder and depression among consecutive patients seen in an emergency department with acute chest pain. J Gen Intern Med 8:231–235, 1993.

68. THE MANAGEMENT OF CHRONIC PAIN

Robert N. Jamison, Ph.D., and Sharon L. Elliott, M.S.

1. What is the difference between acute and chronic pain?

Acute pain is generally associated with tissue damage and is a warning of injury to the individual. It is expected to be directly proportional to the sensory input of the tissue damage and to continue until the damaged tissue and/or afferent pathways have returned to normal functioning. Chronic nonmalignant pain is a persistent condition often associated with an initial episode of acute pain but continuing long past the time when healing would normally take place. Chronic nonmalignant pain serves no beneficial purpose and is resistant to medical intervention.

Pain syndromes may be categorized according to the character and history of the symptom. *Acute pain* is self-limiting, is usually of less than 6 months' duration and is generally adaptive in nature (e.g., post-surgical pain, dental pain, pain following injury). *Recurrent acute pain* consists of a series of intermittent episodes acute in character but chronic insofar as the condition persists for longer than 6 months (e.g., migraine headaches, trigeminal neuralgia, temporomandibular disorder). *Chronic nonmalignant pain* persists beyond 6 months and is intractable. Pain severity varies over time and may or may not have a known relationship to active pathophysiologic or pathoanatomic process (e.g., chronic mechanical low-back pain, diffuse myofascial pain syndrome). *Chronic progressive pain* increases in severity over time and often is associated with malignancies and degenerative disorders (e.g., skeletal metastatic disease, rheumatoid arthritis). This chapter is concerned mostly with chronic nonmalignant pain.

2. What is the difference between psychogenic and organic pain?

Chronic pain has a complex interaction of factors. The pain is often related to an initial somatic event but, over time, is increasingly influenced by the patient's personality, beliefs, and environment. Attempts to distinguish reliably between organic and psychogenic pain have been largely unsuccessful. Many practitioners incorrectly believe that chronic pain reflects either organic pathology or psychogenic symptoms. If physical findings are inadequate to account for a patient's report of chronic pain, then the pain is often perceived to be largely psychological. However, whether or not an individual presents with organic pathology may be independent of significant psychopathology. For example, a person may have both a major psychiatric illness and clinical low back pain. It is generally unwarranted to assume that psychological factors are the primary cause of pain.

3. What are the best ways to assess chronic pain?

The process of evaluating the chronic pain patient is much like piecing together parts of a puzzle and then using the resulting information to assess prognosis and determine the best course of treatment. A semistructured interview is useful in identifying information pertinent to treatment. Before meeting with the patient, it is helpful to review all referral information, including discharge summaries, psychological testing results, physicians' notes, and medical history reports. Important areas of information which should be included in a semistructured interview are presented in the table below. Structured-interview measures have been published for the assessment of alcoholism and drug abuse (e.g., the CAGE Questionnaire, the Michigan Alcoholism Screening Test [MAST], and the Self-Administered Alcoholism Screen Test [SAAST]) and for psychiatric diagnosis (the Structured Clinical Interview for DSM–III–R [SCID]). Whenever possible, the patient's family members and/or significant other should also be interviewed.

Components of a Semistructured Interview

• Relevant medical history	• Compensation status
• Pain description	• History of drug and alcohol abuse
• Aggravating factors	• History of psychiatric disturbance
• Daily activity level	• Current perceived support
• Past and current treatments	• Motivation to take an active role in treatment
• Education and employment history	

4. Which measures are useful in assessing pain intensity?

Pain intensity can be measured by subjective numerical pain ratings, visual analogue scales (VAS), verbal rating scales, pain drawings, and combined standardized questionnaires. Numerical pain ratings often consist of asking the patient to rate his or her pain on a scale from 0 to 10 or 0 to 100. Ideally, descriptive anchors offered to help the patient gain an understanding of the meaning of each numeric value improve the external validity of the measure. Another popular means of measuring pain intensity is the visual analogue scale (VAS), which uses a straight line with extreme limits of pain on either end of the line. Often the line is ten centimeters long. The pain patient is instructed to place a mark on the line which best indicates the severity of the patient's present pain. Scores are obtained by measuring the distance from the end labeled "no pain" to the mark which is provided by the patient. Evidence exists for the validity of the VAS. Despite its frequent use in measuring chronic pain, scoring VAS is time-consuming, and its validity is questionable for older patients.

Several verbal rating scales exist. These scales consist of words chosen by the patient in describing the pain. Verbal scales not only measure pain intensity, but also assess sensory and reactive dimensions of the pain experience. These scales may consist of as few as four or as many as 15 words ranked in order of their severity, ranging from "no pain" to "excruciating pain." Verbal scales can also measure pain description. The patient chooses words from a list to best describe the pain experience. Examples of these words may include piercing, stabbing, shooting, burning, and throbbing. Of all of the self-report measures, numeric rating scales are most popular. However, no evidence suggests that VAS or verbal rating scales are any less sensitive to treatment effects. All of these measures have been shown to be acceptable in the quantification of clinical pain.

The McGill Pain Questionnaire (MPQ) is a popular comprehensive questionnaire which includes 20 subclasses of descriptors as well as a numeric pain intensity scale and a dermatomal pain drawing. The MPQ has become a frequently used clinical tool in the subjective measurement of pain. A short form of the MPQ also has been published. The MPQ allows for measurement of different aspects of the pain experience and is sensitive to treatment affects and differential diagnosis.

Averaging multiple measures of pain intensity over time increases the reliability and validity of the assessment and is preferable to a single rating. Baseline measures are essential to any decision on the overall impact of treatment for pain.

5. What will assess psychopathology?

Most chronic pain patients do not have a history of premorbid psychiatric disturbance, but show reactive emotional distress in response to their pain. However, when present, major psychopathology is indicative of a poor prognosis for pain therapy. Mental health professionals have an ongoing debate about the best ways to measure psychopathology in chronic pain patients. Pain patients frequently endorse somatic complaints in response to their condition. Thus, there is always a need for caution in interpreting psychological tests in which somatic complaints are considered indicative of psychopathology in pain patients. The measures most commonly used to evaluate psychopathology and emotional distress in chronic pain patients include the Minnesota Multiphasic Personality Inventory (MMPI), the Symptom Checklist 90 (SCL–90–R), the Millon Behavior Health Inventory (MBHI), the Illness Behavior Questionnaire (IBQ), and the Beck Depression Inventory (BDI).

The MMPI is the most popular instrument used in assessing chronic pain patients. This measure consists of 561 true-false items. It has the capacity to determine distinct profiles of pain patients. Studies have shown that profile patterns are able to predict return to work dates as well as response to surgical treatment. A revised version of the original MMPI is now used (MMPI–2). Studies have shown that profile patterns in the original MMPI can be replicated with the MMPI–2. Although this is a very popular test to measure the presence of psychopathology, profiles of chronic pain patients can be misinterpreted because of the physical symptoms frequently endorsed by these patients.

Another measure used to determine emotional distress is the SCL–90. This is a 90-item checklist using a five-point scale which offers a global index score as well as nine subscale scores. The SCL–90 offers a general assessment of emotional distress. It is a relatively brief measure and offers some face validity for the pain patients. It is easy to inspect individual items which may pertain specifically to persons with chronic pain. Its disadvantage is that all subscales are highly correlated and no validity scales exist to determine the presence of subtle inconsistencies in responses.

The MBHI is another popular measure for assessing mood and personality. The MBHI contains 150 true and false items and offers 20 subscales which measure: (1) styles relating to providers; (2) psychosocial stressors; and (3) response to illness. The advantage of the MBHI is that the scales are not subject to misinterpretation resulting from physical symptoms. Unlike the other measures, the MBHI emphasizes medical rather than emotional concerns.

The IBQ is commonly used to determine emotionality and illness behavior in chronic-pain patients. The IBQ contains 62 true-false items and consists of seven subscales measuring symptom complaints and abnormal illness behavior. Patients who are not known to have organic pathology which would account for their pain tend to produce higher IBQ scores. The IBQ is also correlated with anxiety measures.

The BDI assesses depressive symptoms in chronic pain patients. This is a 21-item self-reporting questionnaire that provides a measure of severity of depression. It is commonly used to determine outcome from treatment; and is easy to administer and score. One limitation is the possible misinterpretation of an elevated depression score resulting from frequent endorsement of somatic items by chronic pain patients such as fatigue, sleep disturbances, and loss of sexual interest.

6. Can pain-related beliefs be factored in?

A person's beliefs about pain are important in predicting the outcome of treatment. Negative thoughts about an ongoing pain problem may contribute to increased pain and emotional distress, decreased functioning, and greater reliance on medication. Certain chronic-pain patients are prone to maladaptive beliefs about their condition that may not be compatible with its physical nature (e.g., "This pain will make me lose my mind." "Soon I will become an invalid."). The most popular tests used to measure maladaptive beliefs include the Coping Strategies Questionnaire (CSQ), the Pain Management Inventory (PMI), the Pain Self-Efficacy Questionnaire, the Survey of Pain Attitudes (SOPA), and the Inventory of Negative Thoughts in Response to Pain (INTRP).

Patients who demonstrate an elevated score on the Catastrophizing Scale of the CSQ, who endorse passive coping on the PMI, who demonstrate low self-efficacy regarding their abilities to manage pain, who perceive themselves to be disabled by their pain on the SOPA, and who have frequent negative thoughts about their pain on the INTRP are at greatest risk for poor treatment outcome. It is suspected that patients who have unrealistic beliefs about their condition are also poor candidates for pain treatments.

7. What is the importance of functional capacity?

The assessment of functional capacity and interference with activity is important because third-party payors frequently judge treatment outcome on the basis of improved function and return to work. Reliable instruments used to measure function include the Sickness Impact Profile (SIP), the Short-Form Health Survey (SF–36), the Multidimensional Pain Inventory (MPI), and the Pain Disability Index (PDI).

The SIP is a 136-item checklist which contains 12 subscales measuring levels of physical and psychosocial functioning. Each item is weighted and the scales have been shown to be correlated with other functional capacity measures. Shorter versions of the SIP (Roland and Morris Disability Questionnaire) have been shown to be suitable in assessing function in chronic-pain patients.

The SF–36 was initially developed from the Medical Outcomes Study to survey health status. The SF–36 includes eight scales which measure (1) limitations in physical activities due to health problems, (2) limitations in social activities due to physical and emotional problems, (3) limitations in usual role activities due to physical health problems, (4) bodily pain, (5) general mental health, (6) limitations in usual role activities due to emotional problems, (7) vitality (energy and fatigue), and (8) general health perceptions. The SF–36 is favored over the SIP because it is a shorter test with excellent reliability and validity. The SIP is preferred if the population of patients includes those with extreme physical limitations.

The Multidimensional Pain Inventory is a 56-item measure using 7-point scales. The subscales assess activity interference, perceived support, pain severity, negative mood, and perceived control. The advantage of this self-report instrument is that it was created specifically for chronic pain patients and can be useful in classifying patients into three patient types: Dysfunctional, Interpersonally Distressed, and Adaptive Copers. Strong evidence has been found for a taxonomy of these three chronic pain patient groups.

Other functional measures include The Chronic Illness Problem Inventory, The Waddell Disability Instrument and The Functional Rating Scale. Automated measurement devices such as the portable up-time calculator and the pedometer are useful ways to obtain accurate measures of activity. These devices should be used in conjunction with self-monitoring assessment techniques.

Assessment Categories and Frequently Used Psychometric Measures

Psychosocial History
  Comprehensive pain questionnaire
  The CAGE Questionnaire
  The Michigan Alcoholism Screening Test (MAST)
  The Self-administered Alcoholism Screen Test (SAAST)
  The Structured Clinical Interview for DSM–III–R (SCID)

Pain Intensity
  Numerical rating scales
  Visual analogue scales (VAS)
  Verbal rating scales
  Pain drawings

Mood and Personality
  Minnesota Multiphasic Personality Inventory (MMPI)
  Symptom Checklist 90 (SCL–90)
  Millon Behavior Health Inventory (MBHI)
  Illness Behavior Questionnaire (IBQ)
  Beck Depression Inventory (BDI)

Pain-Related Beliefs and Coping
  Coping Strategies Questionnaire (CSQ)
  Pain Management Inventory (PMI)
  Pain Self-Efficacy Questionnaire
  Survey of Pain Attitudes (SOPA)
  Inventory of Negative Thoughts in Response to Pain (INTRP)

Functional Capacity
  Sickness Impact Profile SIP)
  Short-Form Health Survey (SF–36)
  Multidimensional Pain Inventory (MPI)
  Pain Disability Index (PDI)

8. What is an interdisciplinary pain treatment program?

Chronic pain involves a complex interaction of physiologic and psychosocial factors, and successful intervention requires the coordinated effort of a treatment team with expertise in a variety of therapeutic disciplines. Although some pain centers offer a unimodal treatment approach, most programs use a blend of medical, psychological, vocational, and educational techniques.

Most interdisciplinary pain-treatment programs have as their core staff one or more physicians, a clinical psychologist, and a physical therapist. Other health professionals who may play important roles include clinical nurse specialists, occupational therapists, vocational rehabilitation counselors, and exercise physiologists. Physicians from specialty areas (e.g., psychiatry, neurology, rheumatology, orthopedic surgery, physical medicine, and internal medicine) should be available for consultation. An interdisciplinary staff coordinates efforts to rehabilitate the pain patient and provides a comprehensive discharge and follow-up plan designed to meet the patient's short- and long-term needs.

Treatment Modalities for Chronic Pain

• Medical assessment	• Biofeedback
• Medication management	• Physical therapy
• Pain-reduction treatments	• Psychotherapy
• Didactic instruction	• Vocational counseling
• Relaxation training	

9. How are outpatient pain programs typically structured?

Multidisciplinary pain programs administered on an outpatient basis are often highly structured, time-limited, and organized along a specific treatment schedule (e.g., 5 to 7 days per week for 4 weeks; 1 day per week for 10 weeks). The patient is expected to attend clinic sessions and to participate actively in all aspects of the program. These expectations must be made clear. Patients frequently sign a treatment contract that spells out the general program requirements as well as their individual treatment goals. In addition to helping patients to understand exactly what is expected of them, such a contract provides a mechanism for identifying those patients who, before treatment, lack motivation or may have difficulty conforming to the structure of the program. Patients are asked to keep a daily written record of their pain intensity, medication use, and activity levels.

10. What are the desired outcomes of interdisciplinary treatment?

The therapeutic aims of interdisciplinary interventions for chronic nonmalignant pain include decreased pain intensity, increased physical activity, decreased reliance on pain medication, a return to work, improved psychosocial functioning, and reduced use of health-care services.

11. What are the objectives of cognitive-behavioral therapy for patients with chronic pain ?

The first objective is to help patients change their view of their problem from overwhelming to manageable. Patients who are prone to "catastrophize" benefit from examining the way they view their situation. What could be perceived as a hopeless condition can be reframed as a difficult yet manageable one over which they can exercise some control.

The second objective of cognitive-behavioral therapy is to help convince patients that the treatment is relevant to their problems and that they need to be actively involved in treatment and rehabilitation. They need to understand how relaxation training, cognitive restructuring, adaptive coping skills, and pacing behaviors can help decrease their pain. They also need to reorient their view away from that of passive victim to that of proactive, competent problem-solver. When people are successful in managing difficult painful episodes, their views change. Patients eventually begin to believe themselves capable of overcoming any acute flare-up of pain.

The third objective is to teach patients to monitor maladaptive thoughts and substitute positive ones. Persons with chronic pain are plagued, either consciously or unconsciously, by negative thoughts about their condition. These negative thoughts have a way of perpetuating pain behaviors and feelings of hopelessness. Demonstrating how and when to attack these negative thoughts and when to substitute positive thoughts and adaptive management techniques for chronic pain is an important component of cognitive restructuring. Patients are encouraged to attribute success to their own efforts; they need to feel that they are responsible for the gains they make. Finally, anticipation of problems and lapses needs to be discussed so that the patient will have a "game plan" to manage short-term setbacks.

12. What is the role of group therapy for pain patients?

Pain patients frequently show signs of emotional distress, with evidence of depression, anxiety, and irritability. Group therapy with a cognitive-behavioral orientation is designed to help patients gain control of the emotional reactions associated with chronic pain. Specific problem-solving strategies can be offered during group therapy sessions, including: (1) identifying maladaptive and negative thoughts; (2) disputing "irrational" thinking; (3) constructing and repeating positive self-statements; (4) learning distraction techniques; (5) working to prevent future catastrophizing; and (6) examining ways to increase social support. In addition, group therapy presents an opportunity to discuss any concerns or problems that patients may have in common. Unlike psychotherapists in traditional group sessions, group therapists in a pain-management program are encouraged to be active facilitators. They may need to redirect the discussion so that every member has an opportunity to speak and no individual monopolizes the session.

Certain group members may initially be reluctant to discuss personal problems related to their pain. The group therapist must prevent other group members from being overly judgmental and negative. Group members should be told that they are there to learn from each other and to support each other in gaining control over their condition. In order to maintain a positive group atmosphere, certain participants who show excessive negative behavior may be asked to leave. Participants should be offered individual therapy sessions in which to deal with personal relationship issues.

13. How important is family involvement in therapy?

Chronic pain significantly impacts all members of a family. Family members need to be educated about the goals of therapy and should have an opportunity to share their worries and concerns. Moreover, active involvement of family members helps ensure the patient's long-term success. Therefore, both patients and members of their families should be invited to attend family therapy sessions. At these sessions, the facilitator should encourage family members to ask questions about the pain management program, to discuss their concerns and expectations, and to express their feelings. Besides enhanced communication, important outcomes of these sessions are that family members learn how to help the person in pain to achieve and maintain goals and that they come to understand that they are not alone in their dealings with the person in pain.

14. What are the benefits of relaxation training for chronic pain patients?

Chronic pain patients tend to experience substantial residual muscle tension as a function of the bracing, posturing, and emotional arousal often associated with pain. Such responses, maintained over a long period, can exacerbate pain in injured areas of the body and increase muscular discomfort. For example, it is common for patients with low back pain or limb injuries to develop neck stiffness and tension-type headaches. Relaxation training can lead to pain reduction through the relaxation of tense muscle groups, the reduction of symptoms of anxiety, the use of distraction, and the enhancement of self-efficacy. In addition, this training can increase the patient's sense of control over physiologic responses. In a pain management program, patients are taught and encouraged to practice a variety of relaxation strategies, including diaphragmatic breathing, progressive muscle relaxation, autogenic relaxation, self-hypnosis, and cue-controlled relaxation techniques. Biofeedback training is also common. Live demonstrations of the techniques are preferable to verbal explanations. All participants should be encouraged to practice each of the techniques during the group relaxation sessions and at home. Cassette tapes can be made or purchased for practice purposes.

15. How can vocational rehabilitation help chronic-pain patients?
The goal of vocational rehabilitation is the return of a patient with chronic pain to work. After an extended period out of work, patients become both physically and psychologically deconditioned to the demands and stresses of the workplace. Working together, a vocational rehabilitation counselor and the patient can develop a plan that incorporates both long-range employment goals and short-term objectives based on medical, psychological, social, and vocational information. Vocational rehabilitation counselors are specialists in the assessment of aptitudes and interests, transferable skills, physical capacity, modifications in the workplace, skills training, and job readiness.

16. Which variables predict a low probability of the patient's returning to work?
The most relevant predictor of return to work is the duration of unemployment. After 6 months of unemployment due to chronic pain, the probability of return to work is 50%; the likelihood decreases to 10% after 1 year. Other factors with negative impact on the likelihood of returning to work include limited formal education, limited transferable skills, poor perceived social support, ongoing litigation, a poor relationship with the employer, and job dissatisfaction.

Many chronic pain patients receive workers' compensation benefits or social security disability income. Thus, patients may fear that their benefits will be jeopardized if they return to work. A vocational rehabilitation counselor can help a patient negotiate with an employer in setting up a return to work trial which would not jeopardize the patient's income. Also, through counseling strategies and assessment tools, a patient's suitability for returning to work or retraining can be determined.

17. What is the role of activity and exercise for persons with chronic pain?
Most patients lose physical stamina and flexibility because of a reluctance to exercise and a perceived need to protect themselves from additional physical injury. Some patients have been medically advised to restrict activity when pain increases. Patients with chronic pain need to know that exercise is important. Some stretching, cardiovascular activity, and weight training should be encouraged. An exercise plan should be initially determined by the patient, and reviewed and supervised by a physical therapist or exercise physiologist. Any attempt at an exercise program with chronic-pain patients is bound to produce some disappointment and perceived failure. Patients are encouraged to begin cautiously and setbacks should be anticipated. Ways to improve compliance such as organizing an exercise period with others, joining a health club, or combining exercise with another everyday activity should be explored.

18. Under what circumstances should opioid therapy be prescribed?
Considerable controversy exists about the use of opioid analgesics for chronic nonmalignant pain. Much of this controversy is related to concerns about efficacy, adverse effects, tolerance, and addiction. Some clinicians and researchers believe that long-term opioid use contributes to psychological distress, poor treatment outcome, impaired cognition, and reliance on the health care system. Others argue that chronic opioid therapy for nonmalignant pain is sometimes appropriate. They cite the relatively low incidence of abuse and addiction among chronic-pain patients given opioids, and report that tolerance often does not develop in patients with stable pain pathophysiology.

Current guidelines suggest that the administration of opioids should be considered only after all other reasonable attempts at analgesia have failed. Opioid therapy is contraindicated by a history of substance abuse, a major psychiatric diagnosis, the seeking of drugs from more than one physician, uncontrolled dose escalation, and/or evidence of lack of compliance. Patients with significant adverse reactions to low-dose opioid therapy are also poor candidates. Other *red flags* include excessive pain intensity ratings, extreme ratings of emotional distress, poor perception of coping effectiveness, use of multiple pain descriptors, poor perceived social support, multiple pain sites, poor employment history, and long-term reliance on health care professionals. The decision to use opioid therapy often rests on clinical judgment and treatment orientation. The significance of the factors just discussed is speculative at best, and—until controlled clinical trials are conducted—they cannot be considered reliable predictors of the efficacy of chronic opioid therapy for nonmalignant pain.

19. How can relapse be avoided?

Most chronic-pain patients need support after completing a pain treatment program in order to maintain the gains achieved. Patients should be encouraged to identify and anticipate situations that place them at risk for returning to previous maladaptive behavior patterns. They should also be encouraged to rehearse problem-solving techniques and behavioral responses that will enable them to avoid a relapse. The goals of relapse prevention are to help the patient: (1) maintain a steady level of activity, emotional stability, and appropriate medication use; (2) anticipate and deal with situations that cause setbacks; and (3) acquire skills that will decrease reliance on the health care system. Follow-up has been shown to be vital in helping to prevent relapse. A specific written follow-up plan should be made for each patient which may include participation in individual and group sessions.

20. What criteria are important in the evaluation of a pain treatment program?

An important component of any group-based pain program is its ability to measure its own effectiveness. A number of recommendations for effective program evaluation have been put forward by the Commission on the Accreditation of Rehabilitation Facilities (CARF). A system should be in place for obtaining follow-up information from patients on the use of medications, use of health care services, return to gainful employment, functional activities, ability to manage pain, and subjective pain intensity. Provisions should also be made for periodic contact after discharge. A data-based system should be developed from which information on patients who have completed a program can be obtained on a regular basis. This type of system not only helps determine how a program meets the needs of individual patients, but also offers substantive information on overall efficacy. Program evaluation should encompass achievable goals and objectives and measurable end results. A program evaluation report should include primary objectives, measures, time of measurement, source of information, and expectancies as well as outcome. Finally, program evaluation helps identify which types of services are most effective in the treatment of chronic pain patients.

BIBLIOGRAPHY

1. Commission on the Accreditation of Rehabilitation Facilities: Standards Manual for Organizations Serving People with Disabilities, Tucson, AZ, 1994.
2. Follick MJ, Ahern DK, Aberger EW: Behavioral treatment of chronic pain. In Blumenthal JA, McKee DC (eds): Applications in Behavioral Medicine and Health Psychology: A Clinician's Source Book. Sarasota, FL, Professional Resource Exchange, 1987, pp 237–270.
3. Fordyce WE: Behavioral Methods for Chronic Pain and Illness. St. Louis, Mosby, 1976.
4. Jamison RN: Psychological assessment of chronic pain. Pain Digest 1:230–237, 1991.
5. Jamison RN: Mastering Chronic Pain: A Manual for Persons with Chronic Pain. Sarasota, FL, Professional Resource Press, 1995.
6. Karoly P, Jensen MP: Multimethod Assessment of Chronic Pain. New York, Pergamon Press, 1987.
7. Loeser JD, Egan KJ (eds): Managing the Chronic Pain Patient: Theory and Practice at the University of Washington Multidisciplinary Pain Center. New York, Raven Press, 1989.
8. Nigl AJ: Biofeedback and Behavioral Strategies in Pain Treatment. New York, Spectrum Publications, 1984.
9. Philips HC: The Psychological Management of Chronic Pain: A Treatment Manual. New York, Springer Publishing Company, 1988.
10. Sternbach R: Pain Patients: Traits and Treatments. New York, Academic Press, 1974.
11. Turk DC, Meichenbaum D, Genest M: Pain and Behavioral Medicine: A Cognitive-Behavioral Perspective. New York, Guilford Press, 1983.
12. Turk DC, Melzack R: Handbook of Pain Assessment. New York, Guilford Press, 1992.
13. Wright G: Total Rehabilitation. Boston, Little-Brown, 1980.

69. ASSESSMENT AND TREATMENT OF SEXUAL DYSFUNCTION

Thomas D. Stewart, M.D.

1. Sexual dysfunction can be a symptom of medical illness. Name some examples.
Sexual dysfunction is a neglected vital sign in medical history taking. It can be the first presenting symptom for conditions as diverse as diabetes mellitus, temporal lobe epilepsy, multiple sclerosis, and thyroid dysfunction.

2. Describe a framework for the clinical evaluation of sexual dysfunction.
Masters and Johnson's well known sexual response cycle provides a paradigm for understanding and treating sexual dysfunction. This cycle is as follows:

Appetitive phase—This first step involves noticing attractive people and having an intact libido. There are no specific physiologic responses for this part.

Excitement—This stage is marked by vascular engorgement and lubrication in women and penile erection in men. These responses, associated with flushed skin, intensify and reach a plateau phase before orgasm.

Orgasm—This phase is associated with pelvic muscle contraction and pleasure and is accompanied by ejaculation in men.

Resolution—During this last step genital vascular engorgement gradually abates. This phase is the only one associated with sweating, caused by the response cycle itself. Namely, the exercise involved in sex can cause perspiration in all phases, but only the resolution phase has sweating as a finding specific to it regardless of exercise levels.

Sexual dysfunctions are connected with each phase in this response cycle.

3. Name medical conditions that disrupt the appetitive phase and describe what can be done to correct them.
Hypoactive sexual desire disorder can be caused by temporal lobe epilepsy, hyperprolactinemia, and hypogonadotropic hypogonadism. Carbamazepine can stabilize temporal lobe input to the anterior pituitary gland disrupted by the complex partial seizures of temporal lobe epilepsy. This stabilized input allows the anterior pituitary to increase luteinizing hormone (LH) release, leading to increased production of testosterone from Leydig cells found in the testicles. Testosterone regulates libido in both sexes.

Bromocriptine, a D_2 agonist, can reduce prolactin levels coming from pituitary microadenomas. Intramuscular testosterone offsets low testosterone levels resulting from low LH production in hypogonadotropic hypogonadism. These medications can restore sexual desire by correcting the medical problem underlying this loss. Other medications, such as alpha methyldopa, can impair libido. Libido is reduced in psychiatric conditions such as depression, anxiety, and post-traumatic stress disorder. Psychotropic medications can restore libido lost through mental illness. Proper use of psychotropics helps improve mood and reduce apprehension that underlies loss of desire.

4. What are the analogies between the excitement phases in men and women?
Erections, vaginal engorgement, and lubrication are analogous. They are similar from both embryologic and physiologic perspectives. The work-up for disorders of the excitement phase in men and women (see questions 7–9) is virtually identical.

5. Review factors in the medical history that might contribute to an impaired excitement phase.

Here is a rule of thumb. If something is bad for the heart, it is bad for erections, lubrication, and engorgement. For example, smoking, diabetes, alcohol abuse, hypertension, and hyperlipidemia are all associated with excitement phase dysfunction.

6. Name some physical findings connected with erectile dysfunction.

Gynecomastia, hypogonadism, hyperreflexia, reduced peripheral pulses, and loss of sensation.

7. What is involved in an endocrine work-up for impairment of the sexual excitement phase?

Thyroid function, liver function, glucose tolerance tests, and serum testosterone and prolactin levels.

8. Which vascular studies shed light on the etiology of impairment in sexual arousal?

There are several. They include Doppler determination of penile blood flow and penile blood pressure compared to brachial blood pressure. Penile angiography can spot arterial occlusion. Venous cavernoscopy can pinpoint the venous valvular incompetence that leads to impotence. Internal iliac angiography can identify arterial occlusions that impair erections or lubrication.

9. Describe some medication categories that can disrupt the excitement phase.

Beta blockers, anticholinergics, low-potency phenothiazines, and diuretics.

10. What is a nocturnal penile tumescence (NPT) study?

The NPT is a sleep study usually done over at least 2 nights. A doughnut-shaped plethysmographic device is placed over the penis. It transduces erectile pressure changes into graphic data. The sleep EEG records rapid eye movement sleep associated with firm erections in healthy subjects. This study can demonstrate physiologically intact erectile function that may be undermined by psychogenic factors such as anxiety in the waking state.

11. Is the NPT really the gold standard to separate organic from psychogenic sexual dysfunction?

The NPT *is* susceptible to false positives. Consider the format for the NPT study. Men sleep in a strange bed with electrodes glued to their hair. They have a gel-filled doughnut around their penis. Should they have the good fortune to have an erection while sleeping in the EEG lab, a technician emerges and checks the buckling pressure. Is it any surprise that there are false positives? In addition, clinical anxiety and depressive disorders cause abnormal results in men known to be physiologically intact. Furthermore, results of the NPT may not correlate with known functional capabilities. Although the NPT is sometimes a helpful diagnostic tool, it is not an absolute standard.

12. Name antihypertensive medication categories that do *not* appear to cause excitement phase dysfunction.

ACE inhibitors (enalapril, captopril), calcium channel blockers (verapamil, diltiazem), and alpha antagonists (terazosin, prazosin) may help potency and lubrication.

13. Describe some practical suggestions that can help sexual functioning during the excitement phase.

Water-soluble lubricants can help women with problems in arousal. These lubricants do not linger and do not dissolve diaphragms and condoms as oils can. Men can enhance their erections by pushing down their index and third finger at the base of their penis, thus partially occluding venous return. This method requires females to be in a superior position for intercourse with their bodies at a 45° angle to their partner's, and their weight on their own arms.

14. Which medications can restore erectile function?

As with the appetitive phase, bromocriptine, carbamazepine, and intramuscularly injected testosterone can help some people. No convincing evidence proves yohimbine is useful.

15. What is a vacuum constriction device?

It is a plastic tube, closed at one end, that is placed over the penis, with petroleum jelly forming a seal between the device and the mons pubis. Air is pumped out of the tube, creating a partial vacuum. Within 5 to 10 minutes, an erection develops. A constriction band is then placed at the base of the penis, and the vacuum is released to allow removal of the tube. This erection will allow vaginal penetration for 20 to 30 minutes. Erections produced by these devices are wider and shorter than natural erections. The devices are light blue and cool to touch. Complications include pain and bruises. Several studies have, however, demonstrated their safety and effectiveness.

16. What does a psychodynamic approach to excitement disorders involve?

Psychodynamic psychotherapy can help resolve unconscious conflicts over sexual expression, thus leading to restored responsiveness. This method involves exploring the meaning of potency and arousal along with those fears which are being avoided through not being able to have sexual intercourse.

17. Give an example of a behavioral approach to arousal dysfunction.

Masters and Johnson described a behavioral approach that emphasizes deconditioning stress-related responses that impair sexual functioning. Couples are encouraged to stop attempting relations and to start sensate focus explorations of how to please each other without genital contact. As they become more comfortable, they progress to more overtly sexual contact following a protocol designed to enhance feelings of safety and control. Helen Singer Kaplan modified this technique to include more exploration of individual and couple dynamics and their patterns of communication. Kaplan uses deconditioning techniques to treat sexual dysfunction, similar to those emphasized by Masters and Johnson. Her method includes greater evaluation and treatment of maladaptive patterns of communication that interfere with a couple's relationship in or out of bed. It also considers the individual psychodynamic, and those conflictual issues germane to sexual dysfunction. Couples benefit from an understanding of each other's irrational fears of sexual activity as discovered using Kaplan's approach.

18. What are some vascular interventions to restore excitement phase function?

Balloon angioplasty can open the internal iliac arteries, leading to restored potency or lubrication. Repair of incompetent venous valves, the most common vascular cause of impotence, can restore erectile function.

19. Describe the penile intracavernosal injections used to restore erectile function.

Vasodilators, such as phentolamine and yohimbine, or prostaglandin E, are injected through 29-gauge needles into the corpora cavernosum at 3 o'clock and 9 o'clock positions. The urethra is at 6 o'clock and the dorsal artery of the penis at 12. Injection at 12 or 6 would cause injury, whereas injection at 3 or 9 would allow safe entry into the corpora cavernosa. Prostaglandin E is locally metabolized in the corpora cavernosa and thus is less apt to cause priapism than the other agents which must enter systemic blood flow to be metabolized in the liver. Dosage of prostaglandin E can also be adjusted to control the duration of erection. It may, however, cause a burning sensation at the injection site.

20. What are complications of these injections?

There is a low risk of priapism. There can be painful bruising and the development of fibrosis leading to adhesions with Peyronie's disease, a condition with painful curvature of the penis during erections.

21. Describe penile prostheses as well as their advantages and disadvantages.
Penile prostheses are now in widespread use with over 100,000 having been installed. Implants vary in design. Some have wire inside silastic to allow the penis to be moved into position. Others are inflatable to allow a more normal appearance. Surgical complication following the insertion of prostheses are remarkably rare, even in diabetics. Post-operative infection and erosion through the skin are the main complications. Several studies indicate that patient and partner satisfaction with these devices exceeds 80%.

22. Which expectations men have about these devices can lead to disappointment?
Here are a few examples: "It will make her respond." "I will regain my self-esteem." "I will now have something to offer her." If a urologist should recommend placement of a phallic prosthesis, the patient's expectations regarding the operation should be explored carefully by the consulting psychiatrist. These expectations are likely to lead to disappointment if they are not combined with a concern about the quality of relationship these men want to achieve with their partners. These patients should be strongly encouraged to discuss the prosthesis with their partners so as to gather their feelings about the use of this device. One woman surprised her partner by saying, "Your message is more important than your method." She was clear that she wanted him and not a prosthetic device.

23. Are there sexual dysfunctions specific to the plateau phase?
No. Disruptions of this phase are secondary to malfunctions in other phases. Disorders of excitement will undermine the evolution of the plateau phase. Orgasmic dysfunction will prolong the plateau phase in both genders, leading to discomfort and irritability secondary to lack of release of sexual tension and genital engorgement through an orgasm.

24. What are some causes of orgasmic phase dysfunction?
Peripheral neuropathy, psychodynamic conflict, and medications.

25. What are some medications that cause orgasmic dysfunction?
Selective serotonin reuptake inhibitors (SSRIs), such as fluoxetine, paroxetine, and sertraline, monoamine oxidase inhibitors (phenelzine, tranylcypromine), and anticholernergic agents (low potency neuroleptics, tricyclic antidepressants), can inhibit orgasm. Alpha 2 blockers such as trazodone, prazosin, and thioridazine can impair sperm emission by paralyzing the vas deferens.

26. What helps restore orgasm in patients taking SSRIs?
Cyproheptadine, a serotonin antagonist, has been reported to help, with a 4-mg dose taken 30 minutes before sexual activity.

27. What are some treatments for premature ejaculation?
SSRIs have been reported to help. Masters and Johnson describe behavioral methods designed to help a couple master timing of ejaculation. This technique features deconditioning the anxiety that leads to premature ejaculation. This result is achieved by the male communicating to his partner that he is close to ejaculation. The partner then stops the stimulation and squeezes the glans with the index and third fingers and presses the urethra with the thumb. Using this method the couple can gradually prolong sexual activity before orgasm.

28. Is there a disorder of the resolution phase?
Yes, priapism is an erection that does not go away. It can be caused by alpha blockers such as trazodone and by penile injections as described in questions 19 and 20.

BIBLIOGRAPHY

1. Condra M, Morales A, Owen J, et al: Prevalence and significance of tobacco smoking in impotence. Urology 27:495–498, 1986.

2. Condra M, Morales A, Surridge D, Owen J, et al: The unreliability of nocturnal penile tumescence recording as an outcome measurement in the treatment of organic impotence. J Urol 135:280–282, 1986.
3. Cumming J, Pryor JP: Treatment of organic impotence. Br J Urol 67:640–643, 1991.
4. Drugs that cause sexual dysfunction. The Medical Letter 34:73–78, 1992.
5. Kaplan HS: The New Sex Therapy: Active Treatment of Sexual Dysfunction. New York, Bruner/Mazel, 1974.
6. Lue TF, Tanagho EA: Physiology of erection and pharmacological treatment of impotence. J Urol 137:829–836, 1987.
7. Masters W, Johnson V: Human Sexual Response. Boston, Little, Brown, 1970.
8. Masters W, Johnson V: Human Sexual Response. Boston, Little, Brown, 1966.
9. Morales A, Condra M, Owen J, et al: Is yohimbine effective in the treatment of organic impotence? Results of controlled trial. J Urol 137:1168–1172, 1987.
10. Nadig PW: Vacuum constriction devices in patients with neurogenic impotence. Sexuality and Disability 12:99–105, 1994.
11. Nafzinger EA, Thase ME, Reynolds CF, et al: Sexual function in depressed men. Arch Gen Psychiatry 50:24–30, 1993.
12. Rajfer J, Rosciszewski A, Mehringer M: Prevalence of corporeal venous leakage in impotent men. J Urol 140:69–71, 1988.
13. Segraves RT: Effects of psychotropic drugs on human erection and ejaculation. Arch Gen Psychiatry 46:275–284, 1989.
14. Spark RF, Wills CA, Royal H: Hypogonadism hyperprolactinemia and temporal lobe epilepsy in hyposexual men. Lancet 1:413–416, 1984.
15. Stachl W, Husun R, Marberger M: Intracavernous injection of prostaglandin E1 in impotent men. J Urol 140:66–68, 1988.

70. PSYCHIATRIC ASPECTS OF AIDS

Carl Clark, M.D.

1. What are HIV and AIDS?

Human immunodeficiency virus (HIV) is a retrovirus that infects humans and causes various clinical problems ranging from an asymptomatic carrier state to fatal immune deficiency. Acquired immunodeficiency syndrome (AIDS), the most serious form of HIV infection, results from progressive destruction of the immune system. HIV propagates best in lymphocytes and leads to the destruction of its host cell, primarily the CD4 helper-inducer cells. Destruction of CD4 helper-inducer cells impairs the body's ability to mount an effective immune response. HIV also infects the central nervous system cells and leads to dysfunctions such as peripheral neuropathies and encephalopathies. HIV antibodies, which develop in most people in response to HIV infection, can be detected by two standard laboratory tests, the enzyme immunoassay (EIA, formerly ELISA, or enzyme-linked immunosorbent assay) and the Western Blot. The EIA uses a reactive serum and is regarded as positive if measured absorbance is equal to or greater than a defined cut-off value. The EIA has a sensitivity of 99.7% but a specificity of only 98.5% (for double reactive EIAs). Therefore, the EIA is used as a screening test for HIV antibodies. A positive EIA result is confirmed with the Western Blot test, an immunoblot test that detects antibody to specific viral proteins and glycoproteins. The Western Blot is highly specific. In general, patients are diagnosed with AIDS if they are positive for HIV antibodies and have an opportunistic infection or cancer, HIV encephalopathy, or a helper T-cell (CD4) count < 200 cells/mm^3. The Centers for Disease Control (CDC) developed the original case definition for AIDS in 1981 before understanding of its etiology or pathophysiology.

2. What interventions decrease transmission of HIV?

HIV is transmitted by three routes: sexual, parenteral, and perinatal.

1. **Sexual transmission of HIV.** It is important to get an accurate sexual history to assess a patient's risk of HIV transmission or infection. Sexual transmission may occur when genital secretions and blood are transferred from one partner to another. Risk is decreased by using latex protective barriers (e.g., condoms). Lubricants must be water-based; petroleum or oil-based lubricants damage latex condoms. Use of condoms alone will not decrease transmission. Attitudes and feelings about safe sexual practices must be explored and discussed before meaningful and lasting changes occur. Sexual behaviors considered to contribute to HIV transmission include the following (by order of risk):

    • Unprotected anal intercourse. HIV transmission may occur when the virus comes in contact with the rectal mucosa. The rectal mucosa may sustain small rectal tears that allow HIV direct entry into the blood stream. Activities that increase the risk of damaging the rectal mucosa prior to intercourse may increase the risk of HIV transmission (e.g., enemas, manual rectal manipulation or "fisting"). Unprotected receptive anal intercourse is more risky than unprotected insertive anal intercourse.

    • Oral ingestion of semen. HIV may enter the blood stream through breaks in oral or gastrointestinal mucosa. Epidemiologic studies of gay men do not support the ingestion of semen as a risk for HIV infection.

    • Oral contact with feces.

2. **Parenteral transmission.**

    • Before it was possible to screen the blood supply for HIV, transmission occurred through blood products. The primary route of parenteral transmission currently is through the sharing of needles by intravenous drug users. Needle exchange programs have been shown effective in reducing HIV transmission. Cleaning needles also reduces risk for drug users who share needles. The additional step of cleaning a needle before injecting a drug is unreliable because of the intensity of addiction and difficulty in delaying the desired drug effect.

3. **Perinatal transmission.** In the United States less than 30% of HIV-infected mothers transmit the virus to their infants. The primary prevention for HIV transmission to infants is to prevent infection in women. Breast feeding may result in HIV transmission to the infant. HIV-infected mothers reduce the risk of transmission by using safe alternatives to breast feeding. The U.S. Public Health Service Task Force recommends the use of zidovudine (AZT) to reduce perinatal transmission of HIV.

3. Describe the epidemiology of HIV infection and AIDS.

In the United States the AIDS epidemic has occurred in all social groups. The largest number of AIDS cases have been in gay and bisexual men, followed by intravenous drug users. HIV disease occurs disproportionally in certain racial and ethnic groups. Three-fourths of pediatric cases and four-fifths of cases associated with IV drug use occur in minorities. The AIDS epidemic has paralleled the drug epidemic. Primary prevention efforts have resulted in a decrease in new cases of HIV infection in gay men; however, prevention efforts have been less successful in reducing transmission rates in other populations. Knowledge of the sociocultural aspects of each group is important if primary prevention efforts are to be successful.

4. Describe the psychological and emotional impact of HIV infection.

Patients should receive education about HIV and AIDS before being tested for HIV antibodies. Despite this education, however, one is rarely fully prepared for the emotional impact of learning that one is HIV-positive. This information disrupts the psychological state of the patient and may lead to a stress response that includes a process of denial (refusal to believe or hear the information about being HIV-positive), disorganization (being flooded with thoughts, fantasies, and feeling about being HIV-positive), symptom formation (e.g., anxiety, sadness, depression, anger), and an adaptive or maladaptive response. Examples of adaptive responses include incorporation of the information into personal lifestyle and active attempts to promote well-being and health. Examples of maladaptive responses include denial, avoidance of medical care, impulsive behaviors, suicidal behavior, or other behaviors that do not help patients to attend to their health needs, including continued high-risk sexual behavior. Anxiety, depression, and disturbances in behavior may occur. Symptoms are assessed for severity, and for their impact on the person's ability to deal with the current situation.

Anxiety may produce somatic symptoms, nervousness, sweating, tremors, gastrointestinal disturbances (diarrhea, nausea), or visual impairments. Such symptoms may be attributed to HIV illness or anxiety; thus a careful history is elicited to determine the cause of the dysfunction. Reactions to being HIV-positive rarely result i specific anxiety disorders such as phobias, generalized anxiety disorder, or panic disorder. A form of posttraumatic stress disorder has been described. Treatment interventions include supportive therapy and referral to community support groups and agencies that can assist with both the physical and emotional impacts of the illness. Family members (both biologic and chosen) should receive education about the disorder and supportive counseling.

Depression ranges from mild symptoms with little interference in the person's functioning to major depression. Treatment is indicated if the depression interferes with the person's functioning and does not depend on the underlying medical condition. The psychiatric consultant should differentiate between major depression and the cognitive deficits that may accompany early signs of dementia. Treatment interventions include cognitive therapy, group therapy, and antidepressant medications or psychostimulants. People with HIV infection can be especially vulnerable to the memory impairments caused by the anticholinergic side effects of antidepressants. Therefore, selection of antidepressants with the least anticholinergic side effects is recommended (e.g., venlafaxine, fluoxetine). People in support groups may become demoralized when members of the group die. In general, groups are more effective if the members of the group have a similar stage of HIV infection (e.g., grouping individuals who are asymptomatic or individuals with AIDS).

Psychosis may result from the direct effect of HIV infection in the brain. The differential diagnosis includes acute CNS infections, drug reactions, untreated psychiatric disorders (e.g., bipolar disorder or psychotic depression), and continued effects of drug abuse in the drug-using population. Treatment includes low-dose neuroleptics, behavior management, and, in severe cases, electroconvulsive therapy.

5. When does a patient need a psychiatric evaluation?

Patients who experience a disturbance in mood, cognition, or behavior that interferes with their ability to care adequately for themselves or to keep themselves safe warrant a psychiatric consultation. Emergency intervention is necessary when patients are suicidal, homicidal, or unable to care for themselves. Suicide rates are higher for people with chronic illnesses than for the general population. People with AIDS have a 7.4-fold higher rate of suicide than the general population; people who are HIV-positive also have higher rates of suicide. HIV seropositivity may be a significant risk factor for suicide in general hospital patient populations. Some communities of People Living with AIDS consider suicide a legitimate response to the debilitation of the disease and dementia. This view has been supported by the Hemlock Society in *Final Exit* (1991). Patients with suicidal ideation must be carefully evaluated for major depression and organicity.

6. Describe HIV dementia.

AIDS dementia or HIV-related organic brain disease is a syndrome of progressive dementia that results from direct infection of the brain with HIV. The diagnosis is difficult to make and requires documentation of HIV infection accompanied by decrements in abstract reasoning, difficulties in learning and memory, self-reports of changes in cognition and motor functioning, and observations of such changes by friends and family. The differential diagnosis includes other neurologic diseases associated with HIV (such as CNS infection, neoplasms), medication-induced cognitive impairments, alcohol- and drug-induced impairments, and malnutrition or other metabolic imbalances.

Clinical Manifestations of HIV-Related Dementia

Cognitive impairments	**Generalized systemic symptoms**
Short-term memory deficit; forgetfulness rather than amnesia	Fatigue, sleep changes (hypersomnia)
Decreased concentration and attention	Anorexia, weight loss
Confusion and disorientation	Enuresis
Overall intellectual ability generally well preserved until late in the disease	Hypersensitivity to medications and alcohol
Visuospatial perception deficits	**Cognitive symptoms associated with advanced dementia**
Changes in personality or behavior	Global cognitive impairment
Apathy, decreased interest	Rudimentary or impaired social relationship
Impaired judgment, erratic behavior	Disorientation
Social withdrawal	Psychomotor retardation, decreased spontaneity
Rigidity of thought	Agitation, "sundowning" (e.g., nighttime delusions)
Speech impairment: slow dysarthria, hypophonia; difficulty in following other speakers	Coma
Psychotic symptoms	**Motor symptoms associated with advanced dementia**
Hallucinations	Ataxia
Suspiciousness and delusions	Spastic weakness
Agitation and inappropriate behavior	Paraplegia, quadriparesis
Motor symptoms	Hyperreflexia, myoclonus, seizures
Ataxia, loss of coordination, weakness	Bladder and bowel incontinence
Tremors	

Safety is a concern for demented patients and their caregivers. Caring for a patient with dementia is physically and emotionally demanding. Often significant others try to care for the severely demented patient for longer than they can reasonably do so. Hospice and nursing home care should be considered. The patient and family may struggle with such options, feeling that they represent surrender to the disease. Work is needed to help them to understand that getting assistance with the symptoms of the illness is not the same as giving up on the patient.

7. What is the risk of acquiring HIV infection in a health care setting?
For health care providers the fear of infection is a complex response based on personal history and development, including cultural and emotional components. Health care workers should educate themselves about the risk of acquiring an infection from blood-borne pathogens. Universal blood and body fluid precautions protect health care workers from the probability of infection with HIV, hepatitis B, or other blood-borne pathogens. HIV is not acquired through casual contact such as hand shaking or physical examination.

8. What is safe sex?
Safe-sex practices decrease the risk for acquiring HIV infection through sexual transmission. The goal is to modify sexual behaviors that increase risk of HIV transmission. Most educators of safe-sex practices currently use a risk reduction model when working with sexually active adults who want to decrease unsafe sexual behaviors. This model encourages people not to give up modifying their behaviors if they have an episode of unsafe sex. Safe-sex education has been successful in decreasing transmission rates of HIV in the gay community; recent reports, however, show that some gay men have begun to disregard safe-sex practices. Safe sex may be difficult for some women to negotiate if they feel that discussing safe sex with their partner may threaten other aspects of the relationship or influence self-perception. This issue may be particularly difficult for adolescents.

Safe Sex Guidelines

SAFE	POSSIBLY SAFE	UNSAFE
Mutual masturbation	Anal or vaginal intercourse with a condom	Receptive anal intercourse without a condom
Social (dry) kissing		
Body massage, hugging	Fellatio (sucking; stopping before climax)	Insertive anal intercourse without a condom
Body-to-body rubbing (frottage)	Mouth-to-mouth kissing (French kissing, wet kissing)	Manual-anal intercourse (fisting)
Light S & M activities (without bruising or bleeding)	Urine contact (water sports)	Fellatio (sucking to climax)
		Oral-anal contact (rimming)
Using one's own sex toys	Oral-vaginal contact (cunnilingus)	Any activities involving bruising or bleeding (heavy S & M)
		Using someone else's sex toys

Alcohol and drug use decrease adherence to safe-sex guidelines and have been associated with behaviors that transmit HIV.

9. How should the clinician teach patients about prevention of HIV transmission?
Patients must understand that they cannot be given absolute assurance that their sexual activities are safe; they must assess the relative risk of their sexual behaviors. Although HIV has been detected in saliva, there are no documented cases of transmission through saliva. Patients must assess whether they will alter their kissing behaviors based on this information and how they judge the relative risk of each behavior. Safe-sex education addresses the emotional impact of changing sexual behaviors (for example, the need to eroticise the use of condoms). Many communities offer courses on safe-sex practices through public health departments or

community-based AIDS organizations. Questions from physicians or medical personnel about sexual practices may be the first opportunity for patients to discuss openly their concerns about HIV infection.

10. How does HIV infection affect the patient's sexual self-image?
Some HIV-infected patients come to view themselves as pariahs who no longer deserve sexual feelings or expression. Fear of transmitting the virus may stop all sexual activities. Fear of rejection by a sex partner may interfere with self-disclosure about HIV status. Issues of sexuality need to be addressed to help HIV-positive patients to make informed decisions about future sexual activities. Risk assessment should be based on current knowledge, not on uninformed fears and misconceptions.

11. How does discrimination interfere with the treatment of a person with AIDS?
HIV and AIDS have affected large numbers of gay and bisexual men. Especially in the earlier years of the epidemic, discrimination against people with AIDS was based on homophobia, prejudice, and fear of contagion. Discrimination also occurs because people fear transmission of HIV. Homophobia is the fear and rejection of homosexuality or homosexuals, the attitude that homosexuality is undesirable, hateful, or evil, and a condensation of various negative cultural stereotypes bout gay men and lesbians. As the epidemic has continued, education about gay men and lesbians in the U.S. has helped to decrease the negative stereotypes of gay people. Gay men and lesbians may be reticent to disclose their sexual orientation to health care providers for fear of receiving inferior care. Health care providers may be uncomfortable treating a gay man or lesbian because of strong cultural beliefs, feelings, or views about homosexuals. Health care providers must address such issues so that patient care is not compromised. HIV-infected people may have concerns about confidentiality and fear discrimination in the workplace, from both employers and employees. Each state has its own statutes concerning the reporting of HIV status to the health department. In confidential reporting of HIV status a person's name is kept on record at the health department in confidential files. Health departments with such approaches try to assure the public that records are safe from public disclosure. In states with anonymous testing for HIV, information about the number of HIV positive tests is known, but no record of the HIV-positive person is kept. Drug users have experienced similar discrimination and prejudice from health care providers. The largest rise in new cases of HIV infection is among minority groups. Racism and culturally inappropriate educational materials contribute to the ineffective preventive efforts among ethnic populations.

12. How should the clinician teach intravenous drug users about prevention of HIV transmission?
Needle exchange programs have been shown to be effective in decreasing HIV transmission. Complex social barriers prevent real implementation of this intervention. Clean needles must be used to decrease transmission of HIV and hepatitis. Some states have programs that teach drug users to clean needles with bleach and/or water. Cleaning of needles is somewhat effective. Bleach may cause blood to clot in needles, and clots may lead to transmission of HIV. Addicts may have difficulties in taking time to clean needles, especially when they are withdrawing from their drug of choice.

13. How may the clinician introduce the topic of HIV and AIDS in history taking?
The mnemonic AIDS may be used to facilitate interviewing and to identify patients at risk for HIV infection. The mnemonic begins with a general and less threatening question before moving to more specific questions that deal with sensitive areas.

    A = **A**re you afraid you may have been exposed to AIDS?
    I = **I**ntravenous drug use
    D = **D**iagnostic signs and symptoms of HIV infection
    S = **S**exual behaviors

A "yes" answer to any question signals the need for further exploration and consideration of serologic testing for HIV.

14. What are the particular issues of discrimination for families?

Children with AIDS frequently come from families in which multiple members may be infected with HIV. Complex social problems often face such families, including drug addiction, poverty, and social ostracism. Communication among family members may be thwarted by the need to keep HIV infection a secret. This need often is a result of the family's fear of discrimination for the child in nursery or school settings. HIV-positive children are confronted with the deterioration of developmental skills, social isolation, and the possibility of imminent death. HIV-infected mothers are often confronted with how their child became infected. HIV-infected mothers must cope with illness, motherhood, disclosure of information about the illness to her children, and the effect of HIV infection on her reproductive choices.

BIBLIOGRAPHY

1. Alfonso CA, Cohen MA, Aladjem AD, et al: HIV seropositivity as a major risk factor suicide in the general hospital. Psychosomatics 35:368–373, 1994.
2. Chung JY, Magraw MM: A group approach to psychosocial issues faced by HIV-positive women. Hosp Community Psychiatry 43:891–894, 1992.
3. Cote TR, Biggar RJ, Dannenberg AL: Risk of suicide among persons with AIDS—a national assessment. JAMA 268:2066–2068, 1992.
4. Mahler J, Stebinger A, Yi D, et al: Reliability of admission history in predicting HIV infection among alcoholic inpatients. Am J Addictions 3:222–226, 1994.
5. Mueller TL, Swift RM: Screening for risk of HIV exposure using the A-I-D-S mnemonic. Am J Addictions 1:203–209, 1992.

71. PSYCHIATRIC CONSULTATION IN PATIENTS WITH CARDIOVASCULAR DISEASE

Andrew B. Littman, M.D.

1. What is the current status of type A behavior?

The best known psychosocial risk factor for the development of coronary artery disease is the type A behavior pattern. Type A behavior is defined as the habitual response to perceived demands with impatience and easily provoked aggravation, anger, and/or aggression. The global type A concept includes components of hard-driving nature, perfectionism, and low self-esteem. These global factors have waned in importance as hostility has been found repeatedly to be the toxic element of the type A syndrome. Hostility is linked to coronary artery disease outcomes by numerous mechanisms: increased atherosclerosis and sudden death, precipitation of myocardial ischemia and coronary vasospasm, and persistent cigarette smoking.

2. What other psychosocial factors are associated with poor outcomes for patients with coronary artery disease?

Lack of social support	Phobic anxiety
Social isolation and/or alienation	Anxiety disorders
Low socioeconomic status	Vital exhaustion
Lack of economic resources	Depressive symptoms
Job strain (low control and high demand)	Major depressive disorder

3. What is the impact of major depressive disorder and depressive symptoms in patients with coronary artery disease?

Both major depressive disorder and depressive symptoms have significant impact on patients with coronary artery disease. Major depressive disorder is common in patients with coronary artery disease; 20% of coronary patients have depressive disorder before their diagnosis. Only around 10% of these depressed patients are diagnosed or treated. In a recent study, 18% of patients hospitalized for myocardial infarction had major depressive disorder, and depression predicted mortality at 6 months with a relative risk of 4.3, equivalent to left ventricular dysfunction and history of previous myocardial infarction, the most potent prognostic measures known.

In the past, depressive symptoms in the absence of full-blown major depressive disorder were considered to be self-limited and of minimal importance. However, depressive symptoms are common in coronary patients (18–40%), in addition to the 20% of coronary patients who have major depressive disorder. Depressive symptoms and disorder commonly predate the onset of the initial clinical manifestations of coronary artery disease. Besides the important impact of depressive symptoms and disorder on functional status and quality of life, depressive syndromes are related to poorer adherence to medical treatment, lack of improvement of exercise functioning in coronary patients undergoing an exercise program, and increased risk of coronary atherosclerotic morbidity and mortality in studies of patients with preexisting coronary disease as well as population-based studies.

4. What is known about the behavioral treatment of stress in patients with coronary artery disease?

A number of treatments seem effective in reducing type A behavior and anger in patients with coronary artery disease (CAD), including yoga, emotional support, and group therapy. The most effective techniques were comprehensive in scope, involving education, training in coping methods with either a relaxation or cognitive focus, and frequent training with behavioral techniques.

The earliest studies of group cognitive behavioral therapy for stress modification in patients who have had a myocardial infarction show a reduction of 50% in 3-year combined rate of mortality and recurrent myocardial infarction. A more recent study by Frasure-Smith of patients with myocardial infarction evaluated the effect of stress monitoring and reduction. The mortality rate was three times higher for highly stressed patients who did not receive treatment than for highly stressed patients who received stress reduction treatment.

In addition to studies of the effect of stress reduction on mortality and recurrent infarction, Ornish used a multimodal treatment of comprehensive lifestyle change, low fat vegetarian diet, stress management, and moderate exercise in an attempt to reverse coronary atherosclerosis with lipid-lowering drugs. Both 1- and 4-year follow-ups show continued progression of atherosclerosis in the usual care group compared with regression of atherosclerosis in the comprehensive intervention group.

5. What is known about the pharmacotherapy of type A behavior, anger, and hostility?

The psychopharmacologic treatment of type A behavior, anger, and hostility is still in its infancy. In contrast to behavioral treatment, no currently available studies evaluate the effect of psychopharmacotherapy on CAD morbidity and mortality. Beta blockers are effective in reducing mortality in coronary patients with myocardial infarctions. In addition, beta blockers have been shown to be effective in reducing aggression in the elderly and in patients with organic brain syndromes. However, trials of beta blockers have not been successful in reducing type A behavior or hostility in patients with CAD. Benzodiazepines do not alter type A behavior or hostility but have reduced duration of silent ischemia in a very small number of patients with CAD.

Only recently has a coherent hypothesis about the neurobiology of the hostility syndrome emerged. According to this hypothesis, the hostility, anger, and aggression that are considered to be risk factors for CAD constitute a syndrome produced by low levels of central serotonin. An increasingly large body of literature demonstrates that patients with mood and personality disorders as well as normal volunteers with low levels of central serotonin have a lower threshold for aggressive responses or urges to act angrily.

Serotonergic agents have been used to treat anger in both patients with comorbid mood disorders and patients without a current diagnosable psychiatric condition. Anger attacks are common (44%) in individuals with major depressive disorder. Treatment with fluoxetine reduced such expressions of anger by 70%. In addition, in patients with CAD and hostility but with no axis I psychiatric condition, hostility was reduced by treatment with buspirone, a serotonin 1-A partial agonist.

6. What is known about the pharmacotherapy of depression in patients with CAD?

The pharmacotherapy of depression has been improved by the newer classes of antidepressants. Tricyclic antidepressants have widespread cardiovascular effects, including effects on tachycardia, orthostatic hypotension, conduction delays, and cardiac rhythm. Desipramine is the least anticholinergic tricyclic compound and thus produces the least tachycardia. Orthostatic hypotension is most common (up to 50%) in patients with congestive heart failure, and nortriptyline produces orthostatic hypotension less frequently than any other tricyclic. Preexisting defects of the His-Purkinje conduction system, such as bundle branch blocks, put patients placed on tricyclic antidepressants at risk for serious second- or third-degree blocks. Tricyclics also increase the P-R and Q-T intervals as well as the QRS segment and shorten T-wave height.

Newer antidepressants such as amoxapine produce conduction abnormalities and atrial arrhythmias. Maprotiline has caused torsade de pointes, a characteristic malignant ventricular arrhythmia, at the high end of the therapeutic range. Trazodone has little effect on cardiac conduction, produces beneficial hemodynamics, and rarely exacerbates ventricular ectopy. Buproprion has no cardiotoxicity or anticholinergic effects. Fluoxetine, sertraline, and paroxetine appear to have little cardiotoxicity, no anticholinergic effects, no effect on the electrocardiogram, and in initial studies no effect on cardiac function. Thus, such inhibitors of serotonin reuptake may be especially safe among patients with CAD.

7. What is the effect of denial on patients with CAD?

Many patients with CAD have been found to deny their emotional reactions, characteristically during the acute phases of a hospitalization for cardiac illness. Many patients with CAD deny the presence of cardiac symptoms, such as angina. Recent studies demonstrate that patients with emotional denial more frequently deny cardiac symptoms and delay seeking treatment. Early studies evaluating the effect of emotional denial on morbidity and mortality during acutely stressful hospitalizations for cardiac disease suggest that denial is adaptive. However, follow-up studies show that emotional denial is deleterious to patients' health over the long term. One mechanism appears to be that patients with emotional denial have a greater difficulty modifying cardiac risk factors and resume deleterious health behaviors, especially smoking.

8. Does serum cholesterol have an effect on behavior?

Recent studies have demonstrated that lowering serum cholesterol reduces mortality from coronary atherosclerosis but does not improve overall survival because of an increase in deaths due to accidents, suicide, and violence. One study demonstrated that lowering dietary fat increased aggression and lowered levels of central serotonin in monkeys. Other studies of cholesterol lowering showed an increased risk of violent death only for patients using medications to lower cholesterol; depressive symptoms were more common in coronary patients treated for hyperlipidemia than in untreated patients. The possible effect of lipid lowering on behavior is currently receiving a great deal of attention. No firm recommendations can be given except to be observant for behavioral changes in patients treated for hyperlipidemia.

9. What is the effect of physical activity on patients with coronary artery disease?

Regular aerobic exercise appears to reduce mortality from CAD by 25%. Less recognized is the fact that lower levels of everyday exertion can be very beneficial for coronary patients. Moderate levels of leisure physical activity (30–69 minutes of light-to-moderate activities per day) are enough to reduce CAD mortality by 63%; increased levels of leisure activity do not provide more risk reduction.

Aerobic exercise appears to reduce both the cardiovascular and sympathoadrenal responses to mental stress. Yet despite such benefits, adherence to regular exercise is poor; over one-half of patients who initiate an exercise program drop out of the program after several months. Two-thirds of Americans do not exercise regularly. For patients with preexisting CAD, entry into a comprehensive, structured cardiac rehabilitation program with a credible psychosocial component can help with long-term adherence. A structured long-term maintenance program with active social support is now a common feature of many cardiac rehabilitation programs. For patients who do not have a chronic medical illness, adherence to an exercise program is enhanced by joining employer-sponsored and conveniently located exercise programs.

10. What is the effect of obesity? How can it be treated?

Obesity has a negative effect on hypertension, diabetes mellitus, lipid abnormalities, physical inactivity; it is also an independent risk factor for development of coronary atherosclerosis. Around one-third of overweight individuals who attempt to lose weight maintain the loss; whereas two-thirds regain the weight. Weight reduction programs that are successful focus on long-term change in dietary behavior with restriction of dietary fat intake and behavioral modification of eating habits and dietary urges; exercise four times per week is also an essential element.

Pharmacologic interventions to reduce weight have not been used for 20 years since amphetamines were in common use. Recent research has shown that dexfenfluramine, an indirect and direct serotonergic agent, and selective inhibitors of serotonin reuptake are efficacious in producing long-term weight loss. Some European clinician-researchers consider pharmacologic treatment of obesity in patients with serious medical conditions equivalent to the pharmacologic treatment of hypertension or hyperlipidemia. See chapter 78 for a fuller discussion of methods for obesity treatment.

11. Can systemic arterial hypertension be treated with behavioral techniques?

Many studies have shown that psychosocial stress is associated with elevated arterial blood pressure. Although relaxation training and biofeedback can significantly reduce both systolic and diastolic blood pressures and apparently generalize this effect to nontraining periods for some time, only one study demonstrated the effectiveness of stress management in reducing blood pressure. Nine other studies demonstrated only a minimal (2-mmHg) drop in diastolic blood pressure in nonmedicated patients. A recent study comparing the effects of dietary sodium restriction, stress management, nutritional supplementation, and weight reduction showed beneficial effects only from weight reduction and secondarily from sodium restriction. Thus the behavioral technique of choice for reducing blood pressure appears to be weight reduction in addition to assisted compliance with antihypertensive medication.

12. How can one assist compliance with antihypertensive medication?

There are several components to successful treatment of noncompliance in patients with hypertension or medical illness. A drug profile with minimal negative effect on quality of life is a critical element. This process involves matching the drug profile of side effects to the patient's pathophysiologic state (e.g., congestive heart failure, persistent tachycardia, sleep disturbance) as well as the patient's priorities and values concerning physical and mental functioning. In studies of quality of life among patients receiving antihypertensive drugs, captopril was shown to be superior to other agents in use. Since this study, the advent of numerous new antihypertensive agents with better side effect profiles has made this process easier. It is also important for patients to have a dosing regimen that matches their current one or minimizes the number of doses per day. Patient education and recognition of the risk/benefit relationship of their medication are also important. Finally, it is important to assess carefully psychiatric elements that may impair compliance, such as subtle mood disorders, anxiety, posttraumatic stress, substance abuse, or organic cognitive disorders. Often the patient's past experiences with illness, dependency, or loss helps to explain the lack of compliance. Treatment of disorders or recognition of the coping style of the patient may dramatically improve compliance.

13. How can I help my patients to stop smoking?

If one is working in a primary care setting, keeping track of patients' smoking status, briefly discussing the hazards of smoking in a personalized way, and working with smokers to agree on a specific date for attempting to quit double the quit rate from 4% to around 8% per year. For patients who have failed this approach or who wish to get further help, standard behaviorally based smoking cessation programs have long-term quit rates of around 30%. Such smoking cessation programs are psychoeducational, with didactic information about nicotine addiction and the process of quitting, specific behavioral coping techniques for withdrawal symptoms, relapse prevention, assertiveness and relaxation training, and group social support.

Nicotine chewing gum improves long-term quit rates, but its effectiveness depends on several elements. It appears to have minimal effect if used outside specialized smoking cessation programs, without clear instructions about use or adequate social supports. The effectiveness of smoking cessation programs is maximized when behavioral skills are taught in contrast to a strictly didactic approach. Transdermal nicotine patches are now in common use. Patients should not smoke while using the nicotine patch.

New findings have linked depressive disorders with cigarette smoking. Individuals with higher smoking rates, a history of regular smoking, or difficulty with quitting smoking have a history of major depressive disorder more frequently than those who find it relatively easy to quit smoking. In addition, when patients with a history of depression quit smoking, depressive symptoms or disorder commonly recurs. When these symptoms occur, such individuals are much less likely to mount a successful quit attempt. Doxepin improves rates of quitting smoking in healthy young persons. Studies of the effectiveness of selective inhibitors of serotonin reuptake are currently under way.

Other mood states, such as anger, impatience, and tension, and sleep disturbance are predictive of inability to quit smoking. Our current clinical practice is behavioral treatment for smokers who have high baseline levels or develop such symptoms in the process of quitting. If the symptoms do not improve with behavioral treatment, psychopharmacologic treatment is undertaken. Studies have shown that buspirone reduces craving, irritability, restlessness, and dysphoria during nicotine withdrawal and that smokers with high anxiety have significantly improved quit rates compared with placebo. In addition, buproprion has been shown in initial studies to improve quit rates in smokers who do not have depressive disorders.

14. What are the causes of disability in patients with CAD?

The sequelae of the physical manifestations of CAD have a profound negative effect on functional status and quality of life. It is less recognized that depressive symptoms and depressive disorder contribute to the same degree as the physical manifestations of CAD in reducing functional status and quality of life in an independent manner. This additional negative effect can be ameliorated by direct treatment of the depressive disorder itself. In addition, approximately 25% of patients with CAD do not return to work after a myocardial infarction. Work disability is predicted by low educational level, number of previous myocardial infarctions, and degree of depression. In addition, level of depression is the best predictor of job loss after a myocardial infarction. Current clinical practice dictates referral to a cardiac rehabilitation program for patients whose functional or work status is impaired and further psychiatric evaluation for patients who fail to improve to a level clearly explained by their physiologic status during the rehabilitation program.

15. How is sexual function altered in patients with CAD?

The majority of patients with CAD have diminished sexual desire and frequency of sexual activity; impotence is not uncommon. There are numerous causes for sexual dysfunction, but cardiac function alone is a relatively rare cause. Physiologic capacity to resume sexual activity has been reached when the patient can climb two flights of stairs at a brisk pace. The occasional patient with angina during sex frequently can use prophylactic nitroglycerine or change positions so that there is less isometric muscular tension. It cannot be overemphasized that permission to resume sexual activity and unambiguous information about patient's and partner's concerns and fears are critical to successful recovery of sexual function. Patients with CAD also may have medication-related, neurogenic, or vascular causes for sexual dysfunction. Beta blockers are commonly the culprit. Often overlooked is the serious and common marital conflict during convalescence after a serious cardiac event that has been followed by poor sexual adjustment.

16. What are important psychiatric causes of noncardiac chest pain?

A common presenting symptom of patients in general medical as well as specialty cardiology settings is chest pain without objective organic findings to explain the symptoms. Historically such patients have been labeled as having neurocirculatory asthenia, syndrome X, or hyperventilation syndrome. They frequently have demonstrated psychiatric symptoms, such as anxiety, mood, and somatization disorders. Some series have demonstrated a 50% incidence of panic disorder in patients in cardiology clinics with noncardiac chest pain. Controlled trials of cognitive-behavioral therapy as well as antidepressant treatments, such as imipramine, have shown persistent reduction of pain, psychosocial limitations, and distress for patients with atypical noncardiac chest pain, even in the absence of panic disorder.

BIBLIOGRAPHY

1. Beitman BD, Basha I, Flaker G, et al: Atypical or nonanginal chest pain, panic disorder or coronary artery disease? Arch Intern Med 147:1548–1552, 1987.
2. Fava M, Rosenbaum JF, Pava JA, et al: Anger attacks in unipolar depression. I. Clinical correlates and response to fluoxetine treatment. Am J Psychiatry 150:1158–1163, 1993.
3. Frasure-Smith N, Lesperance F, Talajic M: Depression following myocardial infarction: Impact on 6-month survival. JAMA 270:1819–1825, 1993.

4. Hlatky MA, Haney T, Barefoot JC, et al: Medical, psychological and social correlates of work disability among men with coronary artery disease. Am J Cardiol 58:911–915, 1986.

5. Littman AB: Prevention of disability due to cardiovascular diseases. Heart Dis Stroke 2:274–277, 1993.

6. Littman AB: A review of psychosomatic aspects of cardiovascular disease. In Fava GA, Freyberger H (eds): Psychosomatic Medicine. Farmington, CT, Karger, in press.

7. Littman AB, Ketterer MW: Behavioral medicine in consultation-liaison psychiatry. In Rundell J, Wise M (eds): American Psychiatric Press Textbook of Consultation-Liaison Psychiatry. Washington, DC, American Psychiatric Press, in press.

8. Milani RV, Littman AB, Lavie CJ: Depressive symptoms predict functional improvement following cardiac rehabilitation and exercise program. J Cardiopulm Rehabil 13:406–411, 1993.

9. Milani RV, Littman AB, Lavie CJ: Psychological adaptation to cardiovascular disease. In Messerli FH (ed): Cardiovascular Disease in the Elderly, 3rd ed. Boston, Kluwer Academic Publishers, 1993, pp 401–412.

10. Ornish D, Brown SE, Scherwitz LW, et al: Can lifestyle changes reverse coronary heart disease? Lancet 336:129–133, 1990.

11. Rosal M, Downing J, Littman AB, Ahern D: Sexual functioning post-myocardial infarction: Effects of beta-blockers, psychological status and safety information. J Psychosom Res, in press.

12. Wells KB, Stewart A, Hays RD, et al: The functioning and well-being of depressed patients: Results from the medical outcome study. JAMA 262:914–919, 1989.

72. CONSULTATION FOR THE CANCER PATIENT

Andrew Roth, M.D., Mary Jane Massie, M.D., and William H. Redd, Ph.D.

1. What are the most stressful times for cancer patients and their families?
Psychiatrists and psychologists are often asked to bolster patients' and families' coping skills during crisis points in cancer treatment. These points include learning of the diagnosis of cancer, beginning any new treatment (surgery, radiation, chemotherapy), waiting for test results, learning that treatment efforts have failed or of recurrence of disease, undergoing painful medical procedures, and struggling with uncontrolled pain. Issues of dying, palliative care and end-of-life decisions (such as health care proxies and "do not resuscitate" orders) must also be dealt with. Patients' families have to manage their own fatigue, put much of the rest of their lives on hold, and tolerate frequent interruptions in work, parenting, social, and school schedules while providing support and practical services for their loved one.

2. Do all cancer patients get depressed?
The reported rates of major depression in patients with cancer vary widely from 1% to 53%, depending on the measures used and the population studied. Although not all cancer patients are depressed, most are distressed at crisis points in illness. Most experience a brief period of denial or despair followed by distress with a mixture of symptoms of depressed mood, anxiety, insomnia, anorexia, and irritability. These patients report having difficulty carrying out daily activities, and having lingering thoughts about the uncertainty of the future. These symptoms last for days to several weeks, after which usual patterns of adaptation return. This normal response is highly variable and is modulated by medical factors, such as extent of disease, physical symptoms, degree of debilitation, and prognosis. About 25% of cancer patients continue to have high levels of anxiety and depression persisting for weeks to months. These disorders are called adjustment disorders with depressed, anxious, or mixed moods depending on the major symptoms. Of course, before making any diagnosis of depression or anxiety, the clinician must first consider whether uncontrolled pain or other cancer symptoms are causing a patient to appear depressed or anxious.

3. Given that many cancer patients are distressed, how is depression diagnosed in patients with cancer?
When a patient's depressed mood is persistent or worsening and is accompanied by hopelessness, despondency, guilty feelings, and suicidal ideation, major depression is the likely diagnosis. Depression is treatable and is not "normal" in most patients with cancer. The patient's mood, physical symptoms (vegetative or somatic) of depression and the severity of depression, including suicide risk, must be assessed. Physical symptoms must be carefully evaluated to determine whether fatigue, insomnia, and decreased libido are caused by depression, by cancer, or by the treatment itself. Doctors often underestimate the morbidity caused by depression, because they themselves tend to believe they would feel depressed, even suicidal, if the roles were reversed.

The biologic correlates of depression, or neurovegetative symptoms (e.g., decreased appetite, insomnia, fatigue, loss of energy, loss of libido, and psychomotor slowing) are the best measures for depression in physically healthy adults. They are, however, unreliable in cancer patients who often have no appetite because of chemotherapy, who sleep poorly because of pain or because they are hospitalized, and who are fatigued because of the cancer, radiation therapy or chemotherapy. When both depression and debilitation are present in patients with advanced cancer, it is often difficult to decide which condition is primary, and a trial of antidepressants is warranted.

Questions Used to Assess Depressive Symptoms in Cancer Patients

QUESTION	SYMPTOM
Mood	
How well are you coping with your cancer? Well? Poorly?	(Well being)
How are your spirits since? Down? Blue?	(Mood)
Since diagnosis? During treatment? Depressed? Sad?	
Do you cry sometimes? How often? Only alone?	
Are there things you still enjoy doing or have you lost pleasure in things you used to do before you had cancer?	(Anhedonia)
How does the future look to you? Bright? Black?	(Hopelessness)
Do you feel you can influence your care or is your care totally under others' control?	(Helplessness)
Do you worry about being a burden to family and friends during treatment for cancer?	(Worthlessness)
Feel others might be better off without you?	(Guilt)
Physical Symptoms (Evaluate in the context of cancer-related symptoms)	
Do you have pain which isn't controlled?	(Pain)
How much time do you spend in bed? Weak? Fatigue easily? Rested after sleep? Any relationship to change in treatment or how you feel otherwise physically?	(Fatigue)
How is your sleeping? Trouble going to sleep? Awake early? Often?	(Insomnia)
How is your appetite? Food tastes good? Weight loss or gain?	(Appetite)
How is your interest in sex? Extent of sexual activity?	(Libido)
Do you think or move more slowly?	(Psychomotor slowing)

4. What medical conditions cause depression in cancer patients?

Uncontrolled Pain	Medications
	Steroids
Metabolic Abnormalities	Interferon and interleukin-2
Hypercalcemia	Methyldopa
Sodium, potassium imbalance	Reserpine
Anemia	Barbiturates
Deficient vitamin B_{12} or folate	Propranolol
	Some antibiotics (amphotericin B)
Endocrinologic Abnormalities	Some chemotherapeutic agents
Hyper- or hypothyroidism	Vincristine
Adrenal insufficiency	Vinblastine
	Procarbazine
	L-asparaginase

Uncontrolled pain is a common cause of depressed mood in cancer patients. It is accompanied by symptoms of anxiety and a sense of anguish that life is intolerable unless pain is relieved. Patients interpret a new or increasingly severe pain as a sign that the cancer has progressed, resulting in greater depression and hopelessness. Suicide is a real risk in these patients, especially if they do not believe that efforts are being made to control the pain or that relief is possible. Suicidal ideation and major depressive symptoms usually abate when the pain is controlled.

When medical conditions are the cause of depressed mood, the mood can usually be reversed when the condition is reversed, or with antidepressant medication.

5. How is depression treated in patients with cancer?

Treatment is directed at helping patients adapt to the stresses they are undergoing and helping to strengthen coping abilities. Individual or group psychotherapy may help clarify the medical situation, the meaning of illness, and support and encourage positive coping strategies. Cognitive therapy, which focuses on how an individual's inaccurate perception or assessment of his situation leads to anxious and depressed feelings, can be used to help patients develop an adaptive perspective on their circumstances.

The level of distress a person experiences, the inability to carry out daily activities, and the response to psychotherapeutic interventions determine when a psychotropic medication is needed. With some severe adjustment disorders with depression, as well as major depressive disorders, antidepressants are used in conjunction with psychotherapeutic interventions.

6. What antidepressants are most useful for patients with cancer?

Dosages in Cancer Patients

MEDICATION	START/DAILY DOSE (MG)*	PRIMARY SIDE EFFECTS/COMMENTS
Tricyclics (TCAs)		All TCAs can cause cardiac arrhythmias; blood levels are available for all but doxepin. Get baseline ECG.
Amitriptyline (Elavil)	10–25/50–100	Sedation; anticholinergic; orthostasis
Imipramine (Tofranil)	10–25/50–150	Intermediate sedation; anticholinergic; orthostasis
Desipramine (Norpramin)	25/75–150	Little sedation or orthostasis; moderate anticholinergic
Nortriptyline (Pamelor)	10–25/75–150	Little anticholinergic or orthostatic; intermediate sedation; therapeutic window
Doxepin (Sinequan)	25/75–150	Very sedating; orthostatic hypotension; intermediate anticholinergic effects; potent antihistamine
Second Generation		
Bupropion (Wellbutrin)	75/200–450	May cause seizures in those with low seizure threshold/brain tumors; initially activating.
Trazodone (Desyrel)	50/150–200	Sedating; not anticholinergic; risk of priapism
Serotonin Specific Reuptake Inhibitors (SSRIs)		SSRIs have few anticholinergic or cardiovascular side effects
Fluoxetine (Prozac)	10/20–40	Sexual dysfunction including anorgasmia Headache; nausea; anxiety; insomnia. Has a very long half life; may be even longer in debilitated patient.
Sertraline (Zoloft)	25/50–150	Nausea; insomnia
Paroxetine (Paxil)	10/20–50	Nausea; somnolence; asthenia; no active metabolites
Psychostimulants		All psychostimulants may cause nightmares,
d-Amphetamine (Dexedrine)	2.5/5–30	insomnia, psychosis, anorexia, agitation, and
Methylphenidate (Ritalin)	2.5/5–30	restlessness. Possible cardiac complications. They should be given in two divided doses at 8 a.m. and noon; can be used as analgesic adjuvant and to counter sedation of opiates
Pemoline (Cylert)	18.75/37.5–150	Follow liver tests
Other		
Venlafaxine (Effexor)	75/225–375	Inhibits reuptake of both serotonin and norepinephrine. Achieves steady state in 3 days. May increase blood pressure.

* Starting doses used in cancer patients differ from those prescribed for physically healthy depressed pateints.

When choosing an antidepressant, it is important to consider secondary effects which may be utilized for their positive value. For example, a sedating antidepressant (such as amitriptyline or trazodone) is useful for an agitated patient who has difficulty sleeping, because it has both calming and sedating effects. A patient's earlier response to a particular medication, or a family member's experience with an antidepressant, can help predict the response.

In the last few years, the SSRIs have become widely used because of their efficacy and low risk of significant side effects. The primary side effects of fluoxetine are gastric distress and nausea, brief periods of anxiety, headache, and insomnia (less common, hypersomnia). A troubling side effect is anorgasmia. The primary side effects of sertraline are nausea, diarrhea, dyspepsia, tremor, dizziness, ejaculatory delay in men, and insomnia. Sertraline's shorter half-life allows for more rapid hepatic clearance or renal excretion than fluoxetine, often a useful effect in the medically ill. Paroxetine has no active metabolites and therefore is also excreted relatively quickly upon discontinuation. Nausea, somnolence, and asthenia are among its more common side effects. Because all these drugs are strongly protein-bound, consideration must be given to their ability to increase blood levels of other medications such as coumadin, digoxin, some anticonvulsants, and cisplatin.

In the past, tricyclic antidepressants, or TCAs (amitriptyline, doxepin, imipramine, nortriptyline, and desipramine), were the most commonly used drugs for depression and for the treatment of neuropathic pain. They are started at a low dose (10 to 25 mg at bedtime), especially in debilitated patients, and increased slowly (by 10 to 25 mg every few days) until symptoms improve. For reasons that are unclear, depressed cancer patients often show a therapeutic response to a tricyclic at much lower doses (75 to 125 mg daily) than are usually required in physically healthy depressed patients (150 to 300 mg daily). Blood levels should be obtained for amitriptyline, imipramine, desipramine, and nortriptyline 5 days after initiating a new dose in order to prevent toxicity, to verify compliance with treatment, and in the case of nortriptyline to target the therapeutic window of 50 to 150 ng/ml.

The choice of a tricyclic also depends on the nature of the depressive symptoms, medical problems present, and side effects of the TCA. The depressed patient with psychomotor slowing will benefit from use of the compounds with the fewest sedating effects, such as desipramine. Patients with stomatitis secondary to chemotherapy or radiotherapy, or with slow intestinal motility or urinary retention, should receive an antidepressant with the fewest anticholinergic side effects. These might include bupropion, trazodone, desipramine, nortriptyline, or an SSRI. Bupropion is less cardiotoxic than TCAs and has an activating effect in withdrawn, medically ill patients. It should be used with caution in patients at risk for seizures or those with brain metastases or primary brain tumors, however, because it is reported to lower the seizure threshold more than other antidepressants.

Patients who are unable to swallow pills may be able to take an antidepressant in an elixir (amitriptyline, nortriptyline, doxepin, or fluoxetine) or in an intramuscular form (amitriptyline or imipramine). Intramuscular (IM) administration causes discomfort because of the volume of the vehicle; hence 50 mg is usually the maximum dosage that can be delivered per IM injection. Parenteral administration of TCAs can be considered for the cancer patient unable to tolerate oral administration (because of absence of swallowing reflex, presence of gastric or jejunal drainage tubes, or intestinal obstruction). Three TCAs are available in injectable form: amitriptyline, imipramine, and clomipramine. All three have been given intravenously; however, only imipramine and amitriptyline are available for IM injection. The intramuscular route may cause excessive bleeding in the cancer patient with low platelet levels. Close monitoring of cardiac conduction by electrocardiogram is recommended when these medications are used intravenously. Hospital pharmacies can also prepare some TCAs (i.e., amitriptyline) in rectal suppository form, but absorption by this route has not been studied in cancer patients.

Imipramine, doxepin, amitriptyline, desipramine, and nortriptyline are frequently used in the management of neuropathic pain in cancer patients. Dosing is similar to the treatment of depression, and analgesic efficacy, if it occurs, is usually observed at a dose of 50 to 150 mg daily; higher doses are needed occasionally. Although the initial assumption was that analgesic effect resulted indirectly from the effect on depression, it is now clear that these tricyclics have a separate specific analgesic action probably mediated through several neurotransmitters, most prominently norepinephrine and serotonin. The newest antidepressant, as of this writing, is venlafaxine, which effects both norepineprhine and serotonin neurotransmitter systems.

The psychostimulants (methylphenidate, pemoline, and dextroamphetamine) are useful in low doses for patients who are suffering from depressed mood, apathy, depressed energy, poor concentration, and weakness. They promote a sense of well-being, decrease fatigue, and stimulate appetite. They are helpful in countering the sedating effects of morphine, and they produce a rapid effect in comparison to the other antidepressants. Side effects include insomnia, euphoria, and mood lability. High doses and long-term use may produce anorexia, nightmares, insomnia, euphoria, or paranoid thinking.

Treatment with dextroamphetamine and methylphenidate is usually initiated at a dose of 2.5 mg at 8:00 A.M. and noon, and increased by 2.5 mg as needed. Typically, patients are maintained on the medication for 1 to 2 months, after which approximately two thirds will be able to be withdrawn without a recurrence of depressive symptoms. Pemoline, a less potent psychostimulant, comes in a chewable tablet so patients who have difficulty swallowing can absorb the drug through the buccal mucosa. Pemoline should be used with caution in patients with renal impairment; liver function tests should be monitored periodically with longer term treatment.

7. How common is anxiety in patients with cancer?

More than two-thirds of cancer patients who have a psychiatric disorder have reactive depression or anxiety (adjustment disorder with depressed or anxious mood). About 4 to 5% have preexisting anxiety disorders. These disorders can cause severe suffering and can compromise clinical care. Early recognition and treatment is essential to optimize patient care. A careful search for etiology is essential for appropriate treatment.

Reactive anxiety is the most common type of anxiety in cancer patients. It is an exaggerated form of a normal anxious response. It is distinguished from normal fears of cancer by the duration and intensity of symptoms, and the degree of functional impairment, especially compliance with treatment. Fearfulness, accompanied by symptoms of anxiety, is expected and *normal* before painful or stressful procedures (e.g., bone marrow aspiration, chemotherapy, radiation therapy, wound debridement); before surgery; and while awaiting test results. Many anxious patients respond to reassurance and support; some require aggressive treatment. Patients who are extremely fearful, are unable to absorb information, or to cooperate with procedures, usually require psychotherapy, medication and/or behavioral interventions to reduce symptoms to a manageable level.

8. What are the medical causes of anxiety in cancer patients?

The second most frequent cause of anxiety in the cancer patient is a set of medical factors: uncontrolled pain, abnormal metabolic states, medications that produce withdrawal states, and, less frequently, hormone-producing tumors. These types of anxiety are classified as anxiety disorders of medical origin.

Anxious patients may present with a wide variety of symptoms such as nervousness, tremulousness, palpitations, shortness of breath, diarrhea, diaphoresis, numbness and tingling of the extremities, feelings of imminent death, and phobias. Patients in severe pain appear anxious and agitated and usually respond to adequate pain control with analgesics. Analgesics should never be ordered on an as-needed basis for significant pain because such dosing generates anxiety about control of the pain. Analgesics ordered around the clock reach a steady state which allows the patient to relax and trust that the pain will not return between doses, though rescue doses should be made available.

The acute onset of anxiety may herald a change in metabolic state or an impending catastrophic event. Sudden anxiety accompanied by chest pain or respiratory distress suggests a pulmonary embolus. Patients who are hypoxic are anxious and fearful that they are suffocating or dying. Sepsis and delirium can also cause anxiety symptoms. Many drugs can precipitate anxiety in the medically ill. Corticosteroids can produce motor restlessness and agitation, as well as depression and suicidal ideation. Symptoms tend to develop on high doses or during rapid tapering-off.

Bronchodilators and beta-adrenergic receptor stimulants used for chronic respiratory conditions can cause anxiety, irritability, and tremulousness.

Akathisia, motor restlessness accompanied by subjective feelings of distress and hyperactivity, is a side effect of several neuroleptic drugs (e.g., prochlorperazine and metoclopramide) used to control emesis. Metoclopramide also causes depression and suicidal ideation in some patients. Ondansetron and granisetron produce few side effects of this kind.

Withdrawal from narcotics, benzodiazepines, barbiturates, and alcohol results in anxiety, agitation, and behaviors which may be problematic in the patient being treated for cancer. Withdrawal after hospital admission often occurs in patients with cancers of the head and neck who frequently have histories of heavy alcohol use.

Questions to Ask about Symptoms of Anxiety

Have you experienced any of the following symptoms since your cancer diagnosis or treatment? If yes, when do they occur, i.e., days before treatment, during procedures, at night, no specific time? How long do they last?

Do you feel nervous, shaky, or jittery?

Have you felt fearful, apprehensive, and tense?

Have you had to avoid certain places or activities because of fear?

Have you experienced your heart pounding or racing?

Have you had trouble catching your breath when nervous?

Have you had any unjustified sweating or trembling?

Have you felt a knot in the pit of your stomach?

Have you felt a lump in your throat when getting upset?

Do you find yourself pacing back and forth?

Are you afraid to close your eyes at night for fear that you will die in your sleep?

---

9. What are some other anxiety syndromes seen in cancer patients?

The stress of cancer may reactivate a preexisting phobia, panic disorder, generalized anxiety disorder, or posttraumatic stress disorder. These disorders are described in detail elsewhere in this book. Some patients become very anxious before surgery, chemotherapy, and painful procedures or dressing changes (anticipatory anxiety), which can be a conditioned anxiety response.

10. How is anxiety treated in cancer patients?

The initial management of anxiety entails providing adequate information and support to the patient. Psychological approaches include combinations of cognitive-behavioral therapeutic techniques, brief supportive therapy and crisis intervention, insight-oriented psychotherapy, and behavioral interventions. Behavioral approaches such as progressive relaxation, guided imagery, meditation, biofeedback, and hypnosis can be used to treat anxiety symptoms associated with painful procedures, pain syndromes, waiting for results of tests (i.e., prostate specific antigen levels), and anticipatory fears of chemotherapy and radiation therapy or other cancer treatments.

11. What forms of drug therapy are appropriate?

An anxiolytic medication is usually prescribed along with a psychological approach. Choice of a benzodiazepine depends on the duration of action best suited to the patient, desired rapidity of onset, route of administration available, presence or absence of active metabolites, and metabolic problems to be considered. Dosing schedules depend on patients' tolerance and requires individual titration. The short-acting benzodiazepines (alprazolam and lorazepam) are given three to four times per day. Short-acting benzodiazepines, particularly those that can be administered by multiple routes, have become widely used with medically ill patients. Alprazolam can be absorbed sublingually for patients who have difficulty swallowing. Clonazepam, a longer-acting drug with antiseizure properties, is quite useful for panic symptoms and associated insomnia. A drug with a rapid onset of effect (e.g., lorazepam, diazepam) is effective for high levels of distress. Benzodiazepines decrease daytime anxiety and reduce insomnia. The most common side effects of benzodiazepines are dose-dependent and are controlled by titrating the dose to avoid drowsiness, confusion, motor incoordination, and sedation. All benzodiazepines can cause respiratory depression and must be used cautiously (or not at all) in the presence of respiratory impairment. The respiratory depressant effects are additive or even synergistic in the presence of other drugs such as antidepressants, antiemetics, and analgesics. Low doses of the antihistamine, hydroxyzine, or of the neuroleptic chlorpromazine, can be used safely and relatively effectively in situations where concern exists about depressing central respiratory mechanisms. In patients with hepatic dysfunction, it is best to use short-acting benzodiazepines which are metabolized primarily by conjugation and excreted by the kidney (e.g., oxazepam and lorazepam) or those which lack active metabolites (e.g., lorazepam).

Buspirone, a nonbenzodiazepine anxiolytic, is useful for elderly patients, for those who have not previously been treated with a benzodiazepine, or for those at risk of habituation with benzodiazepines. It is started at 5 mg t.i.d. and can be increased to 15 mg t.i.d. Low dose neuroleptics (e.g., thioridazine 10 to 25 mg t.i.d.) are also used to treat severe anxiety when an adequate dose of a benzodiazepine cannot be reached or is not helpful, or when the patient has a mild confusional state accompanied by symptoms of anxiety.

Akathisia can be quickly controlled by stopping or changing the causative drug (if possible) or by the addition of a benzodiazepine, a beta-blocker such as propranolol, or an antiparkinsonian agent such as benztropine. Treatment of withdrawal states depends on the particular agent. Sometimes the goal is to stabilize the patient on the agent (i.e., a benzodiazepine) and sometimes a suitable substitute can be given (i.e., a benzodiazepine for ethanol or for a barbiturate). Anxiety before chemotherapy or painful procedures and dressing changes is controlled by a short-acting benzodiazepine such as lorazepam, which also provides anterograde amnesia. Given intravenously, lorazepam also reduces vomiting in patients receiving emetogenic chemotherapy. Both oral lorazepam and alprazolam reduce nausea and vomiting related to chemotherapy.

In general, cancer patients need to be encouraged to take sufficient amounts of medication to relieve anxiety and pain. Medications are readily discontinued when symptoms subside; concerns about addiction are far exaggerated in cancer patients who have no history of drug abuse (see question 26 on pain control).

12. What is the most likely psychiatric diagnosis of a patient who was reported as being disoriented and agitated when his family was visiting an hour ago, but who now seems calm?

The most likely diagnosis is delirium (also called encephalopathy). Often psychiatric consultations are requested for patients who appear depressed, angry, psychotic, or anxious, but who, after further evaluation, are found to be delirious. These are important distinctions, because treatment recommendations are quite different for these disorders. Untreated delirium can lead to death. Delirium, dementia, and other cognitive disorders caused by medical conditions or substances occur in roughly 15 to 20% of hospitalized cancer patients and in more than 75% of terminally ill cancer patients. Delirium is an etiologically nonspecific, global, cerebral dysfunction characterized by an inability to maintain or shift attention properly. Other symptoms include decreased levels of consciousness; disturbance in the sleep-wake cycle, disorientation to person, place or time; abnormal perceptions such as visual or auditory (less frequent) hallucinations; and problems with cognition, such as memory impairment and language disturbance (i.e., dysnomia or dysgraphia). An important diagnostic feature of a delirium is the waxing and waning of the above symptoms. Delirium is distinguished from dementia by the more rapid onset, fluctuation in symptoms, the potential for reversibility, and the degree to which memory problems are prominent (more prominent in dementia).

13. Which metabolic disorders may cause confusional states and other psychiatric symptoms?

ABNORMALITY	MOOD DISORDER	MANIA	DELIRIUM	DEMENTIA	PSYCHOTIC DISORDER	ANXIETY DISORDER	PERSONALITY CHANGES
Hypercortisolism	+++	++	++	+	+++	+	+
Hypocortisolism	++	—	+	+	+	—	+
Hyperthyroidism	+	+	++	+	++	+++	+
Hypothyroidism	+++	—	++	+	++	—	—
Hypercalcemia	++	—	++	++	++	—	—
Hypoglycemia	++	+	+++	++	++	+++	+
Hyponatremia (SIADH)	++	—	++	++	+	—	—
Hypokalemia	++	—	++	++	+	+	—
Hypophosphatemia	+	—	++	+	—	++	++
Pheochromocytoma	—	—	—	—	—	+++	++

+++ = Frequent; ++ = Common; + = rare; SIADH = sustained inappropriate antidiuretic hormone.
Adapted from Breitbart WB: Endocrine-related psychiatric disorders. In Holland JC, Rowland JH (eds): Handbook of Psychooncology: Psychological Care of the Patient with Cancer. New York, Oxford University Press, 1989, pp 356–366; and Breitbart W, Holland JC: Psychiatric Aspects of Symptom Management in Cancer Patients. Washington, APA Press, 1993, p 29.

14. Which chemotherapeutic agents may cause confusional states and other psychiatric symptoms?

AGENTS	DEL	LET	HALL	DEM	DEP	PER	MAN	PSY	EPS	COG
Aminoglutethimide										X
L-Asparaginase	X	X	X							X
5-Azacytidine										X
Bleomycin	X									
Carmustine	X				X					
Cisplatin	X									
Cytosine arabinoside	X	X								X
Dacarbazine					X					
Fludarabine	X				X					X
Fluorouracil	X								X	
Hexylmethylamine			X							
Hydroxyurea			X							
Imidazolecarboxamide (DITC)										X
Interferon	X	X	X		X			X		
Interleukin	X	X	X							X
Isophosphamide	X	X	X							
Methotrexate	X	X		X		X				
Prednisone	X		X		X	X	X	X		X
Procarbazine	X	X	X		X		X			
Vinblastine	X	X	X		X					
Vincristine	X	X	X							

Note: Del = delirium; Let = lethargy; Hall = hallucination; Dem = dementia; Dep = depression; Per = "personality change"; Man = mania; Psy = psychosis; EPS = extrapyramidal symptoms; Cog = cognitive dysfunction.
Adapted from Breitbart W, Holland JC: Psychiatric Aspects of Symptom Management in Cancer Patients. Washington, APA Press, 1993, p 33.

15. What is the treatment for delirium?

Treatment of delirium includes maintenance of the patient's safety and symptomatic therapy. The underlying etiology must be determined, and if possible, reversed. Work-up should include metabolic studies (sodium, potassium, calcium, magnesium, renal functions, liver functions), medication review, and, if a CNS infection or hemorrhage is suspected, lumbar puncture. Brain imaging may be necessary. With drug-induced delirium, the drug (e.g., steroids) often cannot be discontinued or tapered and the clinical syndrome must be managed with psychotropic medication. Environmental manipulation and a low dose of a neuroleptic are useful for a patient who has a mild delirium without agitation. If the patient is a danger to himself or to others because of a confused or disinhibited state, observation by a one-to-one companion is indicated. Frequent reminders by staff or family of location, day, time, and outside events help distract patients from their thoughts, hallucinations, or delusions, and can afford them appropriate orientation.

Haloperidol, a high-potency neuroleptic, used in low dose orally, is the preferred drug for treatment of mild organic mental disorders in patients with cancer. It can also be used safely parenterally. The usual starting dose of 0.5 mg once or twice daily (PO, IV, IM, SC) is administered initially, with doses repeated every 45 to 60 minutes and titrated against symptoms. Haloperidol provides mild sedation and amelioration of the behavioral problems. Lower potency neuroleptics such as thioridazine and chlorpromazine are used in low doses when a more sedating medication is desired; however, they carry increased risk of postural hypotension and anticholinergic effects. Benzodiazepines and barbiturates should be avoided because they paradoxically worsen the patient's confusion as active metabolites accumulate.

Management of a severe delirium with agitation, accompanied by combativeness and paranoid thinking, requires immediate recognition and rapid collaborative intervention by oncologic, psychiatric, nursing, and security staffs. The patient should be moved to a quiet, but visible, area on the unit with a companion, away from potentially dangerous objects, such as scissors, needles, glassware, knives, and other sharp objects. Neuroleptics may be given in oral concentrate form or parenterally, for faster absorption and to assure administration of the drug. The minimal effective dose should be used and titrated to achieve sedation but with minimal autonomic and extrapyramidal effects. Relatively low doses of haloperidol (1 to 3 mg/day) are usually effective in treating agitation, paranoia, and fear. Parenteral doses are roughly twice as potent as oral doses. The addition of intravenous lorazepam, 0.5 mg to 1 mg every 1 to 2 hours PO or IV, adds to the sedation produced by haloperidol and may reduce the risk of extrapyramidal effects. Once stabilized the patient may then be maintained on an oral or intravenous dose of haloperidol that is equivalent to half to two-thirds of the dose required to calm the patient over the initial 24 hours. This may be given in a two to three times per day regimen.

Methotrimeprazine (IV or SC) is often used to control confusion and agitation in terminal delirium. Dosages range from 12.5 mg to 50 mg every 4 to 8 hours up to 300 mg per 24 hours for most patients. Hypotension and excessive sedation are limitations of this drug. Midazolam, given by subcutaneous or intravenous infusion in doses ranging from 30 to 100 mg over 24 hours, is also used to control agitation related to delirium in terminal stages. The goal of treatment with midazolam and methotrimeprazine is quiet sedation only.

16. What should you do if a patient tells you that he has suffered long enough with his illness and now wants to kill himself?

Sit down and talk with the patient. You should determine whether the suicidal statement is an offhand comment resulting from frustration or disgust (such as, "If I have to have one more MRI this year, I'll jump out the window") or whether the patient is communicating despair ("I can no longer bear what this disease is doing to all of us"). The house officer needs to explore the seriousness of the thoughts. Does the patient have an immediate plan or thoughts that if in the future there is a recurrence he might kill himself; or is the patient stockpiling medication; or does he own or have access to a weapon? Note also whether there are psychological predictors (e.g., prior psychiatric disorder, particularly depression or substance abuse; recent bereavement; few social supports) or medical predictors (e.g., poorly controlled pain, advanced stage of disease with debilitation, mild delirium with poor impulse control, or hopelessness or helplessness in the context of depression) that may be contributory. The latter two categories involve issues which, if reversed or addressed with proper therapy, would facilitate resolution of the suicidal ideation.

Questions to Ask to Assess Risk of Suicide

Open with this statement (asking does not enhance risk):
"Most patients with cancer have passing thoughts about suicide, such as 'I might do something if it gets bad enough'"

Have you ever had thoughts like that?	(Acknowledgment)
Any thoughts of not wanting to live or that it would be easier if you died?	
Do you have thoughts of suicide? Plan?	(Seriousness)
Have you thought about how you would do it?	
Have you ever been depressed or made a suicide attempt?	(Prior history)
Have you ever been treated for other psychiatric problems or have you been psychiatrically hospitalized before getting diagnosed with cancer?	
Have you had a problem with alcohol or drugs?	(Substance abuse)
Have you lost anyone close to you recently? (family, friends, co-patients)	(Bereavement)

Management of the suicidal patient includes maintaining a supportive relationship, giving the patient a sense of control by helping him to focus on that which can still be controlled, conveying the attitude that much can be done to improve the quality, if not the quantity, of life, even if the prognosis is poor. Aggressively treat symptoms such as pain, nausea, insomnia, anxiety, and depression. If the patient is actively suicidal, a 24-hour companion must be provided to establish constant observation, monitor the suicidal risk, and reassure the patient.

17. What should you do if this patient wants you to help him kill himself?
Often we say, "We have failed you if suicide seems to be your only alternative." The clinician explores medical and psychological issues that can be reversed. For instance, continuous uncontrolled pain can lead to a desire to be "put out of my misery." Aggressive treatment of pain, depression, insomnia, and anxiety, or at least making an alliance to try to resolve these problems, can help turn the tide for a patient. Patients who are thinking about dying often have specific issues that are frustrating them, and clinicians have an opportunity to find out how to help them regain some hope. Perhaps a patient would be more comfortable at home than in the hospital. Staff sometimes arranges for weddings to be moved to the hospital so that a patient can participate in an important family event. This call for help by the patient is also an opportunity for clinicians to help mobilize his support systems (i.e., family, colleagues, and members of his religious community). For patients who are lonely and have no family, volunteers who visit the patient in the hospital or at home can provide welcome distraction from medical issues.

The issue of physician-assisted suicide is controversial for legal as well as ethical reasons. Discussion of these issues and realistic alternatives for the patient with attending physicians, hospital clergy, and the psychiatrist are strongly encouraged.

18. If a patient wants to join a support group, what should the physician's attitude be?
Supportive and encouraging! Support groups for cancer patients are present in a variety of locales and settings. They are often distinguished by site of disease, by the professional nature of those running the group, and by different schools of therapeutic theory. Not all patients want to have therapy (either individual or group) and not all patients will benefit from it. Variables which

affect one's benefit from a group include a person's previous involvement in therapy, psychological mindedness, current social supports, extent of physical disease or limitations, and cognitive deficits.

Two studies have shown that participation in cancer therapy groups improved the quality of patients' lives. Some data suggest that participation in groups may also increase longevity. The number of subjects in these studies were, however, small and so they need to be replicated. Still, they are an encouraging avenue of hope for cancer patients.

Patients can find out about existing support groups by contacting their local American Cancer Society Chapter, The National Coalition of Cancer Survivors, Cancer Care, Cansurmount or their local hospital or oncologist.

19. A patient wants to try an alternative cancer therapy. What can you say?

Many alternative cancer treatments are available to patients both in the United States and abroad. They range from treatments which are outright frauds and can be lethal, to others that are aimed at improving well-being and are therefore assumed to enhance the body's ability to fight the cancer. These treatments include nutritional approaches, psychological-spiritual approaches, and immunotherapeutic approaches, or some combination of all of these. As individuals assume more responsibility for their own health and hold more holistic health beliefs, interest will continue in these alternative approaches among patients. Physicians are becoming increasingly informed about alternative treatments and are usually supportive of their use so long as they do not interfere with more traditional therapy. Staff should respect patients' consideration of alternative therapies. Clinicians should encourage questions and offer information regarding risks and benefits.

20. A patient wants to know more about guided imagery and how it can help. What can you tell him?

Guided imagery is a technique that facilitates and deepens relaxation. It adds a component of distraction to other methods of symptom control like medication. Guided imagery is also used by some patients with the expectation of treating their cancers and controlling tumor growth. This latter method involves visualizing the body's own physiologic defenses fighting cancer cells. For example, the patient may visualize his white blood cells as "pac-men" which ingest cancer cells in a particular part of the body. It is, however, important to point out that at this time no compelling scientific evidence indicates that any specific visualization technique has anticancer effects. Patients ought to discuss these issues with their primary physician. Clinicians do support patients' attempts to cope with their disease, so long as these attempts to not compromise ongoing medical care.

21. Seeing children with cancer is so overwhelming. What is important to understand about how a child copes with cancer?

Cancer in a child is difficult for the patient, and devastating for the family and the health care professional. Specific developmental tasks at different ages affect the response to the need for procedures, adjustment to strangers, and to the use of machines of advanced medical treatment.

From birth to 2 years of age, important developmental milestones include an appreciation that people will respond to the child in a certain fashion, and that they will meet the child's needs. Most often the mother is the primary caretaker, and from whom the child develops a basic sense of trust and hope. The child also learns an ability to interact with and explore the environment. By the end of this phase children are beginning to master a sense of autonomy and independence. When parental ties are disrupted by hospitalization during this phase, there is a profound effect. Inconsistency in parenting may result in a sense of mistrust, with an exaggerated sense of stranger anxiety. Painful procedures and handling by strangers often lead to helpless feelings, fears, and mistrust. Parents question their competence as caregivers when illness strikes their children. Older siblings are likely to feel guilty, angry, sad, and neglected. A child treated for cancer before age 3 will have virtually no recollection of the experience; his parents will never forget.

22. Does the child react differently at 3 years?

In early childhood, from 3 to 5 years of age, children are experimenting with their autonomy and interacting in the world. A transition to symbolic thought evolves with language development. Fantasy and imaginative play are possible. Cognitive and affective aspects of development predominate. Health and illness are seen as two separate states, not on a continuum, as viewed by older children and adults. Separation from both parents and siblings by hospitalizations and other time-occupying treatments are acutely felt. The sick child may show jealousy of healthy siblings and friends. Parents are tempted to protect their children and reassert a level of control more appropriate to earlier periods of life. Having parents "room in" during hospitalizations can be very useful, but exhausting, which leads to a decreased parenting ability.

Play is the primary form of intervention in this period, because of its link with normal growth activity. Rehearsal of procedures, such as pretending to take blood pressures or blood with a play kit, is also helpful. Information given to a child should be concrete, nontechnical, and at the appropriate developmental level for the child, such as: "We need to take a picture of your head and you need to lie on a table. There will be a great big doughnut surrounding your head, and you'll need to lie very still," rather than, "You are going for an MRI scan of your brain."

23. How can you help a child between the ages of 6 and 11 handle cancer treatment better?

The middle childhood and latency years (ages 6 to 11) are characterized by entry into school, a major socializing force in children's lives. Children compare themselves with others and master important developmental tasks.

Cancer during this period often causes parental conflicts over caretaking, difficult emotions for siblings, and isolation of the sick child from peers. There can be a major impact resulting from school disruption on the child's sense of competence and self-esteem. At this age, children are aware of the gravity of their disease even if they do not yet have a full appreciation of the irreversibility of death.

The child's reintegration into school can be aided by discussions with the hospital social worker or nurse clinician and workshops for teachers and classmates. It is important to help the patient master various tasks by setting realistic and attainable goals, by increasing caretakers' flexibility, by modifying tasks, and by providing additional support and encouragement.

Treatment for cancer in children can be extremely aggressive and, for many, can be more painful than the disease itself. Repeated infusions of highly emetic chemotherapeutic agents, bone marrow aspirations, lumbar punctures, and venipunctures can be painful and frightening to a child who may not be able to understand their purpose. Some children believe that they can die from procedures. As with younger children, those who are experiencing hair loss or loss of limbs because of their cancer treatment may think that doctors and nurses are punishing them for some wrong deed. Ask the child about such thoughts and see if the child understands what is happening. Try to correct misperceptions.

Parents' level of distress will play a large role in modulating children's expressions of emotional distress. Therefore support and education of parents is crucial to treatment of children. Anxiolytic medications can be useful in children; however, many children do not like being sedated, and will resist this type of intervention on a regular basis. Behavioral interventions such as breathing exercises, attentional distraction, reinforcement, imagery, and behavioral rehearsal have been shown to be useful in a variety of problems facing children and their parents, including pain, anxiety, and nausea.

24. Adolescence can be a difficult time for a healthy teenager. What are some things to know that can help a teenager deal with cancer?

In adolescence, major changes are occurring in the physical, cognitive, social, mood, and sexual spheres simultaneously. Each of these areas must be acknowledged when designing interventions to help a teenager cope better. Dramatic physical and physiologic changes occur in puberty, accompanied by significant psychological changes. Adolescents try to achieve a stable self-identity, to enter into mature relationships with peers of both sexes, and to gain independence from their parents and family. Illness or treatment during this period will likely lead to disturbances in some of the areas of functioning mentioned. Hospitalizations and prolonged separations from friends may lead to feelings of isolation and of missing out on important life activities.

Support from peers is crucial to the adolescent. It is usually desired from other sick adolescents, rather than from "well friends," who are perceived by patients as not being able to understand what they are going through. Because support groups are popular in this age group, encouraging participation can be helpful. "Veteran patients" are also useful to demonstrate effective coping strategies. The more independence and control of treatment decisions and responsibilities that can be given to the adolescent patient, the better the long-term adjustment to illness. For instance, patients should be encouraged to participate in self-care. Parents still may provide an important source of support, though they may appear less important in the communication process than at earlier ages.

25. You find a staff member getting teary while talking with a patient, crying openly when leaving the room, and visiting the patient on a day off. What is going on?

One explanation is that this patient is having a difficult time, and the staff member is extremely empathetic. Likely, however, this behavior has more to do with the staff member's life and his overinvolvement with the patient than with the patient's life. For instance, memories of a family member who was in a situation similar to the patient's, or recollection of losses experienced by a clinician at an earlier time may be triggered by an interaction with a patient.

These types of feelings may also be related to the staff person's current mood state; for instance, he or she may be feeling depressed or overwhelmed by work issues (e.g., many recent deaths on a particular ward) or may be having difficulty with work and receiving few rewards at home. Medical students, house staff, and nurses usually do not want to admit that they are having a hard time. Yet support can be made available by administrative and counseling staffs and peers to help understand the situation and to help get through it.

Particular situations which may signify trouble include, "the need to try to save the patient," resulting in adversarial relationships with other health professionals involved in a patient's care. Overinvolvement with, or avoidance of, a patient and angry feelings toward a patient whose condition is deteriorating or toward other staff involved in the care of the patient may also indicate problems. Another common reaction is "the need to protect the patient," which involves not bringing up for discussion, even when appropriate, topics that may be painful or emotionally distressing for the patient (e.g., health care proxies, resuscitation orders, failed treatments, or worsening prognosis).

Recognition of our limitations and vulnerabilities is as important as being aware of the common reactions noted. If you find that this or a similar set of circumstances is occurring to you or to someone you are working with, talk it over with an advisor or supervisor to get help with the situation.

26. Is cancer always associated with pain?

Unfortunately, almost always. Pain can be related to the disease, to treatment for the disease, and to procedures. Psychological variables such as the meaning of pain, perceptions of control, fear of death, depressed mood, and hopelessness are recognized as contributing to the cancer pain experience and may increase the likelihood of a patient reporting pain. It is estimated that about 15% of patients with localized disease and between 60% and 90% of those with advanced cancer report debilitating pain.

Today, more attention is being given to alleviating and preventing pain. In cancer patients, however, pain is often undertreated. Factors contributing to the undertreatment of pain include lack of proper assessment of the pain, the assumption that psychological rather than medical variables are the cause of pain, lack of knowledge of current therapeutic approaches, focus on prolonging life and cure versus alleviating suffering, the belief that opioids should be "saved in case you need them later," inadequate physician-patient relationship, fear of respiratory depression, and fear of addiction. Both patients and physicians share this fear. Although tolerance and physical dependence commonly occur, addiction (i.e., psychological dependence) is rare and almost never occurs in individuals who do not have a history of drug abuse before cancer.

A useful approach to treatment of cancer pain is the step ladder approach advocated by the World Health Organization. Mild pain is treated with nonopioids, such as nonsteroidal antiin-flammatories and doses are increased to dose-limiting toxicity or relief. Moderate pain is treated with weak opioids (codeine or oxycodone), and severe pain is treated with strong opioids (morphine) regardless of stage of disease. Adjuvant analgesics (i.e., tricyclic antidepressants, phenothiazines, psychostimulants, and benzodiazepines) can be used with any of the above choices, when therapy is limited by dose-related side effects.

Adjuncts to the treatment of pain include the provision of support, knowledge, and skills using a crisis intervention model. Cognitive-behavioral therapy techniques, such as relaxation, distraction, and desensitization, are also useful in the treatment of cancer pain.

BIBLIOGRAPHY

1. Breitbart W, Holland JC: Psychiatric Aspects of Symptom Management in Cancer Patients. Washington, DC, American Psychiatric Press, 1993.
2. Derogatis LR, Morrow GR, Fetting J, et al: Prevalence of psychiatric disorders among cancer patients. JAMA 249:751–757, 1983.
3. Holland JC, Rowland JH: Handbook of Psychooncology. New York, Oxford University Press, 1989.
4. Massie MJ, Heilgenstein E, Lederberg MS, Holland JC: Psychiatric complications in cancer patients. In Holleb AI, Fink DJ, Murphy GP (eds): Clinical Oncology. Atlanta, American Cancer Society, 1991.
5. Mermelstein HT, Lesko L, Holland JC: Depression in the cancer patient. Journal of Psycho-oncology 1:199–216, 1992.
6. Shuster JL, Stern TA, Greenberg DB: Pros and cons of fluoxetine for depressed cancer patients. Oncology 6:45–55, 1993.
7. Roth AJ, Holland JC: Psychiatric complications in cancer patients. In Brain MC, Carbone PP (eds): Current Therapy in Hematology-Oncology. St. Louis, Mosby, 1995.
8. U.S. Department of Health, Management of Cancer Pain, Clinical Practice Guidelines. Washington, DC, U.S. Government Printing Office, 1994.

73. PSYCHOLOGICAL PERSPECTIVES IN THE CARE OF PATIENTS WITH DIABETES MELLITUS

Alan M. Jacobson, M.D.

1. Why are psychological perspectives so important for the treatment of diabetes mellitus?

Both type I and type II diabetes demand considerable change in lifestyle and learning of complex information, pose threats of future complications, and may lead to premature death. Diabetes also involves enforced role change, potential for suffering pain, and numerous insults to the person and family, including bias in hiring, problems in getting insurance, embarrassment, and living with fear of the future. The treatment of diabetes rests on a strong foundation of knowledge on the part of the physician, other health care professionals, and the patient and his or her family. Type I diabetes requires learning the complex task of using insulin, whereas patients with type II diabetes are forced to make major lifestyle changes well after a period in which they have developed consistent habits. In addition, patients with type II diabetes are often obese and must take a new approach to diet in the face of well-ingrained behaviors. Furthermore, later in the course of type II diabetes patients may need to take insulin at the very time when it is more difficult to see and manipulate small objects. Because of the need for behavior change, the psychological management of the patient and the identification of emotional problems may be critical for successful treatment of diabetes mellitus.

2. What is the starting point for a psychological approach to care?

Successful treatment of a complex chronic condition such as diabetes mellitus rests on the therapeutic relationship developed between the patient and his or her healthcare provider(s), including physicians, dietitians, psychologists, and nurse educators. The strengths of a therapeutic relationship can be conceptualized through a term derived from psychotherapy: the therapeutic alliance. The therapeutic alliance refers to the underlying level of agreement about the goals of and approaches to treatment. The nature and strength of the alliance often go unaddressed during the course of most treatment. Indeed, the exact strength of the therapeutic alliance may remain entirely hidden to the clinician. Yet it may have important positive and negative effects on the course of treatment.

For example, a therapy group for patients with diabetes had been meeting for several weeks when a new member entered treatment. The group therapist had been concerned in previous meetings that the patients had not developed clear understanding of the objectives and methods of treatment. The new patient posed immediate problems because he was suspicious and frightened of the patients and therapist. In his first session the other patients spontaneously responded to these feelings by explaining carefully and repetitively the purpose of the group therapy, the style of approach that would be taken, and their own hopes for benefit. The new patient, relieved and reassured by the other patients' explicit and thoughtful explanations that addressed his worries, went on to use the group treatment effectively. The explanations were given with such accuracy that they virtually mirrored what the therapist herself might have said, thus reflecting a strong but previously latent alliance that was firmly in place during treatment.

In this instance, as in medical treatment, the strength of the relationship or alliance may not be readily apparent to the physician. Furthermore, temporary breaches in the alliance may mask underlying strengths that can be shored up over time. Such breaks in the alliance are typically noticeable when patients fail to follow through with treatment recommendations, e.g., repeatedly forgetting to bring the results of metabolic monitoring to a medical appointment. The same patient may follow through at other times with other requests, reflecting clear agreement and comfort with treatment objectives. Such variations represent the fluidity of the therapeutic alliance. From visit to visit the strength of the alliance may vary, depending on the task. For example, the patient failing to bring home glucose testing records may have particular discomfort with this aspect of treatment. Such discomfort suggests that the strength of the alliance may not be sufficient to work on an especially upsetting problem. In a sense, the additional stress temporarily overwhelms the working alliance. This fluidity suggests an important principle of treatment: The therapeutic alliance should not be taken for granted. Continual attention is required to buttress the alliance and to address provocative treatment issues over the course of follow-up. Indeed, treatment often moves in a direction from easier to more difficult tasks. Thus the alliance may be sufficiently strong for the patient to learn the basic technique of insulin treatment but not sufficiently strong to address the more difficult challenges of decreasing fat and carbohydrate intake or beginning to make changes in an otherwise erratic lifestyle to stabilize metabolic control.

3. What can the physician do to strengthen the therapeutic alliance? How is it weakened?
The patient and/or his or her insurance pays for a service that the clinician with special expertise provides. Equally essential to the physician's technical expertise is knowledge of how to engage patients in a joint exercise of decision making and treatment. Whereas technical and medical expertise brings the patient to the clinician, transactional expertise builds an effective alliance and facilitates behavior change.

Some patients may wish and even demand directly and/or indirectly shared responsibility for setting the agenda for each medical appointment, whereas other patients initially may prefer the physician to assume complete responsibility. However, recent studies from typical clinical practices in the United States suggest that encouraging patients to take an active role in setting the agenda for the meeting may improve adherence to the clinician's recommendations. For example, one study of a group of patients with diabetes demonstrated that an intervention designed to activate patients to take more responsibility for directing the medical interview led to better glycemic control and improved adherence. Encouraging patient activity does not mean abrogating responsibility for providing clear, coherent direction. It simply means that sharing control appears to enhance respect for the clinician's advice. The shift in orientation proposed by the activation of patients mirrors a widely espoused change in the workplace. This approach gives added responsibility for decision making to employees. In factories, for example, teams of workers on the assembly line are given more opportunity to suggest and implement ideas about improving efficiency and quality in the manufacturing process.

One approach to improving the therapeutic alliance, conceptualized by Lazare and colleagues, focuses on the identification of hidden patient requests and negotiation between patient and clinician. Asking questions not only gives patients the opportunity to help set the agenda of the meeting but also brings out new information that can be used in planning treatment, including hidden patient requests, concerns, and goals. Often clinicians have clear, predetermined goals for their intervention. The nurse educator's job is to educate or train the patient about injection techniques and handling insulin; the dietitian must teach the patient how to select appropriate foods; and the physician diagnoses and treats intercurrent problems and directs treatment (e.g., insulin regimen and dosage). This often involves recommending changes in the treatment regimen. For example, recognizing that the patient with type II diabetes has not been able to maintain adequate glycemic control on diet plus an oral agent may lead to a recommendation for using insulin. However, the patient may come to the same appointment with entirely different requests and goals that remain unexpressed. In many transactions it is sufficient for the clinician to make recommendations that the patient will follow. This does not imply inadequate attention to the needs of the patient; it means simply that the therapeutic alliance is strong and that the patient is comfortable and ready to follow the recommendations of the expert.

In other instances the therapeutic alliance is weakened by patient distress about the particular aspect of treatment, prior problems in the relationship, inadequate communication between clinician and patient, or psychological problems on the part of either. In such instances, the recommendations may not be acceptable. The physician must ask sufficient questions to identify patient concerns and goals and thus to negotiate the next step in treatment. However, the patient may not be ready to begin insulin even then. He or she may want to try again a previously failed diet. How should the clinician react? The clinician knows that on past occasions the patient has tried to lose weight to decrease insulin resistance and thus to improve the likelihood of better glycemic control. The patient is terrified of insulin injections and is not yet ready to start. If the clinician insists by making a strong recommendation, the patient often will not follow through. At this juncture, after identifying the patient's hidden concerns and requests, the clinician has the opportunity to negotiate a settlement. This approach has two benefits. First, it strengthens the therapeutic alliance by reassuring the patient that he or she retains some sense of control over the future. Of even greater importance, he or she knows that the clinician has listened and comprehended the underlying concerns. This recognition can be a remarkably reassuring and comforting experience for patients. Being heard may calm anxiety to the point that the patient accepts the original recommendation. On the other hand, it may be necessary for the patient to try again the failed diet before beginning insulin. It is clear that such interactions can be frustrating, because the patient may wish to try many times something that obviously is no longer working. But each attempt provides an opportunity for rediscussion and strengthening of the bond that eventually will allow the patient to begin something that is terrifying.

The uncovered concerns may seem indirectly related to treatment. Examples include requests to write a letter to support an application for special housing, wishes to discuss work problems, or demands for apparently unwarranted treatment. An approach that uncovers hidden concerns is the first step in engaging the patient in negotiating the next steps in the treatment program.

Certainly, there may be emergency situations in which something must be done. The patient's glycemic control is so poor that he has been in ketoacidosis and hospitalized. A change must be made. Previous identification of hidden requests and negotiation of settlements let the patient know that he or she can be heard. When a crisis is reached, forceful direction based on fundamental trust can lead to acceptance of a confronting recommendation that "it is now time; we can't wait any longer."

If patient and clinician have not agreed on a model for interaction, the therapeutic alliance may be weakened. Patients have implicit models for the way in which clinicians should act. For example, some patients may not value a treatment recommendation unless it includes a prescription. Furthermore, underlying beliefs about the value of certain types of treatments may be derived from traditional views of medicine and treatment. Cultural factors typically play an important role in determining such assumptions. The clinician may anticipate such differences when patients from distinct cultures come for help, but important cultural variations in attitude may be found even among members of different cultural groups from the same country. In addition, personality, family up-bringing, and past experiences with illness may engender different views of the nature of therapeutics.

4. What role can the psychiatrist play in the care of patients with diabetes?

In the most difficult of situations, when the physician has difficulty in maintaining objectivity and a comfortable relationship with the patient, psychological consultation and conjoint treatment approaches may be extremely helpful. The psychiatrist can provide the patient a time and place to consider the expectations of the physician and to help negotiate between patient and physician the steps of treatment. Sometimes such consultations are initiated by the patient, but more often they are initiated by the physician who feels loss of control. This may occur early in treatment when the therapeutic alliance is often weak.

For example, a 25-year-old man was hospitalized in diabetic ketoacidosis with previously undiagnosed type I diabetes mellitus. After initial stabilization in the intensive care unit, he was transferred to a medical floor, where the first steps of teaching and diabetes treatment were instituted. The patient was terrified of taking insulin by injection and refused all but two injections over the first few days on the unit. A psychiatric consultation was requested, because the physician believed that the patient was not ready to accept treatment recommendations and required immediate transfer to an inpatient psychiatric unit. The patient, according to the medical team, had recognizable signs of diabetes for several months but had been avoiding contact with a physician. He had a history of hospitalization for an apparent psychotic disorder and had remained marginally functional in the community. He had a supportive family but was unable to maintain independent living. The psychiatrist found that the patient was guarded and frightened but not overtly psychotic or clinically depressed. He had denied the possibility of diabetes until transfer to the medical unit, where he made the first struggling attempts to accept the notion of taking insulin. During the consultation he asked questions about the course of diabetes and its treatment and expressed some optimism because he had given himself one injection. The patient wanted the staff to give him more time to get used to shots. The psychiatrist answered each question, suggested further discussions with the nursing staff, and indicated to the staff that the patient was beginning to acknowledge his need for insulin. He indicated that transfer to a psychiatric unit was not needed and suggested that the team give the patient another few days to grapple with the reality of his new diagnosis. During follow-up sessions he allowed the patient to vent feelings about his new medical condition. Over the next few days the patient accepted twice daily injections and started to learn self-injection and self-monitoring techniques. When the patient was discharged, he was taking his own injections. The patient's fears decreased as he came to experience the actuality of diabetes care. In turn he gradually accepted treatment without forced change through confrontations. In essence, the illness did the confronting, and the staff, once comfortable with the patient's participation in decisions to start treatment in a less than optimal manner, provided expert support.

5. What role does the family play in the treatment of diabetes?
Many studies have addressed the effects of diabetes on patients and their families, with specific focus on child and adolescent patients. Although studies of children with diabetes have failed to show consistent effects on personality and psychological maturation, there is little doubt that diabetes increases stress in parents and patients with diabetes. It is not clear whether there are distinct changes in most families of patients with diabetes, but evidence now suggests that children of families that adapt more successfully in terms of increased successful organization, cohesiveness, and maintenance of a warm, nurturing environment are more likely to cope effectively in the care of their diabetes. Thus family factors are critical influences on the course of illness, and involvement of the family is an important feature of the care of patients with diabetes. For example, a spouse may contact the physician about her husband, who tests infrequently, because he feels "okay," even though he has had periodic hypoglycemic episodes that required assistance. The consciousness-raising process is entered jointly by the medical professional and appropriate loved ones. In all instances, such confrontations must be carried out nonjudgmentally with great care to avoid backlash that may lead to even greater problems with self-care.

6. Is there an important link between depression and diabetes?
It now appears that major depression is more common among adult patients with type I diabetes than in the general population; this increase in prevalence is greatest among men. The relationship of diabetes and depression is not unique. It has been widely recognized that depressive disorders are more common in many groups with chronic illness than in community samples. The indication that affective disorders are common in diabetic patients is important. Depression may influence profoundly functional health status to as great or greater extent than chronic medical illnesses. Furthermore, the presence of depression in diabetic patients is associated with problems with glycemic control. The magnitude of the effect of depression on glycemic control suggests that depression places diabetic patients at risk for the well-recognized sequelae of chronic hyperglycemia—more rapid progression of microvascular complications.

7. Does diabetes influence the methods of diagnosis and treatment of depression?

The diagnosis and treatment of depressive disorders in patients with diabetes should follow the same general principles as in patients without a concomitant medical condition. However, certain issues deserve special consideration. The diagnosis of clinical depression rests on identification of a specific set of symptoms that may involve physical, cognitive, affective, and attitudinal changes. Physical symptoms may include fatigue, psychomotor retardation, insomnia or excessive sleeping, and weight loss; cognitive symptoms may include decreased concentration and poor recent memory; and affective symptoms may include depressed mood, loss of interest in activities, and increased guilt, shame, fear, or anxiety. In addition, patients with depression may present with altered attitudes such as pessimism about the future and a sense that actions cannot lead to positive consequences. Most patients present with only a few such symptoms. If the presentation consists predominantly of physical symptoms, the diagnosis of depression in a patient with diabetes may be difficult. Poorly controlled diabetes with persistent hyperglycemia and ketonuria may present with physical symptoms similar to the physical symptoms of depression. Thus it may be important to evaluate the patient's status after a short period of improved glycemic control. If after 2 weeks of improved control physical symptoms persist, a diagnosis of depression may be warranted. If physical symptoms are accompanied by depressive attitudes and affective symptoms, it is unlikely that poorly controlled diabetes accounts for the problem. In such instances earlier treatment for depression should be considered.

Despite suggestions that antidepressants and lithium carbonate may affect blood glucose levels, in practice this is rarely a significant clinical problem. Patients starting antidepressants should be alerted to the possibility of more irregular control of blood glucose levels. Because lithium carbonate appears to have an insulinlike action, lower blood glucose levels may be anticipated. Possible long-term side effects of lithium (e.g., renal toxicity and hypothyroidism) should not be considered an absolute contraindication to its use in patients with diabetes. As with all patients treated with lithium, regular follow-up of medical status is necessary.

The commonly used antidepressants have side effects that may complicate treatment. In patients with diabetes such side effects may be especially problematic. For example, tricyclic antidepressants may cause orthostatic hypotension. In patients with autonomic neuropathy such side effects may be exacerbated. The possible cardiac side effects of tricyclic antidepressants may increase the risk for arrhythmias in diabetic patients with advanced coronary vessel disease. The newer antidepressants, such as the selective serotonin reuptake inhibitors (SSRIs) have fewer cardiovascular side effects. However, their use may pose specific problems in patients with gastroparesis; one of the common side effects of SSRIs, nausea and vomiting, may be especially problematic. Because of such complexities, patients with diabetes may require several trials of antidepressants. Moreover, slow titration to optimal doses may be needed to initiate successful treatment. As with all depressed patients, it is important to recognize that the single most common reasons for treatment failure are inadequate length of treatment and inadequate dosing. Patients presenting with side effects at low doses may be able to tolerate the medication if the dose is increased slowly.

Patients with depression may have symptoms that limit learning ability and confidence in self-treatment. Thus, treatment of depression in patients who have problems with glycemic control or other aspects of self-care should be accompanied by appropriate counseling. For example, pessimistic attitudes may inhibit willingness or ability to care for diabetes and patients may need reeducation about material that was either not learned or forgotten during the depressed period.

8. Are eating disorders common in patients with diabetes?

Given its considerable requirements for changes in diet, diabetes mellitus, especially type I, may pose a special risk for the development of eating disorders. Diabetes in the population at greatest risk, women aged 15–35 years, may precipitate the development of clinical eating disturbances. To date, available studies do not answer this question clearly. Some evidence suggests increased rates of anorexia nervosa and bulimia in young women with diabetes. It is quite evident that ideals of body weight, which lead women to strive for weight loss, have problematic consequences in patients with diabetes. Polonsky and colleagues have shown that 30% of women with type I diabetes across the adolescent and adult age range acknowledged at least some omission of insulin and that 9% of all women acknowledged frequent omission of insulin. As expected, omission occurred even more commonly in women aged 15–30 but was found even in older women.

Binging and purging are often experienced as shameful and may be hidden. Because of the likelihood of underreporting, current rates may underestimate the frequency of insulin omission. A significant minority of women who acknowledge omitting insulin do so explicitly to lose weight. Omission of insulin to lose weight is associated with a high level of psychopathology and is linked to significant problems with glycemic control. A history of eating disorder is also predictive of early development of retinopathy. Such findings underline the importance of identifying possible problems with body weight ideals and their association with habits of self-care.

Many patients with diabetes do not fully develop an eating disorder, although they discover the "merits" of occasional insulin underuse to control weight. Such patients, who do not meet threshold for diagnosis, may be the most difficult to identify, yet they represent an important high-risk group.

9. What are special considerations for the treatment of diabetic patients with eating disorders?

The treatment of eating disorders and associated conceptions of body weight is often difficult and time-consuming. Physician and patient may find themselves struggling to agree on goals for treatment. Thus, eating-related problems are particularly fruitful areas for collaborative models of treatment and for identifying specific areas of change that the patient is prepared to address.

The most important special considerations in the treatment of eating-related problems in diabetic patients revolves around the availability of self-administered insulin and its underuse as a method of "purging." Because many patients fear weight gain, underdosing with insulin becomes the preferred method of regulating weight. Underdosing may be present without other methods of purging. The identification of this form of eating disorder may require repeated questioning in a nonjudgmental manner. Because shame frequently accompanies eating-related problems, the clinician may uncover such problems only when the patient has sufficient comfort and senses that she will not be chastised.

The treatment of eating disorders in which underuse of insulin plays an important role is made more complex by the water-retaining effects of insulin. In such instances, reinsulinization may require considerable negotiation between patient and physician. The patient often does not differentiate between sources of weight gain or body size change. A 10-pound weight loss is a 10-pound weight loss, and a 10-pound weight gain is a 10-pound weight gain, whether the change is due to changes in water volume, fat stores, or muscle mass. Thus reinsulinization accompanied by rapid weight gain and overt edema may be a terrifying experience for patients with intense beliefs about excessive weight.

For example, a 23-year-old woman presented with bulima that included binge eating and extensive underdosing with insulin. When hospitalized because of diabetic ketoacidosis and restarted on insulin, she rapidly regained the weight lost through dehydration and experienced pitting edema of the ankles. She became increasingly depressed and panicked by the weight gain to the extent that she requested a lower dose of insulin to control the terrifying spiral of weight. Despite careful explanation about the source of added weight, the patient could not differentiate between water gain and gain in fat stores. Thus, as part of the treatment plan, the dose of insulin was lowered and gradually increased to an optimal level. Hospitalization was extended until her weight stabilized; only then could the patient return home without threat of continuing weight gain from fluid retention.

In rare instances, gastroparesis that causes vomiting and weight loss may mimic or complicate anorexia and bulimia. Among young women with relatively short durations of diabetes and complicated family histories, eating disorders and gastroparesis may be difficult to differentiate. Functional gastrointestinal investigations suggesting slowed gastric emptying may be used to identify the gastroparetic component but effective treatment usually requires intervention in a family, individual, and medical level. In some instances symptoms may be secondary to psychological and family conflicts, whereas in others psychological and family conflicts may stem in part from the severe early onset of the confusing and frightening diabetic complication of gastroparesis.

10. Are anxiety disorders readily diagnosable in patients with diabetes?

As with affective disorders, anxiety syndromes may be confused with diabetes-related symptoms. Most commonly, patients may not be able to differentiate between symptoms of panic anxiety and hypoglycemic states. Anxiety syndromes may include physical symptoms such as palpitations, sweats, and headaches as well as physical and emotional feelings of trembling, foreboding, and panic. In most instances repeated self-testing of blood glucose levels can be used to help the patient discriminate between hypoglycemic and anxiety-related symptoms. When emotional symptoms predominate, the patient probably is experiencing a form of anxiety disorder. Thus patients whose presentation includes increased obsessive thoughts, compulsive acts, fear, or obsessive worry are more likely to have an underlying anxiety disorder. Treatment with currently available antianxiety agents usually poses no special problems in patients with diabetes. As in patients with depression, treatment should incorporate counseling to help patients deal with underlying concerns that may be important causes of the anxiety syndrome. In some instances such concerns are diabetes-related; however, the problem may relate only partially to the patient's illness.

For example, a 45-year-old patient with type I diabetes presented with increased fear, obsessional thoughts, and panic anxiety. Initially the symptoms were associated with worries about future complications that began soon after the patient increased his frequency of home glucose testing and insulin injections. Heightened awareness of diabetes appeared to be the critical trigger for the psychological reaction. On further inquiry it became clear that the patient was also experiencing considerable marital difficulties, which played an important role in bringing out the anxiety disorder. Treatment that addressed both diabetic and marital issues was therefore instituted.

11. Can psychological screening measures be useful in the care of patients with diabetes?

Given the practical problems of caring for patients in busy clinical practices, psychosocial screening can help clinicians to identify problems for further assessment. Three measures may be of some use in identifying at-risk patients:

1. The Beck Depression Inventory is a widely used, brief, self-report inquiry into symptoms of depression. It may be used by the primary care physician and/or the diabetologist to identify areas for further inquiry as well as to document the level of depressive symptoms. Many other screening measures also have been developed for assessing anxiety and depression.

2. Quality of life measures may be useful in identifying the level of impact of illness on the patient's perception of well-being. Assessment can be used to identify the overall level of quality of life as well as particular areas of patient concern. The Diabetes Quality of Life Measure developed for the Diabetes Control and Complications Trial (DCCT) is one such measure. Prior studies suggest a high degree of reliability and validity. Such quality of life measures can be augmented by specific questions that the practitioner finds helpful or shortened by selection of a subset of especially relevant questions from the scale. This measure includes particular questions oriented toward adolescents and young adults with diabetes; although designed for type I patients, it also may be used in older patients with type II diabetes.

3. The Problem Areas in Diabetes Scale (PAID) scrutinizes specific concerns about diabetes and the distress level associated with their presence. The measure is designed as a screen and covers multiple issues. It may be used to identify particular problem areas in the emotional experience of diabetes and behavioral problem areas that can be targeted for special attention and intervention. Practitioners are encouraged to add to the list for clinical use.

Such screening measures may be considered as guides for the clinician. They can be used to stimulate discussion, to identify hidden patient concerns, and to guide the clinician toward an improved understanding of the patient's emotional life.

12. Summarize key features of the psychological care of patients with diabetes.
The most important feature of many chronic diseases, like diabetes, is the requirement for developing new attitudes and behaviors. Maintenance of such behaviors requires repeated effort from patients, family members, and health care providers. A strong, close working relationship with the healthcare provider is the base on which treatment rests. The psychological management of patient problems begins with recognition of the importance of this relationship. The more the clinician understands about the psychological themes embedded in the life of a patient with diabetes and the more that the clinician integrates these themes into the treatment process, the more likely that care will succeed. Thus it is critical that the doctor's office is what Hemingway described as a "clean, well-lighted place"; that is, a place which appeals in the darkest of night and at the moment of greatest despair. Even if behavior change has been minimal, the patient seeing that light will be comforted throughout the process of adaptation to diabetes.

BIBLIOGRAPHY

1. Beck AT: The Beck Depression Inventory. Psychological Corporation. Harcourt Brace Jovanovich, 1978.
2. Curry S: Commentary: In search of how people change. Diabetes Spect 6:34–35, 1993.
3. DCCT Research Group: The effect of intensive treatment of diabetes on the development and progression of long-term complications in insulin-dependent diabetes mellitus. N Engl J Med 329:886–977, 1993.
4. Dunn SM, Turtle JR: The myth of the diabetic personality. Diabetes Care 4:640–646, 1982.
5. Gavard JA, Lustman PJ, Clouse RE: Prevalence of depression in adults with diabetes: An epidemiological evaluation. Diabetes Care 16:1167–1178, 1993.
6. Hemingway E: The Complete Short Stories. New York, Scribners, 1987.
7. Jacobson A, de Groot M, Samson JA: The evaluation of two measures of quality of life in patients with type I and type II diabetes mellitus. Diabetes Care 17:267–274, 1994.
8. Jacobson AM, Hauser S, Anderson B, Polonsky W: Psychosocial aspects of diabetes. In Kahn C, Weir G (eds): Joslin's Diabetes Mellitus, 13th ed. Philadelphia, Lea & Febiger, 1994.
9. Jacobson AM, Hauser ST, Lavori P, et al: Family environment and glycemic control: A four-year prospective study of children and adolescents with insulin-dependent diabetes mellitus. Psychosom Med 56:401–409, 1994.
10. Kaplan S, Greenfield S, Ware J: Assessing the effects of physician-patient interactions on the outcome of chronic disease. Med Care 27(Suppl):S110–S127, 1989.
11. Lazare A, Cohen F, Jacobson AM, et al: The walk-in patient as a customer: A key dimension in evaluation and treatment. Am J Orthopsychiatry 42:872–873, 1972.
12. Lustman PJ, Griffith LA, Clouse RE, Cryer PE: Psychiatric illness in diabetes mellitus. Relationship to symptoms and glucose control. J Nerv Ment Dis 174:736–742, 1986.
13. Polonsky W, Anderson B, Lohrer P, et al: Assessment of diabetes specific distress. Diabetes Care 18:754–760, 1995.
14. Polonsky W, Anderson B, Lohrer P, et al: Insulin omission in women with IDDM. Diabetes Care 17:1178–1185, 1994.
15. Rodin GM, Daneman D: Eating disorders and IDDM: A problematic association. Diabetes Care 15:1402–1411, 1992.
16. Rodin G, Rydall A, Olmstead M, et al: A four-year follow-up study of eating disorders and medical complications in young women with insulin-dependent diabetes mellitus. Psychosom Med 56:179, 1994.

XI. Special Treatment Problems

74. ASSESSMENT AND MANAGEMENT OF THE SUICIDAL PATIENT
Randall D. Buzan, M.D.

1. Define suicide.
Suicide is the act of intentionally killing oneself, but patients often use the term differently. For instance, patients who repeatedly cut themselves superficially to assuage severe anxiety may describe themselves as "suicidal," but with further questioning they often can distinguish these acts from more ominous injuries inflicted with the intent to kill. It is thus important to clarify what patients mean when they say they are feeling "suicidal."

2. How common is suicide?
One percent of Americans will die by suicide, and over 30,000 people take their own lives each year in the United States, making suicide the eighth leading cause of death. The U.S. suicide rate has averaged 12.5 per 100,000 over the past century; it peaked at 17.4 during the Depression in 1932, dipped to a nadir of 9.8 in 1957, and has hovered at 12.4 over the past decade. Adolescent rates have tripled over the past 40 years from 4 per 100,000 to 13.2 per 100,000, making suicide the third leading cause of death in this group. Eight to ten people attempt suicide for every one who completes it. Although suicide in preadolescent children is rare, more than 12,000 children under the age of 13 years are hospitalized each year for self-destructive acts.

3. Name four demographic risk factors for suicide.
Age. Among Caucasians the suicide rate has correlated with age for the past 40 years; Caucasians aged 75–84 kill themselves twice as often as those aged 15–24. Among black Americans rates are highest in men aged 25–34, which is still lower than the rate of their white same-age counterparts.

Race. Overall, whites complete suicide twice as frequently as do blacks or Hispanics. Suicide rates in American Indians and Alaskan Natives are 1.7 times higher than in whites, occurring predominantly in the young.

Sex. Although the relationship between age and suicide varies among races, male rates consistently exceed female rates across races, with an overall male:female ratio of 3:1 to 4:1. On the other hand, women make 60–70% of suicide attempts, which exceed completed suicides by a ratio of 23:1.

Marital status. Divorced or widowed people clearly have the highest rates, followed by single people and finally by married people. Among women, the more children they have, the lower the suicide rate.

4. List the most commonly used suicide methods in order of frequency.
Men: Firearms, hanging, gasses–vapors, drug ingestion
Women: Drug ingestion, firearms, gasses–vapors, hanging

5. Which psychiatric patients are at risk? Why is this important?
Ninety to 95% of suicide victims suffer from a psychiatric illness at the time they die; therefore, defining subgroups at risk may help to focus prevention efforts. Whereas 45–70% of victims suffer from clinical depression at the time of death, making depression an important risk factor,

several studies demonstrate that the degree of *hopelessness* is even more predictive of future suicidal behavior than the severity of depression. Listed below are suicide rates by psychiatric diagnosis. Others at increased risk include those with a previous suicide attempt, depression accompanied by severe anxiety or panic attacks, anorexia nervosa, and a history of child abuse or incest.

Diagnosis	Suicide Rate (%)
Major depression	15
Bipolar disorder	10–15
Schizophrenia	10
Alcohol dependence	2
Borderline personality disorder	4–9.5
Antisocial personality	5

Up to 60% of psychiatric inpatients who kill themselves do so within 6 months of discharge, and the month immediately after discharge is a particularly high-risk period. Careful planning of discharge for suicidal inpatients is therefore essential.

6. **What medical illnesses are associated with an increased suicide risk?**

Acquired immunodeficiency syndrome (AIDS) (21- to 36-fold increase)	Multiple sclerosis
	Porphyria
Gastrointestinal cancers	Delirium tremens
Head injury	Cushing's disease
Epilepsy (5-fold increase)	Renal failure on hemodialysis
Temporal lobe epilepsy (25-fold increase)	(5-fold increase)
Peptic ulcer disease	Huntington's chorea
Spinal cord injuries	Klinefelter's syndrome

Most studies do not describe the mental status of the patients, and thus it is unclear whether the increased suicide risk is due to comorbid depression, organic brain disease, or some specific factor from the medical condition itself.

7. **Describe the biologic findings in suicide victims.**

The most compelling data thus far indicate a relative deficiency of serotonin (5-hydroxytyramine [5-HT]) in the central nervous system (CNS) of suicide victims. Postmortem studies reveal decreased presynaptic inhibitory 5-HT receptors and increased postsynaptic 5-HT receptors in the prefrontal cortex. 5-Hydroxyindoleacetic acid (5-HIAA), the major metabolite of serotonin, is reduced in the cerebrospinal fluid of depressed patients and is even further reduced in depressed patients who are suicidal or have attempted suicide. This finding is particularly robust in patients who have attempted suicide by violent means (such as with firearms).

Compared with those who have died by other causes, suicide victims have (1) increased beta and decreased alpha-1 adrenoreceptors and (2) reduced numbers of corticotropin-releasing–factor receptors in the frontal cortex. These findings suggest dysregulation of CNS adrenergic function and the hypothalamic-pituitary-adrenal axis, respectively, but they may represent the neurophysiology of depression rather than being specific to suicidal behavior.

Studies of the dexamethasone suppression test, thyrotropin-releasing hormone stimulation test, and platelet monoamine oxidase levels in suicidal patients have yielded mixed results.

Recent metaanalyses of cardiovascular disease prevention trials have shown that although decreasing serum cholesterol by diet or medication reduces mortality due to coronary heart disease, overall mortality was unchanged, partially because of an increase in suicides. The possible relationship between serum cholesterol and suicide awaits further study. Preliminary findings of low levels of magnesium in cerebrospinal fluid and low plasma testosterone in suicide victims have yet to be replicated.

8. **Is suicide hereditary?**

Maybe. Adoption studies demonstrate a suicide incidence of roughly 4% in the biologic relatives of adoptees who killed themselves, with an incidence of less than 1% in adoptive relatives and in biologic relatives of matched nonsuicidal adoptees. The difference is significant. Twin studies show a roughly six-fold greater concordance for suicide in monozygotic than in dizygotic twins. Such findings may represent inheritance of predisposing psychiatric illnesses rather than a specific genetic susceptibility for suicide, although heritability of suicide per se cannot be ruled out.

A related issue is the possibility that patients may copy the behavior of a loved one who has committed suicide; knowing a suicide victim is in fact a risk factor for suicidal behavior. This element of family history is thus important to elicit when one evaluates a suicidal patient.

9. Why do people kill themselves?

Suicide has many determinants, but it is always an attempt to solve a problem, albeit in a maladaptive way. Wondering with the patient why he or she is feeling suicidal helps to define the problem. Asking patients to describe what they think would happen if they killed themselves may elicit wishes for revenge, power, control, punishment, atonement, sacrifice, restitution, escape, sleep, rescue, rebirth, reunion with the dead, or a new life.

10. Do antidepressants, especially fluoxetine (Prozac), increase suicide risk?

Over 50% of depressed patients have suicidal feelings, and thus it is not surprising that some patients taking antidepressants report suicidal feelings or kill themselves. In 1990 Teicher et al. described 6 patients who appeared to have become more suicidal after starting Prozac. This report spurred a public controversy over the safety of Prozac and other antidepressants. Subsequent carefully conducted studies have found that the suicide rate of patients on Prozac is actually less than that of patients on other antidepressants, and sound evidence suggests that treatment of depression with antidepressants or electroconvulsive therapy decrease mortality from suicide.

Antidepressants, however, are the most commonly used drugs in fatal overdoses and therefore must be prescribed carefully. The therapeutic index of a drug is derived by dividing the dose that is lethal to 50% of subjects (LD50) by the dose that is effective for 50% of subjects (ED50). In laboratory animals the therapeutic indices of neuroleptics, tricyclic antidepressants, and lithium are 100, 10, and 3, respectively. In humans, neuroleptics alone rarely kill in overdose, but it may take only a 10-day supply of an antidepressant or a 3-day supply of lithium to kill 50% of patients. Thus, when a patient is in the midst of a suicidal crisis, it is sensible to prescribe no more than a week's worth of medication and often less. Perhaps because of their effects on cardiac conduction, tricyclic antidepressants are more lethal in overdose than Prozac and some of the newer antidepressants. Some clinicians therefore prefer to use the newer drugs in suicidal patients.

11. Does asking patients about suicidal feelings "put the idea into their heads"?

No. No evidence supports this commonly held misconception. Suicidal patients typically are relieved to find someone who wants to help.

12. How does one ask a patient about suicidal feelings?

Communicating a genuine interest in the patient's feelings is far more important than the exact wording that one uses to find out about suicide potential. The following list of questions proceeds from general to more specific queries:

- Have you ever wished you (weren't here) were dead?
- Have you ever thought about hurting or killing yourself?
- Have you ever acted on those feelings? (When, how, what precipitated each attempt? Was there an actual intent to die? Who rescued/found you? What treatment was obtained?).
- When is the last time you felt suicidal?
- Have you been feeling suicidal lately?
- How have you thought you might go about killing yourself?
- Do you currently have the means to carry out this plan (e.g., rope, pills, gun)?
- Do you have easy access to a gun? Is it at home? Is it loaded? Guns should always be discussed with suicidal patients, even if they are not part of the divulged plan, because of their high lethality and frequent use in suicide.

- How close have you come to actually carrying out this plan?
- Do you wish you were dead now?
- Have you thought about killing anyone else? (Homicidal and suicidal feelings often coexist, and homicidal thoughts can be explored much like suicidal thoughts.)

13. Describe the next steps in the evaluation of the suicidal patient.

Once the suicidal patient has been identified and the issues above have been explored, the evaluation proceeds as follows:

- Answer the question "Why now?" That is, try to understand what recent experience gave rise to the patient's suicidal feelings and what problem the patient is trying to "solve."
- Make a diagnosis. Psychological factors aside, suicide is an indication of an underlying disorder. Most patients are depressed, alcoholic, or character-disordered, and diagnosis of the underlying condition guides arrangement of appropriate treatment.
- Perform a mental status examination. The presence of delirium or psychosis may make the history unreliable and predispose the patient to impulsive and unpredictable behavior.
- Meet the family (or most important social support/best friend). Evaluating the patient's resources for support and contacting collateral sources (such as the patient's therapist or physician) are the key steps in deciding how reliable the patient may be and in corroborating the patient's account of his circumstances. Collateral contacts are often instrumental in discerning the actual problem the patient is trying to solve and in designing alternative sensible solutions.

14. What is the SAD PERSONS scale?

SAD PERSONS is an acronym for the important risk factors for suicide:

S Sex
A Age
D Depression

P Previous attempts
E Ethanol abuse
R Rational thinking loss (particularly psychosis)
S Social supports lacking
O Organized plan
N No spouse
S Sickness (with attention to medical disorders that have been shown to increase risk).

15. List five immediate treatment objectives in the management of acutely suicidal patients.

1. Protect the patient from self-abuse until the suicide crisis has passed. Suicidal feelings are always episodic, and thus the task is to keep the patient safe while helping to defuse the crisis.
2. Anticipate and treat any medical complications of a suicide attempt.
3. Define and solve, if possible, the acute problem that precipitated the crisis.
4. Diagnose and arrange treatment of the underlying problem that predisposes the patient to suicidal behavior.
5. Deal with the acute grief reactions of bereaved family members of the suicide victim.

16. List criteria that should be fulfilled before considering discharge of the suicidal patient from the emergency room or doctor's office.

1. The patient no longer feels suicidal.
2. The patient is medically stable.
3. The patient is able to promise believably to return to the emergency room or doctor's office before harming him- or herself if suicidal thoughts recur.
4. The patient is not intoxicated, delirious, demented, or psychotic.
5. All firearms at home have been removed.

6. The acute precipitants to the crisis have been identified, addressed, and in some way resolved.

7. Treatment for the underlying psychiatric illness has been arranged.

8. The physician believes that the patient will follow through on the treatment plan.

9. The patient's social supports have been contacted and agree with the discharge plan.

Patients who do not meet these criteria generally must either (1) remain in the emergency room or doctor's office until the issue in question is resolved or (2) be admitted to a psychiatric facility.

CONTROVERSY

17. Do patients have a right to kill themselves?

For:

1. People have a fundamental right to self-determination as long as exercising that right does not impinge on anyone else's rights.

2. Prevention of suicide represents misguided paternalism that inappropriately violates individual rights.

Against:

1. In all but terminally ill patients, suicide is symptomatic of treatable mental illness. Evidence for this position is commonplace in that almost all suicide attempters are subsequently grateful that they did not succeed. Even in one study of terminally ill patients, the few patients who wished for death to come early suffered from clinical depression.

2. Opinions that suicide is an act of free will sometimes derive more from antipathy toward these frequently provocative and covertly furious patients than from an objective, well-considered desire to further their best interests.

3. Religious and moral objections (e.g., suicide is against God's will).

BIBLIOGRAPHY

1. Beck AT, Steer RA, Beck JS, Newman CF: Hopelessness, depression, suicidal ideation, and clinical diagnosis of depression. Suicide Life Threat Behav 23:139–145, 1993.
2. Blumenthal SJ, Kupfer DJ (eds): Suicide Over the Life Cycle: Risk Factors, Assessment, and Treatment of Suicidal Patients. Washington, DC, American Psychiatric Press, 1990.
3. Brent DA, Perper JA, Moritz G, et al: Firearms and adolescent suicide. A community case-control study. Am J Dis Child 147:1066–1071, 1993.
4. Brown JH, Henteleff P, Barakat S, Rowe CJ: Is it normal for terminally ill patients to desire death? Am J Psychiatry 143:208–211, 1986.
5. Buzan RD, Weissberg MP: Suicide: Risk factors and prevention in medical practice. Annu Rev Med 43:37–46, 1992.
6. Buzan RD, Weissberg MP: Suicide: Risk factors and therapeutic considerations in the emergency department. J Emerg Med 10:335–343, 1992.
7. Carpenter BD: A review and new look at ethical suicide in advanced age. Gerontologist 33:359–365, 1993.
8. Diekstra RF: The epidemiology of suicide and parasuicide. Acta Psychiatr Scand Suppl 371:9–20, 1993.
9. Filteau MJ, Lapierre YD, Bakish D, Blanchard A: Reductions in suicidal ideation with SSRIs: A review of 459 depressed patients. J Psychiatry Neurosci 18:114–119, 1993.
10. Goldacre M, Seagroatt V, Hawton K: Suicide after discharge from psychiatric inpatient care. Lancet 342:283–286, 1993.
11. Lewis B, Tikkanen MJ: Low blood cholesterol and mortality: Causality, consequence and confounders. Am J Cardiol 73:80–85, 1994.
12. Pfeffer CR: Suicidal behavior among children and adolescents: Risk identification and intervention. In Frances AJ, Hales RE (eds): American Psychiatric Press Review of Psychiatry, vol. 7. Washington, DC, American Psychiatric Press, 1988, pp 386–401.
13. Roy A: Suicide and psychiatric patients. Psychiatr Clin North Am 8:227–241, 1985.
14. Teicher MH, Glod CA, Cole JO: Antidepressant drugs and the emergence of suicidal tendencies. Drug Saf 8:186–212, 1993.
15. Yehuda R, Southwick SM, Ostroff RB, et al: Neuroendocrine aspects of suicidal behavior. Neurol Clin 6:83–102, 1988.

75. ASSESSMENT AND MANAGEMENT OF THE VIOLENT PATIENT

Jane L. Erb, M.D.

1. How common is violent behavior?

Up to 60% of patients in health care settings have been reported to exhibit physically aggressive behavior. The rate depends on a number of variables, including the clinical site of the study, how one defines "violent" behavior, and the manner in which the incidence of such behavior is tracked. Although extrapolation from these studies to the general clinical population is difficult, violence is clearly common and probably increasing. Most acts of aggression fortunately do not result in serious injury, yet an understanding by the clinician of their causes and management is imperative.

2. What causes aggression?

It is generally believed that an act of violence implies a psychiatric disturbance. Although numerous studies, including studies of violent offenders, support this relationship, not all acts of aggression occur in conjunction with psychiatric or medical disease. Premeditated acts of violence, particularly those that are not recurrent, may occur in the absence of definable illness. Conversely, not all psychiatric illness has the same potential for violence. Violent behavior, therefore, is a nonspecific symptom that may or may not reflect underlying medical or psychiatric illness.

3. Which specific disorders are associated with violent behavior?

Schizophrenia	Intermittent explosive disorder
Manic phase, bipolar disorders	Organic disorders
Substance and alcohol abuse	Organic personality disorder
Personality disorders	Organic delusional disorder
Antisocial personality disorder	Organic mood disorder
Borderline personality disorder	Dementia
Childhood disorders	Delirium
Conduct disorder	
Oppositional disorder	
Mental retardation	

4. Which major mental disorder is associated must commonly with violent behavior?

Probably the major mental illness most commonly associated with violent behavior is schizophrenia. Whether in response to command hallucinations or to paranoid delusions, schizophrenia is aggravated by disorganization of thought and behavior and may manifest with aggressive behavior. Signs of impending violence may or may not be present; violent behavior may occur precipitously, without warning, in response to internal stimuli. This awareness is essential for clinicians evaluating schizophrenic patients.

5. What causes violent behavior in manic patients?

The combination of agitation, impulsivity, and often delusional ideation or hallucinations puts manic patients at risk for violent behavior. Their violence is often markedly sudden because of the lack of inhibitions. An inadvertent challenge to their control, especially in light of their grandiosity, often provokes such an outburst.

6. How does alcohol abuse lead to violence?

Alcohol abuse, with or without comorbid psychiatric disorders, correlates highly with violence, both through the disinhibition of intoxication and the agitation, delirium, or hallucinosis of withdrawal.

7. Which other drugs of abuse are associated with violence? Describe briefly their effects.

Both stimulants and hallucinogens have been frequently incriminated in acts of violence. Cocaine and amphetamines may lead to agitation, emotional lability, and psychosis, particularly once the initial euphoria dissipates or with chronic use. Amphetamines, in particular, are known to effect mental status up to 2 weeks after use. Phencyclidine (PCP) is probably the hallucinogen most often associated with severe violence because of its effect on thinking, judgment, and perception. The presence of horizontal or vertical nystagmus in association with agitation should alert the clinician to the possibility of PCP intoxication. Barbiturates and benzodiazepines may cause aggression in two instances: (1) during the withdrawal phase agitation may be associated with violent behavior and (2) elderly, mentally retarded, and certain other persons with central nervous system dysfunction may respond paradoxically to sedatives with agitation and violence. The mechanisms are presumed to be similar to those of alcohol withdrawal and pathologic intoxication, respectively. Opiates are associated indirectly with violence, probably through behaviors related to drug acquisition rather than psychogenic effect.

8. Describe the relationship between personality disorders and violence.

In **borderline personality disorders,** traits of intense anger, impulsivity, and turbulent relationships often occur in conjunction with substance abuse and other self-destructive behaviors. Such patients are especially at risk for both suicidal and assaultive behaviors. Given their tendency toward affective instability, **mood disorders** are inevitably an important part of the differential diagnosis. In **antisocial personality disorder,** the patient violates many societal norms; violence is but one manifestation.

9. Describe the relationship between childhood disorders and violence.

Conduct disorder, by definition, is the childhood antecedent to adult antisocial personality disorder, although not all children with conduct disorder later develop the adult counterpart. Children with **oppositional disorder** display frequent temper outbursts, anger, and defiant behavior; physical aggression is not a prominent problem but may occur. Finally, **mentally retarded children** and adults clearly are at risk for violent behavior. Their threshold for aggression appears to be lower because of (1) a tendency toward impulsivity and (2) difficulty in communicating their needs effectively.

10. Define intermittent explosive disorder.

Intermittent explosive disorder, formerly called episodic dyscontrol, is a disturbance of impulse in which acts of aggression occur out of proportion to the stimulus. Interepisode behavior is not marked by impulsivity. The diagnosis requires that all other potential causes and disorders associated with violence must be ruled-out. Although some authors suggest that the incidence of such dyscontrol may be higher among patients with seizure disorders, no evidence indicates that ictal or postictal states cause such behavior.

11. Which neurologic and medical diseases are associated with organic disorders that may lead to violence?

Violence may be seen in a host of organic disorders, such as organic personality disorder, organic delusional disorder, organic mood syndrome, dementia, and delirium. By definition, one must be able to identify a specific organic cause. Neurologic and medical diseases associated with violent behavior are listed below:

Neurologic diseases

Dementias (e.g., Alzheimer's, Pick's, normal pressure hydrocephalus)

Stroke syndromes
Anoxic encephalopathy
Wilson's disease
Infections of the central nervous system (syphilis, human immunodeficiency virus, herpes
    simplex virus, other encephalitides, and meningitis)
Ictal, postictal, and interictal states
Tumors, especially of temporal and frontal lobes
Multiple sclerosis
Huntington's disease
Head trauma
Parkinson's disease
Systemic disorders affecting CNS function
    Metabolic disease (e.g., hypoglycemia, electrolyte disturbance)
    Toxic agents (e.g., drug, alcohol, heavy metal, poisons)
    Infectious disease
    Vitamin deficiencies (B12, folate, thiamine)
    Endocrine disturbances (thyroid, Cushing's disease)
    Hepatic and uremic encephalopathy
    Acute intermittent porphyria
    Lupus erythematosus

12. What are the risk factors for violence?

Obviously, any disorder associated with an increased incidence of violence is a risk factor. In addition, studies of violent behavior have revealed other specific risk factors, many of which occur in conjunction with the disorders listed in question 11.

A history of physical abuse as a child or witnessing such abuse is an increasingly publicized correlate of adult violence.

Present environment also should be considered; for example, subcultures in which physical aggression is an accepted expression of anger or frustration may place a person at higher risk for aggressive behavior. Such cultures are often associated with an increased rate of unemployment, physical crowding, and poverty, all of which are independent risk factors. Ethnicity has not been found to be among the risk factors of violence.

Men are generally more often involved in aggression than women, although the sex ratio equalizes in inpatient settings, perhaps because of the diversion of violent men into the prison system.

Young age groups have been consistently found to be more apt to display aggression. However, when one examines the full spectrum of the population, the incidence of violence increases in the elderly, presumably because of the aggression associated with dementia and delirium.

As is the case with suicide, a history of violence or impulsivity or an articulated plan with access to a weapon increases the risk of violence immensely. These are critical elements in the history, as noted below.

13. What is the neurobiologic substrate of aggression?

It is commonly believed that patients with temporal lobe epilepsy are at increased risk of violent behavior. This is an area of heated debate, with proponents claiming that surface electroencephalography is inadequate in identifying ictal rhythms. Clearly, when patients with complex partial seizure disorders display violent behavior during an ictus, the violence is not directed at an individual or focused within the environment. Despite the possibility of interictal aggression, studies designed to determine whether patients with temporal lobe epilepsy carry a higher risk compared with patients without epilepsy are inconclusive. Postictal aggression is related to the presence of encephalopathy and may be seen after any type of seizure associated with altered awareness.

Although there is no strict correlation between aggression and site of lesion, experiments of nature and animal studies support an association of such behavior with lesions of the medial temporal lobe, hypothalamus, and septum. The disinhibition that may occur with frontal lobe pathology also may result in violent and other impulsive behaviors.

Numerous researchers have attempted to identify the neurochemical substrate of aggression. Although testosterone, norepinephrine, and dopamine have a putative role, probably the largest body of consistent data implicates serotonin. Decreased levels of serotonin metabolites in the cerebrospinal fluid appear to relate to violent behavior, particularly when committed impulsively.

14. What are the subtle cues to potential violence?
Impending violence is not always preceded by warning signs. However, clinicians should be familiar with certain common indicators. Any of the diagnostic groups in question 3 or risk factors in question 12 should be considered, particularly in conjunction with the following:
- In the emergency room, staff refusal of medications or services sought by the patient is a common precipitant of aggression.
- The first few days in the hospital, a time during which the patient is unclear about acceptable limits on behavior or treatment plans, involve a higher risk.
- A sudden change in behavior, evidence of intoxication, or use of sunglasses indoors should serve as potential warning signs of impending violence or at least draw attention to potential paranoia or possible use of drugs.
- Certainly agitation, pacing, loud or pressured speech, and anger should be monitored closely.
- Above all, verbal threats of violence must always be taken seriously and follow-up with further questioning.

15. What is the work-up of violent behavior?
Violence is a symptom and therefore should be evaluated much like any other presenting symptom:
- Thorough history of violent behavior
  Present and past behavior
  Other impulsive behaviors
- Detailed questioning of violent threats
  Onset, duration, frequency
  Specific methods
  Intent
- Access to weapons
- Mental status and cognitive examinations
  Agitation
  Signs of psychosis, mania, or intoxication
  Attentional and memory functioning
- Physical and neurologic examination
- Laboratory studies
  Screening chemistries and hematologic tests
  Thyroid function studies
  Assessment of B_{12}, folate, calcium, magnesium, PO4, rapid plasmin reagin
  Serum and urine toxicology
  Other studies as clinically indicated (e.g., imaging study of brain, specialized studies of cerebrospinal fluid, serum, or urine)
- Imaging studies of brain
- Electroencephalogram
- Documentation
  Direct quotations from patient
  Detailed rationale for treatment or referral
  Conversations with third parties

16. How may one facilitate a thorough history?

A thorough history of the behavior by the patient as well as by other informants is essential. It is often helpful to begin by eliciting the history of the patient's chief complaint and to shift into the history of the violent behavior later in the interview, when a rapport is established.

17. How should one respond verbally to violent behavior?

One should try to maintain at all times a calm, controlled demeanor. Anger is a common response when one is threatened, but such expression by the clinician inevitably leads to further escalation by the patient. Escalation is also the likely result if the clinician challenges the patient through any display of condescension or counterattack. The clinician must remain as conscious as possible of inappropriate responses and maintain restraint. One gains the upper hand in such situations through the assumption of the submissive position. The clinician should admit that he or she feels frightened by the patient's behavior; this admission usually leads to a deescalation of rage and provides a useful reality check for the patient. Also useful is identifying the emotion that the patient appears to be experiencing in the form of an inquiry (e.g., "you seem quite upset?"). The patient should be encouraged to talk about what is upsetting him or her. If threats of violence continue, the clinician should tell the patient that he or she is going to call for help—and do so immediately. If violence appears imminent, the clinician should leave the room, mobilize staff, and arrange for the safety of staff and other patients.

18. Describe the appropriate behavioral response to a violent patient.

Verbal management of potentially violent patients usually should be attempted first, but such intervention is not always sufficient, especially with patients who have organic or psychotic disorders. Hence, the clinician should have a well-organized behavioral strategy established with associated staff that can be implemented efficiently when necessary. In high-risk settings, such as emergency rooms or psychiatric outpatient clinics, offices should be set up with an emergency buzzer, code word, or signal that can discreetly alert other staff of a potentially volatile patient. Staff should be clear on how to respond, including whom to call (e.g., security, police) and how to provide for the safety of other staff or patients in the area. Occasional drills to practice such responses may be life-saving. Whenever violent behavior is a concern, the patient should be seen with staff (clinical or security) located either nearby or in the same room. Clinicians who work in high-risk settings should set up their interviewing space so that both the clinician and the patient have easy, unobstructed access to the door. One should never sit behind a desk. Heavy or sharp objects should be removed. Similarly, the clinician should be careful and perhaps avoid wearing jewelry and neckties when working with such patients. In the event the patient escapes, the clinician should not run after him or her. If a weapon is revealed, the clinician should not attempt to retrieve it; instead, the clinician should attempt to engage the patient in conversation, signal for help, and encourage the patient to place the weapon in a neutral place.

19. What is the appropriate role of seclusion and restraint?

A specific form of behavioral management that provides for the safety of the patient and staff when all else fails is the use of physical restraint and seclusion. Implementing such restraints requires access to staff who undergo regular inservice training in the application and monitoring of restraints or seclusion. A restraint team typically has a designated leader who directs the application of restrains as well as talks to the patient as the restraints are applied. The staff must understand the experience of the patient undergoing such restraint; in some states, staff are required by law to be personally placed in restraints as part of their training. Whether physical or chemical restraint is preferred continues to be controversial; in general, the choice depends on the individual case and availability of resources in the treatment setting. When the cause of the aggression is unclear or when frank delirium is present, one should consider minimizing exposure to psychotropic medications, because they may confuse or exacerbate the clinical picture.

20. Describe the proper use of drugs and chemical restraint in treating violent behavior.
First and foremost, the underlying disorder should be treated pharmacologically whenever possible. The use of chemical restraints in controlling acutely violent behavior is another form of therapeutic intervention. Pharmacologic restraint may be used after verbal and behavioral interventions have failed, either alone or in combination with physical restraint. Medications are an ideal intervention when it has been determined that the underlying cause of the aggression is a psychiatric disturbance that is pharmacologically responsive. All patients should be given an opportunity to take the medication voluntarily, in either the oral or intramuscular form.

21. Which psychotropic agents should be considered for chemical restraint?
Benzodiazepines. Through their sedative action, benzodiazepines usually have a calming effect and may provide a speedy and effective response, particularly when administered intramuscularly. Close observation of the patient is essential, with frequent monitoring of vital signs, because of the potential for respiratory depression. Paradoxical responses, including increased anger and agitation, also may occur, particularly in mentally retarded, elderly, and personality-disordered patients. Organic brain syndromes are also thought to increase the risk of paradoxical response.

Neuroleptics. Although the antipsychotic effects of neuroleptics may be especially beneficial for treating psychotic patients who are assaultive, such effects may not take place for up to 1 week or more. It is more likely that the tranquilizing properties of the neuroleptics are responsible for the sedating effects. Again, close observation of the patient is necessary, including monitoring for extrapyramidal side effects, dystonic reactions, and akathisia. A pattern of increasing agitation should immediately trigger the question of whether the clinician is ensnared in a vicious cycle of chasing akathisia, which may manifest as mounting agitation, with increasing doses of neuroleptics. If akathisia is suspected, one should first try lowering the dose of the neuroleptic. If this leads to a further increase in agitation, benzodiazepines or beta blockers should be tried, because they often are more effective against akathisia than are anticholinergics.

Barbiturates. The respiratory depression and risk of laryngospasm precludes the use of barbiturates in most instances, given the relative advantages of benzodiazepines and neuroleptics.

22. What are the recommended doses of benzodiazepines and neuroleptics for emergency treatment of assaultive behavior?
Benzodiazepines
    Lorazepam: 0.5–2 mg orally or intramuscularly every 1–4 hr
        Use lower doses for elderly or medically ill patients.
        Watch for respiratory depression or laryngospasm (rare).
        Watch for paradoxical agitation.
Neuroleptics
    Haloperidol: 0.5–5 mg orally or intramuscularly every 1–4 hr
    Droperidol: 5 mg intramuscularly or slow intravenous push every 15 min until sedated, not to exceed 50 mg/24 hr
    Chlorpromazine: 10–25 mg every 1–4 hr
        Watch for orthostatic hypotension, especially with chlorpromazine.
        Monitor regularly for extrapyramidal signs; treat with anticholinergics (e.g., benztropine, 1–2 mg orally or intramuscularly every 4 hr).
        Be especially attentive to signs of akathisia; treat with dose reduction or propranolol, 10–20 mg orally every 4 hr, lorazepam, 0.5–2 mg every 4 hr.

23. What should be done if a staff member or another patient is hurt?
If there is any question of physical contact, an immediate physical examination should be performed by the physician on call if the victim is a patient. If the victim is a staff member or visitor, the nearest emergency department or employee health office is usually appropriate. Documentation of any findings or the absence of injury is important both in the examining physician's medical report and in an incident report form, which is available in most institutions.

Once physical injuries are clarified and treated, the victim must be supported emotionally not only at the time of the incident but also throughout the following weeks. Emotional sequelae may take several weeks to surface and also may be quite severe. Often the symptoms take the form of a posttraumatic stress reaction with easy startle, autonomic hyperactivity, sleep disturbance, and even avoidance behaviors. In addition, a tremendous amount of self-blame, anger, and guilt often emerge as the sense of vulnerability intensifies. Complicating matters is the response, or lack thereof, of the institution. The dynamics of institutional systems may involve, in part, a contagious spread of fear and unconscious threat; peers as well as administrators may inadvertently pathologize the victim. Such a reaction further entrenches the self-blame. Because of this potential, some hospitals establish a committee that routinely interviews and offer limited support services to staff who are assaulted. Such committees are equipped to refer for more intensive counseling, if necessary.

24. Is long-term treatment available for violent patients?

Yes. If a definable underlying medical or psychiatric condition causes the aggression, it should be identified and treated. When addressing the underlying condition fails to control fully the violent behavior, the following strategies may be considered:

Pharmacologic strategies. Mood stabilizers, including lithium, carbamazepine, and valproate, have been found to be effective in some violent patients, probably through their tendency to dampen impulsivity. Mood or seizure control doses should be used, with appropriate laboratory monitoring. Propranolol also has been effective for some cases of aggressive behavior, in divided doses of up to 800 mg/day. The effect on blood pressure is not significant when the dose is titrated slowly. The standard starting dose is 20 mg, up to 3 times/day. Dose adjustment both upward and downward should be gradual because of the effect on blood pressure, and the trial ideally should last 4–6 weeks because of the latency of response. Clozapine, an atypical antipsychotic, has been reported to ease aggressive impulses in chronically psychotic and aggressive inpatients. Possibly through its effects on serotonin receptors, buspirone also may possess antiaggressive effects.

Behavioral strategies. Particularly in hospital inpatient settings or in other institutional settings with the potential for structure, modification of aggression through behavioral strategies may be useful. Treatment may include the use of rewards in exchange for self-control of aggression. It is essential to avoid reinforcing negative behaviors through attention to the patient. Of course, chemical or physical restraints are imperative if physical danger is imminent or assault has occurred. However, staff members should be conscious of the attention that they pay to the patient in the process of restraining him or her, because such attention may serve as a reinforcer. An important addition to the behavioral strategy is social skills training, particularly for regressed, psychotic, or retarded individuals who may be aggressive out of frustration at not getting their needs met. Educating such individuals about more socially appropriate ways of meeting their needs may be extremely useful.

Psychotherapy. Individual, family, and/or group psychotherapy may be useful for individuals who are genuinely invested in trying to change their violent behavior and who can maintain sufficient control of their impulses to allow the therapist and others involved in the therapy to feel safe. It is especially critical that the therapist be able to monitor accurately both his or her emotional responses to the patient and shifts in the affective expression of the patient. Dealing with mounting fear, as described above, is crucial. The therapist also must be aware of the potential for anger toward the patient as an expression of vulnerability. Unattended anger may indirectly influence the therapy in destructive ways.

BIBLIOGRAPHY

1. Beck JC: The potentially violent patient: Legal duties, clinical practice, and risk management. Psychiatr Ann 17:695–699, 1987.
2. Blair DT: Assaultive behavior. Does provocation begin in the front office? J Psychosoc Nurs 29(5):21–26, 1991.

3. Davis S: Violence by psychiatric inpatients: A review. Hosp Community Psychiatry 42:585–590, 1991.

4. Eichelman B: Aggressive behavior: From laboratory to clinic. Quo Vadit? Arch Gen Psychiatry 49:488–492, 1992.

5. Elliot FA: Violence. The neurologic contribution: An overview. Arch Neurol 49:595–603, 1992.

6. Franzen MD, Lovell MR: Behavioral treatments of aggressive sequelae of brain injury. Psychiatr Ann 17:389–396, 1989.

7. Lanza ML: The reactions of nursing staff to physical assault by a patient. Hosp Community Psychiatry 34:44–47, 1983.

8. McNiel DE, Myers RS, Zeiner HK, et al: The role of violence in decisions about hospitalization from the psychiatric emergency room. Am J Psychiatry 149:207–212, 1992.

9. Miller RJ, Zadolinnyi K, Hafner RJ: Profiles and predictors of assaultiveness for different psychiatric ward populations. Am J Psychiatry 150:1368–1373, 1993.

10. Randolph LB: When a patient becomes violent. Psychiatr Resident, May/June 1992, pp 18–22.

11. Ratey JJ, Leveroni C, Kilmer D, et al: The effects of clozapine on severely aggressive psychiatric inpatients in a state hospital. J Clin Psychiatry 54:219–223, 1993.

12. Stevenson S: Heading off violence with verbal de-escalation. J Psychosoc Nurs 29(9):6–10, 1991.

13. Tardiff K: Concise Guide to Assessment and Management of Violent Patients. Washington, DC, American Psychiatric Press, 1989.

14. Tardiff K: The current state of psychiatry in the treatment of violent patients. Arch Gen Psychiatry 49:493–499, 1992.

15. Yudofsky SC, Silver JM, Schneider SE: Pharmacologic treatment of aggression. Psychiatr Ann 17:397–404, 1987.

76. NEUROLEPTIC MALIGNANT SYNDROME

James L. Jacobson, M.D.

1. Describe neuroleptic malignant syndrome.

Neuroleptic malignant syndrome (NMS) is an acute, potentially fatal, idiosyncratic reaction to neuroleptic medications (which primarily are antipsychotic medications). The principal manifestations are due to disorders of thermoregulation and skeletal muscle metabolism mediated via central mechanisms. The usual presentation consists of four primary features: (1) hyperthermia, (2) extreme generalized rigidity, (3) autonomic instability, and (4) altered mental status. The overall appearance is of a profoundly ill individual with an alert, frightened stare.

2. What are the specific criteria for diagnosis of NMS?

The diagnosis of NMS requires the presence of specific historical information, physical signs, symptoms, and exclusionary criteria. There must be a **recent history of exposure** to neuroleptic medication. Usually this exposure is acute and occurs within 7–10 days of onset of the syndrome. However, NMS can occur in chronic usage. **Temperature elevation** can be mild or severe. **Autonomic instability** is indicated by labile hypertension (less often hypotension) and tachycardia. **Mental status** is always **altered**, typically in the form of delirium, which may progress to stupor, obtundation, and coma. Extreme **muscular rigidity** has been characterized as "lead-pipe rigidity" and is present in all skeletal muscle. **Diaphoresis** is always present. **Sialorrhea** is often present, as is **dysphagia**. Alternative etiologies for these symptoms must be excluded by history, examination, and laboratory studies.

3. Are there specific laboratory findings for NMS?

No laboratory findings are pathognomonic for NMS, but certain studies are important both to support the diagnosis of NMS and to exclude other systemic illnesses. Common laboratory findings are creatinine phosphokinase (muscle fraction) often massively elevated, and leukocytosis. Electrolyte disturbances that may occur secondarily, as well as hypocalcemia, hypomagnesemia, and hypophosphatemia, may require therapy. Urinalysis often reveals proteinuria and myoglobinuria from rhabdomyolysis. Cerebrospinal fluid (CSF) studies should be normal. An EEG may show diffuse slowing without focal abnormalities. To evaluate a patient with suspected NMS, the following studies should be done to exclude a systemic illness: CBC with a differential WBC; serum electrolytes; creatinine and BUN; muscle and hepatic enzymes; thyroid function tests; urinalysis; EKG; appropriate cultures for infection; and brain imaging, EEG, CSF studies (when indicated).

4. What is the differential diagnosis of NMS?

The differential diagnosis includes several processes that can cause increased temperature due to abnormal thermoregulation. These are divided into primary CNS disorders and systemic disorders.

Differential Diagnosis of NMS

PRIMARY CNS DISORDERS	SYSTEMIC DISORDERS
Infections (viral encephalitis, post-infectious encephalitis, HIV)	Infections
	Metabolic conditions
Tumors	Endocrinopathies (thyrotoxicosis, pheochromocytoma)
Cerebrovascular disease	Autoimmune disease (SLE)

Table continued on following page.

Differential Diagnosis of NMS (Cont.)

PRIMARY CNS DISORDERS	SYSTEMIC DISORDERS
Head trauma	Heat stroke
Seizures	Toxins (CO, phenols, strychnine, tetanus)
Major psychoses (lethal catatonia)	Drugs (salicylates, dopamine inhibitors and antagonists, stimulants, psychedelics, MAOIs, anesthetics, anticholinergics, alcohol or sedative withdrawal)

From Caroff SN, et al: Neuroleptic malignant syndrome: Diagnostic issues. Psychiatr Ann 21:130–147, 1991, with permission.

5. What causes NMS?

The specific antidopaminergic activity of antipsychotic medications appears to be the predominant cause of NMS. Central dopaminergic systems are involved in thermoregulation as well as regulation of muscle tone and movement. The relatively infrequent occurrence of NMS, however, suggests the concurrence of other factors. Speculations have included imbalances with other neurotransmitter systems, abnormalities in second messenger systems, and the presentation of particular risk factors. Currently, all of the antipsychotic medications have been reported to cause NMS, including a recent report implicating the atypical antipsychotic medication clozapine and the recently released neuroleptic risperidone. NMS also has been reported with some antiemetic medications such as prochlorperazine maleate and metoclopramide, which are also neuroleptics.

6. Which risk factors predispose to the development of NMS?

Suggested risk factors include dehydration, a primary diagnosis of affective disorder (especially bipolar disorder and psychotic depression), concurrent presence of an organic brain syndrome, use of other neuroactive medications, higher relative doses and parenteral administration of neuroleptics, prior history of NMS, electrolyte disturbances, any medical or neurologic illness, and a recent history of substance abuse or dependence.

7. How common is NMS?

Rates as low as 0.02% and as high as 2.5% have been reported, but overall the rate appears to be about 1%.

8. What is the mortality associated with NMS?

Mortality from NMS has been declining since its original description in 1968. The earliest reports suggested mortality rates as high as 75%. In the early 1980s mortality rates declined to 20–30%. Current studies suggest that the mortality rate declined further, probably to less than 15%. Early recognition and familiarity with the syndrome are the most likely reasons for this hopeful trend.

9. Discuss the treatments for NMS.

Early recognition is crucial. Increased temperature, elevated blood pressure, tachycardia, muscle stiffness not responsive to antiparkinsonian agents, clustering of risk factors, dysphagia, and severe diaphoresis early in the course of treatment with neuroleptic medication should alert the physician to the possible emergence of NMS. Neuroleptic and other potentially neurotoxic medications must be stopped. Supportive measures to lower temperature and ensure good fluid intake are essential. Electrolyte disturbances must be corrected. The patient should be closely monitored for signs of impending respiratory failure secondary to severe muscle rigidity and inability to handle oral secretions. Renal function should be monitored closely. Although there is no evidence that osmotic diuresis hastens recovery from NMS, it may help to maintain renal function.

Pharmacologic intervention has tended to be reserved for severe cases. Dopamine agonists (bromocriptine and amantadine) and/or direct muscle relaxants (dantrolene) have been used;

decreased mortality rates have been reported with both types. Dosages vary widely, but doses of bromocriptine have been documented between 2.5 and 35 mg/day. Generally bromocriptine has been started at 2.5 to 5 mg three times daily given orally (or via nasogastric tube in patients with dysphagia or severely compromised mental status). Dopamine agonists, particularly in higher doses, can cause psychosis and/or vomiting, which clearly can complicate the picture and compromise the patient. The only data available on direct-acting muscle relaxants are for dantrolene. Doses of up to 10 mg/kg have been used. The goal is to decrease muscular rigidity in order to decrease the hypermetabolic state in skeletal muscle, which is partially responsible for the hyperthermia in NMS. Dantrolene can cause hepatoxicity, which can lead to overt hepatitis and death. Combinations of dantrolene and dopamine agonists have been used, although there is no evidence that they further decrease mortality when used in combination. Anticholinergic medications commonly used to treat pseudoparkinsonism have little benefit. Although there is no clear evidence to support the use of benzodiazepines in the treatment of NMS, they can be useful in managing an agitated hyperactive patient once NMS has begun to resolve. No currently available drug therapy has been shown to shorten the course of NMS. One study suggested that therapy may prolong the total period of disability from NMS. However, because only the most severe cases have been treated with medication, the apparently longer disease course may be a manifestation of the initial severity of the illness.

10. Will NMS recur with subsequent use of neuroleptic medication?

The risk of recurrence decreases with time. Of patients rechallenged with neuroleptics prior to 2 weeks after resolution of NMS, there is a high recurrence rate. Those cautiously rechallenged 2 weeks or longer after resolution of NMS often tolerated neuroleptics without difficulty. A low-potency neuroleptic agent is chosen for the rechallenge. Dosing should be conservative and increased gradually. Recent interest in the concurrent use of the calcium channel blocker nifedipine has also shown promise in prevention of recurrence, although the data are still incomplete. Some individuals are prone to NMS and, of course, close attention to early symptoms is crucial.

Guidelines for Managing Patients with NMS

---

1. History of a previous episode of NMS confirmed?
   Yes: Go to (2)
   No: Speak with patient, family, and treating physician(s). Retrieve pertinent medical records to confirm the diagnosis of NMS.

2. Based on careful review of the psychiatric history and previous response to treatment, is neuroleptic therapy essential?
   Yes: Go to (3)
   No: Treat accordingly, without neuroleptics

3. Two or more episodes of NMS with more than one neuroleptic?
   Yes: Go to (4)
   No: Wait 2 weeks after recovery from NMS. Rechallenge with a low-potency neuroleptic. If a low-potency neuroleptic originally caused NMS, rechallenge with a low-potency neuroleptic from a different chemical class.

4. Have prophylactic agents—bromocriptine, dantrolene, or nifedipine—been used in conjunction with neuroleptics?
   Yes: Go to (5)
   No: Consider such a trial, or go to (5)

5. Alternatives to conventional neuroleptic therapy:
   (a) clozapine, (b) benzodiazepines, (c) electroconvulsive therapy, (d) anticonvulsants, and (e) lithium.

From Lazarus et al: Beyond NMS: Management after the acute episode. Psychiatr Ann 21:165–174, with permission.

11. Is there any way to prevent NMS?
No. Early recognition and, when clinically warranted, lower dosing, avoidance of parenteral neuroleptic medication, avoidance of rapid increases in dosages, and minimization of the other risk factors (e.g., good hydration) may decrease the incidence of NMS.

12. Are there alternatives to neuroleptic treatment for the acutely psychotic patient?
There are a number of treatment options. Benzodiazepines may help in the management of the hyperactive psychotic patient and lower the absolute dose of neuroleptic needed. When the primary diagnosis is affective disorder (as in a significant percentage of patients developing NMS), aggressive treatment of the manic or depressive illness with antidepressants, lithium carbonate, valproate, or carbamazepine is indicated. It is usually necessary to administer neuroleptic medications concomitantly when psychotic symptoms are present. Electroconvulsive therapy is a viable alternative for manic psychosis and depressive psychosis, and may alleviate catatonia.

In chronic psychotic disorders (e.g., schizophrenia) there may be no alternative to the use of neuroleptic medications. Hence, cautious rechallenging with different classes of neuroleptics is virtually always necessary.

ACKNOWLEDGMENT

This chapter is adapted with permission from Critical Care Secrets, Philadelphia, Hanley & Belfus, 1991.

BIBLIOGRAPHY

1. Addonizio G, Susman VL: Neuroleptic Malignant Syndrome: A Clinical Approach. St. Louis, Mosby, 1991.
2. Caroff SN (ed): Neuroleptic malignant syndrome. Psychiatr Ann 21:128–180, 1991.
3. Castillo E, Rubin R, Holsboer-Truacster E: Clinical differentiation between lethal catatonia and neuroleptic malignant syndrome. Am J Psychiatry 145:324–328, 1989.
4. Coons PJ, Hillman FJ, et al: Treatment of neuroleptic malignant syndrome with dantrolene sodium: A case report. Am J Psychiatry 139:944–945, 1982.
5. Levenson JL: Neuroleptic malignant syndrome. Am J Psychiatry 142:1137–1145, 1985.
6. Pope HG Jr, Aizley HG, Keck PE, McElroy SL: Neuroleptic malignant syndrome: Long-term follow-up of 20 cases. J Clin Psychiatry 52:208–212, 1991.
7. Pope HG Jr, Keck PE Jr, McElroy SL: Frequency and presentation of neuroleptic malignant syndrome in a large psychiatric hospital. Am J Psychiatry 143:1227–1232, 1986.
8. Shalev A, Heresh H, Munitz H: Mortality from neuroleptic malignant syndrome. Clin Psychiatry 50:18–22, 1989.
9. Susman VL, Addonizio G: Recurrence of neuroleptic malignant syndrome. J Nerv Ment Dis 176:234–241, 1988.
10. Rosebush P, Stewart T: A prospective analysis of 24 episodes of neuroleptic malignant syndrome. Am J Psychiatry 146:717–725, 1989.
11. Rosebush PI, Stewart TD, Gelenberg AJ: Twenty neuroleptic rechallenges after neuroleptic malignant syndrome in 15 patients. J Clin Psychiatry 50:295–298, 1989.
12. Zubenko G, Pope HG: Management of a case of neuroleptic malignant syndrome with bromocriptine. Am J Psychiatry 140:1619–1620, 1983.

77. TREATMENT-RESISTANT DEPRESSION

Marshall R. Thomas, M.D.

1. How is treatment-resistant depression defined?

Treatment resistance is a relative term. A frequently used definition is failure to respond to an adequate trial of a standard antidepressant. Even this seemingly straightforward definition presents several problems, however. What constitutes an "adequate" drug trial in terms of dose and duration is still debated, and the drugs most commonly used today (second-generation agents such as the selective serotonin reuptake inhibitors [SSRIs]) are not considered "standard." Even definitions of what constitutes treatment response differ. One commonly used definition, a 50% or greater reduction in Hamilton Depression Rating Scale, defines as responders some patients with significant residual depression.

In recent years the notion of the time required for an adequate trial has been extended from 3–4 weeks to 6–10 weeks in light of studies showing a high rate of response conversion in the second month of treatment. What constitutes an adequate dosage of an antidepressant has been complicated by the introduction of a whole new array of second-generation agents for which antidepressant blood levels are either unavailable or uninterpretable. Previous experience with tricyclic antidepressants (TCAs) demonstrated a 10–40-fold interindividual variability of blood levels for a given dose of drug. Accordingly, many clinicians became convinced of the importance of serum drug level monitoring for drugs such as nortriptyline, desipramine, and imipramine, especially when faced with treatment-resistant conditions.

One definition of treatment-resistant depression is any depression for which the clinician has not yet found a treatment that works.

2. How are patients with treatment-resistant depression different from other depressives?

In general, patients with affective disorders have greater rates of recurrence, relapse, and chronicity than previously appreciated. Of patients with affective disorders,15–20% do not recover fully and have a chronic course. A past history of chronicity or relapse is the strongest predictor of future chronicity and relapse. Chronicity itself may represent the inadequacy of previous treatment rather than treatment resistance. Patients with secondary depressions and comorbid conditions have high rates of both chronicity and treatment resistance.

An older age at onset, failure to normalize a nonsuppressed dexamethasone suppression test (DST) or a blunted thyrotropin-releasing hormone (TRH) stimulation test are biologic markers that predict chronicity and relapse. Treatment-resistant patients are also more likely to show decreased cortical mass and ventricular enlargement on neuroimaging studies.

3. What psychiatric conditions are commonly comorbid with treatment resistance?

Substance abuse, anxiety, and eating and personality disorders are associated with treatment resistance. Substance-abusing depressives are less likely to respond to treatment, more likely to relapse, and more likely to attempt suicide. Patients with panic disorder and comorbid depression have more severe depressions and a poorer response to standard treatments. Depression is common among bulimics and sometimes complicates anorexia. A comorbid personality disorder is seen in 40–60% of depressives. Depressives with comorbid personality disorders have a younger age of onset, more lifetime episodes, more suicidal ideation, and a decreased response to treatment.

4. How do medical disorders affect treatment resistance?

Medical disorders may affect the course of depression in a variety of ways. Medical causes of depression should be sought out and treated when possible. Some conditions, such as chronic pain syndromes, interact reciprocally; worsening or improvement in one leads to parallel worsening or improvement of the other. In general patients with comorbid medical conditions are less likely to receive adequate treatment and to respond to the treatment that they receive.

5. What is the most common cause of supposed "treatment-refractory" depression?
Inadequate treatment is probably the most common cause of chronicity and relapse. An estimated two-thirds of the patients treated in the community receive treatment that is inadequate in terms of dosage (e.g., < 200 mg of imipramine) or duration (e.g., < 4–6 weeks).

6. What is the importance of depressive subtypes?
Depressive subtypes such as psychotic-nonpsychotic, typical-atypical, bipolar-unipolar, and geriatric depressions have differential responses to treatment and require subtype specific treatment strategies.

Depressive Subtypes
Psychotic-nonpsychotic
Bipolar-unipolar
Atypical-typical
Geriatric-late onset

Unrecognized psychotic depression is a common cause of treatment resistance. Patients with psychotic depression respond poorly to antidepressants and antipsychotic drugs when used alone but respond well to electroconvulsive therapy (ECT) or a combination of drugs in adequate dosages. Depressive delusions are more common than hallucinations, although both may occur. Often psychotic symptoms are subtle and revealed only after careful and specific questioning of the patient.

Atypical depression is characterized by mood reactivity (e.g., mood varies with nature of interpersonal interactions), leaden fatigue, rejection sensitivity, and the reversed vegetative signs of increased sleep and increased appetite. These depressive symptoms are common in patients with bipolar depression, hysteroid dysphoria, and borderline states. Such patients respond poorly to tricyclic antidepressants and have a qualitatively superior response to monoamine oxidase inhibitors (MAOIs). Atypical depressives also may respond to the newer agents such as the serotonin reuptake inhibitors (fluoxetine, sertraline, and paroxetine), bupropion, and venlafaxine, but this issue has yet to be settled.

The treatment of bipolar depression is discussed elsewhere (see chapters 12 and 49). Failure to recognize a depression as bipolar may lead to inappropriate treatment strategies that contribute to failed treatment or worsening of the long-term course of the disease.

Geriatric depressives are more likely to experience masked depression and to have symptoms of anxiety, memory problems, and bodily complaints. Late-onset depression, defined as having an onset after age 65, is more likely to be associated with a dementing illness, delusions, and complicating medical conditions. Many elderly depressives have difficulty in tolerating medication trials and respond preferentially to ECT.

7. How does one assess a treatment-resistant patient?
The patient presenting with purported treatment-resistant depression warrants a careful review of psychiatric and medical condition, including a detailed history of past treatment. First, the clinician clarifies whether the patient has a subtype of depression that requires special treatment interventions. Next the dosage and duration of past treatment trials are reviewed in detail to determine whether past treatment trials were optimal. If tricyclics have been used, one should ascertain whether blood levels were obtained and, if so, whether therapeutic levels were reached.

Another review of the patient's medical condition may reveal an overlooked medical problem, such as subclinical hypothyroidism, that needs attention. The clinician also attempts to detect covert comorbid conditions such as substance abuse, anxiety, eating, and obsessive-compulsive disorders. Lastly, personality factors, coping style, social supports, psychosocial stressors (especially the presence of a chronically troublesome marriage), and type of and response to previous psychotherapy are assessed.

Common Causes of Treatment Resistance

Inadequate dosages	Comorbid conditions
Inadequate duration	Medication noncompliance
Inaccurate subtype	Medical causation

8. What role do psychosocial issues play in treatment resistance?
Premorbid personality traits such as chronically low self-esteem and high levels of neuroticism are associated with longer-term treatment resistance, although such symptoms may represent subsyndromal or prodromal expressions of the depressive illness. Patients with borderline conditions present a special challenge to clinicians. Many such patients also have childhood histories of physical and sexual abuse and emotional neglect. How a history of abuse or neglect affects treatment is a subject of some debate and probably varies from patient to patient.

Several studies indicate that a nonsupportive spousal relationship correlates with treatment refractoriness, especially for women. Unemployment is associated with increased rates of depression for men, although having a job outside the home appears protective against depression for women as well. Financial impoverishment, in general, is associated with an increase in severity and chronicity for a variety of psychiatric conditions for both men and women.

9. How does one proceed if the previous antidepressant trials appear to have been adequate?
Once genuine treatment resistance is established, no firm scientific grounding dictates what would be a logical next step. Given this lack of clarity and the fact that serial drug trials are often required, it is important to develop a collaborative relationship with the patient, who is helped to understand the advantages and disadvantages of various treatment options and then becomes an active partner in the decision-making process. The clinician often has countertransference feelings of frustration and helplessness and must be careful not to take such feelings out on the patient. The clinician's role in providing an ongoing sense of hopefulness as various interventions are attempted is extremely important. In general interventions at this point involve either switching or augmentation strategies.

Intervention Strategies for Treatment-Resistant Depression

1. Switching
   - Tricyclic antidepressant (with blood levels)
   - Serotonin or mixed reuptake inhibitor
   - Monoamine oxidase inhibitor
   - Electroconvulsive treatment
2. Augmentation
   - Combinations of tricyclics and serotonin reuptake inhibitors
   - Lithium
   - Thyroid (T_3 or T_4)
   - Buspirone
   - Stimulants
   - Phototherapy
3. Psychosocial
   - Reassess therapeutic strategy
   - Couples/family therapy
   - Substance abuse treatment
   - Cognitive, behavioral, and interpersonal techniques

10. What is a switching strategy?

Switching strategies involve the abandonment of one medication or treatment strategy and replacing it with another. The literature concerning switches to a drug in the same class is mixed. There is little literature to support a switch from one tricyclic to another unless it is a matter of changing side-effect profiles. Some evidence suggests that SSRIs have overlapping but somewhat different efficacy profiles; thus a patient may respond to one SSRI after failing to respond to another. Switching to a new class of agents has the most support in the literature; studies tend to show 50–65% response rates to a subsequent trial of a new class of antidepressant or ECT. Previously it was thought that an estimated 70% of treatment-refractory cases will respond to adequate trials of either a tricyclic antidepressant, MAOI, or ECT. The addition of the SSRIs, bupropion, and venlafaxine to the armamentarium should increase these numbers even further.

11. What is an augmentation strategy?

Augmentation strategies involve adding a new intervention to an ongoing treatment. Augmentation strategies are most frequently used when a patient has had a partial response to the current intervention. The augmentation strategy is an attempt to augment and improve this response by adding to it rather than risking loss of current gains by using a switching strategy.

Lithium augmentation has the most support from research. Lithium augmentation is effective in the treatment of unipolar as well as bipolar depression with response rates of 30–75% in previously refractory patients. The use of thyroid augmentation is more complicated and more controversial. Depressives as a group show increased rates of clinical (grade I) and subclinical (grades II and III) hypothyroidism. Replacement of thyroxine (T_4) may improve antidepressant response. Conversely, some investigators feel that triiodothyronine (T_3) (25–50 μg/day) may augment antidepressant response in some euthyroid nonresponders, but research data are less consistent. Other augmentation strategies involve SSRI/TCA combinations, buspirone, stimulants, phototherapy, anticonvulsants, and calcium channel blockers. MAOIs and TCAs are sometimes used in combination, but this approach must be done by a knowledgeable psychopharmacologist because certain combinations are potentially lethal (e.g., imipramine and an MAOI).

12. What is the role of ECT?

ECT is still the single most potent treatment for severe depression. ECT may be the treatment of first choice in patients with:
- Severe depression with suicidal intent
- Depression associated with life-threatening medical debilitation
- Patients with a history of nonresponse to medication and a positive response to ECT.

Overall the 85–90% response rates to ECT drop to 50% if rigid criteria for previous treatment resistance are applied. As with medication nonresponse, some patients with a history of ECT nonresponse have had inadequate dose (inadequate electrical stimuli or unilateral stimulation only) or duration (inadequate number of treatments). In patients who do not respond, bilateral treatment with a stimulus intensity 150% greater than seizure threshold is warranted.

One problem with ECT is the high rate of relapse (50–60%) in the year after treatment, even if a supposedly adequate medication regimen is resumed. This finding suggests that either novel pharmacologic strategies or maintenance ECT are needed to prevent relapse in previously treatment-resistant patients who respond to ECT.

CONTROVERSY

13. What is the role of psychostimulants in treating treatment-refractory depression?

Issue: Psychostimulants, such as methylphenidate and dextroamphetamine, appear to be effective antidepressants for some patients. Clinicians, however, remain hesitant to use them because of concerns about abuse, tolerance, and side effects.

Discussion: The concern about abuse of stimulants arises in part from an era when stimulants were prescribed at times injudiciously as "pep" and diet pills. When monitored carefully, however, stimulants may be effective and well-tolerated antidepressants for some patients. It remains unclear how the antidepressant response to stimulants compared with the response to other antidepressants.

Patients with a history of depression and attention deficit hyperactivity disorder may be particularly good candidates for the use of stimulants. Bipolar disorder needs to be ruled out, because the use of stimulants in bipolar patients may contribute to mania, cycling, and a general worsening of their condition.

In the past medically ill patients were frequently better able to tolerate stimulants than TCAs such as imipramine, amitriptyline, or even desipramine. The advent of SSRIs (e.g., fluoxetine, sertraline, paroxetine, and fluvoxamine) and other newer antidepressants (e.g., bupropion, venlafaxine, and nefazodone) has expanded the range of antidepressant and provided better-tolerated alternatives (other than stimulants) to the TCAs.

In patients with a history of treatment refractoriness as opposed to antidepressant intolerance, controlled trials of stimulants are lacking, although clinicians note significantly positive effects in some patients. In terms of side effects, stimulants may worsen hypertension in adults and cause tics in children. Another concern is that chronic use of high-dose stimulants may worsen psychosis in psychosis-prone individuals.

BIBLIOGRAPHY

1. American Psychiatric Association: Diagnostic and Statistical Manual of Mental Disorders, 4th ed. Washington, DC, American Psychiatric Association, 1994.
2. Amsterdam JD (ed): Pharmacotherapy of Depression. New York, Marcel Dekker, 1990.
3. Clayton PJ: Bipolar illness. In Winokur G, Clayton PJ (eds): The Medical Basis of Psychiatry, 2nd ed. Philadelphia, W.B. Saunders, 1994, pp 47–67.
4. Nierenberg AA, White K: What next? A review of pharmacologic strategies in treatment resistant depression. Psychopharmacol Bull 26:429, 1990.
5. Phillips KA, Nierenberg AA: The assessment and treatment of refractory depression. J Clin Psychiatry 55(Suppl):20, 1994.
6. Thase ME, Rush AJ: Treatment-resistant depression. In Bloom FE, Kupfer DJ (eds): Psychopharmacology: The Fourth Generation of Progress. New York, Raven Press, 1995, pp 1081–1097.
7. Winokur G: Unipolar depression. In Winokur G (ed): The Medical Basis of Psychiatry, 2nd ed. Philadelphia, W.B. Saunders, 1994, pp 69–86.

78. OBESITY

Rena R. Wing, Ph.D., and Mary Lou Klem, Ph.D.

1. When should a patient be encouraged to lose weight?

Body mass index (BMI) is the currently recommended method of determining a patient's weight status. BMI is calculated by the following formula:

$$\frac{\text{weight in kg}}{(\text{height in meters})^2}$$

BMI correlates well with other measures of body fatness, such as hydrostatic weighing. Patients with a BMI of 19 and 24 are typically defined as within the optimal weight range. Patients with a BMI between 25 and 29 are considered moderately overweight (approximately 15–30% above ideal body weight), whereas a BMI greater than 27.3 in women and 27.8 in men constitutes an established health risk.

A second method of determining weight status is to calculate the patient's degree of deviance from his or her **ideal weight,** which is determined by examining normative weight tables such as those developed by the Metropolitan Life Insurance Company in 1983. Such charts indicate by gender, age, and body frame size the weights at which patients should have the greatest longevity (hence the term ideal weight). Obesity is defined as a body weight at least 20% or more above ideal weight.

In addition, it is important to obtain a measure of **body fat distribution.** Recent studies show that the risk of disease (including diabetes and heart disease) and mortality is related to the location of body fat in addition to total amount. Patients with primarily upper body (abdominal) fat appear to be at significantly higher risk for medical problems than patients with fat located primarily in lower body (femoral-gluteal) areas. Body fat distribution may be determined by the waist-to-hip ratio (WHR), which is calculated by the following formula:

$$\frac{\text{waist in centimeters}}{\text{hip in centimeters}}$$

Ratios of 1.0 or greater for men and 0.80 or greater for women (which indicate a relatively higher distribution of fat in the abdominal area than in the femoral-gluteal area) are associated with increased risk of morbidity and mortality.

In determining when to encourage weight loss, the patient's BMI and body fat distribution should be considered, along with other risk factors for coronary heart disease and whether the patient has a positive family history of obesity-related disease.

2. How common is obesity?

If obesity is defined as BMI ≥ 27.8 for men and 27.3 for women, it is estimated that 31.4% of men and 35.3% of women in the United States are obese. Minority and low socioeconomic status as well as older age are associated with higher prevalence rates; the most striking example is African-American women aged 45–75 years, among whom a prevalence rate of 60% has been observed.

Whereas prevalence rates provide a clear picture of who is currently obese, incidence rates are helpful in understanding when a patient may be at risk for *becoming* overweight. A recent prospective study of adults aged 25–74 years concluded that the risk of major weight gain (defined as an increase of 5 kg/m², or about 14 kg within a 10-year period) was highest in adults aged 25–34 years; women were twice as likely as men to experience a major weight gain. Thus, although the greatest number of currently overweight adults is found among individuals aged 45 and above, the process of becoming overweight is likely to have begun years earlier.

3. Are social and cultural pressures increasing the prevalence of dieting and concerns about being overweight?

Every period of history develops its own standards of beauty and attractiveness. American society places a strong emphasis on thinness as beauty, and the ideal body weight has become increasingly lower. For example, researchers who followed the body weights of Miss America contestants over time found significant decreases in contestants' body weights and measurements in a 20-year period. Concomitant with changes in ideal body weight are rising levels of discontent with body size among the general public. At any one time, 20% of Americans report that they are dieting to lose weight. Given the enormous social pressures to lose weight and individuals' sometimes unrealistic beliefs about weight loss (e.g., that a "perfect body" is achievable), it is important to discuss the purpose of weight loss (to prevent future health problems or to avoid exacerbation of existing problems) and healthy methods of achieving reasonable weight loss goals with all patients seeking to lose weight.

4. What causes obesity?

Obesity results from the combination of genetic predisposition and environmental influences. Studies of twins and adoption studies have shown a strong genetic component to obesity. The body weight of adults who were adopted as infants has been found to resemble the weight of their biologic parents, rather than the weight of their adoptive parents. Moreover, the ability to gain weight is under genetic control. When pairs of monozygote twins were overfed by 1,000 kcal/day for 84 days, the amount of weight gain differed among the pairs (range: 4.3–13.3 kg) but was extremely similar within a pair.

Environmental factors, particularly the amount of food available, the fat content of the food, and the amount of exercise, also contribute to the development of obesity. Migration studies have clearly shown that weight increases as people move from rural to urban environments or from non-westernized to westernized lifestyles. For example, Japanese living in Japan are thinner than Japanese who migrate to Hawaii, who in turn are thinner than Japanese living in the continental United States.

In discussing with a patient the cause of his or her obesity, the practitioner should explain that a genetic predisposition for obesity is an inherited tendency to become overweight and does *not* mean that the patient is doomed to be obese for his or her entire life. This genetic tendency probably can be blunted by regular physical activity and a low-fat diet.

5. What are the medical and psychological consequences of obesity?

Obesity is one of the most serious health problems in the United States. Among adults aged 20–75 years, excessive weight increases the relative risk of hypertension 3-fold, the risk of hypercholesterolemia 1.5-fold, and the risk of diabetes 3-fold. The increased risks associated with obesity are even greater in people aged 20–45 years. The association of obesity with hypertension, diabetes, cardiovascular disease, orthopedic disorders, gallbladder disease, cancer, and other illnesses is estimated to cost $40 billion/year in health care expenditures.

The impact of obesity is not limited to physical health, however. Psychosocial studies of overweight people suggest that obesity also has significant social and economic consequences. For example, overweight women are less likely to marry than normal-weight peers and have lower annual incomes and higher rates of household poverty. Overweight men are also less likely to marry than their normal-weight peers.

6. Are there psychological differences between obese and lean people?

Although overweight people clearly face a number of social and economic disadvantages, current research does not support the hypothesis that in general they exhibit higher levels of psychopathology than normal-weight counterparts. The earliest studies used highly select (and thus unrepresentative) samples of obese patients who were seeking treatment for weight and psychological problems; not surprisingly, the studies found that such patients indeed showed high levels of psychological distress. Later studies that used nonclinical samples found no such differences between obese and normal-weight people on measures of depressive symptoms, general psychopathology, assertiveness, and self-consciousness.

Although obese people in general do not exhibit higher levels of psychopathology than normal-weight counterparts, a subset of overweight patients report frequent episodes of binge eating and increased levels of psychological distress. Such patients typically report consuming large amounts of food in a short period, during which they feel that they are unable to stop eating. They are also likely to report marked distress over episodes of binge eating and to display elevated scores on measures of depressive symptoms. Such patients may require individualized treatment or a program specifically designed for obese binge eaters.

7. What are the benefits of weight loss? How much does the patient need to lose to achieve such benefits?

Weight loss significantly reduces many of the health risks associated with obesity, including diabetes, hypertension, dyslipidemia, cardiovascular disease, and postoperative complications. In obese people who develop diabetes, weight loss is associated with increased insulin sensitivity and improved serum glucose levels; in many cases, weight loss may allow reduction or elimination of oral medication or insulin. Weight loss also may lead to significant improvements in hypertension, with a 10% decrease in systolic blood pressure among men who achieve a 15% decrease in body weight. Obesity often is associated with elevations in serum triglycerides and decreases in high-density lipoprotein (HDL) levels. A significant weight loss may reverse both lipid abnormalities and thus reduce atherogenic risk. Other health-related benefits of weight loss include improved pulmonary function, lower surgical risk, and risk of postoperative complications, and improved functional capacity in patients experiencing low back pain and osteoarthritis of the knee. Weight loss also has been shown to decrease the level of self-reported depressive symptoms.

In discussing with patients the role of weight loss in treatment of their medical problems, it is important to emphasize that many improvements in health can be achieved with relatively small losses. For example, a decrease in body weight of as little as 10% has been reported to normalize blood pressure in overweight patients, and improvement in HDL levels has been observed in people losing only 5–10% of initial body weight. Modest weight losses also produce long-term benefits in obese patients with type II diabetes. Thus, even severely overweight patients or patients with a history of unsuccessful attempts to lose weight should be encouraged to achieve modest losses.

8. What are the main components of an effective weight loss program?

The most successful weight loss programs involve a combination of diet, exercise, and behavior modification. The diet is usually set at 1,000–1,500 kcal/day, depending on initial body weight. Weight loss programs increasingly emphasize low fat intake, with 20–30% of calories consumed as fat. Walking is usually recommended as the form of exercise, with gradually increasing goals until the patient is walking 2 miles/day 5 days/week. Strategies for behavior modification are typically taught in a group format with weekly meetings for about 6 months, followed by periodic booster sessions. The goal of behavioral programs is to teach patients to modify eating and exercise behaviors by changing the environmental stimuli (cues) and reinforcers that control such behaviors. Strategies include the following:

Examples of Strategies Used in Behavioral Treatment Programs

Strategies focusing on behavior	
Self-monitoring	Patients are asked to record eating and exercise in a daily diary, to indicate the calories and fat grams in each food, and to note the calories expended through physical activity.
Goal setting	Patients are given short- and long-term goals for intake, exercise, and weight loss (e.g., to lose 2 lb/week). Goals are set at attainable but challenging levels.

Table continued on following page.

Examples of Strategies Used in Behavioral Treatment Programs (Cont.)

Strategies focusing on changing antecedents (cues)	
Stimulus control	Patients are taught to remove cues for inappropriate behaviors and to increase cues for appropriate behavior (e.g., to refrain from bringing ice cream into the house, to put the exercise bike where it can be more easily seen and used).
Cognitive restructuring	Patients learn to counter negative self-statements with more positive ones (e.g., instead of thinking, "I ate that candy; now I might as well eat the whole box," patients learn to say to themselves, "Eating candy is no big deal. I'll just make sure I follow my meal plan closely for the rest of the day").
Strategies focusing on changing consequences (reinforcers)	
Self-reinforcement	Patients are taught to reward themselves for behavior changes (e.g., putting aside $1.00 each time they take a walk and saving for a new blouse).
Contingency contracts	Patients sign a written statement with a therapist or friend, indicating a specific behavior or short-term weight loss and a specific reward if and only if they achieve their goal.

Obesity is a chronic disease that requires chronic, ongoing treatment. Thus, it is important to identify programs that provide ongoing care and combine diet, exercise, and behavior modification. Initially such programs produce weight losses of 20–40 lbs, and approximately 50–60% of this loss is maintained 1 year after the program.

9. What is the role of very low calorie diets?
Very low calorie diets (VLCDs) allow < 800 kcal/day and are usually given as liquid formula or as lean meat, fish, and fowl with appropriate vitamin and mineral supplements. Intake of 1 g/kg ideal body weight of protein of high biologic value is important in VLCDs to help preserve lean body mass. VLCDs appear to be safe when used with proper medical supervision in carefully selected patients who are moderately to severely overweight (BMI ≥ 30). Moreover, they are effective in producing substantial initial weight losses and concomitant improvements in obesity-related conditions. Patients find the rigid structure of VLCDs helpful and on average lose 20 kg in 12 weeks. Such diets may be helpful to patients who require immediate weight loss and amelioration of medical conditions; they also may be highly motivating to patients who feel that they cannot succeed at weight loss.

The long-term outcome of VLCDs is no better than what can be achieved with balanced low calorie diets of 1,000–1,500 kcal/day. To limit weight regain, which may be rapid, a gradual refeeding program must be implemented after the VLCD, and all participants must receive behavior therapy and guidance on increasing physical activity. Although such approaches limit weight regain, they do not prevent it; at 1-year follow-up, there are no significant differences in weight loss with VLCDs vs. other dietary regimens.

10. Are any drugs useful in the treatment of obesity?
The primary treatment for obesity is diet, exercise, and behavior modification. For some patients, however, adding medication to this regimen may be helpful. Currently two types of drugs are used in the treatment of obesity: noradrenergic (e.g., diethylpropion, mazindol, and phentermine) and serotonergic (e.g., fenfluramine and fluoxetine) drugs.

Results of controlled trials with noradrenergic drugs show that treated patients lose on average 0.23 kg/week more than placebo patients over a 4-week period. After this time, weight loss continues at decelerating speed; the long-term effects of noradrenergic drugs have not been adequately studied. Fenfluramine partially inhibits reuptake of serotonin and releases serotonin from nerve endings. Fenfluramine has been shown to inhibit food intake and produces weight losses of approximately 20lb.; weight loss occurs between months 1–8, followed by a plateau in patients who remain on medication. Fluoxetine is an inhibitor of serotonin reuptake; its use also has been shown to produce greater weight loss than placebo through 6 months; however, after 6 months, some patients regain weight while still on medication, and differences between placebo and drug-treated patients become nonsignificant by 1 year. Thus, these drugs have relatively modest effects on long-term weight loss. Subgroups of patients may respond better to each type of drug, but as yet such subgroups have not been defined.

A recent study reported more promising results from the combination of a serotonergic (d, 1-fenfluramine) and a noradrenergic drug (phentermine). The combination increased weight loss over that achieved with placebo by 17 kg; more importantly, the effect appeared to be maintained over 3 years, but further research is needed to confirm this finding.

Several points should be noted about drug treatment:

1. Most drug regimens have modest effects on weight loss.

2. Drug treatments for obesity work only if the drugs are continued over time; once treatment stops, the weight is regained. Thus, a patient probably will need to be maintained on drug treatment for life.

3. The most effective way to use any drug is in combination with education about diet and exercise and training in behavior modification.

11. How important is exercise for weight loss and maintenance?

Exercise alone (e.g., without diet) appears to produce only minor weight losses. However, in conjunction with modest caloric restriction, exercise produces a greater loss of body weight and body fat and greater improvements in waist-to-hip ratios than either technique alone. Several randomized controlled trials have also shown that the combination of diet and exercise produces better long-term maintenance of weight losses than diet only. Moreover, the single best predictor of long-term maintenance of weight loss is habitual exercise. Given such data, as well as data indicating that regular exercise (independent of weight loss) decreases the incidence of non–insulin-dependent diabetes mellitus and coronary disease in overweight persons and has a positive effect on mood, it is reasonable for physicians to recommend moderate physical activity for all overweight patients.

The best type of exercise for weight loss is low-intensity, long-duration activity such as walking. A 150-lb individual expends 100 calories by walking 1 mile. Overweight people should increase their physical activity gradually to prevent injury. Eventually they should build up to a goal of walking 2 miles/day 5 days/week.

12. What are the risks of weight cycling?

Recently, a great deal of attention has been given to possible adverse effects of weight cycling, i.e., repeated episodes of weight loss followed by weight regain. Weight cycling has been said to decrease metabolic rate and to alter body composition, thus making subsequent efforts at weight loss more difficult. However, the majority of animal and human studies do not support such statements. In general, weight cycling appears to have no consistent negative effects on body composition, energy expenditure, or future attempts at weight loss.

Another concern was that weight cycling may affect cardiovascular morbidity and mortality. People with marked variability in body weight have been shown to have greater morbidity and mortality than people whose weight remains stable. Such data come mainly from large epidemiologic studies that were not originally designed to analyze this issue; unfortunately, no information is available about whether the weight cycles involved voluntary or involuntary weight loss (i.e., was the cycling due to prior illness or to voluntary effort to lose weight?). In addition, many such studies do not address the question separately for obese and normal-weight people. Weight cycling may have negative effects in thinner people (in whom it is likely to be unintentional), but little or no effect in overweight people. Moreover, no evidence suggests that weight cycling has negative effects on cardiovascular risk factors, such as blood pressure, lipids, or body fat distribution.

On the basis of present findings about weight cycling, physicians should encourage nonobese patients to maintain a stable weight. Obese patients should be encouraged to lose modest amounts of weight and to use strategies that promote long-term weight control (namely, diet, exercise, and behavior modification). Fear of weight cycling, however, should not deter efforts at weight loss among obese people, because the risks of remaining obese are greater than the risks of weight cycling.

13. Is obesity a major problem in children?
The prevalence of obesity among children is increasing at alarming rates in the United States, and many overweight children will become overweight adults. The chances that an overweight child will remain overweight are increased in families in which the parents are also overweight and in children who remain overweight through adolescence.

Treatment of obesity in children appears to be far more effective than treatment of obesity in adults. A behavioral treatment program in which both the overweight child (age 8–12 years) and his or her overweight parent are treated together and taught to modify diet and exercise habits has been shown to be successful in reducing obesity in overweight children through a 10-year follow-up interval.

BIBLIOGRAPHY

1. Blair SN: Evidence for success of exercise in weight loss and control. Ann Intern Med 119(7 pt 2): 702–706, 1993.
2. Bray GA: Obesity: Basic considerations and clinical approaches. Disease-A-Month 18:449–540, 1989.
3. Bray GA: Use and abuse of appetite-suppressant drugs in the treatment of obesity. Ann Intern Med 119 (7 pt 2):707–713, 1993.
4. Epstein LH, Valoski A, Wing RR, McCurley J: Ten-year follow-up of behavioral, family-based treatment for obese children. JAMA 264:2519–2523, 1990.
5. Kanders BS, Blackburn GL: Reducing primary risk factors by therapeutic weight loss. In Wadden TA, VanItallie TB (eds): Treatment of the Seriously Obese Patient. New York, Guilford Press, 1992, pp 213–230.
6. National Task Force on the Prevention and Treatment of Obesity: Very low-calorie diets. JAMA 270:967–974, 1993.
7. Stunkard AJ, Wadden TA (eds): Obesity—Theory and Therapy. New York, Raven Press, 1993.
8. Van Itallie TB: Health implications of overweight and obesity in the United States. Ann Intern Med 103:983–988, 1985.
9. Wadden TA: The treatment of obesity: An overview. In Stunkard AJ, Wadden TA (eds): Obesity Theory and Therapy. New York, Raven Press, 1993, pp 197–218.
10. Wing RR; Weight cycling in humans: A review of the literature. Ann Behav Med 14:113–119, 1992.
11. Wing RR: Behavioral treatment of obesity: Its application to type II diabetes. Diabetes Care 16:193–199, 1993.

XII. Ethical and Legal Issues in Psychiatry

79. CONFIDENTIALITY AND PRIVILEGE

Jeffrey L. Metzner, M.D.

1. Define confidentiality.

Confidentiality refers to the ethical duty of the physician not to disclose information learned from the patient to any other person or organization without the consent of the patient or under proper legal compulsion. The Hippocratic Oath described the duty of confidentiality as follows:

> Whatsoever I shall see or hear in the course of my profession as well as outside my profession in my intercourse with men, if it be what should not be published abroad, I will never divulge, holding such things to be holy secrets.

This duty is described by the American Medical Association in section 4 of the *Principles of Medical Ethics:*

> A physician shall respect the rights of patients, of colleagues, and of other health professionals, and shall safeguard patient confidences within the constraints of law.

The Principles of Medical Ethics with Annotations Especially Applicable to Psychiatry (1993) elaborates in section 4, annotation 1:

> Confidentiality is essential to psychiatric treatment. This is based in part on the special nature of psychiatric therapy as well as on the traditional ethical relationship between physician and patient.

2. Is confidentiality a legal duty of the psychiatrist?

The existence of a legal obligation to protect the confidentiality of communications arising from the physician-patient relationship has evolved primarily through court decisions, although statutory regulations may also be pertinent. Successful lawsuits against physicians for breach of confidentiality have been based on the following legal theories:
1. Implied contract to keep information confidential
2. Invasion of privacy
3. Tortious breach of duty of confidentiality
4. Statutory regulations

Courts have awarded damages for breach of confidentiality based on the contractual relationship between the physician and patient, which was determined to include an implied agreement that the physician would keep confidential any information received from the patient. Recovery also has been based on invasion of privacy, which has been defined as an unjustified disclosure of a person's private affairs with which the public has no legitimate concern in such a fashion to cause humiliation and/or emotional suffering to ordinary persons. The nature of the physician-patient relationship has been determined to create for the physician a fiduciary duty (i.e., to act primarily for the benefit of another) to keep information obtained through such a relationship confidential. Therefore, a tort action can be used to recover damages. A tort is a civil wrong, other than breach of contract, for which the court will provide a remedy in a form of an action for damages. Finally, courts have occasionally allowed recovery based on licensing statutes that focus on issues of privileged communications.[9]

3. When are physicians' disclosures legally justified?

A valid consent for a release of information protects the psychiatrist ethically and legally. State law and/or relevant rules and regulations often specify the requirements for such a release. A valid consent minimally means that the patient was competent to provide such authorization and did so knowingly and voluntarily. Written consent that specifies the purpose and scope of information to be released is recommended. Written consent often clarifies to the patient the nature of the disclosure and provides documentation for the physician for risk management.

Many evaluations for medicolegal (i.e., forensic) purposes, which are performed at the request of third parties to address issues such as impairment ratings for worker's compensation purposes, disability insurance payments, and appropriateness of treatment, are not confidential. The *Ethical Guidelines for the Practice of Forensic Psychiatry* developed by the American Academy of Psychiatry and the Law state that

> [t]he psychiatrist maintains confidentiality to the extent possible given the legal context. Special attention is paid to any limitations on the usual precepts of medical confidentiality. An evaluation for forensic purposes begins with notice to the evaluee of any limitations on confidentiality. Information or reports derived from the forensic evaluation are subject to the rules of confidentiality as apply to the evaluation and any disclosure is restricted accordingly.

Reports and/or information obtained from such examinations can be disclosed to the third party that requested the examination without risk of a successful lawsuit by the evaluee on the basis of breach of confidentiality. Consent is implied when the person proceeds with the evaluation after having been provided appropriate information about its nature and the lack of or limits to confidentiality.

Disclosures without consent from the patient have been found to be permissible by courts when an overriding public interest (e.g., public safety) was at issue. However, a careful risk-benefit analysis needs to be made before such disclosures. Consultation with a colleague and/or attorney should be part of the risk-benefit analysis. Information released under such circumstances should be relevant to potential public harm and provided only to those in need of such information.

Many state court decisions and/or statutes have adopted the principle of a psychotherapist's duty to protect as described in the Tarasoff II decision *(Tarasoff v. Regents of the University of California,* 551 P.2d 334 [1976]). In certain circumstances this duty may be legally discharged by warning the patient's intended victim, whether or not the patient consents to releasing such information. However, jurisdictions differ concerning recognition and discharge of such a duty, and the clinician must be familiar with the law in his or her state. In states without such a duty, a physician may be liable for breach of confidentiality if a warning to a third party is provided without obtaining valid consent from the patient.

State statutes often require physicians to report to various governmental agencies certain conditions such as infectious diseases (e.g., sexually transmitted diseases, tuberculosis), suspected child abuse, and gunshot wounds. States have taken very different approaches to confidentiality and reporting issues relevant to infection with the human immunodeficiency virus (HIV) and acquired immunodeficiency syndrome (AIDS). Physicians need to be familiar with pertinent statutes in their own states concerning both conditions that are to be reported and threshold criteria for making such reports.

4. Are there any reporting requirements about patients who may have a medical or psychiatric condition that may impair their driving ability?

Most states clearly indicate in their statutes and in the information provided to licensed motorists that the driver is primarily responsible for his or her own safety and the safety of others. Ten states have clearly written guidelines under which drivers must inform the state of medical conditions. However, few states have written criteria for determining driver safety, and physician reporting of unsafe drivers is generally not required by state law.[10] There generally has not been a great impetus to interfere with the physician-patient relationship, although physicians are encouraged to report patients who they believe would be unsafe behind the wheel to the Department of Motor Vehicles. Physicians generally are granted some form of immunity from liability when making such reports in good faith.

Physicians in Pennsylvania appear to have the strictest reporting requirements. Judicial decisions have held physicians liable for injuries in motor vehicle accidents involving their patients who drive. Several significant precedents involving psychiatrists' duty to warn and/or to protect a third party arose from driving cases. Physicians should be familiar with pertinent statutes and case law within their jurisdiction.

5. Are any statutes other than reporting statutes pertinent to confidentiality?

A number of states have enacted mental health confidentiality statutes that establish a rule of confidentiality and describe exceptions. For example, the Colorado statute that establishes procedures for involuntary commitment provides that "all information obtained and records prepared in the course of providing any services [for the care and treatment of the mentally ill] . . . shall be confidential and privileged matter" (C.R.S. 27-10-120). The law specifies various exceptions, such as peer review, communications between qualified professional personnel in the provision of services or appropriate referrals, information released to the courts as necessary to the administration of the provisions of this article, certain circumstances for releasing confidential information to family member(s) of an adult with mental illness, and appropriate research (C.R.S. 27-10-101, 102, 116, 120, 120.5 as amended).

Legislation often requires that rules and regulations about confidentiality be promulgated by the state's Division of Mental Health or equivalent agency. The physician should be familiar with such rules and regulations within his or her jurisdiction because they vary significantly among states. Federal rules and regulations regarding confidentiality are applicable to substance abuse treatment programs that receive federal funds (42 U.S.C. §§ 290dd-3 and 290ee-3 (1988), amended by 42 U.S.C. §§ 290dd-3 (e) and 290ee-3 (e) and (g) [Supp. III, 1991]). Records and information from such programs can be released only under conditions specified in the regulations, which provide detailed information about the nature of the written release required. Access to information about patients and records in the Veterans Administration Hospitals is determined by various federal laws and regulations, such as the Freedom of Information Act and Privacy Act.

6. How do ethical guidelines address issues relevant to confidentiality?

The Principles of Medical Ethics with Annotations Especially Applicable to Psychiatry emphasize that

> [t]he continuing duty of the psychiatrist to protect the patient includes fully apprising him/her of the connotations of waiving the privilege of privacy. . . . Ethically the psychiatrist may disclose only that information which is relevant to a given situation. He/she should avoid offering speculation as fact.

It is good practice, both clinically and from the perspective of risk management, to provide the patient with a copy of the information (e.g., report, completed insurance form) to be disclosed before its release. Generating the report in the presence of the patient and/or with direct input from the patient is often therapeutic and contributes to good treatment planning. The most frequent request for information comes from insurance companies, which often inquire about diagnosis, treatment progress and planning, or issues relevant to disability and/or insurability.

Confidentiality may be breached ethically in the interest of protecting the patient:

> Psychiatrists at times may find it necessary, in order to protect the patient or the community from imminent danger, to reveal confidential information disclosed by the patient (American Psychiatric Association Ethics Committee, 1993).

Thus it is often clinically and ethically appropriate for the physician to inform a depressed patient's relative or roommate about suicide risk to protect the patient from dangerous behavior. The physician's legal liability under such circumstances is low if his or her assessment was reasonable. Although physicians do not have a legal duty to warn others of a potential suicide attempt by a patient, the physician does have a duty to provide reasonable care to his or her patients; this duty includes implementing appropriate steps to decrease the risk of suicide. A psychiatrist should not release information to family members or others without appropriate authorization from the patient or an overriding interest of protecting the patient. For example, confidential information should not be given to a spouse who requests information or help about problems that may affect the marriage unless the patient provides appropriate authorization.

7. How does confidentiality apply to the treatment of minors?

The general and forensic psychiatric literature about issues specific to confidentiality with children and adolescents was sparse until the 1990s. From a legal perspective, the psychiatrist can generally assume that a parent has the legal right to full information about the treatment of a minor if the parent is legally entitled to authorize treatment for a minor child. However, full implementation of such a legal principle would often cause significant clinical problems. Such problems can be minimized by establishing ground rules of confidentiality and exceptions with patients and parents before beginning treatment. The ground rules generally are different for adolescents than for younger minors because of developmental differences and an increased right to privacy. State statutes often provide guidance about issues of confidentiality in the treatment of minors. The American Academy of Child and Adolescent Psychiatry Code of Ethics (1980) and articles by Macbeth,[8] Benedek,[6] and Weintrob[12] provide detailed discussions of legal, clinical, and ethical considerations relevant to confidentiality and treatment of minors.

8. What is the physician-patient privilege?

Most state legislatures have created a testimonial privilege that prohibits a physician from disclosing in a judicial or quasijudical proceeding (with certain exceptions) any confidential information learned during the course of treatment. Thus, testimonial privilege is an evidentiary rule created by statute, applicable to judicial settings, and limited in scope. The privilege belongs to the patient—not to the physician. A breach of privileged communication may result in a lawsuit against the physician. Physician-patient privilege statutes have been enacted because of the recognition that confidentiality is needed to maintain the therapeutic relationship, which also may have benefits for the community (e.g., people receive necessary treatment for illness). The recognition of the importance of a patient's privacy also has been a justification for such statutes.

Although there is no federal privilege statute, some federal courts have recognized a physician-patient privilege under certain circumstances. The state law on privilege applies in federal court when an element of a claim or defense is governed by state law (Rule 501, Federal Rules of Evidence).

9. What are the exceptions to privilege?

1. When a valid waiver of privilege is executed by a competent adult patient or his or her legal guardian
2. When the patient has initiated litigation in which his or her mental or emotional condition is an element of a claim or defense in a legal proceeding
3. Most court-ordered examinations involving a wide range of legal issues
4. Malpractice proceedings initiated by the patient against the physician
5. Involuntary civil commitment proceedings
6. Contesting of a will
7. Certain criminal proceedings
8. Reports required by various mandatory reporting statutes

The above list is not inclusive, and the type of exceptions differs from state to state. For example, some state statutes allow for the waiver of a physician-patient privilege, at the discretion of the judge, in child custody disputes. The physician needs to be familiar with the appropriate law in his or her state. Disclosures made to the physician for purposes other than obtaining treatment are not covered by privilege. States vary regarding the presence of privilege if disclosure occurs when third parties (e.g., family members) are present during the communication. Jurisdictions also differ about whether communications arising in the course of couples' and/or group psychotherapy are privileged. Nonphysician providers supervised by physicians generally are not covered by the patient-physician privilege statute, although they may be covered by a statute specific to their profession.

10. How should the psychiatrist respond to a subpoena?
A subpoena duces tecum is a subpoena issued by the court at the request of one of the parties to a lawsuit; it requires a physician to bring (i.e., produce) pertinent medical records. In contrast, a subpoena ad testificandum requires the attendance of the physician for testimony purposes. Neither subpoena compels the physician either to testify or to release records to the attorney who requested the subpoena. Ethical and legal principles may properly prevent the psychiatrist from either testifying or disclosing the subpoenaed medical records.

The psychiatrist may release medical records and/or testify when the subpoena is accompanied by a valid consent form signed by the patient. Reasonable attempts should be made to inform the patient or the patient's attorney about the subpoena to verify the validity of the consent and to discuss relevant issues.

The psychiatrist should contact the patient or the patient's attorney when a signed consent form is not attached to the subpoena to determine whether the patient has consented, explicitly or implicitly, to waive the privilege. It is important to remember that the privilege belongs to the patient and not to the physician. However, the physician has an ethical and legal obligation to withhold information obtained during the course of treatment as privileged from disclosure in a legal context unless an exception clearly exists (e.g., signed consent) or the physician is directed by the court to testify and/or to release the record. The psychiatrist should discuss with the attorney, when appropriate, issues about disclosure of highly sensitive information that appears not be be pertinent to the issues under litigation. The patient's attorney or the psychiatrist has the option of filing a motion to quash the subpoena or to limit the nature of the information to be disclosed on the basis of physician-patient privilege and the duty to maintain confidentiality, when the patient has not consented to waive the privilege. A hearing is held in which the judge rules on the motion. The psychiatrist can ethically testify and/or release medical records when ordered to do so by the court, despite lack of consent from the patient. The psychiatrist should not rely on the statements or opinions of the attorney who requested the subpoena about issues relevant to waiver of the privilege.

11. What are the principles of confidentiality after a patient's death?
According to the Ethics Committee of the American Psychiatric Association, confidentiality ethically survives a patient's death unless disclosures are required by statute or case law. Some state statutes allow the executor or administrator of the deceased patient's estate or certain relatives to have access to the patient's medical record. The physician-patient privilege also may be waived in certain states after the patient's death. The psychiatrist should obtain guidance from legal counsel or the court about questions concerning the waiver of privilege.

Similar issues arise in circumstances that are not addressed by statute or case law. The psychiatrist may be questioned by the police during the course of an investigation involving the death of a patient or may be asked specific questions by grieving family members. The psychiatrist should not disclose specific information obtained from the patient, although answering questions in terms of general psychiatric principles may be appropriate. The psychiatrist's liability for breach of confidentiality is minimized by obtaining authorization from the patient's legal representative and close family members.[9]

12. Is it a breach of confidentiality to use a collection agency or attorney in an attempt to collect unpaid bills?
No ethical principles preclude psychiatrists from using the legal system or collection agencies for bill collection. The physician-patient privilege does not prevent a doctor from suing to collect proper fees. However, the legal and ethical obligations of the psychiatrist to protect the patient's confidentiality continues despite breach of the treatment contract when the patient fails to pay the bill. Patients may sue for breach of confidentiality when the psychiatrist discloses their status as patients to an attorney or collection agency. In general, the only information that needs to be disclosed to the collection agency or attorney is the patient's name, balance due, and dates of services. Confidentiality is best preserved by describing the dates of services as office visits rather than visits for psychotherapy or medication management.

Because of issues of confidentiality and risk management, the psychiatrist first should use methods of recovering fees other than a collection agency or small claims court. A matter-of-fact letter to the patient requesting either payment in full within a specified time frame or a proposal from the patient for a payment schedule is a useful alternative. If there is no response to such a letter within a reasonable period, another letter should be sent that requests a similar response within a specified period and informs the patient that referral will be made to an attorney or collection agency for initiation of appropriate legal action if the patient does not respond. It is important to select a collection agency or attorney who acts in a responsible fashion, both for professional reasons and to minimize the risk that the patient will retaliate by filing a counterclaim for malpractice, an ethical complaint, or a complaint to the Board of Medical Examiners or equivalent agency. Physicians need to be informed about any pertinent laws within their states that specify procedures that must be followed before using a collection agency or attorney to recover unpaid bills.

13. What confidentiality issues are involved with new technology?
The availability of voice mail, cellular telephones, and fax machines may lead to unintentional breaches of confidentiality. Voice mail messages may be played back by persons other than the patient; cellular telephone conversations may be heard by other parties; and records sent via fax machines may be sent to the wrong number. Therefore, detailed voice mail messages should not be left for patients unless assurances have been given by them that other persons do not have access to their voice mail. Patients should be told when a cellular telephone is used and reminded that confidentiality is not guaranteed under such circumstances. Fax machines should not be used for routine transmission of confidential information, and procedures should be implemented to ensure safeguarding of confidential information that needs to be sent in a prompt fashion.

14. What practical pointers about confidentiality and privilege may help the clinician?
The concepts of confidentiality and privilege are often confusing because of overlapping principles and numerous exceptions. Confidentiality is an important element in developing a therapeutic alliance with patients. A breach of confidentiality may result in legal liability, ethical complaints, adverse actions pertinent to a physician's license to practice medicine, and criminal prosecution in certain circumstances. Practical pointers for the clinician include the following:

Practical Pointers

1. Follow the general principle to honor a patient's confidences unless a legally cognizable exception applies.
2. Have your own form for written "Authorization for Release of Medical/Mental Health Information," which can be tailored to specific circumstances. If requested to release AIDS/HIV information, check with legal counsel or the state Department of Health to ensure that the authorization is specific enough to meet legal requirements.
3. When in doubt about the validity of consent to release information, call your patient to discuss information and to verify consent.
4. When performing an evaluation (e.g., worker's compensation), clarify limits of confidentiality at the outset. Explain who will and will not receive a copy of the report.
5. Obtain competent advice before releasing information to anyone after a patient's death.
6. Apprise group therapy members about parameters of confidentiality.
7. When subpoenaed to testify or release records, seek advice from legal counsel. Generally, you want to ensure that the patient executes written, informed consent or that a court order is obtained.
8. Do not automatically assume that a managed care company has obtained patient consent for release of information. Try to discuss such authorization with the patient at the outset of treatment. Obtain written consent.
9. If using a collection agency or small claims court to collect an unpaid bill, make sure that you send the patient appropriate advance notice in writing and reveal the least amount of information necessary. (Caveat: collections often lead to malpractice counterclaims.)

From Macbeth JE, Wheeler AM, Sither JW, Onek JN: Confidentiality and privilege. In Legal and Risk Management Issues in the Practice of Psychiatry. Washington, DC, Psychiatrist's Purchasing Group, 1994, with permission.

BIBLIOGRAPHY

1. American Academy of Child and Adolescent Psychiatry: Code of Ethics. Washington, DC, American Academy of Child and Adolescent Psychiatry, 1980.
2. American Academy of Psychiatry and the Law: Ethical Guidelines for the Practice of Forensic Psychiatry. Washington, DC, 1991.
3. American Psychiatric Association Ethics Committee: The Principles of Medical Ethics with Annotations Especially Applicable to Psychiatry. Washington, DC, American Psychiatric Association, 1993, pp 1–19.
4. American Psychiatric Association Task Force Report 31: Disclosure of Psychiatric Treatment Records and Child Custody Disputes. Washington, DC, American Psychiatric Association, 1991.
5. Applebaum PS, Gutheil TG: Clinical Handbook of Psychiatry and the Law. New York, McGraw-Hill, 1991.
6. Benedek EP: Ethical issues in practice. In Schetky DH, Benedek EP (eds): Clinical Handbook of Psychiatry and the Law. Baltimore, Williams & Wilkins, 1993, pp 75–88.
7. Council on Ethical and Judicial Affairs: Code of Medical Ethics: Current Opinions with Annotations. Chicago, American Medical Association, 1994, p xiv.
8. Macbeth JE: Legal issues in the psychiatric treatment of minors. In Schetky DH, Benedek EP (eds): Clinical Handbook of Child Psychiatry and the Law. Baltimore, Williams & Wilkins, 1992, pp 53–74.
9. Macbeth JE, Wheeler AM, Sither JW, Onek JN: Confidentiality and privilege. In Legal and Risk Management Issues in the Practice of Psychiatry. Washington, DC, Psychiatrists' Purchasing Group, 1994, pp 2-1–2-31.
10. Metzner JL, Dentino AN, Godard SL, et al: Impairment in driving and psychiatric illness. J Neuropsychiatry 5:211–220, 1993.
11. Simon RI: Clinical Psychiatry and the Law. Washington, DC, American Psychiatric Press, 1987.
12. Weintrob A: Confidentiality and its dilemmas in child and adolescent psychiatry. In Rosner R (ed): Principles and Practice of Forensic Psychiatry. New York, Chapman & Hall, 1994, pp 323–330.

80. LEGAL RESPONSIBILITIES WITH CHILD ABUSE AND DOMESTIC VIOLENCE

Ronald Schouten, J.D., M.D.

The discussion of physicians' legal responsibilities in any area of medicine can cause considerable anxiety. This poses a significant problem, because legal issues arise in all aspects of medical practice. Physicians need not have an intricate knowledge of the law, however, any more than lawyers who encounter medical problems need to study medicine. Instead, a general knowledge of legal issues and a sensitivity to situations in which such issues arise are sufficient.

The key to handling medicolegal questions is a willingness to seek consultation from attorneys and colleagues familiar with medicolegal issues. All physicians have access to legal advice through their malpractice insurers, hospital, medical society, or private attorneys familiar with health care matters. The reluctance of physicians to ask for help may be the largest obstacle to anxiety reduction and successful resolution of medicolegal issues. For that reason, the response to each of the questions below includes the general advice to ask for help from legal advisors. Such a step provides the maximum protection, the greatest relief from anxiety, and the widest freedom to practice good clinical medicine.

Child abuse and domestic violence are significant social problems. Physicians are in a position to detect and prevent such acts of violence as well as to treat the victims. Society has realized the role that physicians can play in dealing with these problems and has placed obligations on physicians to respond.

CHILD ABUSE

1. What obligations does a physician have when child abuse is suspected?

Every state in the United States has passed legislation that makes physicians and other professionals mandatory reporters of child abuse and neglect. The obligation usually arises at a low level, e.g., when the health care professional believes or has a reasonable basis to believe that a child under 18 is a victim of abuse or neglect. Statutes vary with regard to the types of abuse to be reported and whether or not the child must have been seen as a patient by the reporter. The report is made to the state social service agency responsible for child welfare. Hospital social service offices and attorneys have the name of this agency and should be able to advise the physician on when and how the report is to be made. The penalties for failure to report vary from state to state, but usually they involve a substantial fine and may include criminal penalties. Failure to report also may become the subject of disciplinary actions by the state agency responsible for physician registration.

2. What malpractice risks arise in the area of child abuse?

A physician who fails to diagnose or report child abuse may be held liable for injury or wrongful death of the child as the result of subsequent abuse. Such suits may allege failure to diagnose, failure to report, or failure to conduct a proper investigation. When the child is removed from the home because of suspected child abuse, malpractice suits may arise from negligent selection of placement for the child or failure to monitor the placement. Suits also may arise from alleged wrongful removal of the child from the home, although such suits are unsuccessful when the removal was carried out in good faith.

3. What is child abuse?

Child abuse is broadly defined, although state statutes may have different specific definitions. The Child Abuse Prevention and Treatment Act of 1973 defines child abuse and neglect as

> . . . the physical treatment and mental injuring, sexual abuse, negligent treatment, or maltreatment of a child under the age of 18 by a person who is responsible for the child's welfare under circumstances which indicate that the child's health and welfare is harmed or threatened thereby.

Physical abuse may be defined as any injury to a child that is not accidental. Physical neglect refers to a failure to provide for a child's emotional or physical needs. Neglect may include failure to obtain needed medical treatment, even when the failure is consistent with the parents' religious beliefs. Physical neglect is the most common form of physical abuse.

Sexual abuse includes any nonconsensual or consensual sexual activity between an adult and a child. It includes exhibitionism, oral-genital contact, and fondling as well as intercourse.

4. What are the indicators that a child may be suffering from physical abuse or neglect?

There is no single profile of the abused child or the abusive adult. Child abuse should be included as part of the differential diagnosis of all childhood injuries and unexplained illness. Green[7] has suggested that the following elements of the history may indicate that an injury was inflicted rather than accidental:

- Unexplained delay in bringing the child for treatment after an injury.
- The supervising adult offers an explanation which is implausible or contradictory.
- The explanation of the injury is incompatible with the physical findings.
- The child has had a series of similar or otherwise suspicious injuries, e.g., repeated burns from "touching a hot stove."
- The injury is blamed on a sibling or is attributed to self-injury, e.g., "He keeps throwing himself down the stairs."
- The child has a history of treatment for injuries at various hospitals.
- When interviewed, the child accuses the supervising adult of having caused the injury.
- The parents seem to have unrealistic and premature expectations of the child, e.g., "She (a 1-year old) should know that crying in the middle of the night really upsets me."
- The supervising adult minimizes the injury or seems unconcerned about it.
- The supervising adult has a prior history of having been abused as a child.

Adapted from Green AH: Forensic evaluation of physically and sexually abused children. In Rosner R (ed): Principles and Practice of Forensic Psychiatry. New York, Chapman & Hall, 1994.

Findings on physical examination that may indicate physical abuse include bruises on the buttocks and genitals, burns to the perineum, cigarette burns, abdominal trauma, head injury, multiple fractures of different ages, spiral fractures of long bones, eye injuries, and ear injuries.

The signs of physical neglect may be more subtle but are best summarized by children who present with malnutrition or poor hygiene or merit a diagnosis of failure to thrive. Children who do not meet psychological or physical developmental milestones may be suffering from physical neglect.

5. What is Münchhausen's by proxy?

Münchhausen's syndrome is a disorder in which an individual feigns or induces physical illness for the apparent purpose of becoming a patient. Such individuals are often willing to undergo invasive, painful, and debilitating medical procedures, including amputation, as part of the patient role. Indeed, undergoing such procedures may be a motivating force for their behavior. The goal of the behavior is psychological gratification, perhaps by getting attention from physicians, rather than the pursuit of disability claims or monetary reward. When confronted with their behavior, such individuals generally sign out of the hospital against medical advice or drop out of treatment with the confronting physician.

Münchhausen's by proxy refers to the situation in which a parent simulates illness, exaggerates actual illness, or induces illness in a child. The reasons for such behavior are unclear, but they most commonly arise from a desire to get attention from members of the medical profession. The behavior of such parents can range from benign and deceptive to fatal. For example, some parents put cranberry juice in a child's diaper to simulate vaginal bleeding. Others put drops of blood into the child's urine sample to simulate hemorrhagic cystitis. At the other end of the spectrum are parents who have smothered their children to simulate apnea or injected fecal material subcutaneously to cause fever. Such behavior is a form of child abuse and is reportable to the appropriate agency.

Failure to identify a child who is the victim of Münchhausen's by proxy may lead to a malpractice action against the treating physicians.

Signs and Symptoms of Münchhausen's by Proxy

- Medical illnesses which are unusual and for which there is inconsistent explanation.
- Repeated episodes of medical illness in a child with no apparent underlying medical problems, e.g., repeated urinary tract infections in children with normal anatomy.
- Treatment of the child for illness by a number of different physicians at different institutions.
- The child has been treated for these illnesses in different parts of the country.
- The child's parent resists or refuses release of information from previous treating physicians.
- The parent has a history of odd, unexplained injuries or illnesses.
- Siblings with a history of odd, unexplained injuries or illnesses.

Adapted from Schreier HA, Libow J: Hurting for Love: Münchhausen's by Proxy Syndrome. New York, Guilford Press, 1993.

6. What resources are available for parents who have difficulty with controlling their temper or other problems with parenting skills?
Many state social service agencies and private child welfare programs offer parenting classes, support groups, and day care. In addition, many states have toll-free telephone numbers for parents who feel that they are at risk of physically abusing their children.

7. What are the signs and symptoms of sexual abuse of a child?

- The child reports a pattern of repetitive, escalating behavior, beginning with exposure of genitals and extending from mutual touching to intercourse or attempted intercourse.
- The child identifies someone well known to him or her as the abuser who told them that the act was "our secret."
- Physical injuries to the perineum and genitalia.
- Occurrence of sexually transmitted diseases or repeated genitourinary infections.
- Anxiety disorders, including symptoms of posttraumatic stress disorder.
- Increased aggression and impulsivity, including sexually oriented aggression against other children.
- Precocious sexual behavior, compulsive masturbation, and promiscuity may occur. Conversely, adolescents and adults who have been sexually abused may avoid all heterosexually oriented activities.

Adapted from Quinn KM, White S: Interviewing children for suspected child abuse. In Schetky DH, Benedek EP (eds): Clinical Handbook of Child Psychiatry and the Law. Baltimore, Williams & Wilkins, 1992.

Estimates from the U.S. Department of Health and Human Services suggest that in 1987, 2.5/1,000 children were sexually abused.

8. If a patient confides that he or she has abused a child in the past, is the physician required to report this information?

In most jurisdictions, confidentiality requires that information about past misdeeds, including criminal acts, not be disclosed. Some states require that distant as well as recent acts of abuse be reported. In any jurisdiction, however, if the physician has a reasonable basis to believe that the patient is about to repeat the abuse, there may be an obligation to intervene. Clinical intervention, before a repeat offense occurs, is most helpful. This may include a voluntary request for services from a child welfare agency or entering into structured psychiatric treatment for the individual and family.

9. If an adult patient reports that he or she was sexually abused in the past, does the physician have an obligation to report such information to public authorities?

Generally, states require that such information be reported only if other minor children are in the home and the physician has reason to believe that they also may be at risk of abuse. In addition, some jurisdictions may require the reporting of child abuse even if it occurred in the distant past.

Allegations of past sexual abuse have become the subject of civil litigation over the past several years. Law suits against alleged perpetrators of sexual abuse, brought by individuals who report recent recovery of repressed memories, have generated a great deal of controversy. Zealous clinicians have been sued successfully on the basis that they convinced the patient of such "memories" of sexual abuse. Good patient care and informed risk management dictate that the physician receiving such information be supportive of the patient's statements, while at the same time remaining neutral about their accuracy. Documentation of the reports should not comment on the veracity of the claim of abuse. The physician should avoid the use of words such as "alleged" and "claimed," using instead words such as "said" and "reports." The clinician has no way of knowing whether or not the abuse occurred, short of an admission by the accused perpetrator. Hypnosis and narcotherapy (such as amytal interviews) may be helpful therapeutically but are not valid methods of establishing an historically accurate account of abuse.

10. Can a physician be sued successfully for breach of confidentiality if suspected child abuse is reported?

Threats to sue clinicians who report suspected abuse are to be expected. The child abuse-reporting statutes protect reporters from liability by providing an exception to confidentiality requirements. The exceptions apply when the decision to report is reasonable and made in good faith.

DOMESTIC VIOLENCE

11. What obligations does a physician have when domestic violence is suspected?

In contrast to situations involving child abuse, the physician's legal obligations with regard to domestic violence are unclear. Society has tended to view domestic violence as a private matter into which the state should not intrude. As a result, legislators have begun to address this issue only recently.

Most states do not specifically require physicians or others to report suspected domestic abuse. There is a growing trend, however, toward enactment of broad-based prevention statutes that impose a requirement to report suspected domestic abuse in a range of cases. For example, the Kentucky Adult Protection Act requires that

> Any person, including but not limited to, physician, law enforcement officer, nurse, social worker, department personnel, coroner, medical examiner . . . , having reasonable cause to suspect that an adult has suffered abuse, neglect, or exploitation, shall report or cause reports to be made in accordance with the provisions of this chapter.

The reports are to be made to the Department of Adult Services. The reporting requirements are not specific to situations of domestic violence; they cover all types of abuse, neglect, or exploitation. Failure to report is considered a criminal misdemeanor.

In 1994 California passed a new mandatory reporting statute that imposes broad reporting requirements on "any physician or surgeon who has under his or her charge or care any person" whom he or she knows, or reasonably should know, has suffered a wound or other physical injury "where the injury is the result of assaultive or abusive conduct." The statute also recommends documentation of comments about past domestic violence, mapping of injuries, and referrals to local domestic violence services for victims. Failure to report is a misdemeanor "punishable by imprisonment in a county jail for not exceeding six months, or by a fine not exceeding one thousand dollars ($1000), or by both that fine and imprisonment."

California's reporting statute is unusual in specifically mentioning domestic violence. Physicians in most states have a legal obligation to report gunshot wounds, suspicious puncture wounds, and unexplained deaths. Thus, the physician who fails to report such events in the context of a domestic dispute may face legal repercussions. State requirements for the reporting of child abuse, elder abuse, or abuse of people with mental or physical disabilities also may come into play.

Although few states have mandated specifically the reporting of domestic violence, many states have been aggressive in enacting and enforcing laws against domestic violence. In addition to criminal penalties, the states provide for restraining orders that prohibit the perpetrator from approaching the victim and either threatening or committing violent acts.

One of the biggest barriers in the fight against domestic violence has been the belief that assault and battery within the home is somehow permissible as a "private matter" between the individuals. That attitude has led perpetrators of domestic violence to believe that their behavior is acceptable. It has led victims to believe that no one will help them and that reporting such violence is useless. Paradoxically, when victims speak out, their complaints are often minimized by those who assume that the situation could not have been too bad if the victim failed to complain for so long.

The physician's legal obligations in domestic violence may be defined by case law arising from situations in which a patient poses a risk of harm to others. Physicians treating patients with infectious diseases have been found liable for failure to warn nonpatients of the risk of infection. Psychiatrists and other mental health professionals have been found to have a duty to protect third parties against the violent acts of their patients in certain situations. This duty is often called the Tarasoff duty, after the California case that first laid out such obligations. The steps taken to protect the third party need not include breach of the patient's confidentiality.

In some jurisdictions, a history of violence and indications that the patient presents a clear risk of violence against an identifiable person in the near future is enough to give rise to the Tarasoff duty. Possibly this obligation could be extended to nonpsychiatrists. Physicians should check with local authorities to determine obligations in their state.

Even when the threat is not explicit, psychiatrists may have an affirmative duty to commit involuntarily a patient who poses a reasonable risk of violence as a result of mental illness. Finally, a physician potentially could be sued for negligence when he or she knows, or should know, that a patient is a victim of domestic violence but takes no steps to intervene.

12. How common is the problem of domestic violence?

Estimates of the incidence and prevalence of domestic violence vary, but they are all dramatic. Between two and four million women per year are believed to be victims of partner violence, including 1 in 7 women seen in general office practices for medical care, 1 in 3 women presenting for care in emergency rooms, 1 in 4 women who commit suicide, and 1 in 4 women who are pregnant. An estimated 50% of the mothers of abused children are victims of domestic violence. Domestic violence is believed to be the most common single cause of traumatic injury to women.

13. What constitutes domestic violence?

Domestic or partner violence involves actual or threatened physical injury, sexual assault, psychological abuse, economic control, and progressive social isolation. States differ as to what relationships qualify as "domestic." Massachusetts, for example, takes a broad view. Its domestic violence statute covers current or previous relationships between parties of any combination of genders who are or were married, related by blood, share or shared a residence, or are or were involved in "a substantial dating relationship." "Substantial" has been interpreted as a single episode of sexual activity. Other states are more restrictive in defining the relationship.

14. How can domestic violence be detected?

As with other medical conditions, the simplest way to determine whether a patient has been a victim of domestic violence is to ask. Just as we ask simple, nonjudgmental questions about sexual activity as part of a routine screening history, physicians should include a question about domestic violence in the history. This inquiry must be conducted privately, away from the partner or other family members.

A question such as "Has a partner ever hit, kicked, or otherwise hurt or frightened you?" is a good starting point. If the answer is positive, more details should be elicited in a nonjudgmental, confidential fashion. The Massachusetts Medical Society suggests the questions below:

- How were you hurt?
- Has this happened before?
- When did it first happen?
- How badly have you been hurt in the past?
- Have you needed to go to an emergency room for treatment?
- Have you ever been threatened with a weapon, or has a weapon ever been used on you?
- Have the children ever seen you threatened or hurt?
- Have the children ever been threatened or hurt by your partner?

Adapted from Alpert EJ, Freund KM, et al: Partner Violence: How to Recognize and Treat Victims of Abuse. Waltham, MA, Massachusetts Medical Society, 1992.

When interviewing potential victims of partner violence, it is important to avoid using terms such as "domestic violence," "abused," or "battered," which can be seen as judgmental. In addition, many individuals who are victims of violence do not see themselves as belonging in such categories. Questions about what the patient did to provoke the violence, why she has not left the batterer, or why she returned to the relationship after leaving should be avoided. If the answer to the initial question is negative, the physician should still look for physical indications of violence.

Physical Signs and Symptoms of Domestic Abuse

- Contusions, abrasions, minor lacerations, fractures, and sprains.
- Neck, head, chest, breast, and abdominal injuries.
- Injuries during pregnancy, especially to the breasts and abdomen.
- Numerous injuries at multiple sites without adequate explanation.
- Chronic pain, psychogenic pain, or pain due to diffuse trauma without visible evidence.
- Physical symptoms related to chronic posttraumatic stress disorder, anxiety disorders, major depression, or stress.
- Gynecologic problems, including frequent genitourinary infections, pelvic pain, and dyspareunia.
- Evidence of rape or other sexual assault.
- Delay between time of injury and arrival at the hospital.
- Previous use of emergency services for trauma.

Adapted from Alpert EJ, Freund KM, et al: Partner Violence: How to Recognize and Treat Victims of Abuse. Waltham, MA, Massachusetts Medical Society, 1992.

It is important that observations suggesting partner violence be documented carefully in the medical record. Photographs are excellent for documenting injuries and are particularly useful if the patient or state prosecutor pursues legal action against the batterer.

15. What should the physician do when domestic violence is suspected?

Victims of domestic violence are often reluctant to reveal the causes of their injuries. The reasons for this reluctance include fear of the batterer, lack of alternatives to the violent living arrangement, lack of economic resources, and failure of previous attempts to get help from physicians, law enforcement, and courts.

The physician may take a first step toward overcoming such obstacles by indicating to the patient, "I am concerned for your safety." This expression of concern, along with a clear indication that the violence is unacceptable, against the law, and deserving of action, may be the first support that the patient has received.

The patient should be referred for treatment of injuries and for support and counseling. Battered women's programs often have lists of mental health professionals who provide treatment. In addition, such programs may provide shelters for victims and children. The physician should discuss contraception and safe sex practices with the victim. If possible, the victim should not be given sedating medication. Such medication may limit the patient's ability to escape in the event of further violence; it also may be used to question the patient's credibility in the event of legal proceedings. The physician should consider whether there is a need to report the suspected violence to the appropriate public agency. Finally, the patient should be put in contact with an advocate for victims of domestic violence so that all alternatives can be explored.

BIBLIOGRAPHY

1. Alpert EJ, Freund KM, et al: Partner Violence: How to Recognize and Treat Victims of Abuse. Waltham, MA, Massachusetts Medical Society, 1992.
2. American Medical Association: AMA diagnostic and treatment guidelines concerning child abuse and neglect. JAMA 254:796–800, 1985.
3. Appelbaum PA, Gutheil TG: Clinical Handbook of Psychiatry and the Law. Baltimore, Williams & Wilkins, 1991.
4. California Penal Code Sec. 11160-1153.2; Amended by ABX1 74, Chapter 19.
5. DeAngelis C: Clinical indicators of child abuse. In Schetky DH, Benedek EP (eds): Clinical Handbook of Child Psychiatry and the Law. Baltimore, Williams & Wilkins, 1992.
6. Flitcraft A, Hadley S, et al: American Medical Association Diagnostic and Treatment Guidelines on Domestic Violence. Chicago, American Medical Association, 1992.
7. Green AH: Forensic evaluation of physically and sexually abused children. In Rosner R (ed): Principles and Practice of Forensic Psychiatry. New York, Chapman & Hall, 1994.
8. Kentucky Adult Protection Act. Kentucky Revised Statutes, Chapter 209.
9. Meadow R: Münchhausen syndrome by proxy: The hinterland of child abuse. Lancet 2:343–345, 1985.
10. O'Doherty N: The Battered Child: Recognition in Primary Care. London, Bailliere Tindall, 1982.
11. Ohio State Medical Association: Trust Talk: Ohio Physicians' Domestic Violence Project. Columbus, OH, Ohio State Medical Association, 1992.
12. Ostow A: Child abuse. In Hyman SE, Tesar GE (eds): Manual of Psychiatric Emergencies, 3rd ed. Boston, Little, Brown, 1994.
13. Quinn KM, White S: Interviewing children for suspected child abuse. In Schetky DH, Benedek EP (eds): Clinical Handbook of Child Psychiatry and the Law. Baltimore, Williams & Wilkins, 1992.
14. Reade J: Domestic violence. In Hyman SE, Tesar GE (eds): Manual of Psychiatric Emergencies, 3rd ed. Boston, Little, Brown, 1994.
15. Schouten R: Allegations of sexual abuse: A new area of liability risk. Harv Rev Psychiatry 1:350–352, 1994.
16. Schreier HA, Libow J: Hurting for Love: Münchhausen's by Proxy Syndrome. New York, Guilford Press, 1993.

81. INVOLUNTARY TREATMENT: HOSPITALIZATION AND MEDICATIONS

John A. Menninger, M.D.

1. Why is involuntary hospitalization necessary?

Although the number of involuntary hospitalizations relative to total psychiatric admissions has decreased considerably in the United States from 90% in 1949 to 55% in 1980,[3] civil commitment of the mentally ill remains a frequent route for inpatient treatment. A majority of persons suffering from severe mental illness show limited insight into their illness. Schizophrenic patients, in particular, may show no recognition that they have a mental illness or need treatment. Depressed patients who are unable to envision hope or recall a better time may be suicidal and unwilling to seek treatment. Manic individuals who have become markedly grandiose and deny that they have any kind of problem or illness that needs treatment may display behaviors that put themselves or others in danger. Other patients may recognize their symptoms as part of an illness but disagree with and refuse recommended treatment. Untreated depression, mania, and psychosis can have devastating effects on both the affected individual and those around him or her: suicide, assaults on others, inadvertent tragedies stemming from delusional thinking, financial and social ruin, and inability to adequately care for one's own needs. Because insight is often lacking, civil commitment is often initiated by others who witness or are the brunt of concerning behavior, whether they be family members, police, or mental health providers.

2. What is the legal basis for involuntary commitment?

The state's authority to commit individuals stems from two legal theories: *parens patriae* and the police power of the state.

Parens patriae, which literally means "parent of the country," provides the sovereign power with authority to protect citizens who for reasons of mental or physical disability or because they are unsupervised minors cannot adequately protect or care for themselves. Intervention by the state is indicated for individuals who are deemed unable to make rational decisions for themselves, including the mentally ill who are "gravely disabled" or suicidal. The state is also obligated to make the decision that is in the best interest of the individual and most clearly reflects the choice that the individual would have made if he or she were competent to do so.

The legal theory of **police power** provides the state with the authority to act for the protection of society and the general welfare of its citizens. In the process of such protection, isolation and confinement of dangerous individuals may be necessary. Not only the criminal element and persons with highly contagious diseases may be detained, but also the mentally ill who are a risk to others. Whereas *parens patriae* provides for the protection of the individual, police power is generally invoked on behalf of society against the individual.

3. Who can be involuntarily hospitalized?

The legal standards specifying the criteria for civil commitment vary widely from state to state. The clinician must be aware of the specific criteria for his or her state. The presence of a mental illness is a prerequisite for civil commitment. Other criteria frequently include dangerous behavior toward self or others, grave disability, and the need for treatment. Over the past three decades there has been a general shift among most states from standards based on the individual's need for treatment to standards that require the person to be considered dangerous to self or others. However, some states have recently modified their statutes to allow for involuntary hospitalization of persons who are in need of treatment but are not imminently dangerous to themselves or others.

Less common criteria used by some states include the responsiveness of the mental illness to treatment and the availability of appropriate treatment at the facility to which the patient will be committed; refusal of voluntary admission; lack of a capacity to consent to or refuse psychiatric treatment or hospitalization; future danger to property; and involuntary hospitalization as the least restrictive alternative.

4. What disorders does the term mentally ill include?

The legal definition of the term mental illness, as spelled out in each state's statutes, varies considerably. Except for Utah, the statutes do not include specific psychiatric diagnoses but instead define mental illness in terms of its effects on the individual's thinking or behavior. Some definitions are rather vague; for example, in the District of Columbia mental illness means "a psychosis or other disease which substantially impairs the mental health of a person." Most definitions include some deleterious effect of the illness. For example, in Georgia mentally ill "shall mean having a disorder of thought or mood which significantly impairs the judgment, behavior, capacity to recognize reality, or ability to cope with the ordinary demands of life." Some definitions are qualified by a reference to the need for treatment. Hawaii's statute specifies that a mentally ill person has "psychiatric disorder or other disease which substantially impairs the person's mental health and necessitates treatment or supervision." Many definitions include aspects of dangerousness. Oregon's statute declares that a mentally ill person is "a person who, because of a mental disorder, is either (a) dangerous to himself or others; or (b) unable to provide for his basic personal needs and is not receiving such care as is necessary for his health or safety."

5. Is someone with a developmental disability considered mentally ill?

Although developmental disability (mental retardation) is described in the Diagnostic and Statistical Manual of Mental Disorders, 4th ed. (DSM-IV), it is frequently not considered a mental illness for the purposes of civil commitment. Many statutes completely exclude mental retardation from their definition of mentally ill, whereas others note that such a disorder may not constitute mental illness but does not preclude a comorbid mental illness. A few statutes specifically include mental retardation per se.

6. Are other diagnoses excluded in the definition of mentally ill?

In a few state statutes, the definition of mentally ill specifically excludes other disorders, most commonly alcoholism, drug addiction, and epilepsy. Some exclude "simple intoxication" with either alcohol or drugs. A small number exclude sociopathy, severe personality disorders in general, senility, and organic brain syndrome. Some statutes specifically include alcoholism and drug addiction. Maine's statute includes "persons suffering from the effects of the use of drugs, narcotics, hallucinogens or intoxicants, including alcohol, but not including mentally retarded or sociopathic persons."

7. What is grave disability?

The exact definition of grave disability varies from state to state. In general, the term refers to an inability to care adequately for one's own needs. In some states, a person is gravely disabled if he or she cannot care for basic needs without the assistance of others, even if family or friend are currently providing such care. In other states, the person must be without basic needs of food, clothing, shelter, or essential medical care.

8. What are the differences between emergency detention, observational institutionalization, and extended commitment?

Involuntary hospitalization may be divided into emergency, observational, and extended commitment. Each has a specific purpose, although there is often considerable overlap. All states provide for some form of emergency detention, in which the intent is immediate psychiatric intervention to treat what is currently, or soon to become, an emergency situation. Emergency detention allows for an initial psychiatric assessment and at least temporary treatment for an individual who, for example, has presented a danger to self. Some states include statutes that provide for observational commitment. A person satisfying the appropriate criteria may be hospitalized so that the treatment staff and psychiatrist may further observe him or her to determine the diagnosis and to provide limited treatment. Formal procedures for extended commitment can be found in nearly every state. Such commitment allows for continued psychiatric treatment of individuals who meet one or more of the state's specific criteria (usually dangerousness to self or others or grave disability; less common criteria are discussed above) but would otherwise refuse treatment.

9. Who can initiate involuntary hospitalization?

The specifics of which professionals or persons may initiate civil commitment vary among states, and usually within a state depending on the type of commitment sought (e.g., emergency detention or extended commitment). In general, the application for emergency detention is less formal and extended commitment more formal; observational commitment (where available) is somewhere between.

Emergency detention generally may be initiated by another adult, usually a family member or friend who has witnessed the person's deterioration and dangerous behavior. The police also frequently initiate the process, although some states require judicial approval before the person can be detained. A number of states provide for medical certification; that is, an evaluation from a physician stating that the person meets the statutory criterion is adequate to proceed with hospitalization.

Application for **observational commitment** often may be made by any citizen with good reason, although some states limit the application to physicians or hospital personnel. Most states require court approval.

The procedure to request **extended commitment** is the most formal and usually more detailed than the applications for other forms of commitment. In general, one or more of a specific group of people may complete the appropriate forms to request involuntary treatment. Although this group may include spouses, relatives, friends, guardians, and public officials, it is often limited to physicians, hospital superintendents, and other mental health professionals, such as certain licensed social workers and nurses. Even in states that allow for other persons to initiate commitment, generally only a physician can extend commitment beyond the initial period. Often the application must be accompanied by a certificate or affidavit from a physician in which the person's psychiatric presentation, pertinent history, recent behavior warranting commitment, initial diagnosis, and recommendations for treatment are described in detail. Some states require statements from two physicians or an additional statement from a psychologist, mental health board or similar designee. In virtually all states extended commitment is a judicial process. A hearing is scheduled, and either a judge or a jury decides whether to uphold the request.

10. How long does involuntary hospitalization last?

Emergency detention is designed to provide for an assessment of a dangerous situation. It is generally limited to a brief period, usually 3–5 days; the period ranges from only 24 hours in a few states to 20 days in New Jersey. The length of an observational commitment, in states that allow it, varies from 48 hours in Alaska to 6 months in West Virginia. Before the expiration of the emergency or observational commitment, the patient must either agree to voluntary hospitalization or be discharged; otherwise, civil commitment proceedings must be initiated. Extended commitment is also limited; 6 months is a typical period. If at the end of that period the treating psychiatrist recommends continued involuntary treatment, application for further extension of civil commitment may be made. Again the length of time is finite, often 1½–2 times longer than the initial commitment. The possibility for renewal at the end of each period continues as long as it is requested and the patient continues to meet the statutory criteria.

11. Is mental commitment possible on an outpatient basis?

Yes. Many states explicitly provide for outpatient commitment, whereas others simply do not prohibit the extension of civil commitment to outpatient programs. In states with statutes that specifically address outpatient commitment, the length of commitment is generally limited but somewhat longer than for inpatient commitment. The specific criteria and procedures are similar to those for inpatient commitment and likewise vary from state to state. The goal of outpatient commitment may be continued involuntary treatment in a less restrictive setting than the inpatient unit or an attempt to avoid inpatient treatment for a patient whose condition is deteriorating. If the patient fails to comply with the conditions of treatment, rehospitalization is indicated.

12. Which patients are appropriate for outpatient commitment?

Patients appropriate for outpatient commitment include those who have shown a good response to psychiatric medications in the past but are noncompliant with medications and other aspects of treatment without continued coercion. Involuntary outpatient treatment is also indicated for patients who require considerable structure to their lives and support from others to maintain adequate functioning outside the hospital. For outpatient commitment to be realistically tenable, the facility, often a mental health center, should be capable of adequate outreach. Also needed is a high degree of cooperation and communication between the courts authorizing commitment and the outpatient programs as well as between the outpatient and inpatient facilities.

13. What are the rights of patients who have been involuntarily hospitalized?

Persons involuntarily hospitalized maintain a number of rights, some of which are specifically related to the commitment proceedings and come under the rubric of due process. Such rights usually include notice of commitment, objection to confinement, representation by an attorney, presence at the commitment hearing, trial by jury, independent psychiatric examination, and change to voluntary status. Additional civil rights of the mentally ill, regardless of their legal status, generally include humane care and treatment; treatment in the least restrictive setting; free and open communication with the outside world via telephone or mail; and meetings with visitors, particularly their attorney, physician, or clergy; confidentiality of records; possession of their own clothing and money; payment for any work done in the hospital; absentee ballot voting; and being informed of such rights. Many of these rights may be temporarily restricted by the staff if deemed necessary (e.g., while the patient is in restraints or seclusion).

14. Can one treat an involuntary patient?

Just because a patient is admitted involuntarily, treatment cannot be forced. However, involuntary admission does not preclude treatment either. Many patients, despite being hospitalized on a civil commitment, are both amenable and receptive to treatment. They may disagree that they need to be in a hospital, but ironically they do not disagree that they need treatment. It is important to continue to educate patients who deny the need for treatment about their condition, psychiatric diagnosis, and treatment options. The refusal for voluntary hospitalization and voluntary treatment should be sought, explored, and discussed to foster a therapeutic alliance. Simple education or addressing concerns of the patient may allow him or her to decide to sign into the hospital volitionally and/or to agree to treatment. Severe psychosis, mania, or depression, of course, may result in an impasse that requires the court or judge to decide. However, many patients who are initially brought into the hospital involuntarily may later be willing to sign themselves into the hospital and actively participate in their treatment. It is important to recognize that the same therapeutic approaches that help to foster a therapeutic relationship with voluntary patients also help to engage involuntary patients in treatment.

15. May involuntarily hospitalized patients refuse to take medications?

Generally, yes. A majority of states consider all patients, even mentally ill patients hospitalized involuntarily, competent to make personal decisions, including whether to take psychotropic medications, unless they are specifically found legally incompetent by a court of law. Most states provide that an involuntary patient's refusal of medications may be overridden only by court hearing. Many states allow a legally appointed guardian to consent for the patient. A small number of states specifically recognize the right of voluntary patients to refuse medications.

Although a patient's refusal to take medications may stem from delusional thinking or a denial that anything is wrong, the reasons also may be based in reality. The patient may have previously had an intolerable side effect to the medication in question. It is essential to explain the recommended pharmacologic treatments, including expected benefits and possible adverse effects, and to explore fully the reasons behind the patient's refusal. Negotiation and compromise, such as using an alternate medication of the same class or initiating the medication at a lower dose, may be helpful and allow for treatment to proceed.

16. What is the difference between involuntary medications and emergency medications?

Emergency medications are ordered acutely by the treating psychiatrist or physician for a patient who is considered imminently dangerous to self or others, either physically or psychologically, and refuses to take the medications freely. Examples of such situations include the dehydrated and delirious manic patient who is already in restraints but continues to thrash about and bang his or her head against the bed frame. Emergency medications should work acutely (e.g., neuroleptics and benzodiazepines as opposed to antidepressants and mood stabilizers) and must target the serious presenting symptoms. The clinical need for emergency medications must be reassessed frequently, from every several hours to every 24 hours. Often a second opinion about the appropriateness of the emergency medications must be obtained from another physician. Emergency medications are usually limited to a few days.

Involuntary medications are granted by a court in nonemergent situations. Mentally ill persons who require chronic administration of medication and yet have minimal insight into their need may warrant involuntary medications. The treating psychiatrist or physician generally applies for the administration of involuntary medications with an accompanying affidavit supporting the opinion that the patient is mentally ill and incompetent to participate in treatment decisions and that the medications are clinically indicated. The statement also may need to review the patient's prior noncompliance with medication and expected benefit and potential side effects. Some states require that involuntary medications may be requested only for patients who are currently under a civil commitment. The criteria for involuntary medications vary from state to state but commonly include such aspects as incompetence to participate in decisions about treatment and expected clinical deterioration or dangerous behavior to self or others without the medications. Court-ordered involuntary medications are time-limited, often lasting only as long as the patient's civil commitment or for a period set by the judge. Extension beyond that time requires a reappraisal of the patient's condition, response to treatment, and likelihood of future compliance.

17. Can electroconvulsive therapy be given involuntarily?

Many states have provisions in their statutes that specifically allow for refusal of electroconvulsive therapy (ECT). If the person is considered incompetent, then a court order or a guardian's consent is required. If the situation is viewed as a life-threatening emergency, some states allow for ECT to be administered without consent of either the patient or a guardian; however, such consent or a court order should be obtained as soon as possible. Often a second opinion about the appropriateness of treatment and the person's competency to consent must also be obtained. Some states limit the use of ECT to certain psychiatric disorders or age groups; some also limit the number of treatments that can be administered to a patient each year.

18. What are the proper indications for seclusion or restraints?

Both seclusion and restraints are generally viewed as appropriate and sometimes necessary parts of inpatient psychiatric treatment, given the proper indications. Restraints are defined as the physical incapacitation of the person, either in total or in part, by tying him or her securely to a bed or chair, frequently with leather straps. Seclusion refers to the placement of an individual in isolated confinement. A seclusion room is typically small, securely built, and unfurnished or minimally furnished, with a lockable door. The door usually has a small window for viewing the patient or a mounted camera for close monitoring. The most common clinical indications for the use of such external constraints are (1) prevention of serious injury to self or others when other treatment techniques are unsuccessful or inappropriate and (2) prevention of serious physical damage to the inpatient unit or marked disruption of the ward. Other less common reasons include their use as part of a specific behavior therapy program or the patient's own request.

19. What are the legal constraints on the use of seclusion and restraints?

Most states have either specific statutes or administrative rules that regulate the use of restraints. About one-half of states have similar regulations for the use of locked seclusion. In general, the use of restraints and seclusion requires a physician's written order; is limited in duration (often to 24 hours); and must be accompanied by frequent monitoring of the patient's condition, usually by the nursing staff, with documentation of the assessment and reasons for continued seclusion or restraints. If seclusion or restraints are necessary beyond the initial period, a physician must conduct a direct examination, sign another written order, document the behaviors that necessitate continued external constraints, and establish that such measures are the least restrictive intervention. When restraints or seclusion have been used for several consecutive days, a mandatory review by the medical director or superintendent is common.

20. Which is the most restrictive intervention: seclusion, restraints, or involuntary medication?

There is no clearly established hierarchy of intrusiveness. The choice of the most appropriate treatment of a violent psychotic patient varies with the situation, and different clinicians may give opposing views.

21. Who can authorize psychiatric admission of children?

Statutes detailing the psychiatric admission procedures for children are often convoluted and vary widely. In general, children (i.e., legal minors) are considered legally incompetent. This includes incompetence to make a decision about psychiatric hospitalization. The past two decades have seen a number of changes with increased recognition by many states of certain rights of due process for minors. Most states continue to allow a child's parent or guardian to approve admission to a psychiatric hospital regardless of the child's wishes. They also often provide that a child may not be discharged from a mental hospital without authorization from the parents. A number of states have statutes that provide for parentally authorized admission for younger children (up to the age of 13 or 14 years), but older minors have the rights of due process, including a hearing and counsel, either automatically or if they protest their hospitalization. Once hospitalized, the minor's continued need for inpatient treatment must be reviewed periodically, from every 10 days (in Arizona) to every 60 days in other states. Most states now permit older children to admit themselves voluntarily into a psychiatric hospital. The minimal age ranges from 12 years in Georgia to 17 years in Florida. When a child refuses admission for psychiatric hospitalization and the state does not allow for parental consent, emergency commitment proceedings must be initiated.

22. Do the criteria for civil commitment of children differ from those for adults?

The clinical indications for the commitment of minors may differ from those for adults in particular states. In general, if a child is suicidal or homicidal or has a severe mental illness, he or she may satisfy criteria for involuntary hospitalization. Some state statutes include "being in need of treatment," which allows admission of children who do not respond adequately to intensive outpatient intervention. As with the statutes for adults, the specific criteria and procedures vary markedly among states. Usually a psychiatrist must conduct an examination to determine the appropriate services for the child. The assessment must include an interview with the child alone and a thorough review of the child's history. The evaluation should use as many possible sources of information as possible, such as parents, school, and social agencies.

23. Can a child's parents authorize involuntary psychotropic medication?

Many states consider a parent's consent for psychiatric treatment adequate to overrule a minor's refusal to take medication. However, if the treatment is considered unusual or hazardous, such as electroconvulsive therapy or high doses of medications, parental consent may be inadequate; in such cases, the clinician should obtain authorization from a court.

24. May a patient who was admitted voluntarily and then wishes to leave be converted to an involuntary patient?
Yes. When a person who has admitted him- or herself voluntarily wishes to be discharged against the recommendations of the physician and treatment team, the staff are provided time to assess whether the patient meets criteria for civil commitment. If such criteria are met, the process of emergency detention must be initiated at once.

25. What is the difference between incompetence and civil commitment?
  Competence is divided into legal competence and clinical competence. Legal competence refers to a declaration by a court of law that the person is unable to manage adequately his or her assets or to make decisions about personal care and welfare. All adults, including those with severe mental illness, are presumed legally competent until found otherwise. Clinical competence, also called **decision-making capacity,** refers to the ability to comprehend a situation and the consequences of decisions and to communicate such comprehension to others. It refers to a particular question and depends on the patient's understanding and the risks of the proposed intervention. A person may be considered incompetent in one sphere but not another; e.g., the person may be competent to concur with psychiatric hospitalization, but incompetent to consent to ECT. Patients may be subject to **civil commitment** because they fulfill the particular criteria in that state; e.g., they have a mental illness that renders them markedly delusional with paranoia and suicidal thoughts. However, if they fully understand the risks and benefits of a particular treatment or procedure, whether it is receiving medications, having their teeth pulled, or having surgery for gallstones, they remain competent to accept or refuse, regardless of the decision they make. Conversely, an individual with dementia or mental retardation may not have a major psychiatric illness requiring hospitalization but still be clinically incompetent to make a particular decision.

26. Can mentally ill patients who appear to be incapable of understanding their legal rights with regard to hospitalization be admitted voluntarily?
For the most part, unless someone has already been declared legally incompetent, he or she is presumed to be legally competent to make decisions about personal welfare, including psychiatric admission. Some states, however, specify that a patient's decision for voluntary admission must be competent. In such states, the patient would require civil commitment.

27. Is the person who initiated involuntary hospitalization liable for false imprisonment?
A patient claiming to have been negligently hospitalized may seek malpractice litigation for false imprisonment. Such litigation is rare because of the legal protections that ensure due process. Important guidelines for clinicians involved in civil commitments include the following: they should (1) be familiar with both the commitment statutes of their state and the appropriate administrative policies for their facility; (2) act in good faith; (3) conduct a comprehensive psychiatric examination of the person in question; (4) complete all aspects of the necessary commitment forms; (5) describe the specific behaviors and symptoms that support the presence of mental illness and the need for treatment, including behaviors fulfilling commitment criteria such as dangerousness; (6) outline the recommended treatment for the person's condition with consideration for the least restrictive setting; and (7) obtain consultation for equivocal cases.

BIBLIOGRAPHY

Civil commitment in general
  1. Appelbaum PS, Gutheil TG: Clinical Handbook of Psychiatry and the Law, 2nd ed. Baltimore, Williams & Wilkins, 1991.
  2. Bittman BJ, Convit A: Competency, civil commitment, and the dangerousness of the mentally ill. J Forensic Sci 38:1460–1466, 1993.

3. Brakel SJ, Parry J, Weiner BA: The Mentally Disabled and the Law, 3rd ed. Chicago, American Bar Foundation, 1985.
4. Hiday VA: Coercion in civil commitment: Process, preferences, and outcome. Int J Law Psychiatry 15:359–377, 1992.
5. Miller RD: Need-for-treatment criteria for involuntary civil commitment: Impact in practice. Am J Psychiatry 149:1380–1384, 1992.
6. Munetz MR, Geller JL: The least restrictive alternative in the post institutional era. Hosp Community Psychiatry 44:967–973, 1993.
7. Weiner BA, Wettstein RM: Legal Issues in Mental Health Care. New York, Plenum Press, 1993.

Involuntary medications
8. Appelbaum PS: The right to refuse treatment with antipsychotic medications: Retrospect and prospect. Am J Psychiatry 145:413–419, 1988.
9. Cournos F, McKinnon K, Stanley B: Outcome of involuntary medication in a state hospital system. Am J Psychiatry 148:489–494, 1991.
10. Schwartz HI, Vingiano W, Bezirganian Perez C: Autonomy and the right to refuse treatment: Patient's attitudes after involuntary medications. Hosp Community Psychiatry 39:1049–1054, 1988.

Involuntary ECT
11. Mahler H, Co BT, Dinwiddie S: Studies in involuntary civil commitment and involuntary electroconvulsive therapy. J Nerv Mental Disorders 174:97–106, 1986.

Outpatient commitment
12. Geller JL: Clinical guidelines for the use of involuntary outpatient treatment. Hosp Community Psychiatry 41:749–755, 1990.
13. Miller RD: An update on involuntary civil commitment to outpatient treatment. Hosp Community Psychiatry 43:79–81, 1992.
14. Mulvey EP, Geller JL, Roth LH: The promise and peril of involuntary outpatient commitment. Am Psychol 42:571–584, 1987.

Restraint and seclusion
15. Fisher WA: Restraint and seclusion: A review of the literature. Am J Psychiatry 151:1584–1591, 1994.

Insight into mental illness
16. Amador XF, Strauss DH, Yale SA, Gorman JM: Awareness of illness in schizophrenia. Schizophr Bull 17:113–132, 1991.

Psychiatric diagnoses
17. American Psychiatric Association: Diagnostic and Statistical Manual of Mental Disorders, 4th ed. Washington, DC, American Psychiatric Association, 1994.

82. COMPETENCE AND INSANITY

Harold J. Bursztajn, M.D., and Archie Brodsky, B.A.

1. Are competence and insanity purely medical concepts?

No. In common usage they are considered legal concepts, because they represent specific judgments made by the courts. However, they can also be regarded as distinct medicolegal concepts. Although clinical data contribute to the determination of both competence and insanity, the determination also requires a knowledge of relevant statutes as well as a comprehensive analysis of both subjective and objective data. Such a deep level of analysis is not normally a part of clinical evaluation. Indeed, the standards for determining competence or insanity are multidimensional and somewhat case-specific. Relevant factors include:

1. Applicable laws in the governing jurisdiction (e.g., "insanity" involves judgment of lack of criminal responsibility based on a particular standard specified by statute);

2. The act or decision for which a person is to be judged competent or incompetent, sane or insane; and

3. Contextual factors defining the meaning of the act for that person at a particular place and time.

The following glossary provides a guide to basic terminology used in connection with determinations of competence or insanity:

Burden of proof: The obligation in court of the moving party to demonstrate the existence of certain facts or to suffer loss of the proceeding.

Competence: The legal recognition of an individual's ability to perform a task. The concept is not applied globally. Rather, it is directed at a specific category of demands.

Deposition: A form of legal discovery in civil proceedings in which the litigants may question potential witnesses under oath to discover the testimony that they are likely to present at trial.

* Diminished capacity: The response of a criminal defendant requesting to be partially excused for misconduct on the basis of mental condition.

Expert witness: An individual permitted to present opinion in court on matters of fact that are beyond the expertise of ordinary citizens.

* Imperfect self-defense: The response of a criminal defendant requesting to be excused for misconduct on the basis of a mental state of self-defense which is itself substantially influenced by a mental disorder or defect.

Informed consent: Authorization given by a person who is free from coercion or undue influence, who has been given adequate information on the decision to be made, and who has the capacity to understand the information disclosed.

Insanity defense: The response of a criminal defendant requesting to be [entirely] excused for misconduct on the basis of mental condition.

Jurisdiction: The scope of a specific court's authority. A court's decision in a particular case sets precedent for all similar cases arising within the court's geographic boundaries.

Standard of proof: The degree of probability to which factual assertions must be proven to allow a moving party to prevail in litigation.

From Group for the Advancement of Psychiatry, Committee on Psychiatry and Law: The Mental Health Professional and the Legal System (Report No. 131). New York, Brunner/Mazel, 1991, pp 181–186, with permission. (* indicates additions or modifications by the present authors.)

2. Do clinicians make determinations of competence and insanity?
No. Determinations of competence and insanity are made by the courts with the help of assessments by qualified professionals. Ordinarily, such assessments should not be made by a clinician who is treating the person to be evaluated.

3. What professional guidelines apply to combining the roles of treater and evaluator?
The following excerpts from the ethical guidelines of the American Academy of Psychiatry and the Law (AAPL) make clear that an attempt to combine the roles of treater and evaluator involves the clinician in both a **clash of perspectives** and a **conflict of interest**.

> . . . the psychiatrist should inform the evaluee that although he is a psychiatrist, he is not the evaluee's "doctor." . . . There is a continuing obligation to be sensitive to the fact that although a warning has been given, there may be slippage and a treatment relationship may develop in the mind of the examinee.

> A treating psychiatrist should generally avoid agreeing to be an expert witness or to perform an evaluation of his patient for legal purposes because a forensic evaluation usually requires that other people be interviewed and testimony may adversely affect the therapeutic relationship.

4. Discuss the rationale behind the AAPL guidelines.
The reasons for avoiding duality of roles are evident. On the one hand, the empathic, subjective stance that the clinician takes to relieve the patient's suffering and to promote growth is largely incompatible with objective evaluation. On the other hand, the distancing required to perform an objective evaluation, not to mention the loss of confidentiality, tends to undermine the therapeutic alliance. Therefore, when the treating clinician is asked to perform an evaluation for the court, the appropriate response is to refer the patient for a forensic psychiatric evaluation. Likewise, when a forensic evaluation lapses into a treatment relationship despite one's best efforts to the contrary, the wisest response is to refer the patient for further forensic evaluation, especially if the plan is to continue treatment.

5. What is competence?
Competence is generally understood to be the mental soundness necessary to carry out certain legally defined acts. A person is presumed competent unless it is shown that the person has a mental disease or defect that impairs his or her ability to understand the nature or consequences of the act in question. Competence is a matter of degree, but for most legal purposes it is the minimal rather than maximal standard of competence that must be met.

When one moves beyond general descriptions of the elements of competence (such as "understanding of available choices, capacity to make those choices, and freedom from undue influence") to specific medicolegal applications, the term has no single definition. Competence is selective and compartmentalized and must be assessed in relation to the decision or act in question: "Competent to do what, and in what context?"

6. Distinguish between determination of competence in civil law and assessment of criminal responsibility.
Determinations of competence in civil law include competence to give (or withhold) informed consent to medical treatment and competence to make contracts and wills. In criminal law, psychiatrists are asked to assess a defendant's competence to stand trial, to confess, to waive Miranda rights, or to act as his or her own attorney. Psychiatrists are also asked to act as consultants to probation officers or to the courts in preparation of presentencing and probation reports. A psychiatrist is asked to evaluate other areas of competence only on rare occasions; for example, an often neglected question is the defendant's competence to accept a plea bargain. A psychiatrist who is asked to perform an evaluation in a criminal case must ask the attorney to specify which area of competence is in question.

On the other hand, the **assessment of criminal responsibility** (which may hinge on a determination of sanity or insanity) is different in kind from what is normally referred to as assessment of competence. For example, when a question of diminished capacity arises in relation to criminal responsibility, it refers to a distinct set of faculties such as formation of the intent to commit a particular act, appreciation of moral or legal wrongfulness, or ability to conform one's behavior to the requirements of law. Therefore, the questions of competence and criminal responsibility will be treated separately in this chapter, as they are in everyday usage. At the same time, the deeper connection between the two (i.e., that lack of criminal responsibility by reason of insanity presupposes a generally or specifically disabled and, in some particular sense, incompetent mental state) needs to be understood.

7. What decision by the U.S. Supreme Court had a major effect on the definition of competence?

Classically, competence was defined mainly in terms of cognitive awareness. In 1960, in *Dusky v. U.S.*, the U.S. Supreme Court took this conception to its limit, and perhaps beyond, when it defined competence as "not only a factual but a rational understanding."

8. How has the definition of competence evolved since 1960?

As understanding of human psychology deepened, psychiatrists also took into account an affective dimension. That is, various impairments characterized by overwhelming affect, while not leading to psychosis, may restrict a person's sense of choice or hope for the future. Such conditions include full-fledged posttraumatic stress disorder (PTSD) as well as more subtle but nonetheless real syndromes of trauma response (e.g., pathological grief and survivor guilt; see question 12 for an example). Given the many factors that affect competence, the evaluator who goes beyond global assessments often finds that some capacities are impaired, whereas others are not. The evaluator must be alert for subtle, fluctuating signs of incompetence.

9. Distinguish between intrapsychic and interpersonal dimensions of competence.

Competence has both intrapsychic and interpersonal dimensions. The intrapsychic dimensions are often the ones initially addressed. Thus, a forensic evaluation includes a mental status examination (both formal and informal) to look at the person's biologic and intrapsychic integrity, searching for disorders of cognition (e.g., delusions), affect (e.g., hopelessness), or volition (e.g., impulse disinhibition) that may constrain the relevant judgment or behavior. On the other hand, one cannot fully assess a person's competence to consent to treatment without also taking into account his or her functioning in the interpersonal realm of relationships with the caregivers involved (see questions 10–12). In the case of testamentary capacity (the competence required to make a last will and testament), interpersonal relationships are even more central to the assessment (see question 16). Likewise, a person's state of mind at the time of committing a criminal act is often contingent on the interpersonal context, including the perpetrator's perception of self, victim, and their relationship as well as their actual relationship.

10. What is competence to give informed consent to treatment?

Competent informed consent consists of three elements: decision-making capacity, requisite information, and voluntariness. Although all three elements are usually viewed as individual assessments, they are also a function of the patient-clinician relationship. The fact that information has been given does not mean that it has been received or retained. For example, information may be conveyed in an overbearing way or may be incomprehensible to a patient who is more visually than verbally oriented. Voluntariness may be compromised by coercive pressures, whether from clinicians who believe that they know what is best for the patient or from an institutional culture that promotes cost-containment. Such deficits in information or voluntariness, in turn, may overwhelm the patient's decision-making capacity.

Informed consent, therefore, is not a pro forma response to a checklist; rather, it is a process of mutual engagement in decision making. Thus, the competence to give informed consent includes the capacity to engage in a dialogue about benefits and risks and to apply the discussion meaningfully to one's present situation. This capacity may be either enhanced or diminished by the manner in which clinicians carry out their side of the dialogue.

For instance, a recent Massachusetts malpractice trial revolved around the issue of informed consent even though, as a matter of law, the case was not about informed consent because the pro forma requirements had been satisfied. In *Meador v. Stahler and Gheridian* (1993), two physicians were held liable for the complications resulting from their having ordered and performed an allegedly unwanted cesarean section, although a consent form had been signed and no claim was made that the surgery was performed in a negligent manner. In classical informed-consent cases, patients typically have claimed that the risks of recommended procedures were withheld or understated. In this case, however, the physicians were sued successfully for communicating the risks of an alternative procedure in a manner that misled and frightened the patient, thereby undermining her competence to give informed consent (e.g., by allegedly telling her that her uterus would "explode like a hydrogen bomb" if she attempted to give birth vaginally after a prior cesarean section).

11. When is a psychiatrist likely to be consulted about a patient's competence to give informed consent?

Consultations in this area occur in various ways. Commonly, a psychiatrist may be consulted by a general health care professional when a patient refuses medical treatment. Another common situation occurs when a psychiatrist is consulted by a mental health professional when a patient refuses further psychiatric treatment.

The two situations call for different responses. When consulted by a general health care professional, the consulting psychiatrist typically performs a basic psychiatric evaluation to identify crisis-intervention or treatment issues. Once in this consultation/liaison role, the psychiatrist attends to the patient's suffering in the capacity of a clinician. Therefore, if further evaluation of the patient's competence is needed for medicolegal purposes, referral to a forensic psychiatrist should be made. If, on the other hand, another psychiatrist or mental health clinician already is in the treating role, the psychiatrist who is consulted about the refusal of treatment is in a position to make the actual forensic evaluation a primary focus.

12. Describe common pitfalls in the assessment of a patient's competence to give informed consent.

A common bias of clinicians is to obtain a consultation only when the patient refuses treatment, not when the patient agrees to treatment. In terms of risk management as well as the patient's best interest, however, incompetent consent can be as much an issue as incompetent refusal. The coerced cesarean section in question 10 may be understood as an example of incompetent consent. When a question of competent consent arises, a forensic psychiatric consultation is helpful.

It is also a mistake to try to assess competence to consent to treatment globally rather than in relation to the specific circumstances of treatment. Competence to consent to treatment, like competence in general, is not an indivisible concept. A patient may be competent to consent to treatment in most circumstances, but not to a particular kind of treatment or to treatment offered by a particular clinician.

For example, a man in severe congestive heart failure secondary to a surgically correctable cardiac condition refused consent to surgery despite his ability to recite the risks and benefits of the recommended operation. The patient revealed to the consulting psychiatrist that his wife had died 15 years earlier after what had been considered a minor, low-risk operation. The psychiatric consultation gave the patient an opportunity to work through the unresolved grief that impaired his competence to consent. Subsequently he consented and after surgery was grateful that his treating team did not "quit" on him, despite his initial refusal. He described the effect of the psychiatric consultation as "lifting a dark veil."

13. Is assessment of competence also affected by the examiner-examinee relationship and the circumstances of the examination?

Yes. Assessment of a patient's capacity to give informed consent may be biased by unrecognized fluctuations in competence resulting from the setting, time of day, variable medication side effects, rapid changes in pathophysiology, or other factors. The examination may be performed when the patient is at either his or her worst or best rather than in a usual state. Furthermore, a person may be found falsely competent on the basis of overidentification by the examiner or falsely incompetent on the basis of projection of the examiner's own despair or a breakdown in communication. For example, a patient who is frightened and not fluent in the examiner's language may respond with greater understanding to a visual model of the heart than to a strictly verbal description of a coronary bypass graft.

14. How are questions of patient competence raised in cases of alleged patient-clinician sexual contact?

Now it is rare to hear the argument that a patient has given informed consent to sexual contact with a clinician as part of treatment. Not so unusual is the argument that the patient has consented independently to treatment and to concurrent or subsequent sexual contact. The issue, then, is whether the patient is competent to consent to what may be self-destructive physical intimacy with the treating clinician outside of treatment.

From the clinician's standpoint, alleged patient consent to sexual contact is not a defense to the allegation of sexual misconduct. The clinician's fiduciary duty to refrain from sexual contact with patients makes questions of consent irrelevant as far as civil culpability is concerned. In states where such contact is not specified as criminal by statute, questions of competence to consent, as in the case of a patient who is psychotic or considered to suffer from multiple-personality disorder, may be raised to justify bringing criminal charges.

Nonetheless, questions of consent and of competence to consent often enter implicitly into civil litigation. The degree of damage, as suffered by the plaintiff or as perceived by a jury, often hinges on how competent and active the plaintiff was in initiating and maintaining the alleged sexual relationship. In addressing such questions, a thorough forensic evaluation of the plaintiff must recognize the complex interactions between character defenses and trauma in remembering and communicating.

15. What part does competence play in assessing the risk of suicide or violence?

Clinicians are asked to make decisions involving dangerousness to self or others in various contexts, including involuntary commitment and restriction of freedom during hospitalization. In such decisions, competence is an implicit if not explicit consideration. It becomes explicit in states where the criteria for involuntary commitment (in the presence of mental illness) include the ability to care for oneself as well as dangerousness to self or others. A recent proposal seeks to extend the criteria for temporary civil commitment to include incompetence to refuse hospitalization and the inability to live safely in freedom. The decision-making process that leads to commitment is thus analogous to the seeking of guardianship on the basis of incompetence to give or withhold informed consent to treatment.

An often neglected and yet essential aspect of the assessment of potential violence is the assessment of the patient's competence to engage in a dialogue with the clinician concerning potential harm to self or others and measures to prevent it. Dangerousness in itself is so salient to clinicians that the equally important question of the patient's capacity to participate responsibly in monitoring his or her dangerousness tends to pale by comparison. The multidimensional model of dangerousness presented below, in which competence appears as one dimension, illustrates a mindset useful in many areas of clinical decision making, such as addressing the multidimensional complexity of competence itself.

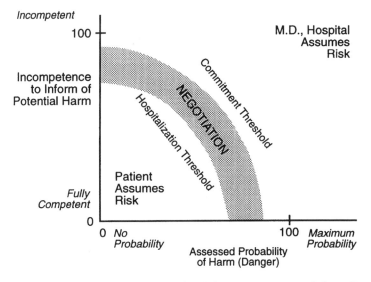

Multidimensional assessment of dangerousness in relation to competence to inform. From Gutheil TG, Bursztajn HJ, Brodsky A: The multidimensional assessment of dangerousness: Competence assessment in patient care and liability prevention. Bull Am Acad Psychiatry Law 14:123–129, 1986, with permission.

16. How do the principles of competence assessment apply to evaluating a last will and testament for testamentary capacity?

Familiarity with state statutes and case law is essential for framing the questions to be answered in the forensic psychiatric evaluation of testamentary capacity. Such questions emphasize functional as opposed to diagnostic considerations. For example, the Supreme Judicial Court of Massachusetts, in *Goddard v. Dupree* (1948), defined testamentary capacity as follows:

> Testamentary capacity requires ability on the part of the testator to understand and carry in mind, in a general way, the nature and situation of his property and his relations to those persons who would naturally have some claim to his remembrance. It requires freedom from delusion which is the effect of disease or weakness and which might influence the disposition of his property. And it requires ability at the time of execution of the alleged will to comprehend the nature of the act of making a will.

Thus, contrary to the all-too-common stigmatization of the mentally ill, a person with schizophrenia cannot be assumed thereby to lack testamentary capacity unless at least one of these specified functions is impaired. In this as in other areas, diagnosis does not by itself determine competence. At the same time, the evaluator must consider numerous possible sources of functional impairment. Often overlooked are impairments resulting from chronic, partially concealed alcohol use, early-onset organic brain syndromes, or drugs, especially pain-relieving drugs such as morphine, that may have subtle but real euphoric and/or dysphoric effects that alter judgment in relatively low dosages (by *Physician's Desk Reference* standards).

Testamentary capacity is customarily considered the lowest level of competence. Even someone who has a guardian of person may have testamentary capacity, despite a rebuttable presumption that she does not. Making a will is considered to require a lesser degree of competence than entering into a contract, for example, in which an adverse party seeks an advantageous position. However, clinicians who work with family dynamics may well find an adversarial relationship between the testator and another party or between two parties contending for the inheritance (in which case the testator must act as judge).

With respect to testamentary capacity, as with other forms of competence, the treating clinician should refer the patient to someone in a position to make an objective evaluation. Especially when deathbed revisions of a will are at issue, the treating clinician's proper concern with relieving the patient's suffering precludes such objectivity. The clinician may confuse competence to consent to treatment with competence to dispose of property, each of which must be assessed independently. A treating clinician may either overestimate or underestimate the deceased person's testamentary capacity. Overestimation may occur if the clinician feels threatened by virtue of having already honored the person's acceptance or refusal of treatment, whereas underestimation may occur if the clinician's most salient memories are of the person in a confused rather than coherent state.

17. Is competence to stand trial equivalent to criminal responsibility?
No. The two assessments have different tests, different time contexts, and different purposes. A person is considered competent to stand trial if he or she understands the nature of the charges and is able to cooperate with counsel. The assessment of competence to stand trial is a present-state examination, whereas determination of criminal responsibility is retrospective and pertains to the person's culpability at the time of the alleged act. Although the criteria for culpability (see question 20) represent a kind of competence at a deep-structural level, the two determinations are entirely separate matters in everyday practice.

Competence to stand trial is usually considered (subject to jurisdictional variations) the lowest level of competence in the criminal realm, because it is seen to require only a minimum of psychological functioning. However, notwithstanding the understandable desire to have defendants stand trial in a speedy, cost-effective way, the question of whether severely impaired clients have the capacity to assist counsel must be assessed on a case-by-case basis.

When clinicians untrained in forensic psychiatry become involved in competence determinations, essential distinctions may be lost. For example, in a prominent murder case (*New Hampshire v. Colbert*, 1992), the suspect was taken to a hospital emergency department. The clinician's finding that the alleged perpetrator was competent to consent to medical treatment was later equated in the courtroom with the suspect's state of mind at the time of the killings. Such extrapolations are clearly unfounded and unreliable. Moreover, when made by the treating clinician in courtroom testimony, they may be both unethical, because they involve a betrayal of the treatment relationship, and prejudicial, insofar as they unduly influence the jury by creating the impression that the accused must be guilty if the treating clinician is willing to testify against his or her own patient.

Of course, the clinician whose testimony is compelled by court order must conform to the requirements of the law. At the same time, the clinician must clarify (through prior notification) the limits of his or her testimony. The treating clinician can testify only as to fact; the primary focus on alleviating the patient's suffering precludes an objective, expert opinion. A referral to colleagues qualified to render an objective opinion may be helpful. Given such prior notification, the court usually is satisfied simply to receive the medical records in lieu of testimony.

18. Why does a person's competence to confess need to be assessed?
Competence to confess may be vitiated by mental disabilities produced by disorders such as psychotic depression, posttraumatic stress disorder, schizotypal personality, obsessive-compulsive disorder, and organic brain syndromes. After hours of hostile questioning, a person who is cognitively competent but made vulnerable by a major mental illness (e.g., schizophrenia, major depression) may come to "remember" committing a crime that he or she did not in fact commit. In Florida, for example, a schizophrenic man spent 9 years in prison for a double murder to which he had falsely confessed. False confessions typically are elicited by coercion and subsequent fear, combined with a conscious or unconscious need to be punished. False confessions also may result from false memory syndrome.

19. Define false memory syndrome.
False memory syndrome is often engendered by overzealous clinicians who cross the boundary between clinical assessment and forensic evaluation—for example, in allegations of child sexual

abuse during custody proceedings. Patients who suffer from immature defenses such as hypochondriasis, conversion hysteria (somatization), splitting (dividing people into saints and sinners), and projection (misattributing to others all personal feelings that are unacceptable to oneself) are especially vulnerable to suggestion by the treating clinician. Such patients often attempt to figure out and then conform to the working hypothesis used by the treating clinician to guide treatment.

Memories—whether reported to a therapist, an attorney, or a courtroom—cannot be accepted as accurate without a careful forensic evaluation of their reliability. People in a state of emotional distress readily remember events that did not occur or forget events that did occur. The pressure to repress traumatic memories or to reestablish control by filling in the gaps in memory is too great for reported memories to be taken at face value. Reported memories may be accurate in general outline but inaccurate in detail or vice versa. They may be further distorted by suggestion and even coaching (by therapists, family members, attorneys, or law enforcement personnel) as well as by a need to maintain a close personal attachment by confirming the other person's construction of past events.

The possibility of deliberate falsification of memory also must be considered. The malingering offender who has not been treated is usually more transparent than the one who has had a chance to practice his or her act during treatment. For example, the forensic psychiatric examiner's finding of multiple personality disorder in an untreated examinee may be prima facie more valid than the same finding in a treated examinee. In addition to possible faking, malingering, or exaggerating, the examiner must consider impairments of memory resulting from displacement (to maintain psychic equilibrium), projection (to maintain self-esteem), or the effects of organic conditions, drugs, or personality disorders.

20. What is criminal responsibility in relation to the insanity defense?

In relation to the classical insanity defense, state statutes may apply some variation of the following historical standards to establish criminal responsibility:

1. The *M'Naghten* **rule** excuses a defendant who, by virtue of a defect of reason or disease of the mind, does not know the nature and quality of the act or that the act is wrong.

2. The *Durham* **rule** excuses a defendant whose conduct is the product of mental disease or defect.

3. The **American Law Institute (ALI) test** excuses a defendant who, because of a mental disease or defect, lacks substantial capacity to appreciate the criminality (wrongfulness) of his or her conduct or to conform his or her conduct to the requirements of the law.

4. The **Federal Insanity Defense Reform Act of 1984** excuses a defendant who, "as a result of a severe mental disease or defect, was unable to appreciate the nature and quality or the wrongfulness of his acts."

Of these tests, the *Durham* rule is broadest in application, the *M'Naghten* rule narrowest. The permissive *Durham* rule, although important historically, is now used only in New Hampshire and the Virgin Islands and is generally referred to as the "product of mental illness" test. The American Law Institute (ALI) test represents an effort to find a middle ground by adding the element of volition to the cognitive standard established by the *M'Naghten* rule. The Federal Insanity Defense Reform Act, by removing the volitional element, essentially reverts to the *M'Naghten* standard. However, although specifying that the mental illness must be "severe," it retains the ALI's term "appreciate," thus allowing the primarily cognitive test to be interpreted as including an affective component.

21. How valid is the public concern that the insanity defense lets dangerous criminals go free?

Especially in highly publicized cases like that of presidential assailant John Hinckley, the insanity defense is used by its critics as a symbol of the failings of the criminal justice system. In fact, however, it is not a real cause of such failings. In an 8-state review, the insanity defense was used in only 1% of felony cases and was successful in only one-fourth of those cases. Indeed, from the point of view of public safety, it may be more effective to treat perpetrators in secure psychiatric facilities than to put them in prison, where they do not have the benefit of treatment and tend to return to the street sooner. In addition, they may either become victims of predatory career criminals or (because often they are easily impressionable) come to imitate them. The high rates of recidivism among previously incarcerated offenders offer little comfort to critics who would abolish the insanity defense.

In any case, partly because of the widespread fear (promoted by sensationalistic journalism) of letting vicious criminals go free, the insanity defense is rarely successful in contested cases. Emotionally evocative characteristics of both victims and perpetrators reduce the likelihood that an insanity defense will be considered nonprejudicially. The Hinckley verdict was the exception, not the rule.

22. What other factors contribute to the difficulty in persuading juries to accept the insanity defense?

Insanity pleas are far more often agreed upon by the prosecution and defense than contested. Largely out of public view, a stipulated "not guilty by reason of insanity" (NGRI) verdict is reached in many cases (more than 80% in one Oregon study) in which the question of sanity is raised. In other cases experts for the two sides agree that the defendant does not meet the jurisdiction's standard of insanity. In the small proportion of cases that actually go to trial—relatively well-publicized cases in which the experts disagree—the popular stereotype of psychiatry as unscientific is reinforced. Ironically, the fact that most cases do not go to trial because of the high interrelater reliability with which most psychiatric diagnoses are made leaves juries with the impression that psychiatrists always disagree. With this impression as a baseline and with two experts in front of them who in fact disagree, jurors naturally tend to disbelieve the field as a whole; this belief leads almost invariably to a guilty verdict.

Besides having to overcome popular stereotypes of mental illness as either fiction or the paradigm of the incoherent "madman," the defense expert has a difficult task from the beginning. Prosecution experts characterize complex acts such as concealment as evidence of rational behavior, even when a deeper analysis may reveal that such concealment is regressive behavior driven by psychosis. Moreover, defense experts often are hampered by limited funds, which make it difficult to budget both a comprehensive forensic evaluation and, where appropriate, the time needed for preparation of testimony to rebut a prosecution expert's negative findings. Finally, gender- and relationship-specific stereotypes, which predispose juries to deliver NGRI verdicts for women who kill their children or for children who kill their parents, result in guilty verdicts for men who kill.

23. What is diminished capacity?

The claim of diminished capacity is a more feasible substitute for the insanity defense in the current climate. Given the limited applicability of the insanity defense and the odds against its prevailing in court, diminished capacity is used with increasing frequency as a flexible (if partial) alternative, filling the need for some assessment of a defendant's mental state as a factor in criminal responsibility. There are two kinds of diminished capacity:

1. The first variant of diminished capacity negates an element of the charged crime by showing that the defendant lacked the requisite mental state to be found guilty of the crime as charged. This defense, when successful, usually results in a conviction on a lesser charge rather than outright acquittal. For example, a person found to have lacked the mental state necessary to commit first-degree murder (i.e., premeditation) may be convicted of second-degree murder. For a person found to have lacked the intent to kill, the charge may be reduced to involuntary manslaughter.

2. The second variant of diminished capacity may be viewed as a partial insanity defense. It is concerned not with whether the defendant entertained a particular mental state, but with why and how the defendant was in a state of mind that precluded full responsibility for his or her actions. This variant, too, is more likely to result in reduction than dismissal of charges. On the other hand, it resembles the insanity defense in that it provides a basis for extenuation (albeit a

controversial one), even if all the elements of the charged crime have been proved. This defense often centers on the impairing effects on decision making of posttraumatic stress disorder and its numerous offshoots, such as battered-woman syndrome. It raises the question of both intrapsychic and interpersonal capacity. Typically, a person's options become subjectively limited in the context of an oppressive relationship. For example, a battered woman who kills her abusive partner may argue that sustained abuse left her feeling that she "had no other choice."

Diminished capacity is also taken into account in the application of the new federal sentencing guidelines, which, after guilt has been determined, allow departures from otherwise mandated sentences if diminished capacity can be shown. Some states—for example, New Jersey—have also adopted this approach to sentencing.

24. Do considerations of diminished capacity form the basis for a claim of imperfect self-defense?
Imperfect self-defense is a prime example of the second variant of diminished capacity. To support a claim of imperfect self-defense, data about the defendant's state of mind at the time of the alleged crime must include the perception that the act was an act of self-defense. For example, a Vietnam War veteran who hears a truck backfire while he is arguing with another driver after a traffic accident may react as if he were under fire. Such a "false-alarm syndrome" may constitute the basis of an imperfect self-defense claim.

25. Are such conditions as battered-woman syndrome, rape trauma syndrome, child sexual abuse accommodation syndrome, and patient-therapist sex syndrome now recognized as legitimate bases for a defense of diminished capacity?
Expert testimony about battered-woman syndrome is admitted with increasing frequency in criminal cases. The courts are also grappling with the admissibility of other such syndromes. Descriptively, all of these labels have some basis in experience. Women are at serious risk of domestic violence, for example, and such abuse (like rape or sexual exploitation in therapy) has traumatic effects. Nonetheless, reliance on putative abuse and trauma syndromes presents serious pitfalls both for the treating psychiatrist and for the expert psychiatric witness. Such diagnoses are not recognized in the Diagnostic and Statistical Manual–IV (DSM–IV) and do not take the place of other diagnoses. They raise questions of unreliability of evidence (including false memories) as well as of stereotyping and stigmatization. Labeling people automatically as victims does not do justice to the enormous range of reactions to adversity of which people are capable. It is necessary, therefore, to evaluate each case individually rather than to assume an a priori syndrome. For example, patient-therapist sex syndrome is merely a hypothetical, schematic construction. A victim of such abuse in fact may suffer from any or all of the claimed symptoms, but each individual case requires careful examination to determine which, if any, of the symptoms are present. Moreover, the presence of such symptoms is not by itself proof that the specifically alleged trauma in fact took place.

26. What impact is DSM–IV likely to have on the assessment of diminished capacity?
DSM–IV may well lead to more frequent claims of posttraumatic stress disorder in both civil and criminal cases; unlike DSM–III–R, it respects the variability of individual response to threatening events. As a result, defenses based on diminished capacity, including imperfect self-defense, may increase.

27. What other mental disorders affect criminal responsibility?
Psychosis, by whatever diagnosis or etiology, is the mental disorder that most commonly serves as a basis for an insanity defense. In addition, people with organic brain syndromes may fail to make the connection between actions and consequences. Multiple-personality disorder also needs to be ruled out. Court decisions in different jurisdictions have been inconsistent about voluntary intoxication as an extenuating factor. In general, mental impairment resulting from either acute voluntary intoxication or chronic substance abuse may result in some degree of diminished

capacity but not in acquittal by reason of insanity. An insanity defense, on the other hand, may be successful in cases of involuntary intoxication, delirium tremens, idiosyncratic intoxication, unpredictable variations in tolerance, or permanent psychosis (such as Korsakoff's psychosis) due to chronic alcohol use.

28. How is a forensic psychiatric assessment conducted?

There is no simple formula for conducting a forensic psychiatric assessment; the method of examination must be tailored to the person being examined and to the factual and legal questions at issue. Although a forensic psychiatrist may be asked to assess a person's current functioning (as in a disability evaluation), more often the forensic psychiatric examination entails reconstruction of a prior mental state. Such an examination is akin to filling in a crossword puzzle; one puts together data concurrent with the events in question and data from the present examination.

It is essential that the examiner maintain objectivity. The examination must be conducted with an openness to evidence and an attitude of informed skepticism. A properly conducted assessment is always an in-depth process and often an extended one. Typically, it includes multiple interviews of the examinee, interviews with others involved in the case, and review of other relevant data such as depositions, police and medical reports, and, when appropriate, site visits and audiotape and videotape reviews. If needed, the examiner may request additional specialized medical consultations and testing, such as a sleep/awake electroencephalograph, which may reveal an underlying seizure disorder. Such data are analyzed with a view toward internal coherence, subtle verbal and nonverbal cues, and corroboration of the examinee's story by other evidence.

As noted in the AAPL ethical guidelines, "An evaluation for forensic purposes begins with notice to the evaluee of any limitation on confidentiality." This so-called Lamb warning serves not only to set the stage for proceeding ethically with a forensic evaluation, but also to prepare the evaluee for hearing a report of the results, as in the context of distressing courtroom testimony.

29. Is it easier to assess someone who has previously been in therapy?

Prior therapy makes the forensic psychiatric examination easier in some ways but more difficult in others. It is easier insofar as a person who has been in therapy may communicate more openly. It is more difficult in that the examinee may respond in line with a preexisting self-concept and a model, conveyed by the treating clinician, of what is appropriate to communicate. Although psychotherapy might be expected to make a person more self-aware, closer examination may reveal that an examinee has been in treatment numerous times with no long-term involvement with any one therapist.

30. Can hypnosis serve as a useful check on the unreliability of an examinee's memories of key events?

Given the heightened suggestibility of hypnotized subjects, under no circumstances should memories uncovered under hypnosis be considered reliable, especially in criminal cases. Rather then decrease the examinee's autonomy through hypnosis, one should strive to enhance the examinee's autonomy—for example, by allowing a portion of the interview to be unstructured and associational. Confrontation has a place, but not to the extent that the examinee will say anything to decrease the anxiety induced by the interview. Advanced training in modes of forensic examination—including the recognition of countertransference, avoidance of subtle cues and suggestions, creation of an atmosphere conducive to open communication, and use of unstructured interview techniques—helps to build expertise in data gathering and evaluation of memories.

31. How useful is psychological testing in the forensic psychiatric assessment?

In selected cases, psychological testing provides useful corroborative evidence, but only if it is used appropriately as an adjunct to—not a substitute for—forensic psychiatric examination. Because testing may disrupt the working alliance needed for the forensic examination, it should be done (when indicated) after rather than before the examination. Tests need to be carefully administered by the examiner to minimize invalid results driven by anxiety, fatigue, reading difficulty, or misunderstanding. Moreover, test results require careful interpretation—first, because a person's state of mind at the time of testing is not necessarily the same as the person's state of mind at the time of the events in question; second, because the results obtained in the forensic context may be invalidated by anxiety and confusion or by attempted manipulation.

32. Is it helpful to visit, photograph, or review photographs of the site of the alleged events?

Sometimes the external reality of the site opens up the internal reality of a person's experience. A site visit may have as many as three stages:

1. The forensic interview may include a reconstruction of the site via remembering. Reporting of memories may serve, in effect, as a metaphorical site visit.

2. The examiner cross-checks the details of the site (by means of a visit or photograph) to assess the accuracy of the account.

3. The examiner visits the site with the witness to observe any physiologic signs or symptoms, verbal or nonverbal, that the person is reexperiencing the feelings associated with the event.

33. Can dreams provide reliable data for medicolegal purposes?

Asking the examinee to communicate dreams (as well as memories, thoughts, and feelings) may yield useful data, but only in the context of a comprehensive forensic psychiatric examination by a psychoanalytically informed examiner with sufficient training and experience. By listening skeptically but carefully to everything communicated by the examinee, including dreams, the forensic psychiatrist gains the required entry into an examinee's internal reality. Dreams cannot be taken as a representation of literal truth; nor can the dream as communicated be assumed to be the dream as dreamt. Rather, one must listen to the dream as one would to any other communication: At what point in the examination was it communicated? Was it communicated spontaneously or at the examiner's inquiry? What associations preceded and followed it? What was the accompanying affect?

Dream communications may contribute to overall assessment of an examinee's credibility, because dreams are hard to fake. People are much more practiced at lying and exaggerating about waking events than about dreams. Specifically, after a genuine trauma (but not a fabricated one), dreams tend to progress from direct representations of the experience to more and more disguised versions. Likewise, the natural progression of emotional reactions in the wake of trauma typically runs from anxiety to depression, whereas a person who is embellishing may emphasize one reaction but not the other.

In DSM–IV, "recurrent distressing dreams" are listed as a possible diagnostic indicator of posttraumatic stress disorder (PTSD). Although vivid dream imagery is sometimes evidence of trauma, as in PTSD, it also may be a manifestation of an underlying hysterical personality disorder or simply a personal characteristic with no diagnostic significance. At the other extreme, the absence of dreams may be significant. For example, a man who had been in an airplane crash reported vivid dreams until the night preceding the anniversary of the crash, at which time he said that he simply felt terrified but had no dreams. Such a detail enables the examiner to explore further the impact of a major life event.

Even when dreams are not reported, it may be worthwhile to inquire about them, especially in the case of people who are not psychologically minded, and, at the extreme, alexythymic. Both characteristics may occur as a result of trauma. When a person has difficulty with expressing feelings, whether for reasons of personality, trauma, or the public nature of the forensic examination, dreams may be a useful vehicle for exploring the examinee's psychic functioning.

34. How does countertransference affect the assessment?

An awareness of how one's own reactions color assessment of another person is essential, regardless of one's subspecialty (e.g., psychopharmacology) or mode or school of treatment. In psychoanalytic terms, this dynamic process is called countertransference. It operates primarily through the mechanisms of projection and identification. One may project one's own competence or incompetence, either in general or in a particular relationship, onto the person being examined. Such projection, as well as overidentification, may affect the assessment of competence in any area discussed in this chapter.

Positive countertransference occurs when one assesses an examinee uncritically—especially an examinee with whom one overidentifies on the basis of similar demographic or personal characteristics—because one wishes to see the examinee as healthy and self-sufficient. A desire to protect the examinee from distress may lead one to avoid exploring emotionally charged areas in which the examinee may be found incompetent. Likewise, a justifiable concern to avoid stigmatization may divert attention from areas of real incompetence.

Negative countertransference occurs when one finds a person competent out of a desire to maintain control and to protect oneself and society from the person's dissembling—so that the defendant, for example, will not "get away with" the crime. On the other hand, one may inaccurately assess someone as incompetent because of failure to establish a communicative alliance for the purposes of the assessment. In this case, the denial of one's helplessness to establish such an alliance may result in projecting the incompetence of the alliance onto the examinee.

The examiner who is retained by one party in a legal action may be susceptible to any of several typical countertransference reactions. It is relatively easy to recognize identification with the attorney (plaintiff, prosecution, or defense) who has retained one's services. More subtle is the reaction-formation by which one identifies with the opposing side. A most insidious (yet common) tendency, especially in response to an anxiety-provoking examinee, is to remove oneself to the safe ground of being the judge. Such detachment may take the form of false certainty in the face of confusing and ambiguous data.

35. What other factors may affect the assessment of criminal responsibility?

The assessment may be biased by "false sanity" resulting from the use of psychotropic drugs or from the setting in which the examination takes place. It is difficult to recognize psychotic states in examinees who have recompensated through medication, psychotherapy, tincture of time, removal from the stressful setting of the events in question, or placement in a structured medical or correctional setting. Conducting an examination in a jail or prison may either mask or induce psychosis, depending on whether the examinee experiences the facility as supportive or stressful. Other factors that may bias the assessment include a restricted emphasis on the appearance of the criminal act (e.g., planning, flagrancy, concealment, flight) without due regard to the psychological facts (e.g., people who are in the midst of a paranoid psychosis often flee or conceal without the requisite intent to obstruct justice).

36. What is "reasonable medical certainty" in the eyes of the law?

In preparing an expert opinion, the forensic psychiatrist initially engages in data gathering and formation of working hypotheses. It is important not to confuse such preliminary opinions with the final product, which, whenever possible, should be formulated to the requisite degree of reasonable medical certainty. Reasonable medical certainty must be distinguished both from absolute certainty, which is unattainable, and from the degree of certainty required to proceed in a clinical context, which is related not to whether a working hypothesis is more likely than not to be true, but to whether it supports a proposed course of treatment that has the optimal risk/benefit ratio among the available alternatives.

Reasonable medical certainty is a term that each jurisdiction defines for itself. A deep understanding of this term is necessary for almost any work in forensic psychiatry. Typically, reasonable medical certainty is taken to mean "more likely than not." However, in Pennsylvania, for example, reasonable medical certainty about the issue of causation means "beyond a reasonable doubt."

When rendering an opinion with the requisite degree of reasonable medical certainty, one must be mindful that the opinion will be used by the court in forming its judgment of which side has met the standard of proof. That standard is often different from the standard for reasonable medical certainty and likewise varies by jurisdiction. In civil cases the standard of proof tends to be "preponderance of evidence," which is another way of saying more likely than not (and thus may be interpreted as a probability of at least 51%). In some civil as well as some criminal actions, the standard of proof is "clear and convincing evidence" (which can be interpreted as a 75% probability). This standard is often used in sentencing hearings and in determining competence to stand trial. In most criminal cases the standard is "beyond a reasonable doubt" (which can be interpreted as 90% or more, depending on the commentator).

In cases involving the insanity defense, depending on the jurisdiction, the defense may have the burden of proving, either by a preponderance of evidence or by clear and convincing evidence, that the defendant has met the insanity standard. In a few jurisdictions the prosecution still has the burden of proving beyond a reasonable doubt that the person was sane at the time of the alleged crime.

An expert witness is sometimes asked whether he or she holds an opinion to a higher standard of proof than that of reasonable medical certainty as defined for that jurisdiction—for instance, whether the opinion is supported by clear and convincing evidence. One may or may not be able to answer such a question. It can be argued, however, that the medical expert's task is only to give an opinion with reasonable medical certainty. If the standard of proof is higher, it is the attorney's job to introduce evidence that, in conjunction with the medical expert's testimony, meets the higher standard.

37. Do special issues arise in the assessment of competence and criminal responsibility in children?

Common areas of competence assessment in children include consent to medical care, such as abortion, and emancipation of minors. In a clearcut instance of the interpersonal dimension of competence, the family must be included in assessments of competence that involve a child or adolescent.

Age is also taken into account in the assessment of criminal responsibility. Age may be an absolute legal barrier to criminal responsibility, as in a state in which children under a certain age are considered incapable of forming the intent to kill. Age also may be a relative barrier in terms of a particular child's capacity to think and make decisions independently.

38. Does competence assessment play a part in product liability suits?

Yes. The forensic psychiatrist may be asked to review package inserts and warning labels or signs with an understanding of how people make choices about potentially dangerous products. Questions of cognitive awareness and affective maturity arise in assessing a person's capacity to assume the risk of using such a product. In the case of children, such questions commonly arise with respect to toys and playground equipment.

39. Do indigent defendants have a right to a court-appointed forensic psychiatric expert in cases in which mental status may be a factor in determining guilt?

According to the U.S. Supreme Court in the landmark case of *Ake v. Oklahoma* (1985), indigent defendants have this right. There is no substitute for a forensic psychiatric evaluation in gathering and interpreting the data needed to determine criminal responsibility. Therefore, recourse to such expertise is essential to a fair trial in cases in which mental status may be relevant. In practice, however, access to court-appointed psychiatric expertise is often restricted in ways that compromise both the expert's independence and the defendant's right to due process. It has been proposed, therefore, that any indigent defendant who shows a reasonable need for forensic expertise be provided with a private psychiatrist of his or her own choosing who is paid for but not controlled by the state. At present, this entitlement must be advocated for, both in individual cases and at the policy level. In the meantime, the forensic psychiatrist must be aware of the dangers of performing an incomplete evaluation because of limited funds. If such a limited evaluation is unavoidable, it should be acknowledged in the psychiatrist's report and/or testimony.

40. How important is an understanding of ethical issues in the practice of forensic psychiatry?
Such an understanding is essential. The AAPL Ethical Guidelines for the Practice of Forensic Psychiatry consider much of what has been discussed in this chapter from an explicitly ethical perspective, with a view toward distinguishing between the methods of forensic and clinical assessment. In forensic psychiatric practice it is not uncommon that issues of competence, consent, and responsibility are intertwined with the ethical and epistemologic issues surrounding agency, autonomy, authenticity, and moral choice. It is often useful, therefore, to seek not only collegial ethical consultation with practicing forensic psychiatrists but also consultation with a trained ethicist for a transdisciplinary perspective.

ACKNOWLEDGMENTS

Phillip J. Resnick and Robert I. Simon contributed highly detailed comments on this chapter, some of which were incorporated essentially verbatim into the text. James C. Beck, Thomas G. Gutheil, Mark J. Mills, Herbert C. Modlin, Jonas R. Rappeport, and Larry H. Strasburger also contributed close readings that much improved the final draft. Alan A. Stone's thought-provoking lectures on the aftermath of the Hinckley verdict and, more recently, Alan M. Dershowitz's exposition of the imperfect self-defense have been most useful. Patricia M.L. Illingworth provided an invaluable perspective on an ethical framework for psychiatric and legal issues. Buz Scherr illuminated with helpful clarity the distinction between "simple intent" and "specific intent" crimes. None of these generous advisers, however, should be held responsible for anything with which readers may disagree.

BIBLIOGRAPHY

1. American Bar Association: ABA Criminal Justice Mental Health Standards. Washington, DC, American Bar Association, 1989.
2. Appelbaum PS, Gutheil TG: Clinical Handbook of Psychiatry and the Law, 2nd ed. Baltimore, Williams & Wilkins, 1991.
3. Beck JC, Parry JW: Incompetence, treatment refusal, and hospitalization. Bull Am Acad Psychiatry Law 20:261–267, 1992.
4. Bursztajn HJ, Feinbloom RI, Hamm RM, Brodsky A: Medical Choices, Medical Chances: How Patients, Families, and Physicians Can Cope with Uncertainty. New York, Routledge, 1990.
5. Bursztajn HJ, Harding HP, Gutheil TG, Brodsky A: Beyond cognition: The role of disordered affective states in impairing competence to consent to treatment. Bull Am Acad Psychiatry Law 19:383–388, 1991.
6. Bursztajn HJ, Scherr AE, Brodsky A: The rebirth of forensic psychiatry in light of recent historical trends in criminal responsibility. Psychiatr Clin North Am 17:611–635, 1994.
7. Group for the Advancement of Psychiatry, Committee on Psychiatry and Law: The Mental Health Professional and the Legal System (Report No. 131). New York, Brunner/Mazel, 1991.
8. Monahan J, Walker L: Social Science in Law: Cases and Materials, 3rd ed. Westbury, NY, Foundation Press, 1994.
9. Perlin ML: Mental Disability Law: Civil and Criminal. Charlottesville, VA, Michie, 1989–1993.
10. Rappeport JR: Reasonable medical certainty. Bull Am Acad Psychiatry Law 13:5–16, 1985.
11. Rosner R (ed): Principles and Practice of Forensic Psychiatry. New York, Chapman & Hall, 1994.
12. Stone AA: Law, Psychiatry, and Morality. Washington, DC, American Psychiatric Press, 1984.
13. Strasburger LH: "Crudely, without any finesse": The defendant hears his psychiatric evaluation. Bull Am Acad Psychiatry Law 15:229–233, 1987.

83. ETHICS AND THE DOCTOR–PATIENT RELATIONSHIP

Claire Zilber, M.D.

> The regimen I adopt shall be for the benefit of my patients according to my ability and judgment, and not for their hurt or any wrong. . . . Whatsoever house I enter, there will I go for the benefit of the sick, refraining from all wrongdoing or corruption, and especially for any act of seduction, male or female.
>
> *Oath of Hippocrates*

1. What is a fiduciary relationship?

A physician has a fiduciary relationship with each of his patients; that is, a duty to act in the patient's best interest and to refrain from exploiting the patient. Respecting the fiduciary relationship and the trust of the patient is a cornerstone of the ethical physician's practice. The Hippocratic oath expresses the essence of the fiduciary relationship.

2. What is a boundary violation?

In the context of the physician–patient relationship, a boundary violation refers to any behavior on the part of a physician that transgresses the limits of the professional relationship. Boundary violations have the potential to exploit or harm patients. The potential areas of exploitation include personal or social boundary violations, business relationships, and sexual activity. Examples of personal or social boundary violations include seeing patients in unorthodox settings for the convenience of the physician, loaning a patient money, or burdening the patient with personal information. Business ventures with a patient or taking advantage of insider information revealed by the patient are examples of unethical business relationships. Any form of sexual activity with a patient is a clear boundary violation.

3. Why is sexual activity with a consenting adult patient considered unethical?

Transference and countertransference are psychiatric concepts that help to explain why sexual activity, even with a consenting patient or former patient, is unethical. Transference is a phenomenon of unconscious displacement of earlier relationship experiences and expectations onto the physician and may cause a wide range of feelings in the patient, from rage to love and sexual attraction. Countertransference is the corresponding unconscious emotional reaction of the physician to the patient. Transference and countertransference may continue even after the termination of treatment; for this reason, psychiatrists may not ethically enter into a sexual relationship with a former patient, no matter how long ago the treatment ended. Many consider the same dynamics applicable to other medical specialists and would extend the prohibition to all physicians. At present, the proscription against sexual activity with a former patient is unique to psychiatry, but sexual activity with a current patient is generally considered unethical in all fields of medicine.

Sexual activity with a patient damages the healing capacity of psychiatric treatment. One survey of psychiatrists found that 65% of those who had been sexually involved with patients felt that they were in love with the patient and 92% believed that the patient was in love with them.[4] In fact, such feelings may have had their origins in transference and countertransference; by acting on the feelings rather than working in therapy to understand them, the psychiatrist harms the treatment and the fiduciary relationship. Freud observed that it is deleterious to the patient if countertransference is acted out: "If the patient's advances were returned, it would be a great triumph for her, but a complete defeat of the treatment. . . . The love relationship, in fact, destroys the patient's susceptibility to influence from analytic treatment."[3]

4. Are feelings of sexual attraction toward a patient unethical?

No. Sexual feelings toward a patient are quite common. In one survey, 87% of psychotherapists (95% of men and 76% of women) acknowledged having been sexually attracted to one or more of their patients.[8] It is important not to act on such feelings. It may be helpful to seek supervision in the treatment of these patients to ensure that the sexual countertransference does not impede the treatment.

5. In the course of discussing a case with a colleague, he tells you that he has been trying a new approach with an emotionally "needy" patient. He has extended the session time beyond the customary 45 minutes, seeing her at the end of the day for $1\frac{1}{2}$ hours. He also begins and ends each session with a hug, which he feels is necessary to assure the patient of his care and concern. Is this behavior ethical?

Sexual transgressions frequently are preceded by such boundary violations. Although some may say that no sexual activity has occurred, others may see the hugs as sexual. It is difficult to know whether the patient experiences the hugs as sexual. Even without the hugs, the circumstances under which the physician is seeing the patient are unorthodox and may harm the treatment. The psychiatrist is also at risk for a formal ethical complaint and a lawsuit. Fifteen percent of lawsuits against psychiatrists involve sexual boundary violations.[10]

6. A patient is looking for financial investors in a project that promises to be lucrative and invites the physician to invest in the project. May the physician ethically participate? The same patient gives a hot stock tip. Is it ethical to act on it?

In the first scenario, participation in a business relationship with the patient may harm the patient's treatment. If the business fails, feelings of anger, guilt, or resentment may emerge between the physician and the patient. The physician may lose the objectivity necessary to provide competent and compassionate treatment if he or she resents having lost money as a result of the business venture. The patient may have similar negative feelings that make it difficult to seek help from the physician for medical problems. Even if the business succeeds, the physician is no longer an impartial and objective person for the patient. In the case of psychiatric treatment, the psychiatrist's relative neutrality and abstinence, central to the healing nature of the therapeutic relationship, cannot be preserved if a business relationship exists between the patient and psychiatrist.

In the second scenario, the physician would be "exploiting information furnished by the patient."[9] In addition, by acting on insider information, the physician may be breaking the law, which in itself is unethical behavior.[9] This applies equally to psychiatrists and other physicians.

7. A patient has just informed the physician of a plan to kill someone. The physician wants to ensure the other person's safety but is also concerned about confidentiality. What may the physician ethically do?

The Principles of Medical Ethics direct physicians to "safeguard patient confidences within the constraints of the law."[9] The law requires the physician to warn the person at risk or to intervene so that no harm may be done. The ethical physician discloses only the information that is necessary and relevant to the situation. Fantasy material, sexual orientation, or other sensitive information usually does not need to be disclosed. The welfare and privacy of the patient should still be protected as much as possible. Whenever possible, it is preferable to involve the patient in the ethical dilemma that the physician faces. For example, by working with the homicidal patient, the physician may be able to obtain a release of information from the patient to warn the person at risk or to persuade the patient to accept hospitalization until the homicidal ideation subsides.

8. A patient has been repeatedly resistant to treatment. He has missed numerous appointments, has not been following treatment recommendations, and is abrasive when the physician raises concerns about such behavior. Frustrated, the physician suggests that the patient seek treatment with someone else. He retorts, "I hired you to be my doctor. I can fire you, but you can't fire me!" Is he right?

A physician may choose not to treat a patient provided that it is not an emergency and that the physician has provided suitable notice and referrals. Generally, the ethical physician works with the patient to achieve as smooth a transition as possible. *The Principles of Medical Ethics* states, "A physician shall, in the provision of appropriate care, except in emergencies, be free to choose whom to serve, with whom to associate, and the environment in which to provide medical services."[9] If a physician has strong and persistent negative feelings toward a patient, he or she will have difficulty providing objective treatment. Likewise, if a physician feels obligated to treat someone regardless of the circumstances, problems with treatment may arise. As an old truism advises, *you can't treat someone who you can't not treat.*

9. A physician suspects that a colleague has been abusing alcohol. One morning, while on hospital rounds, the physician smells alcohol on the colleague's breath. Is the physician obligated to take action?

According to *The Principles of Medical Ethics,* "Special consideration should be given to those psychiatrists who, because of mental illness, jeopardize the welfare of their patients and their own reputations and practices. It is ethical, even encouraged, for another psychiatrist to intercede in such situations."[9] This ethical principle is easily extended to physicians in other specialties. Furthermore, in some states physicians are mandated to report impaired colleagues to the medical licensing board. The bylaws of most hospitals and health maintenance organizations also require reporting of suspected or proved impairments. Once reported, impaired physicians are strongly encouraged to enter into treatment. Every effort is made to assist the physician to get help so that he or she may retain medical license and practice. Physicians are often reluctant to report their impaired colleagues because they do not want to be responsible for jeopardizing another doctor's professional practice; in fact, however, reporting is an excellent way to help impaired colleagues and to facilitate their entry into treatment.

10. A 35-year-old man in the final stages of acquired immunodeficiency syndrome (AIDS) asks for the physician's help. He is in constant pain and homebound, with no appreciable quality of life. He would like to overdose on medications to stop his suffering but does not have enough of a stockpile to ensure a lethal overdose. He informs the physician of his plan and asks the physician, who sympathizes with his plight, to write a prescription for a lethal dose of narcotics. What may an ethical physician do in this situation?

The Principles of Medical Ethics explicitly states, "A physician shall respect the law and also recognize a responsibility to seek changes in those requirements which are contrary to the best interests of the patient. . . . It is conceivable that an individual could violate a law without being guilty of unethical behavior."[9] At present it is illegal to assist in a suicide, although a few states have introduced legislation that would allow physician-assisted suicide. In the above case, the physician may not legally prescribe a lethal dose of narcotics. Many physicians feel strongly that their role is to treat illness and to save lives, not to assist in taking a life. They also raise concerns about the limits of physician-assisted suicide: for whom is it appropriate, who decides it is appropriate, and how is it regulated? The possibility of abuse of the law raises many concerns for physicians who otherwise may have no ethical objections to physician-assisted suicide.

Some physicians may disagree with the prohibition against physician-assisted suicide. Such individuals may ethically organize to change the law. *The Principles of Medical Ethics* allows for the possibility that a physician who assists a suicide may be acting ethically, even though the action is illegal. In fact, many doctors have quietly hastened death in some of their patients with terminal illness, acting on their belief that relieving hopeless suffering is consistent with their role as a physician.

Regardless of a particular physician's stance on the issue of assisted suicide, he or she should do everything else in his or her power to treat the patient's pain and to improve the patient's quality of life. In many instances ameliorable conditions, such as chronic cancer pain, lead patients to seek death. When the pain is treated and the patient feels comforted, suicidal wishes may be alleviated.

ACKNOWLEDGMENT

The author is grateful to David Wahl, M.D., and Michael Weissberg, M.D., for reviewing this chapter.

BIBLIOGRAPHY

1. Appelbaum PS: Statutes regulating patient-therapist sex. Hosp Community Psychiatry 41:15–16, 1990.
2. Carr M, Robinson GE: Fatal attraction: The ethical and clinical dilemma of patient-therapist sex. Can J Psychiatry 35:122–127, 1990.
3. Freud S: Observations on Transference Love (1914), in The Standard Edition of the Complete Psychological Works of Sigmund Freud, Vol. 12. Translated and edited by J. Strachey, London, Hogarth Press, 1958, pp 157–171.
4. Gartrell N, Herman J, Olarte S, et al: Psychiatrist-patient sexual contact: Results of a national survey: I. Prevalence. Am J Psych 143:1126–1131, 1986.
5. Lazarus JA: Sex with former patients almost always unethical. Am J Psychiatry 149:855–857, 1992.
6. Menninger WW, Gabbard GO (eds): Sexual boundary violations. Psychol Ann 21:644–680, 1991.
7. Menninger WW: Inappropriate Doctor-patient Relationships. Presented at the Menninger Winter Psychiatry Conference, Park City, Utah, 1993.
8. Pope KS, Keith-Spiegel P, Tabachnick BG: Sexual attraction to clients: The human therapist and the (sometimes) inhuman training system. Am Psychol 41:147–158, 1986.
9. The Principles of Medical Ethics with Annotations Especially Applicable to Psychiatry. Washington, DC, American Psychiatric Association, 1993.
10. Simon R: Clinical Psychiatry and the Law. Washington, DC, American Psychiatric Press, 1987.

INDEX

Page numbers in **boldface type** indicate complete chapters.

Motor activity
  evaluation of, with mental status examination, 8
  perseveration of, as frontal lobe dysfunction, 11
Motorcycle gang members, amphetamine abuse by, 121
Mourning, 174–179
  definition of, 175
  differentiated from melancholy, 176, 177
Movement disorders, as dementia cause, 186
Movement therapy, for dissociative identity disorder, 140
MSE. *See* Mental status examination
Multidimensional Pain Inventory (MPI), 404–405
Multiple personality disorder. *See* Dissociative identity disorder
Multiple sclerosis
  as bipolar mood syndromes cause, 70
  brain imaging evaluation of, 47
  as depression cause, 182, 396
  as personality change cause, 182
  as psychosis cause, 181
  as suicide risk factor, 452
  as violent behavior risk factor, 458
Mumps, as autism risk factor, 313
Munchhausen's by proxy, 171, 487–488
Munchhausen's syndrome, 171
Muscle relaxants, addiction to, 120
Muscle relaxation, progressive, 255, 257, 259
Mushrooms, hallucinogenic properties of, 126
Music therapy, for dissociative identity disorder, 140
Myoclonus, nocturnal, 157

Nail biting, compulsive, 94
Naltrexone
  as alcohol abuse treatment, 114
  as opioid addiction treatment, 118
Narcanon Family Groups, 343
Narcissistic personality disorder, 202, 204, 216
Narcolepsy, 121, 156, 298
Narcotic analgesics
  abuse of, by adolescents, 340
  as sexual dysfunction cause, 145
  withdrawal from, by cancer patients, 434
Narcotics Anonymous, 133, 343
National Coalition of Cancer Survivors, 439
Negative predictions, as cognitive processing error, 228
Neologism, definition of, 11
Neologistic speech, psychoses-related, 197
Neurobehavioral Cognitive Status Examination, 9
Neurofibromatosis, as autism risk factor, 313
Neuroimaging. See Brain imaging
Neuroleptic malignant syndrome, 273, 274–275, 281, **464–467**
  in bioplar disorder patients, 279
  electroconvulsive therapy for, 303
Neuroleptics, **270–276**
  action mechanism of, 270
  adverse effects of, 271–272, 274, 281, 349. *See also* Neuroleptic malignant syndrome
  as anorexia nervosa therapy, 151

Neuroleptics (*cont.*)
  atypical, 270
  as autism therapy, 314
  as chemical restraint for violent patients, 461
  chlorpromazine equivalent dosage of, 270
  contraindication in bipolar disorder, 281
  contraindication in Parkinson's disease, 389–390
  daily oral doses of, 270
  as delirium therapy, for cancer patients, 437
  as dementia therapy, 189
  as dissociative identity disorder therapy, 141
  drug interactions of, 132–133, 274, 279
  indications for, 271
  as mania therapy, 279
  use during pregnancy, 367–368
  as schizophrenia treatment, in adolescents, 350
  sedative properties of, 297
  as sexual dysfunction cause, 144
  as tardive dyskinesia cause, 274, 281, 348
  therapeutic index of, 453
  therapeutic window of, 273
  trial of, 272–273
  typical, 270
Neurologic disorders
  autism-related, 310
  behavioral presentations of, **180–184**
  as bipolar mood syndromes cause, 70
  as delirium cause, 192
  differentiated from conduct disorder, 324
  as generalized anxiety disorder cause, 89
  psychotic symptoms in, 196–198
  as violent behavior risk factor, 457–458
Neuropathy
  peripheral, alcoholic, 112
  as sexual dysfunction cause, 145
Neuropsychological testing, **26–31**
  components of, 27–28
  effects of psychiatric disorders on results of, 28–30
  referral for, 26–27, 28
Neurosurgery, as obsessive-compulsive disorder therapy, 98
Neurosyphilis
  as bipolar mood syndromes cause, 70
  as depression cause, 182
  as personality change cause, 182
Neuroticism, treatment-resistant depression-related, 470
New Hampshire v. *Colbert*, 507
Nicotine chewing gum, 424. *See also* Smoking cessation
Nicotine dependence. *See also* Smoking
  generalized anxiety disorder-related, 89
Nightmares
  antipsychotic therapy for, 271
  compared with night terrors, 157–158
Night terrors, 157–158, 296
Nocturnal myoclonus, as insomnia cause, 157
Nocturnal penile tumescence (NPT), 411
Noncompliance, stimulant therapy for, 299
Nonverbal learning disability, 316
Noradrenergic drugs, as obesity treatment, 476–477
Norepinephrine levels, in schizophrenia, 55